Australian
Medical Council Limited

GOOD MEDICAL PRACTICE

PROFESSIONALISM, ETHICS AND LAW

5TH EDITION

HELEN MILROY AM
ANNE TONKIN AO
THEANNE WALTERS AM
TIM WILKINSON

Acknowledgement of Country

The Australian Medical Council (AMC) acknowledges the Aboriginal and/or Torres Strait Islander peoples as the original Australians, and the Māori people as the tangata whenua, or original peoples of Aotearoa New Zealand.

We acknowledge and pay our respects to the Traditional Custodians of all the lands on which the AMC works, and their ongoing connection to the land, water and sky.

The AMC acknowledges the past policies and practices that impact on the health and wellbeing of Aboriginal and/or Torres Strait Islander and Māori peoples and commits to working together with communities to support healing and positive health outcomes.

The AMC is committed to improving outcomes for Aboriginal and/or Torres Strait Islander and Māori peoples through its assessment and accreditation processes including equitable access to health services for First Nations peoples.

We note that the language to refer to so many separate and diverse Nations is viewed differently, and wish to note that the language choices made in this book referring to these many Nations are not intended to diminish the individual and unique identities of these Nations. We acknowledge these differences, and our shared knowledge and experience.

Published by the Australian Medical Council Ltd
PO Box 4810
KINGSTON, ACT 2604, Australia
Phone: +61 2 6270 9777 Website: www.amc.org.au

1st edition published 1994
2nd edition published 1997
3rd edition published 2010
4th edition published 2016
5th edition published 2026

Print ISBN: 9781923118430
Digital PDF: 9781923118447
Epub: 9781923118423

Copyedited by SuperScript Writing & Editing
Internal design by Anthouse Communications
Cover and section opener design by Megan Steele-Ferguson
Indexed by Master Indexing

The cover for this publication features the **Rod of Asclepius**, the enduring symbol of medicine and healing, entwined with Australia's national and state floral emblems to reflect the uniquely local context of this text.

Each flower represents a state or territory: **golden wattle** (Australia), **waratah** (NSW), **common heath** (Vic), **Cooktown orchid** (Qld), **Sturt's desert pea** (SA), **kangaroo paw** (WA), **Tasmanian blue gum** (Tas), **royal bluebell** (ACT) **and Sturt's desert rose** (NT).

Woven together, these elements symbolise the interconnectedness of ethics, law and health care across Australia—rooted in diverse traditions, landscapes and legal systems, yet unified by a common commitment to care for the Australian community.

Foreword

In an era of rapid transformation in health care, the fifth edition of Good medical practice: professionalism, ethics and law arrives at a critical juncture. This edition reflects the evolving landscape of medical practice in Australia, shaped by technological innovation, shifting societal expectations, and the growing recognition of the importance of cultural safety and equity in healthcare delivery. It is both a reaffirmation of enduring principles and a forward-looking framework for doctors navigating the complexities of modern clinical practice.

The Australian Medical Council (AMC) has long championed the values of professionalism, ethical integrity and legal accountability as foundational to medical practice. These pillars are not static; they must be continually reinterpreted in light of new challenges, emerging norms, and the lived experiences of patients and practitioners alike. This edition is informed by a broad and inclusive list of contributors, drawing on the insights of clinicians, regulators, educators, legal experts and—most importantly—the communities served by the medical profession.

Professionalism remains the cornerstone of good medical practice. Yet, its meaning and application have evolved. In this edition, professionalism is framed not only as a set of behaviours but as a dynamic relationship between the doctor, the patient and society. It encompasses clinical competence, ethical conduct, and a commitment to continuous learning and reflective practice.

This book explores how professionalism is expressed in diverse contexts—from rural general practice to high-tech tertiary care—and how it must adapt to the realities of interprofessional collaboration, digital health and patient-centred care. It also addresses the challenges posed by burnout, moral injury and systemic pressures, recognising that sustaining professionalism requires institutional support and personal resilience.

Ethical practice is at the heart of medicine's social contract. This edition expands its ethical discourse to include contemporary dilemmas such as artificial intelligence in diagnostics and the ethical use of social media. It recognises that innovation must be balanced with caution, and that new technologies bring new responsibilities. It encourages doctors to critically appraise the tools they use, to remain vigilant about patient safety, and to uphold ethical standards in all forms of care delivery.

Importantly, the guide foregrounds the ethical imperative of cultural safety. It acknowledges the historical and ongoing impacts of colonisation on Aboriginal and Torres Strait Islander peoples and affirms the role of doctors in promoting health equity and respectful care. Ethical practice, in this context, is not merely about avoiding harm but actively contributing to healing and justice.

This edition also revisits enduring issues—confidentiality, informed consent and end-of-life care—with fresh perspectives informed by legal developments and cultural shifts.

Legal knowledge is essential for safe and accountable practice. The fifth edition provides a clear and accessible overview of the legal frameworks governing medical practice in Australia. It covers key areas such as professional regulation, mandatory reporting, negligence and the legal dimensions of consent and capacity.

New chapters address emerging legal concerns, including the regulation of telehealth, data privacy, and the medicolegal implications of working across jurisdictions. The book also offers practical advice on documentation, communication, and navigating complaints and investigations—areas where legal literacy can significantly impact outcomes for both patients and practitioners.

Trust is the foundation of the doctor–patient relationship and of medicine's place in society. This edition reflects the community's evolving expectations of the medical profession—expectations shaped by greater transparency, consumer empowerment and a growing awareness of systemic inequities.

Good medical practice emphasises the importance of communication, empathy and shared decision making. It encourages doctors to listen actively, to respect diverse values and beliefs, and to engage patients as partners in their care. It also addresses the role of doctors in public discourse, including the responsibilities that come with speaking out on health issues and participating in advocacy.

This book is designed to support doctors at every stage of their professional journey—from medical students and trainees to experienced clinicians and those in leadership roles. It is also a valuable resource for international medical graduates, regulators, educators, and members of the public who seek to understand the standards of medical practice in Australia.

Each chapter is structured to provide practical guidance, often containing illustrative case studies and lists of resources to guide further reading on particular topics. The aim is not only to inform but to provoke thoughtful engagement with the principles of good practice. The book encourages readers to consider how professionalism, ethics and law intersect in their daily work and to use these insights to enhance the quality and integrity of their care.

As well as being authored by a diverse range of contributors, the book also reflects feedback from community stakeholders, including patients, carers and consumer advocates. Their voices remind us that good medical practice is not defined solely by professional standards but by the experiences and outcomes of those we serve.

As medicine continues to evolve, so too must our understanding of what it means to be a good doctor. This edition of *Good medical practice* is both a reflection of where we are and a vision for where we might go. It challenges doctors to uphold the highest standards of professionalism, to navigate ethical complexity with integrity, and to engage with the law as a framework for accountability and justice.

It also invites ongoing dialogue. The AMC recognises that no guide can be definitive or final. Professionalism, ethics and law are living domains, shaped by new knowledge, changing contexts, and the collective wisdom of the profession and the community. We offer this edition not as a prescription but as a companion—one that supports doctors in their lifelong commitment to good practice.

Geoff McColl
President
Australian Medical Council

Contents

PART THREE: ROLES AND RESPONSIBILITIES IN THE AUSTRALIAN HEALTH AND LEGAL SYSTEMS 319

List of tables

List of figures

Preface

The primary purpose of this book is to provide information central to the professional, ethical and legal requirements of being a doctor. It is designed to support doctors who have recently completed their training and are commencing independent clinical practice, as well as the many overseas-trained doctors who come to Australia each year. It is also likely to be relevant to medical students and doctors at any stage of their careers. Even highly experienced doctors may find it a valuable reference when specific or practical issues arise in their practice.

This edition represents a change in the process of updating the book, in that it has been written by multiple contributors rather than the three authors who were responsible for the fourth edition, published in 2016. Several of their chapters have been retained with a few updates, others have been significantly updated, and a few are completely new. There have been many changes in the legal frameworks surrounding medical practice since the publication of the previous edition; for example, the introduction of voluntary assisted dying. Ethical approaches to issues such as termination of pregnancy and technology-based consultations have evolved over recent years. Technological developments, including artificial intelligence, have had major impacts on medical practice. Medical regulation has also evolved further since the fourth edition, with recent years seeing new regulatory responses to issues such as boundary crossings by doctors and domestic violence. Cultural safety in health care has become recognised as a key factor contributing to the overall health of Aboriginal and/or Torres Strait Islander peoples.

We began developing the fifth edition by inviting input on its content. The Australian Medical Council surveyed regulatory, professional, legal and community groups on the content of the book, society's expectations of the medical profession, and the ethical, legal and professional requirements for new and emerging practice areas. Australian Medical Council staff engaged with medical complaints authorities and reviewed available complaints data to assist in identifying areas where advice to practitioners might be useful. Chapter contributors also led focused stakeholder engagement sessions on the new chapters to discuss the proposed content.

We have grouped the chapters thematically into three major themes: Being a good doctor; Supporting individuals, groups and communities; and Roles and responsibilities in the Australian health and legal systems. This is not a book intended to be read from cover to cover, and we hope that the groupings will assist doctors who are looking for information about particular aspects of their role.

The cover art work, designed by Megan Steele-Ferguson from the Australian Medical Council, incorporates a stylised version of the Rod of Asclepius, a classical symbol of healing and medicine, surrounded by Australia's national and state and territory floral emblems, providing a thematic connection to the Australian context. The artwork was created using hand-cut paper collage, which was then digitised and refined to provide a memorable identity for this book.

Finally, we acknowledge the work of the authors of the four previous editions and hope that this fifth edition will prove to be a worthy successor. During the writing of this edition, one of the members of the editorial panel, Dr Greg Kesby, died suddenly. We acknowledge the contribution that he made to the book, and have included a tribute to him.

Helen Milroy AM
Anne Tonkin AO
Theanne Walters AM
Tim Wilkinson

A tribute to Dr Gregory John Kesby AM

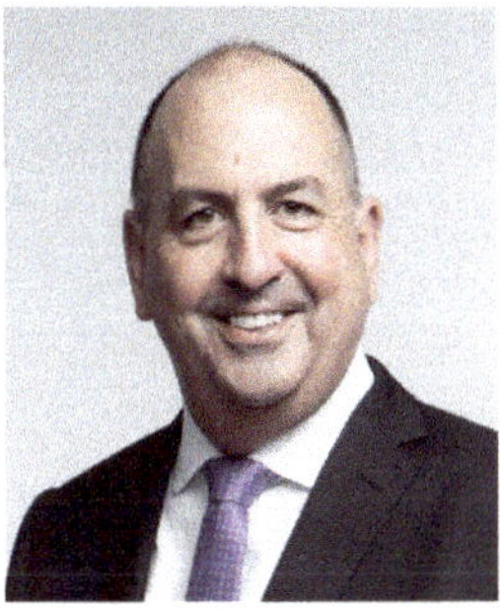

Dr Greg Kesby AM
Courtesy of Ms Vanessa Ballard

The Editorial Panel, authors and contributors of this edition of *Good medical practice* acknowledge the contributions of the late Dr Greg Kesby AM, who was editor-in-chief at the beginning of this project in 2021 and contributed to shaping the publication until his passing on 25 October 2021 at the age of 58.

Dr Greg Kesby BSc(Hons), MBBS(Hons) NSW, PhD(Cantab), DDU, ASUM, FRANZCOG, CMFM, MAICD initially studied for a double degree in science and medicine at the University of New South Wales, and graduated with honours in both fields. Following research at the Physiological Laboratory at the University of Cambridge, Dr Kesby was admitted to the degree of Doctor of Philosophy. His interest in physiology, maternal-fetal medicine, genetics and fetal therapy led Dr Kesby to pursue specialist training in obstetrics and gynaecology in both the UK and Australia. He was a Fellow of the Royal Australian and New Zealand College of Obstetricians and Gynaecologists and a specialist in maternal-fetal Medicine. He worked as a maternal-fetal medicine specialist at both Sydney Ultrasound for Women and the Department of High-Risk Obstetrics and Fetal Medicine at the Royal Prince Alfred Hospital in Sydney. For more than 10 years, Dr Kesby was an examiner and a member of the Council of the Royal Australian and New Zealand College of Obstetricians and Gynaecologists. He was a passionate teacher throughout his career.

Dr Kesby made a significant contribution to medical regulation, and ethics and professionalism in medicine, serving on the Medical Council of NSW for more than 10 years (including 3 years as President), as a Director of the Australian Medical Council, Chair of the NSW Board of the Medical Board of Australia, and Chair of the Professionalism and Ethics Advisory Committee and Professional Standards Committee of the Royal Australian and New Zealand College of Obstetricians and Gynaecologists.

We acknowledge and thank Dr Kesby and hope that this new edition meets the high standards that he would have expected.

Acknowledgements

This publication had its genesis in 1994 with the first edition of *Good medical practice: professionalism, ethics and law*. The book has been updated in three subsequent editions – the most recent fourth edition (published 2016) was written by Kerry Breen, Stephen Cordner and Colin Thomson. The current edition has been written by a large number of contributors, some of whom updated chapters from the fourth edition, while others wrote completely new chapters. The overall scope of the book owes much to the original three authors, and we thank them for their work on the previous editions and their generous gifting of the intellectual property in the fourth edition to the Australian Medical Council to form the backbone of the fifth edition.

We acknowledge, along with the many listed contributors to this edition, many medical and other health professional colleagues, lawyers, academics, administrators and regulators, and others whose help on this project has been invaluable. The publication would not have been able to reach the high standard that it has without their assistance.

They are Katrina Anderson, Sara Bird, Marie Bismark, Kerrie Bradbury, Andrew Brown, Ngiare Brown, Stuart Carney, Dan Corkery, Amanda Frier, Tessa Ho, Sue Kirsa, Caroline Lamb, Kate Leslie, Jennifer Martin, Fiona McDonald, Eleanor Milligan, Patrick Mitchell (UK), Susan O'Dwyer, Maree O'Keefe, Philip Pigou, Kiri Rikihana, Jenny Ryan, John Topfer, Simon Walker, Tamara Weaver and Choong-Siew Yong.

We thank Darlene Cox, Chief Executive Officer, Health Care Consumers' Association of the ACT, who provided health consumers' reflections on good medical practice in this book's introductory chapter.

We thank Anne Tonkin AO, who has not only been a member of the GMP Editorial Panel, but also authored and contributed to several chapters, and acted as content editor of this book. Anne's work has enabled the completion of this edition.

We also thank SuperScript Writing & Editing, Anthouse Communications, Master Indexing and the Editorial Panel and Editorial Project Team led by Caroline Watkin at the Australian Medical Council.

About the Editorial Panel

Helen Milroy AM MBBS, FRANZCP, CATCAP is a Palyku woman of the Pilbara region of Western Australia but was born and educated in Perth. Helen was WA 2021 Australian of the Year and joint winner of the 2020 Australian Mental Health Prize. Currently Helen is the Stan Perron Professor of Child and Adolescent Psychiatry at the Perth Children's Hospital and University of Western Australia. Helen is an Honorary Research Fellow at the Telethon Kids Institute; Chair of Gayaa Dhuwi (Proud Spirit) Australia; and a board member of Beyond Blue. Helen has been a longstanding advocate for cultural safety and the wellbeing of children.

Anne Tonkin AO BSc(Hons), BMBS, M.Ed, PhD, FRACP, FRACMA (Hon) was the Chair of the Medical Board of Australia from 2018 to 2024, having previously chaired the South Australian Board from 2012 to 2018. Anne trained as a general physician with a subspecialty in clinical pharmacology, and practised at the Royal Adelaide Hospital for more than 25 years. She was a clinical academic at the Adelaide Medical School for 22 years, becoming Professor in Medical Education and Director of the Medicine Learning and Teaching Unit. Anne also served the Australian Medical Council as a council member and had longstanding involvement in its accreditation processes for medical schools and specialist colleges until her appointment to the Medical Board of Australia.

Theanne Walters AM is Deputy Chief Executive Officer of the Australian Medical Council. Theanne has worked on standards of health and medical education for more than 20 years. She contributes nationally and internationally to projects and forums to advance good practice in program accreditation and standards of medical education. She is an advisor to the World Federation for Medical Education and in the Western Pacific Region contributes to external evaluations of medical schools and accreditation development through the Western Pacific Association for Medical Education.

Tim Wilkinson MBChB MD, MClinEd, PhD, FRACP, FANZAHPE, FAMEE is Professor in Medicine and Medical Education at the University of Otago, Aotearoa New Zealand. He was the MBChB programme director 2013–2021 and Dean of the Otago Medical School 2022–2024. His research interests are assessment of clinical competence and performance, workplace learning, selection into medical school, career paths, and professionalism. In 2002 he was an inaugural winner of the Minister of Education/NZQA Tertiary Teaching Excellence Award (for sustained excellence in tertiary teaching). In 2016 he was awarded the Australian and New Zealand Association for Health Professional Educators' highest award for outstanding achievement in the field of health professional education in Australia, Aotearoa New Zealand and internationally. He holds editorship roles on several medical education journals, and works as a consultant physician in geriatric medicine.

About the authors and contributors

Vanessa Ballard JD (Hons), GradCertProfLegalPrac, GradDipMedSon, BAppSc(MedImaging) is the Executive Officer at the NSW Health Care Complaints Commission. With a background as a medical radiation scientist and sonographer, she has held several senior leadership roles across both public and private health sectors in NSW. Vanessa is also admitted as a lawyer of the Supreme Court of NSW and has dedicated the past six years to health and medical regulation, primarily in the areas of research, investigations, policy and governance.

Ruanne Brell BA, LLB (Hons) is a senior legal advisor in the Advocacy, Education and Research division at Avant, Australia's largest medical indemnity insurer. Ruanne has more than 20 years' experience in health law, assisting and advising doctors on a wide variety of medical and health law issues. She researches and contributes to medicolegal education and advocacy positions for doctors, including on topics such as medical records, consent and privacy. Previously Ruanne was a civil litigation lawyer and also co-authored the National Disability Insurance Scheme Handbook.

Will Cairns OAM BA, MB BS, FRACGP, FAChPM has retired from clinical practice as a specialist in palliative medicine and remains active in the ongoing development of palliative medicine and palliative care across Australia. He is currently a Member of Queensland's Voluntary Assisted Dying Review Board. He was very active in the palliative care response to the COVID-19 pandemic, with particular reference to the need for advance care planning and triage and resource allocation decision making.

Earlier in his career he worked as a GP before moving across to palliative medicine where for many years he was the sole doctor specialising in palliative medicine in northern Queensland. He was the Founding Director of the Townsville Palliative Care Service, and at various times Clinical Director of the Townsville Cancer Centre, and Clinical Director of Cancer Services for North Queensland. He served two terms as President of ANZSPM and one as President of the Australasian Chapter of Palliative Medicine, during which time he led the successful application for the recognition of the specialty of Palliative Medicine.

Caroline Clarke BM, DM, FRACP, FRACMA, is a retired Medical Administrator and Paediatrician. She has over 40 years' experience in health care. She has held a number of senior clinical and administrative roles in the acute public health sector with responsibilities ranging across clinical workforce, clinical governance and risk, operational management, digital health and research. Her most recent appointment was as Chief Medical Information Officer at the Royal Victorian Eye and Ear Hospital in Melbourne. She practised clinically for many years as a paediatric endocrinologist with a particular interest in diabetes, and as an adolescent physician.

In 2020/21 she chaired the Australian Medical Council's (AMC) Medical Workforce Digital Capabilities Advisory Group. She is currently the Chair of AMC's Recognition of Medical Specialties Committee and a member of the AMC Specialist Education Accreditation Committee. She has been on a number of AMC Specialist College accreditation teams.

Jemma Collova has Italian heritage, and was born and raised on Whadjuk Noongar country (Perth). Jemma is a postdoctoral Research Associate at the School of Indigenous Studies at the University of Western Australia, and works in partnership with Aboriginal and Torres Strait Islander peoples to improve cultural safety in mental health services. Jemma has worked at the intersection between academic research and government, including working for the Australian Government Office of Industry Innovation and Science, and for WA Police.

Darlene Cox is an experienced consumer advocate and has been active in the health consumer movement since the late 1990s. Darlene has been the Executive Director of the Health Care Consumers' Association since 2008. She is an eminent advocate for health consumers with an excellent knowledge of the health system, both locally and nationally. Darlene has a long, strong, practical understanding of community engagement principles. She contributes to local and national health committees including the Australian Commission on Safety and Quality in Health Care, AMC, Australian Health Practitioner Regulation Agency (Ahpra), Australian Digital Health Agency, Capital Health Network and ACT Government.

Brendan Crotty AM MB BS, MD, FRACP is a retired gastroenterologist and general physician. He was the Foundation Dean of the Deakin Medical School (2006–2011) and then Executive Dean of Deakin's Faculty of Health (2011–2019). He is a member of the AMC Prevocational Accreditation Standards Committee and was chair of the AMC working party overseeing the development and implementation of the National Framework for Prevocational Medical Training. He was also a member of the working party that recently reviewed the AMC standards for medical schools. He is a board member of the Barwon Health Board and the board of the Victorian Doctors Health Program.

Sue Dawson LLB, MUrbPl, BSW, is a recognised Australian leader in strategy and public policy, as well as in sector wide and organisational transformation. Prior to her current appointment as Independent Expert Reviewer to lead the review of complexity in the National Registration and Accreditation Scheme for health practitioners, Sue held the position of NSW Health Care Complaints Commissioner. She formerly occupied senior leadership roles in the Commonwealth and NSW public sectors.

Sue has formal qualifications as a lawyer, an urban planner and a social worker. In relation to her recognised qualification in public sector policy and service delivery, Sue is an Executive Fellow of the Australia and New Zealand School of Government (ANZSOG). Her passion is promoting collaboration within and between organisations, to deliver practical and innovative solutions and with the overarching consideration of delivering better outcomes for the community.

Jen Desrosiers works as a Researcher at the AMC. Her background in academic roles and specialist medical colleges is in public health with a focus on cultural safety, health systems science and medical education. Jen's previous experience includes contributing to health equity working with marginalised people and humanitarian response to those affected by conflict, violence or disaster. Jen has published journal articles about global health, cultural safety, HIV, sexual and gender diversity and medical education.

Antonio Di Dio MBBS, DipRANZCOG, FRACGP, GAICD, CHIA, AFACHSM, FAMA is a GP based in Canberra, and is also the Director of the Professional Services Review. He is a past state Australian Medical Association (AMA) president and board member and has served on numerous panels and committees, including for RACGP and Ahpra, and in helping doctors and the profession. He serves on many boards including the national Drs4Drs board and the Medical Benevolent Association of NSW-ACT, and is the Executive Chair of the National Doctors Health & Wellbeing Leadership Alliance. Associate Professor Di Dio has served for 30 years on on-call panels for doctor wellbeing, and is passionate about psychosocial safety and workplace culture. He is devoted to standards, professionalism, respect and care of our colleagues, and promoting good medical practice. He is the current SES Champion for the Public Sector Neurodiversity Community of Practice and is involved in the Australian National University medical school.

Richard Doherty MBBS (Hons), DObst RCOG, FRACP is trained in paediatrics and in paediatric infectious diseases. He is currently joint Deputy Chair of the board of the Royal Children's Hospital in Melbourne, honorary consultant physician in Paediatric Infectious Diseases at Monash Children's Hospital in Melbourne and an Honorary Professor in the Department of Paediatrics, Faculty of Medicine, Nursing and Health Sciences, Monash University. Professor Doherty was previously Dean of RACP, Head of the Department of Paediatrics and Associate Dean for Teaching Hospitals at Monash University, Medical Program Director (Children's Program) at Southern Health, consultant physician at the Royal Children's Hospital in Melbourne and Deputy Director of the Macfarlane Burnet Centre for Medical Research (subsequently the Burnet Institute). He was also Chair of the Board of Examiners and ex-officio Director at the AMC. Professor Doherty has served on a wide range of national committees including National Health and Medical Research Council (NHMRC) grant review panels, the 2016 Intern Review, and the National Medical Training Advisory Network, as well as Victorian Department of Health immunisation, workforce and medical training advisory committees.

Roy Donnelly MBBS, MBA, LLB, FRACMA, FCFM RCPA is a barrister working in medical negligence, health practitioner regulation and health law. Roy is qualified in both medicine and law. Roy worked for many years as a senior medical administrator at Royal Prince Alfred Hospital, Sydney, and later as a legal advisor to the local health district. He was a legal representative and a deputy chair for the RPA Human Ethics Research Committee. Roy has also worked as a senior medical manager and legal advisor to the NSW Justice Health and Forensic Mental Health Network.

Roy was admitted as a NSW legal practitioner in 2007 and as a barrister in 2017. He was called to the bar of England and Wales in October 2023. He currently works at Pump Court Chambers London where he is primarily instructed in health practitioner regulation matters and coronial inquests. He maintains a NSW based practice in medical negligence and health law at 7 Garfield Barwick Chambers Sydney. Roy has particular experience advising on complex matters of health law, and matters at the interface of law, clinical care, and medical ethics.

David Ellwood AO MA, DPhil (Oxon), MB, BChir (Cantab), FRANZCOG (CMFM), DDU is an obstetrician and gynaecologist with a subspeciality qualification in maternal-fetal medicine. He is a past-President of the AMC, and chaired the Medical Schools Accreditation Committee from 2011 to 2017. He is Professor of Obstetrics & Gynaecology at Griffith University, Queensland and until recently was Head of School of Medicine and Dentistry and Dean of Medicine. He is clinically active and is currently the Medical Director of Maternal-Fetal Medicine at Gold Coast University Hospital. He is also the Co-Director of an NHMRC-funded Centre of Research Excellence in Stillbirth at the Mater Research Institute, Brisbane, and has wide-ranging research interests in the prediction and prevention of adverse outcomes of pregnancy.

Michael E Franco MBBS, FRACP, FAChPM, FAIDH is a consultant medical oncologist and palliative medicine specialist. He is an adjunct associate professor in the faculties of Medicine, Nursing & Health Sciences and Information Technology at Monash University in Victoria. Michael played an integral role in establishing the Palliative and Supportive Care Clinical Trials Program at Monash Health; he is an NHMRC Grant Assessor and has been Principal Investigator on national and international trials. He is on the Specialist Committee of the Thoracic Oncology Group of Australasia and was the inaugural Co-Chair of the Supportive and Palliative Medicine Subgroup. Michael is eminent in medical accreditation and is a Fellow of the Australasian Institute of Digital Health, holding positions of national standing with the Postgraduate Medical Council of Australia, Confederation of Postgraduate Medical Education Councils and International Association for the Study of Lung Cancer.

Christine Gee AM is Chair of the Medical Board of Australia's National Special Issues Committee (Sexual Boundaries and Family Violence) which is the delegated committee responsible for regulatory decisions on matters relating to sexual boundary violations and family violence. She was first appointed as a Community Member of the Queensland Board of the Medical Board of Australia in 2014. Christine is also the Chief Executive Officer of Toowong Private Hospital and holds a number of local, state and national board appointments. She is the National President of the Australian Private Hospitals Association and a board member of the Australian Commission on Safety and Quality in Health Care.

In 2023, Christine was appointed as a Member (AM) of the Order of Australia for significant service to the community, particularly through hospital administration. Christine's personal philosophy puts patients at the centre of care, and both acknowledges and values the power of lived experience in the planning, design, delivery, measurement and evaluation of care.

Lynn Gillam AM is a clinical ethicist, and Academic Director of the Children's Bioethics Centre at the Royal Children's Hospital, Melbourne. Lynn provides clinical ethics case consultation and policy advice, and leads research in paediatric clinical ethics. She is also Professor in Health Ethics at the University of Melbourne, in the Department of Paediatrics, where she teaches ethics in the MD course, and ethics and qualitative research design in other health professional courses.

Peter Greenberg OAM MD, PhD, FRACP is a consultant physician in general internal medicine who is currently an Honorary Emeritus Physician in the Department of General Medicine at the Royal Melbourne Hospital, Honorary Principal Fellow in the schools of Medicine and Population & Global Health at the University of Melbourne and Adjunct Associate Professor in the School of Public Health and Preventive Medicine, Monash University. Peter chaired the NHMRC working committee, which developed the 2006 NHMRC toolkit *Making decisions about tests and treatments: principles for better communication between healthcare professionals and healthcare consumers*. Another of his publications is *Difficult physician–patient encounters*, co-authored with Kerry Breen. Peter continues to tutor University of Melbourne medical students in professional practice, which includes aspects of communication and ethics.

Julie Hamblin has worked for more than 30 years as a lawyer and policy consultant in health law, clinical risk, disability and international development. In addition to her own legal practice in health law and ethics, she has served on numerous government and other advisory bodies in the health sector, including the Australian Research Integrity Committee, the NSW Health Ethics Advisory Panel, the MBS Review clinical committees for obstetrics and gynaecology and the Attorney-General's International Pro Bono Advisory Group. She has a particular interest in sexual and reproductive rights, having worked with the United Nations Development Programme and other organisations on projects relating to public health and HIV/AIDS in more than 20 countries in Asia, the Pacific, Africa and Eastern Europe.

Julie is an experienced non-executive director. She chairs the boards of Australian Volunteers International and Maluk Timor Australia and is the Independent Board Director for the Royal Australian and New Zealand College of Obstetricians and Gynaecologists.

Karin Hammarberg RN, BSc, PhD is adjunct senior research fellow at the School of Public Health and Preventive Medicine at Monash University and was senior research officer at the Victorian Assisted Reproductive Treatment Authority from 2011 to 2024. Karin is a registered nurse with 20 years' experience as clinical coordinator of IVF programs. She has significant clinical and research expertise in the psychosocial aspects of reproductive health including fertility health promotion and assisted reproductive technology. Since completing her PhD in 2006, Karin has published two books, nine book chapters and more than 100 peer-reviewed papers.

Amandeep Hansra BMed(Hons), MPH&TM, ACCAM, GlobalEMBA, FRACGP, FAIDH, GAICD is an adjunct associate professor in Biomedical Informatics and Digital Health at the University of Sydney as well as a practising GP in Sydney, Australia. Amandeep is recognised as a leader in telehealth and digital health and has set up telehealth businesses both locally and internationally. She is a board director and adviser to many digital health companies. Amandeep sits on the board of AMA NSW, Healthdirect, the Australian Council on Healthcare Standards (International) and MoleMap New Zealand. Amandeep also leads the Australian Clinical Entrepreneur Program in NSW and is an advocate for healthcare innovation and entrepreneurship among clinicians.

Felicity Hawker AM MBBS, FCICM is an intensive care specialist who worked for over 30 years in intensive care units in NSW and Victoria. She currently works as a Director of Professional Affairs with the College of Intensive Care Medicine of Australia and New Zealand.

Jeremy Hayllar BA(Hons), MB(Hons), MSc, MD, FRACP, FRCP, DTM&H, FAChAM , attended Birmingham Medical School, after a law degree at Oxford. He trained in general medicine and gastroenterology in London. His MD examined the GI effects of NSAIDs. From 1992 he spent 10 years in the hard-drinking mining community of Mount Isa as Director of Medical Services and general physician.

Between 2004 and September 2025 he was Clinical Director, Alcohol and Drug Service, Metro North Mental Health, and since 2018 has been a pre-eminent Senior Medical Officer. He represented the RACP during planning for real time prescription monitoring (QScript) and was a member of the Queensland Medicinal Cannabis Expert Advisory Panel. He helped in updating Queensland Health guidelines into withdrawal management and opioid use disorder, as well as the national pharmacotherapy guidelines and alcohol- and drug-related resources with the Australian College of Rural and Remote Medicine.

Georgie Haysom BSc, LLB(Hons), LLM(Bioethics), GAICD, GC, PsycBM is the General Manager, Advocacy, Education and Research at medical indemnity provider Avant. She is a lawyer and has worked in health law for 30 years, assisting, advising and educating doctors on a wide range of medicolegal issues, including several years representing doctors in medical negligence litigation. For the past 10 years she has worked in the advocacy, education and research division at Avant, which aims to improve quality, safety and professionalism in medical practice. In that role she has written on many topics, including informed decision making and privacy, for a variety of audiences and in a range of formats.

She has a longstanding interest in the interaction between law, medicine and ethics, and the way in which the law impacts on medical practice. She is a member of the Australian Digital Health Agency's Privacy and Security Advisory Committee and the South Eastern Sydney Local Health District's Clinical Ethics Committee.

Philip Hébert MD, PhD, FCFPC is a professor emeritus in the Department of Family and Community Medicine at the University of Toronto. More than 25 years ago he founded and then directed the ethics program at the medical school in Toronto. Although retired, he continues to teach and write. His core interest is in professional ethics and he has written two books on the topic: *Doing right: a practical guide to ethics for physicians and medical trainees* (4th edition, in association with Wayne Rosen, Oxford University Press, 2019) intended for learners and practitioners; and *Good medicine: the art of ethical care in Canada* (Doubleday Canada, 2016) aimed at a wider audience.

Kathryn Sarah Hutt MBBS, BSc(Med), MPH, MA(AppliedEthics), GAICD is a GP working in urban and remote communities in NSW; she is also an experienced medical administrator. Kathryn is currently the Medical Director of Doctors' Health NSW, an independent registered charity providing 24/7 support to doctors and medical students and also delivering education, contributing to research and advocating for doctors' health and wellbeing. In previous roles, Kathryn gained considerable experience at a senior management level in hospitals of all sizes, and as an adviser on medical workforce, training and service planning at a state level. She also has extensive experience in human research ethics and professional regulation. Kathryn recognises the fundamental importance of a healthy and respectful professional culture, and the many benefits of improving doctors' health and wellbeing, for individuals and for the communities in which they serve

Michael Isaacs BSc, BA, MD is a medical registrar for the Department of Medicine at Ipswich Hospital, Queensland. He has a strong background in industrial advocacy in the medical field, as a union delegate for Australian Salaried Medical Officers' Federation Queensland and previous Chair of the AMA Queensland Committee of Doctors in Training (CDT) Industrial Relations Special Interest Group. In these roles he assisted in the negotiation of a new state enterprise bargaining agreement for medical officers (MOCA 6). He also has a keen interest in philosophy and ethics, stemming from his undergraduate studies. He was awarded the Eric W Peet Memorial Prize in Medical Ethics during his medical degree, and is presently the CDT representative on the AMA Ethics and Medicolegal Council.

Louise Johnson GAICD, BSc(Hons), DipEd, DipManagement, MRegulatoryStudies was Chief Executive Officer for the Victorian Assisted Reproductive Treatment Authority for 16 years, involved with the regulation of the assisted reproductive treatment industry in Victoria, management of the donor conception registers and public education about assisted reproductive treatment and the prevention of infertility. Louise is currently a board director of Central Highlands Rural Health, and Chair of the NHMRC Embryo Research Licensing Committee, and a consumer representative on the Australasian College for Emergency Medicine's Council of Advocacy, Practice and Partnerships (CAPP). Louise was previously a panel member on the Victorian Patient Review Panel, a member of the Victorian Board of the Medical Board of Australia and Occupational Therapy Board of Australia, and Chair of Women's Health Victoria.

Joanne Katsoris MBBS has been an experienced medical regulator for more than 25 years, having worked for the Medical Practitioners Board of Victoria before being appointed to the position of Executive Officer to the Medical Board of Australia in 2009.

Joanne is a medical practitioner who previously worked in a range of hospital-based clinical and administrative positions in Melbourne and at the Australian Red Cross blood service.

Margaret Kay AM MBBS(Hons) PhD, FRACGP, DipRACOG, GAICD is a general practitioner with clinical and research expertise in both doctors' health and refugee health. In 2013, she completed her PhD in physician health, focusing on how doctors access health care for themselves, and has published extensively in the area of doctors' health. Dr Kay holds an academic title as Senior Lecturer with the Faculty of Health, Medicine and Behavioural Sciences at the University of Queensland and enjoys teaching doctors and medical students about physician health. She is also the Clinical Lead in Multicultural Health with the Brisbane South PHN. In 2022, she was awarded Membership of the Order of Australia for significant service to medicine, to medical education, and to migrant health.

Ian Kerridge AM BA, BMed(Hons), MPhil(Cantab), FRACP, FRCPA is Professor of Bioethics and Medicine at Sydney Health Ethics at the University of Sydney, Honorary Professor in the Department of Philosophy at Macquarie University and Staff Haematologist/Bone Marrow Transplant physician at Royal North Shore Hospital, Sydney. He is also Chair of the South-Eastern Sydney LHD Clinical Ethics Committee, Steering Committee member of the Australian Ethical Health Alliance and a Director of Praxis Australia—an Australian not-for-profit organisation devoted to education in research and research ethics. He has previously been Chair of RACP's Ethics Committee and a member of the Australian Health Ethics Committee. Ian trained in medicine at the University of Newcastle, in bone marrow transplant (BMT) at the Royal Free Hospital and University College Hospital in London, and in philosophy at the universities of Sydney, Newcastle and Cambridge. He is the author of six textbooks of ethics and over 500 papers on ethics, philosophy, haematology and BMT.

Nicole Lawless BA, PGDip(ForensicPsych), LLB, LLM was the Executive Director of Legal Services at the Health Care Complaints Commission; she commenced at the Commission in October 2021. Nicole also held the statutory role of the Director of Proceedings. Nicole was admitted as a solicitor in 2002. Prior to joining the Commission, Nicole was the NSW Deputy Ombudsman, where she led the Complaints and Investigations Branch. Nicole previously worked in the NSW Ombudsman's Office as a legal advisor and Counsel Assisting the Ombudsman. Nicole has also held roles as a prosecutor at the NSW Office of the Director of Public Prosecutions, as the Deputy Director of the Criminal Law Review Division in the NSW Attorney General's Department, as a policy advisor in the Department of Premier and Cabinet on the prevention of violence against women, and heading up the legal and strategy team representing the Department of Family and Community Services in the Royal Commission into Institutional Responses to Child Sexual Abuse.

Wendy Lipworth BSc(Med), MBBS, MSc, PhD is Professor of Bioethics in the Discipline of Philosophy at Macquarie University, Sydney. Her work sits at the intersection of ethics and epistemology. She has led multidisciplinary research on commercial influences on health care and biomedical science and is an author of RACP's Guidelines for ethical relationships between health professionals and industry (fourth edition, 2018). She is President of the Australasian Association of Bioethics and Health Law and Co-Director of the Macquarie University Ethics and Agency Research Centre. She is a member of the steering committees of the Australian Ethical Health Alliance (representing PRAXIS Australia) and Brain Cancer Australia.

Erw in Loh MBBS, LBB(Hons), MBA, MHSM, PhD, FRACMA, FACLM, FAICD is President of the Royal Australasian College of Medical Administrators (RACMA). He was most recently National Director of Medical Services for Calvary Health Care. He was previously Group Chief Medical Officer at St Vincent's Health Australia, Chief Medical Officer at Goulburn Valley Health and Chief Medical Officer of Monash Health. He has qualifications in medicine, law and management. He is a barrister and solicitor of the Supreme Court of Victoria and High Court of Australia. He has adjunct professorial appointments at Monash University, University of Melbourne and Macquarie University. He has been an invited speaker at local and international conferences, and has published books, book chapters and journal articles on health leadership, health law, clinical governance, AI and health technology. He is a member of the Association of Professional Futurists. He received the Distinguished Fellow Award from RACMA in 2017 for 'commitment to governance, research and publication'.

Tamara Mackean MBBS, MPH, FAPHM is a Waljen woman, Professor of Aboriginal and Torres Strait Islander Public Health Research with the College of Medicine and Public Health and the inaugural Research Lead: Indigenous Research Strategy with the Deputy Vice-Chancellor, Research at Flinders University. Tamara conducts a broad range of public health research on health systems and equity, decolonisation in health research, culturally safe quality health care, workforce development and the multiple determinants of Indigenous health and wellbeing. Through a commitment to decolonisation and working at the interface of knowledge systems, Tamara brings together her public health knowledge and her cultural standpoint to generate new ways of working and new evidence for best practice and policy.

Peter Martin MB BCh BAO, MMed, FAChPM is a professor of clinical communication and end-of-life care. Peter has been involved with communication skills training for almost 30 years and has been a clinician for 35 years. He has taught on numerous postgraduate communication skills courses with a variety of health professional disciplines nationally and internationally over the past 15+ years. He is also involved in whole-of-organisation interventions to improve the quality of clinical communication.

Prudence McEvoy MBBS, DipPsychotherapy, FRANZCP, Cert Accreditation Child and Adolescent Psychiatry is a senior child and adolescent psychiatrist who is currently Lead Psychiatric Director within the Department of Child Protection in South Australia. This position was created in 2019, and has enhanced the interface between child and adolescent psychiatry and child protection. She was previously Clinical Director of the statewide Child and Adolescent Mental Health Service, and has always worked with infants, children and adolescents who have experienced child maltreatment both in private and public practice.

Talila Milroy FRACGP, MBBS, BSc is a Yindjibarndi and Palyku GP and early career researcher. She has research interests in Aboriginal health and women's and children's health. She held an RACGP academic post with the University of Western Australia, where her research project focused on experiences of racism for Indigenous GP trainees. She currently provides primary care services to Aboriginal women and children in a multidisciplinary clinic in Rockingham, WA. She contributes to Aboriginal health and general practice teaching at UWA Medical School.

Dinesh Palipana OAM MD, LLB, GradDipLP, CertEM, GAICD was the first quadriplegic medical intern in Queensland. Dinesh is a doctor, and lawyer. Dinesh works in the emergency department at Gold Coast Health. He is a researcher and senior lecturer at the Griffith University. Dinesh was a senior advisor to the Disability Royal Commission. He is an ambassador to the Human Rights Commission's IncludeAbility program, a co-founder of Doctors with Disabilities Australia, and an advisory board member to Healthylife.

Dinesh was Gold Coast Health's Junior Doctor of the Year in 2018. He was awarded the Medal of the Order of Australia in 2019. He was the third Australian to be awarded a Henry Viscardi Achievement Award. He was the 2021 Griffith University Young Alumnus of the Year. Dinesh was the Queensland Australian of the Year for 2021. His autobiography, *Stronger*, was published in 2022.

Lisa Pritchard LLB(Hons I), GradDipLegalPrac is Deputy Public Guardian at the Office of the Public Guardian (Queensland). Lisa's responsibilities include acting as Statutory Health Attorney to provide consent to health care as decision maker of last resort, and overseeing investigations into allegations of abuse, neglect and exploitation of adults with impaired capacity. Lisa has over 25 years of experience in consumer protection and complaints management in the UK and Australia, including in human services and health regulation and complaints management as Director of the Professional Standards Unit, Queensland Medical Board; Director Ethical Standards Unit, Queensland Health; and Executive Director, Queensland Office of the Health Ombudsman (Assessment and Resolution). Lisa was a foundational member of the executive team at the Office of the Health Ombudsman at its inception in 2014, and established and led the complaints management and dispute resolution functions.

John M Quinn AM MBBS, FRACS, FACS, GAICD is a retired consultant vascular surgeon who worked in public and private practice in Brisbane. Prior to retirement in 2018 he was Director of Vascular Surgery at Princess Alexandra Hospital in Brisbane. John has also been Executive Director for Surgical Affairs at the Royal Australasian College of Surgeons (RACS) since 2005, and in addition is currently Director of Medical Services at St Vincent's Private Hospital Northside (Brisbane). In all of these areas he is exposed to matters of professionalism, ethics and the law, especially transgressions or alleged transgressions in these and related fields. He has been very involved with RACS in the training of vascular surgeons and served as Chair of the Training Board in Vascular Surgery and also as Senior Examiner for Vascular Surgery for RACS.

Dr Quinn was awarded Membership of the Order of Australia (AM) for significant service to medicine in the fields of general and vascular surgery and to professional organisations.

Gary D Rogers MBBS, MGPPsych, PhD, FAMEE, FANZAHPE, PFHEA is a health professions educational leader, learning and teaching scholar, public health researcher and GP with a focus on HIV medicine. He is Professor of Medical Education and Dean of the School of Medicine at Deakin University in Victoria, Australia. Gary is a former President of the Australian and New Zealand Association for Health Professional Educators and a current member of the Executive Committee of Medical Deans Australia and New Zealand. He also serves on AMC's Medical Schools Accreditation Committee. Professor Rogers' educational research focuses on the affective learning associated with the acquisition of professional and interprofessional values among health professional students, as well as widening access to health professional education as a health workforce strategy.

Tim Shaw PhD, BSc is Professor of Digital Health at the University of Sydney and leads the Research in Implementation Science and eHealth Group. He is recognised as an international leader in digital health and focuses on how health data can be used to transform care and how technology can support new models and approaches to care. He specialises in building partnerships across industry, services, government and universities to deliver high-impact research translation and education. Over the past five years he has been a chief investigator on over 30 competitive or commissioned research and development projects totalling more than A$124 million.

Bernadette Tobin AO MA(Melb), MEd(Melb), PhD(Cantab) is the director of the Plunkett Centre for Ethics, located at St Vincent's Hospital in Sydney, and Reader in Philosophy at Australian Catholic University. She has held adjunct appointments in the medical faculties of the University of New South Wales and the University of Sydney. She served for three triennia on the Australian Health Ethics Committee. She has authored more than 50 articles singly or jointly with others in the peer-reviewed literature. In 2016 she was appointed an Officer in the Order of Australia.

Tim Usherwood BSc, MBBS, MD, DMS, FRCP, FRCGP, FRACGP is Emeritus Professor of General Practice at the University of Sydney; Honorary Professorial Fellow at the George Institute for Global Health; and Consultant Emeritus at Westmead Hospital. He was Chair and then Deputy Chair of the Board of Western Sydney PHN (WentWest Ltd) until 2022, having led establishment of WentWest in 2002 initially as the regional general practice training provider for western Sydney. He chaired the General Practice and Primary Care Committee of the 2016–2020 MBS Review, and was Head of Westmead Clinical School 2019–2020. Professor Usherwood's research has focused on the development and evaluation of interventions to improve health outcomes in chronic disease and primary care, with particular application to healthcare access, vascular disease, depression and asthma. He has published more than 250 refereed research papers on these and related topics. Professor Usherwood practised clinically at Western Sydney Community Controlled Aboriginal Health Service for almost 20 years, and subsequently at Western Sydney Sexual Health Centre and Public Health Unit.

Emma Warnecke MBBS(Hons), FRACGP, MMH, Grad Cert LT Health Professionals is a Medical Practitioner and Associate Professor at the University of Tasmania, School of Medicine. Emma has a long-held interest in effective communication and shared decision making, and wrote an article for Australian Family Physician in 2014 on the art of communication. Emma also has an interest in mental health and doctor wellbeing.

Emma found herself on the other side of the doctor–patient relationship after being diagnosed with triple negative breast cancer in 2018, in her 40s. Emma has written an article about her journey (https://insightplus.mja.com.au/2021/42/when-the-doctor-becomes-the-patient-my-breast-cancer-journey/). With this lived experience of the patient perspective through the lens of a doctor, Emma continues to be a passionate advocate for patient empowerment through enhancing communication.

Susan Wearne BM, PhD, MMedSci, FACRRM, FRACGP, MRCGP, DCH, DRCOG, DFFP, GCTEd, GAICD is Senior Medical Adviser, Health Workforce Division in the Australian Government Department of Health, Disability and Ageing. She works on the Australian Government policies and programs that teach and train quality health professionals and promote their distribution to underserved areas. This role capitalises on her experience as a GP and academic in Alice Springs, which included work at an Aboriginal Medical Service and for the Royal Flying Doctor Service.

As a UK graduate, Susan hopes her chapter on the Australian healthcare system gives other international medical graduates the information that she learned opportunistically from generous students and colleagues when she moved from Yorkshire to Central Australia and then Canberra.

Mark Wenitong MBBS has Kabi Kabi and South Sea Islander heritage and holds a significant leadership role in First Nations health and mental health fields covering clinical governance, strategic primary healthcare planning, research and policy. He is a past president and founding member of the Australian Indigenous Doctors' Association, the inaugural Co-Chair of the Queensland Health statewide First Nations Clinical Network. He is currently a National Mental Health Commissioner. He sits on the national Aboriginal and Torres Strait Islander genomics advisory group, and the national advisory group for the implementation of the national Aboriginal and Torres Strait Islander health plan. His main area of clinical interest is Aboriginal and Torres Strait Islander primary health care and translation of research into practice, and has been heavily involved in research translation in remote Aboriginal and Torres Strait Islander primary health care in Cape York and the Torres Strait.

PART ONE

Being a good doctor

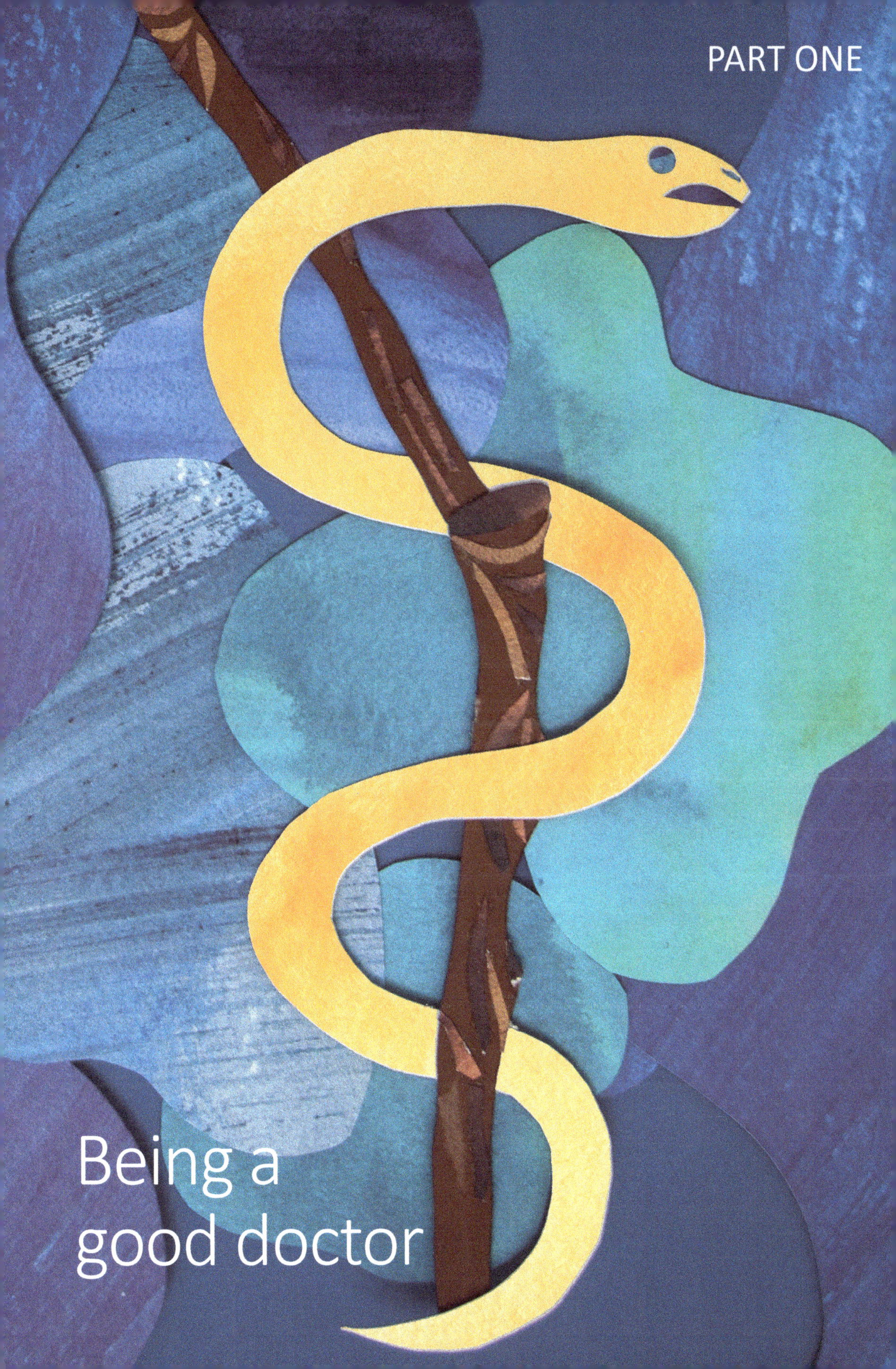

01 Good medical practice in a changing environment: a consumer perspective

Darlene Cox

There have been a great many changes in the healthcare environment since the publication of the last edition of *Good medical practice.*

The most significant, of course, was the COVID-19 pandemic (see Chapters 4, 20, 24 and 29). In addition, we are seeing increasing complexity of disease, compounded by changes in key social determinants of health (see Chapters 16 and 17) and rapid changes in technology including the wide application of artificial intelligence in health care (see Chapter 29).

The need to keep up to date and maintain professional competence is an added pressure with the fast pace of changes in legislation, environmental issues, and scientific and medical knowledge (see Chapter 10). There is an expectation that doctors will know how to update their knowledge and practice, and engage meaningfully in that process.

The pandemic has changed the delivery of health care and community expectations of health care. It has underscored how much value we place on our health professionals. It has reinforced the importance of consent and informed decision making (see Chapter 7) and exposed increasing inequity (see Chapter 16). The pandemic saw an increase in misinformation and disinformation. Addressing disinformation is a particular challenge as it involves people knowingly spreading false information to deceive (see Chapter 5). The pandemic also reminded us of the value of consumer empowerment and the importance of health literacy (see Chapter 7). These are professional, legal and ethical issues that doctors face on a daily basis.

We are seeing more pronounced inequity, and the gap between the haves and have-nots is growing. This includes cost-of-living pressures, and very real housing and homelessness issues. The waiting times to access health care, and the challenge for consumers to access affordable health care, compound this. Many people are faced with hard decisions about how to balance their household budgets, and that includes deciding whether or not to fill prescriptions, have diagnostic imaging or see their GP (see Chapter 30). Social determinants shape our access to and experience of health care, and our health outcomes (see Chapter 16).

As consumers, we are taking a more active role in decision making about our medical care. We have more access to health information, and this has changed the patient–doctor relationship. Consumers and carers are using internet-based search engines to find health information. This is an act of empowerment and enables us to participate actively in our own care and decision making. However, misinformation and low health literacy also make this problematic. Consumers can struggle to identify high-quality health information from reputable sources (see Chapters 5 and 7).

When consumers talk about what good medical practice looks like, we talk about doctors who:

- handle our questions, concerns and fears in an empathetic way
- listen carefully to what we have to say
- explain the purpose of treatments and medications and talk about the side effects in ways we can understand
- provide information we can read at a time of our choosing, to help us manage our health
- will refer to another specialist if our matter is beyond their scope of practice and clinical competence.

Health care is about people. Care is designed and delivered by people to meet the needs of people, and there are emotional aspects of health care that we need to acknowledge. The principles of consumer-centred care reflect this and ensure consumers are seen in their own context. Consumer-centred care maintains a holistic view that respects each consumer's individual circumstances, values and preferences. Specialisation and the emergence of subspecialties bring benefits and risks to health care. The risks are compounded by the fragmentation of the health system. We need doctors to balance specialised and technical skills with the relational aspect of caring for people and providing personal care to individuals. We need to reframe the health system to focus on the needs and experiences of consumers, families and carers (see Chapter 20).

Consumer-centred care is a way of thinking and doing things that sees the people using health and social services as equal partners in planning, developing and monitoring care. This means putting people and their families at the centre of decisions and seeing us as experts about our own lives, working alongside professionals to get the best outcome. It is as much about the way professionals and patients think about care and their relationships, as it is about the actual services available. It is about supporting us as consumers to be more active in our care, which leads to better health outcomes.

For doctors, there are very practical aspects to consumer-centred care:

- Get to know your patients.
- Be mindful of the way you speak to us and the way you speak about us.
- Help us to participate in our own care.
- Be curious and ask questions.
- See us as part of the team—this is about your work and about our lives—we absolutely want to be part of the team.

Health care is relationship-based work. We will always need the technical skills, diagnostic tests, understanding of medications and lifesaving procedures—that is a core part of your training. But overwhelmingly, for consumers, a good relationship with our health practitioner is what makes good health care. A relationship is built on trust and an exchange of knowledge. Those pieces of information we share with you can have a critical impact on the treatment pathway and health outcome. That relationship may be formed in one encounter, or one shift or over a longer period. These relationships are not just an indulgence, they are the foundation of good health care (see Chapters 2, 3, 5, 6, 7 and 21).

Good health care is based on teamwork (see Chapter 11). The teams include health workers as well as patients, families and carers. They can also involve specialist community organisations. While this can add to the complexity of providing health care, community services and social care play an important role in a person's health and quality of life. We saw the value of direct and early engagement with specialist local community organisations in the development and rollout of public health campaigns and services during the pandemic. The involvement of these groups was important to understand and meet the needs of people from multicultural communities, people living with significant disadvantage, people who live in crowded homes or have unstable housing, and people who may have poor mental health and issues with addiction.

Health care is intersectional. This is a growing area of focus in medical education and health policy. It relates to each individual's unique experiences of discrimination and stigma, arising from intersecting layers of oppression or disadvantage from different social identities. This could include race, disability, class, sexuality, gender, spiritual beliefs and citizenship status, which can intersect within a single individual (see Chapters 16 and 17). These intersecting identities can lead to devaluation, stereotyping, judging and discrimination of the patient. This shapes interactions with healthcare providers and can influence treatment options and interventions, and ultimately health outcomes.

Our communities are diverse and there are different cultural understandings of health. The biomedical model may not be consistent with the cultural values and beliefs of people from multicultural communities. This includes consumers, families and carers as well as doctors and healthcare teams. Similarly, there are limitations with the application of the biomedical model to disability, where people with disability are often seen as needing to be 'fixed'. A social model of care is more inclusive. It recognises that people living with impairments live in a world with physical, attitudinal, social and institutional barriers that limit the way a person with disability can move around, communicate and enjoy quality of life.

Understanding the diversity of consumers and families in terms of our communities and characteristics can make it easier to identify barriers to accessing health care. Our willingness to trust is influenced by our perception of doctors' behaviour and whether we feel valued and respected, and whether the things that are important to us are acknowledged. This can impact care as we may not feel safe to share information you need from us to make a diagnosis or identify effective treatment options. An intersectional approach enables doctors to see their patients as a whole person.

Over many years consumers have shared their experiences with doctors, both good and bad. They are clear about what they need:

- 'I need to be listened to.'
- 'I want my clinicians to understand where I'm coming from and see that I am more than my disease.'
- 'I don't want them to judge me.'
- 'I want them to help me to understand what is happening to me.'

This last point is important as it supports and enables shared decision making and empowerment. We rely on doctors to provide advice and information that we understand, and that is relevant to our individual circumstances, to support us to make an informed decision and choose the best option. Consent is ours to give (see Chapter 7).

We want to be listened to, to feel seen and heard, because for consumers—your patients—feeling cared for is part of our experience. For many, it's as important as the treatment we receive. The experience of being cared for by a health professional who has been friendly, generous with their time and knowledge, and considerate of our needs, never leaves us. Kindness and empathy both matter (see Chapter 5).

Be mindful of the barriers many of us experience in accessing health care. Sometimes the barriers may not be obvious but can include things like:

- having difficulty understanding, speaking or reading English
- being concerned about the stigma associated with the condition we have, or the person we are
- being unable to drive or not having access to private transport
- holding different cultural understandings about health care, causes of disease and decision making
- being a carer for someone else with significant or competing needs
- having difficult past experiences in health care
- finding the system difficult to navigate and understand.

Doctors can address inequity by recognising these barriers and going the extra mile for those affected patients to look at ways to make health care more accessible to these groups.

There are increasing expectations of public reporting on the quality and safety of care (see Chapter 23). This is a matter of public interest and can support consumers to make informed choices about their care.

We are also seeing increasing politicisation of health care, which adds pressure to those working in the system. We see leaders clashing over public policy as well as interpretations of medical advice. Many consumers find this confusing, and it makes the public health messages harder to communicate. This underscores the importance of the voice of medical experts in public policy and developing effective responses. Public health and infectious disease physicians, microbiologists and epidemiologists have been at the forefront of the public policy debates. This is consistent with our expectation that doctors will advocate for social policy so that those most at risk of poor outcomes are not forgotten and have their health needs met.

Disinformation is both dangerous and malicious. The pandemic revealed a growing mistrust of doctors by some individuals and communities around the safety and efficacy of vaccinations. This was compounded by constant media coverage and the rise of social media as a source of health information. Doctors are on the front line of dealing with this, in relation to supporting people to find the truth about their health.

One of the most pressing social, moral and ethical issues of our time is climate change. We are living in a changing climate that is impacting human health. We all have a responsibility to do what we can to reduce the environmental cost of health care. This requires a change in models of care and prescribing behaviour from all healthcare providers, administrators and regulators. It also requires changes in expectations of health care from consumers, carers and communities. Climate action needs to achieve mitigation, adaptation and equity. This will include:

- keeping people healthy so our need for health care reduces
- reducing the prevalence of low-value care
- decarbonising the health system to reduce greenhouse gas emissions and minimise its carbon footprint
- protecting the most vulnerable people from adverse effects of global warming, as they will be disproportionately affected.

Think about the health of our planet. Look for ways to reduce the carbon footprint and greenhouse gas emissions in your practice.

You are making lives better. This includes providing care and reassurance, working to diagnose disease, supporting us to make informed decisions about our treatment options, and supporting us in our recovery. Your compassion, reassurance and ability to help us understand what is happening to us at times of deep stress, when we are not feeling well, are afraid and have lost a sense of control, is valued. This is important work. Our communities, our society, value the work you have all been trained to do.

02 On being a good doctor: the changing face of medical professionalism

Tim Wilkinson, Theanne Walters AM, Anne Tonkin AO, Philip Hébert

Introduction

This chapter will explore what it means to be a good doctor and a member of a trusted profession. Recently, there has been a focus worldwide on the importance of medical professionalism. A good doctor is one who strives to practise competently, upholds the ethical standards of medicine, and is committed to all the roles expected of doctors. However, the exact nature of medical professionalism, as expressed in the literature, is not static. We discuss how our understanding of medical professionalism has developed, how professionalism is learned by doctors, how it may be best demonstrated in daily practice, and end with a discussion of the art of medicine.

This chapter has been developed from an earlier version by doctors Kerry Breen, Stephen Cordner and Colin Thomson in the fourth edition of this book [1], with updated literature and concepts reflecting changes in understanding of professionalism over the past decade. It introduces a number of topics that are further explored in other chapters of this book.

2.1 Medical professionalism

2.1.1 What is medical professionalism?

The term 'medical professionalism' can encompass all the desirable attributes of a good doctor by referring to the skills, attitudes and beliefs required for practitioners to successfully respond to the conditions and troubles of patients and their communities. A narrower view can reduce this simply to behaving ethically. Several definitions are explored here.

The UK's Royal College of Physicians (RCP) in 2005 defined professionalism as 'the set of values, behaviours, and relationships that underpin the trust the public has in doctors' [2]. Since that publication, society and health care have undergone significant change, with major implications for professionalism. A more recent and highly recommended report took the RCP's definition as a starting point and expanded and updated it by identifying seven key aspects of doctors' working lives essential to professionalism [3], which position the doctor as:

- healer: the concept at the core of medical professionalism, incorporating the values of compassion, respect and integrity, putting patients first but also attending to self-care
- patient partner: doctor–patient relationships have changed from the traditional structure (in which patients deferred to doctors) to a more equal partnership

- team worker: promoting effective teamwork by fostering communication and building a positive working culture in healthcare teams across different professions
- manager and leader: managing resource allocation and providing clinical leadership, which requires courage, the ability to innovate and improve, and the ability to manage risk and uncertainty
- patient advocate: particularly promoting patient safety in health care but also on broader issues affecting health
- learner and teacher: a commitment to lifelong learning and the ability to reflect on an experience to improve practice, as well as a focus on teaching and training of the next generation
- innovator: achieving the best blend of innovation (using digital technologies and artificial intelligence) with the human elements of patient care.

The Australian Medical Association's (AMA) definition of professionalism refers to the 'values and skills that the profession and society expects of doctors, encapsulating both the individual doctor–patient relationship and the wider social "contract" between the profession and society' [4].

It can be seen that different organisations and academics have varied definitions of professionalism. This plurality can be confusing but is expected. Nevertheless, there are some core features that remain common. A systematic review [5] concluded that professionalism incorporates:

- adherence to ethical practice principles
- effective interactions with patients and with people who are important to those patients
- effective interactions with other people working within the health system
- reliability
- commitment to maintenance, and continuous improvement, of competence in self, others and systems.

Professionalism describes the personal and professional attributes required for effective medical practice that patients, their families and their communities can trust. These traits of professionalism are often considered 'humanistic' [6] and go beyond the 'scientific' skills and attitudes required of doctors. Patients and families—indeed the public in general—take it for granted that modern doctors will be knowledgeable and skilful and will keep that knowledge and those skills up to date [7]. At a practical level, the Medical Board of Australia has published *Good medical practice: a code of conduct for doctors in Australia* [8], which describes the behaviours expected of all doctors registered to practise in Australia.

2.1.2 Professionalism as a social contract

Notwithstanding the plethora of definitions, professionalism should be seen as a mutually agreed contract between the profession and the public. A profession can be defined as

> a disciplined group of individuals who adhere to ethical standards and who hold themselves out as, and are accepted by the public as possessing special knowledge and skills in a widely recognised body of learning derived from research, education and training at a high level, and who are prepared to apply this knowledge and exercise these skills in the interest of others [9].

This approach typically identifies a profession by its capacity for self-regulation, a feature that implies great trust placed in that profession by the community.

The medical profession exists (with the consent of society) to serve the function of maintaining the wellbeing of society and the health of its members [3]. This is a shared responsibility—together medical professionals are expected to act in the public good; to adhere to high ethical and moral standards; to respond to societal needs; to possess core humanistic values, including honesty and integrity; to exercise accountability for themselves and their colleagues; to demonstrate moral discipline; and to reflect upon their actions and decisions [10].

Professional status is not an inherent right, but a privilege granted by society. The maintenance of professional status thus depends on the public's confidence that professionals can be trusted. As societal values and aspects of the practice of medicine and the delivery of health care change over time, the medical profession must strive to keep in step with not only the scientific advances in medicine but also with the expectations of the community.

It is expected that a modern health professional is aware of the social, cultural and environmental causes of health and illness and is prepared to act as an advocate for distinct communities of patients. The modern physician must recognise and manage the upstream causes of illness and the social determinants of wellness and ill health, and be prepared to act, altruistically, as an advocate for the benefit of defined populations of patients and their communities [3] (see also section 2.2 and Chapter 16, Achieving full health potential: health equity).

This is the changing face of medical professionalism and emphasises the growing recognition of the importance of 'cultural humility' to good medical practice, defined as 'a process of being aware of how people's culture can impact their health behaviours and in turn using this awareness to cultivate sensitive approaches in treating patients' [11]. Cultural safety for Aboriginal and/or Torres Strait Islander people is an essential component of effective care for these groups and is explored more in Chapter 17, Culturally safe health care for Aboriginal and/or Torres Strait Islander peoples.

2.1.3 Self-regulation as a defining feature of a profession

As common definitions of a profession include its responsibility and capacity for self-regulation, it is worthwhile examining the changing meaning of the term. For much of the distant past, self-regulation referred to the individual professional's capacity to manage their own conduct, and the profession's responsibility to regulate the professional conduct of its members. In the recent past, this has changed, commencing with the addition of community and legally qualified members to medical boards and medical disciplinary tribunals. With the introduction of national registration in 2010 in Australia, the basis of medical regulation changed again (see Chapter 21, Regulation of the medical profession).

On its website [12], the Medical Board of Australia states that its purpose is 'to ensure that Australia's medical practitioners are suitably trained, qualified and safe to practise. Public safety is our priority.' The role of the Medical Board within its partnership with the Australian Health Practitioner Regulation Agency (Ahpra) is to set standards, including the code of conduct for doctors in Australia [8], issue guidelines, and make decisions about complaints brought to it about individual practitioners.

2.1.4 What does unprofessional medical practice look like?

Professionalism may also be defined in the negative by examining examples of obvious unprofessional conduct such as wilful misconduct, substance abuse, bullying, sexual harassment and unreliability. Unprofessional conduct can be categorised in various ways. Examination of the categories of complaints and notifications received by the Medical Council of New Zealand and the Medical Board of Australia (see Chapter 21, Regulation of the medical profession) and health complaints commissioners (see Chapter 22, Healthcare complaints and complaint systems) reveals that communication breakdown heads the list and is often a contributing factor in other concerns. The Australian Commission on Safety and Quality in Health Care recognises the key role of effective clinical communication with patients and colleagues in reducing patient complaints and improving the safety of health care [13]. Fraudulent and poor record keeping also commonly accompany unprofessional behaviours [14]. It is noteworthy that a small group of doctors (about 3–5%) accounts for almost half of all patient complaints [15], suggesting that there would be benefit for those practitioners and their patients if they adapted their professional approach. Complaints likely to lead to disciplinary action with suspension of registration include sexual misconduct (see Chapter 8, Sexual and other professional boundaries: being a doctor in modern society), gross negligence, issuing fraudulent certificates, illegal prescribing of drugs of addiction (see Chapter 30, Prescribing and administering medicines), and conviction for serious crime (including fraud against Medicare). Practitioners of alternative medicine and those who would offer treatments or diagnostics of unproven efficacy need to be particularly careful that their communication with patients is honest and comprehensive; if not, their practices may lead to complaints about conflict of interest and concerns regarding unprofessional conduct.

Similarly, advances in information technology and electronic communication have led to the development of new approaches to medical practice (see Chapter 29, Professional practice, digital technology and artificial intelligence). Some of these, such as provision of technology-based medical consultations to people living in remote areas or those who have difficulty accessing in-person services, represent important advances. These services were vitally important during the peak of the COVID-19 pandemic, both in Australia and overseas. However, there are others that appear to be motivated by profit rather than good service, and do not represent good medical practice. These include questionnaire-based prescribing or referral services, whereby the doctor providing the service has no real-time interaction at all with the patient. Caution is required if a medical practitioner is invited to provide this type of service, as any adverse consequence may result in regulatory action. All doctors need to be guided by their own sense of ethical responsibility when considering involvement in such enterprises.

2.1.5 Why professionalism matters now

Professionalism is assumed, but must be explicitly articulated and taught because it is not innate. Professionalism matters because societal expectations extend beyond personal beliefs—these expectations shift with time and culture. Doctors need to recognise different frameworks (professional bodies, patients, communities and cultures) and be able to navigate them. This may be particularly important for international medical graduates (IMGs), because different cultures have different conceptions of professionalism. Doctors entering a new country must not only adapt to their new professional identity but potentially also to a new professional culture [16].

2.1.6 What is driving the current focus on professionalism

The focus on professionalism in Europe and North America arose through a number of serious concerns, but the founding event for modern professional ethics was the rise and fall of Nazi medicine [17]. It is well known that Nazi medicine had not the slightest interest either in the welfare of patients or in obtaining consent of the subjects of human experimentation. The Nuremberg war crimes tribunal affirmed that patients were to be included in research *only* with their voluntary consent. This may seem obvious now, but it was not obvious then and was frequently not followed in medical research.

Subsequently, for example, it was discovered that unethical, non-consensual research had been conducted in the UK, the US and Canada in the 1960s and 1970s [18–20]. Patients, both adults and children, were enrolled in research without their consent and subjected to hazardous conditions and denied effective known treatment. This situation was scandalous. As the implicit morality of medicine had failed to protect patient welfare, this led to the birth of institutional research ethics committees and their explicit oversight of medical research [21]. (See also Chapter 31, Medical research, for further discussion of this topic.)

A more recent driver of the interest in professionalism was the recognition of the frequency of unwanted harm occurring during medical treatment, such as adverse drug events and incorrect medication prescribing. It also includes headline-grabbing events such as the preventable deaths of children in the early 1990s undergoing heart surgery in Winnipeg [22] and at the Bristol Royal Infirmary in the UK [23]. An influential 2000 American report identified the frequency of medical errors and identified the commonest cause of error to be unsafe systems of care, rather than individual operator failings [24].

Medical error has been a challenge to the profession. It had an obligation to address the epidemic of errors, but did it also have an obligation to disclose such events to patients? One concern was that focusing on such events might stoke public fears of wide-ranging medical regulatory failures and undermine confidence in health care. The notion that the profession does indeed have a standing obligation to disclose harmful medical incidents created a new higher moral standard for medicine and has had a salutary impact on the profession [25]. Adverse events and patient safety are discussed more in Chapter 23, Patient safety.

2.2 Doctors as advocates and stewards

Doctors need to be advocates for their individual patients and for the more general issue of patient safety, but also must be aware of threats to public health more generally, including the crisis in healthcare spending. The medical profession has often felt excluded from political decisions around healthcare planning and funding. There has been vigorous debate about professionalism and the political implications for physicians of threats to the health of populations [26]. There is an evolving consensus that physicians have a responsibility to manage scarce and expensive medical resources wisely. Campaigns abound to encourage doctors to consider themselves to be careful stewards of the healthcare system [27].

Due to this funding issue, there is bound to be pressure on doctors to alter their primary commitment from individuals to communities and the broader population. Borkan et al. have argued forcefully as to the role they feel physicians ought to play as 'system citizens'.

> Recent evidence highlights the need for a more inclusive approach, from a one-physician plus one-patient model toward a more comprehensive team-based population medicine model… This evolving professionalism demands that each clinician assumes the role of 'system citizens'—viewing one's position within the context of the larger health system and practicing in a manner that is team-based, collaborative, and attuned to the HSS (Health Systems Science) issues inherent to a patient's health [28].

Not all physicians would see themselves in this way, but in its 2015 update, the Royal College of Physicians and Surgeons of Canada's CanMEDS document considers leadership on this issue to be one of seven key roles for physicians: 'As a societal expectation, physicians demonstrate collaborative leadership and management within the health care system' [29]. This is also an expectation of the Australian Medical Council in its accreditation standards [30]. However, as Breen has observed, leadership on this issue will take 'considerable moral courage' [31]. (See also Chapter 24, Resource allocation and rationing in health care, for further discussion of this issue.)

A broader role of stewardship has become more apparent and more essential over the first two decades of the 21st century, as it has become clear that climate change is one of the biggest threats to the planet and to human health. As pointed out by McLean and Singh [32], it is becoming increasingly clear that physicians now need to address the health impacts of climate change and should play a central role in supporting activities related to climate action and environmental sustainability. Stewardship of healthcare resources is an important part of this role, including avoiding the unnecessary provision of services or prescribing of drugs, but planetary health stewardship needs to include consideration of the environmental impacts of decision making, both at the individual patient level and also across health services [32].

The AMA's 2023 position statement declares: 'Doctors have an ethical and professional responsibility to serve as stewards of healthcare resources', and further, that 'the anticipated effects of climate change on community health add an additional layer of urgency to addressing strains on healthcare resources and facilitating good stewardship' [33]. All doctors should consider how they may take action within their own practices to conserve resources and minimise their own impact on the climate, and some may also feel it appropriate to become involved in advocacy for broader actions to reduce climate change, as suggested in the RCP's publication *Advancing medical professionalism* [3].

2.3 Medicine: a science and an art

In recent years, there has been a renewed interest in describing medical practice as an art, as a humanistic enterprise. One example is neurologist Oliver Sacks' traumatic experience of depersonalisation after he received surgery to reattach his torn quadriceps muscle, but his practitioner failed to acknowledge the neuropsychological recovery he also required after he developed psychogenic leg paralysis post-operatively; Sacks recounts the story in his wonderfully wise book, *A leg to stand on* [34].

Doctors may foster a therapeutic relationship by being respectful of patients, being courteous and civil, listening to them and taking their concerns seriously. Indeed, 'minimum standards' of politeness should be expected from *all* doctors—and not only to patients and families but to *each other* and to other healthcare staff and trainees as well. The unwavering interest in and respect for the patient's situation is at the heart of professionalism. A doctor is not only knowledgeable, competent, thorough and conscientious, but also has the capacity to show compassion and empathy for patients that is evident and ever-present, and expressed through highly developed communication skills.

This is not to deny the importance of the scientific basis of much of modern medicine, but instead to portray medicine as a mixture of both art and science [35]. It might seem useful to try to discern what constitutes scientific medicine and what is encompassed in the term 'the art of medicine' but the implied dichotomy is a false one [36].

Advances in knowledge of the science and technology of medicine (embracing pathogenesis, diagnosis, and pharmaceutical, procedural and surgical interventions) represent an extraordinary achievement for modern medicine. While these advances have generally been beneficial for humankind, they have not been without significant downsides. These downsides include escalating healthcare costs (see Chapter 24, Resource allocation and rationing in health care) and accusations of poor care at life's end (see Chapter 19, Advance care planning and end-of-life care), of treating patients as objects and of not considering the whole person. The art of medicine functions to compensate for some of the perceived limitations of medicine's technical prowess.

Saunders has written:

> Most would agree that the Art is what happens between a doctor and a patient that cannot be found in a scientific text. This interaction requires a physician to possess compassion, understanding, and sympathy, while being both supportive and emotionally available. It requires strong communication skills and great listening skills [35].

In arguing strongly for a renewed emphasis on teaching in the humanities for medical students (see section 2.3.2), Halperin also addressed the question of the balance between the science and art of medicine, stating that:

> [I]mmersion in science is a necessary part of medical education but not sufficient ... medical students must come to understand that much of medical knowledge is a function of time and place, that medicine is a profoundly social enterprise and that the practice of medicine is value laden [37].

2.3.1 Fostering and maintaining professionalism

In Aotearoa New Zealand and Australia, as well as in North America, all medical schools and postgraduate training programs include education in professionalism as a core pedagogic responsibility, although how best to fulfil that responsibility remains uncertain [38].

Positive attitudes to professionalism must be inculcated into new doctors and every effort made to maintain these attitudes and attributes over a lifetime of medical practice [39,40]. This may require a lot from training programs, especially if a trainee is unreceptive to the new expectations of medical professionalism. In recognition of the need for more socially aware and patient-sensitive practitioners, medical schools have altered their admission requirements to try to choose applicants who are more likely to be receptive to the evolving moral nature of the medical professional. It is commonly recognised that choosing those who have academically excelled in the sciences is not sufficient for this purpose [41]. But trying to predict who would be the 'best' practitioner is a fraught process and the subject of some debate [42]. There is also increasing attention to the best ways in which professionalism can be assessed—which typically requires multiple assessment tools linked longitudinally [5]. It is certainly true that learning to be a good professional does not end with the successful completion of a medical training program.

2.3.2 How is the art of medicine best taught?

Instruction in the art of medicine is crucial to the education of the medical professional [43]. Role modelling, mentoring and learning from observing doctor–patient interactions are built into medical student and junior doctor training and theoretically should produce good doctors, if the role models are practising good medicine [44,45]. Medical students and doctors who are exposed to (and receptive to) educational approaches that include narrative medicine, communication skills, professionalism, empathy enhancement, and other arts of medicine generally will not only be better doctors but will also be happier doctors.

Summary

The concept of medical professionalism is multifaceted and difficult to define, but vital to good medical practice. This chapter has surveyed a range of definitions, considered professionalism as a social contract (including self-regulation), and examined current drivers of change, doctors' advocacy roles, and the challenges to maintaining professionalism. It has considered unprofessional practice and returned to the enduring importance of medicine as both a science and an art. A number of the themes raised here are considered in more detail in subsequent chapters of this book.

References

1. Breen K, Cordner S, Thomson C. On being a good doctor: professionalism and the art and science of medicine. In: Good medical practice: professionalism, ethics and law (4th edition). Canberra: Australian Medical Council, 2016.
2. Royal College of Physicians, UK. Doctors in society: medical professionalism in a changing world. London: RCP, 2005.
3. Tweedie J, Hordern J, Dacre J. Advancing medical professionalism. London: Royal College of Physicians, 2018. https://core.ac.uk/download/346567562.pdf (accessed Aug 2025).
4. Australian Medical Association. Medical professionalism 2010. Revised 2015. https://ama.com.au/position-statement/medical-professionalism-2010-revised-2015 (accessed Sep 2025).
5. Wilkinson TJ, Wade WB, Knock LD. A blueprint to assess professionalism: results of a systematic review. *Acad Med* 2009; 84: 551–558.
6. Doukas DJ, McCullough LB, Wear S, et al, for the Project to Rebalance and Integrate Medical Education (PRIME) Investigators. The challenge of promoting professionalism through medical ethics and humanities education. *Acad Med* 2013; 88: 1624–1629.
7. Breen KJ, Plueckhahn VD, Cordner SM. Ethics, law and medical practice. Sydney: Allen & Unwin, 1997.
8. Medical Board of Australia. Good medical practice: a code of conduct for doctors in Australia. 2020. https://www.medicalboard.gov.au/Codes-Guidelines-Policies/Code-of-conduct.aspx (accessed Aug 2025).
9. Australian Council of Professions. What is a profession. 2003. https://professions.org.au/what-is-a-professional (accessed Aug 2025).
10. Swick HM. Toward a normative definition of medical professionalism. *Acad Med* 2000; 75: 612–616.
11. Prasad SJ, Nair P, Gadhvi K, et al. Cultural humility: treating the patient, not the illness. *Med Educ Online* 2016; 21: 30908.
12. Medical Board of Australia. https://www.medicalboard.gov.au (accessed Aug 2025).
13. Australian Commission on Safety and Quality in Health Care. Communicating with patients and colleagues. https://c4sportal.safetyandquality.gov.au/communicating-with-patients-and-colleagues (accessed Aug 2025).
14. Thomas J. Medical records and issues in negligence. *Indian J Urol* 2009; 25: 384–388.
15. Bismark MM, Spittal MJ, Gurrin LC, et al. Identification of doctors at risk of recurrent complaints: a national study of healthcare complaints in Australia. *BMJ Qual Saf* 2013; 22: 532–540.
16. Jha V, Mclean M, Gibbs TJ, Sandars J. Medical professionalism across cultures: a challenge for medicine and medical education. *Med Teach* 2015; 37: 74–80.
17. Lifton RJ. The Nazi doctors: medical killing and the psychology of genocide. New York: Basic Books; 1988, updated 2000.
18. Gaw A. Exposing unethical human research: the transatlantic correspondence of Beecher and Pappworth. *Ann Intern Med* 2012; 156: 150–155.
19. Nix E. Tuskegee experiment: the infamous syphilis study. A+E Television Networks—History, 2017. https://www.history.com/news/the-infamous-40-year-tuskegee-study (accessed Sep 2025).
20. Velasquez-Buritica J. MK-ULTRAViolence: or, how McGill pioneered psychological torture. The McGill Daily, 2012. https://www.mcgilldaily.com/2012/09/mk-ultraviolence (accessed Sep 2025).
21. Eckstein S. Manual for Research Ethics Committees. Centre of Medical Law and Ethics King's College Hospital, London UK. Cambridge University Press, 2003.
22. Sinclair M (Chair). The Report of the Manitoba Paediatric Cardiac Surgery Inquest: An inquiry into twelve deaths at the Winnipeg Health Sciences Centre in 1994. http://www.pediatriccardiacinquest.mb.ca/pdf/pcir_intro.pdf (accessed Sep 2025).
23. Kennedy I (Chair). The report of the public inquiry into children's heart surgery at the Bristol Royal Infirmary (BRI) 1984–1995: learning from Bristol. 2001. https://www.bristol-inquiry.org.uk/final_report/the_report.pdf (accessed Sep 2025).
24. Institute of Medicine (US) Committee on Quality of Health Care in America; Kohn LT, Corrigan JM, Donaldson MS, editors. To err is human: building a safer health system. Washington, DC: National Academies Press, 2000.

25. Healthcare Excellence Canada. Canadian disclosure guidelines: being open with patients and families. Ottawa: Canadian Patient Safety Institute, 2011. https://www.healthcareexcellence.ca/en/resources/canadian-disclosure-guidelines/ (accessed Sep 2025).
26. Huddle TS, Maletz KK. Physician involvement with politics: obligation or avocation? *Virtual Mentor* 2011; 13: 757–764.
27. Choosing Wisely campaign. https://choosingwiselycanada.org/ (accessed Sep 2025).
28. Borkan JM, Hammoud MM, Nelson E, et al. Health systems science education: the new post-Flexner professionalism for the 21st century. *Med Teach* 2021; 43 (sup 2): S25–S31.
29. Frank JR, Snell L, Sherbino J, editors. CanMEDS 2015 physician competency framework. Ottawa: Royal College of Physicians and Surgeons of Canada, 2015. https://canmeds.royalcollege.ca/uploads/en/framework/CanMEDS%202015%20Framework_EN_Reduced.pdf (accessed Sep 2025).
30. Australian Medical Council. Standards for assessment and accreditation of primary medical programs. https://www.amc.org.au/wp-content/uploads/2023/08/AMC-Medical_School_Standards-FINAL.pdf (accessed Aug 2025).
31. Breen K. Medical professionalism: is it really under threat? *Med J Aust* 2007; 186: 596–598.
32. McLean R, Singh H. Professional responsibilities for Planetary Health Stewardship. *J Gen Intern Med* 2025.
33. Australian Medical Association. Position statement on doctors' role in stewardship of healthcare resources. 2023. https://www.ama.com.au/sites/default/files/2023-06/AMA-Position-Statement-on-Doctors%27-Role-in-Stewardship-of-Healthcare-Resources-2023_0.pdf (accessed Aug 2025).
34. Sacks O. A leg to stand on. New York: Summit Books, 1984.
35. Saunders J. The practice of clinical medicine as an art and as a science. *Med Humanit* 2000; 26: 18–22.
36. Whitehead C, Kuper A. A false dichotomy. *CMAJ* 2015; 187: 683–684.
37. Halperin EC. Preserving the humanities in medical education. *Med Teach* 2010; 32: 76–79.
38. Hochberg MS, Kalet A, Zabar S, et al. Can professionalism be taught? Encouraging evidence. *Am J Surg* 2010; 199: 86–93.
39. Berger AS, Niedra E, Brooks SG, et al. Teaching professionalism in postgraduate medical education: a systematic review. *Acad Med* 2020; 95: 938–946.
40. Scott I, Phelps G, Rubin G, et al. Putting professionalism and delivery of value-added health care at the heart of physician training and continuing professional development. *Intern Med J* 2012; 42: 737–741.
41. Powis D. Improving the selection of medical students. *BMJ* 2010; 340 :c708.
42. Barr D. Science as superstition: selecting medical students. *Lancet* 2010; 376: 678–679.
43. Rogers DA, Boehler ML, Roberts NK, Johnson V. Using the hidden curriculum to teach professionalism during the surgery clerkship. *J Surg Educ* 2012; 69: 423–427.
44. Batt-Rawden SA, Chisolm MS, Anton B, Flickinger TE. Teaching empathy to medical students: an updated, systematic review. *Acad Med* 2013; 88: 1171–1177.
45. Gordon J. Medical humanities: to cure sometimes, to relieve often, to comfort always. *Med J Aust* 2005; 182: 5–8.

Further reading

Charon R. Narrative medicine: honoring the stories of illness. New York: Oxford University Press, 2006.

Gawande A. Being mortal: illness, medicine, and what matters in the end. London: Profile Books, 2014.

Hayter C. Cancer confidential: backstage dramas in the radiation oncology clinic. Toronto: University of Toronto Press, 2022.

Montgomery K. How doctors think: clinical judgement and the practice of medicine. New York: Oxford University Press, 2006.

Peterkin AD, Skorzewska A. Health humanities in post-graduate medical education. Toronto: Oxford University Press, 2018.

03 Ethical principles for the medical profession

Lynn Gillam AM

Introduction

Ethics is a much-discussed topic in medicine these days, both within and outside the medical profession. But why? Medicine is a helping profession and doctors are good people motivated by a desire to help their patients and the community—so why is there a need to think and talk explicitly about ethics? Reflecting on this question is a good way to develop an overall understanding of the place of ethics in medical practice, before drilling down into the details.

The context in which doctors practise medicine has a number of features that make explicit consideration of ethics important. In Australia and in very many other countries, medicine as a profession has a particular place of power and influence in the community, even if individual doctors do not see this, or do not want to be in a position of power. Through a system of laws and regulation, society has effectively granted doctors special powers and privileges, allowing doctors to do things that others do not have social permission to do. Doctors can ask people to remove their clothes, touch people's bodies and cut into them, and administer potentially harmful substances. This would not be socially or legally acceptable outside the domain of medical care. Doctors also have power over access to medicines and hospitals, and have the authority to exempt people from attending work, doing exams and standing trial in a court of law. None of this is a bad thing. In fact, individuals and the community benefit from this arrangement, which allows high-quality health care to be delivered safely and consistently to the whole population. However, it does mean that people who are injured or unwell are in a vulnerable situation. Not only are they functioning less effectively than usual as a person, but they are also dependent on the goodwill of doctors to get access to treatments. It is not that doctors are choosing to exercise power over patients; the structure of society just gives doctors this power. This is one of the fundamental reasons why awareness of, and commitment to, ethical practice is so important in medicine. Doctors have power over patients for good or ill, life or death, simply because of what medicine is. This situation creates a responsibility for doctors to actively take care to do the right thing. The vulnerability inherent in the patient's position needs to be addressed by affirming particular ethical obligations of doctors to protect and respect patients.

One of the significant changes in Western society over the last 50 years has been a decline in public trust in institutions and the professions, including but not limited to medicine [1]. The model of medical practice which was founded on unquestioning trust in and respect for doctors is no longer tenable. The community expects transparency and accountability from doctors and other professionals. The consumer- and patient-rights movements have been instrumental in this change, and the idea of patients' rights has become a well-established foundation of medical practice in Australia and other countries, supported by government policy and in legislation. So, the internal features of medicine as a profession that drive the focus on ethics are matched by these external developments.

Other features of medicine and health care in Australia and internationally are also significant. There is increasing social diversity in the medical profession and in the community. Doctors and patients come from many different cultural, religious and social backgrounds, and hold different (though often unarticulated) ideas about the nature of health and disease, roles in health care (how doctors and patients should interact and who has responsibility for what), how families work, what counts as good parenting, and what is a good way to live. Doctors cannot assume that they and their patients have shared values and world views—which makes explicit articulation of the values of the medical profession very important. Alongside this is the increasing complexity of medicine—the range and technical difficulty of possible investigations and treatments is expanding rapidly, which means more options for medical management, but often less clarity about which option is best. Even if patients wanted doctors to make all the decisions about their treatment, that would not be straightforward in many instances.

So now what? Ethics matters, but how to know what constitutes ethical practice in medicine with all this diversity and complexity? This chapter presents the account of ethical practice in medicine that is standard in the profession. This understanding of ethics is the foundation for the World Medical Association's Declaration of Geneva [2], the Medical Board of Australia's *Good medical practice: a code of conduct for doctors in Australia* [3], and national codes of medical ethics in many countries around the world. The standard account is based on some basic principles and values that are held to transcend personal, cultural and religious differences. The classic source for these principles is the work of Tom Beauchamp and James Childress, authors of the hugely influential *Principles of biomedical ethics* [4]. The principles are universal and fundamental in the way that human rights are universal and fundamental. While there has always been contention among moral philosophers about the ultimate basis for ethics, the theoretical debate tends to focus on differences between moral theories such as utilitarianism and deontology. When it comes to matters of ethical practice, however, much of the theoretical debate fades away. There may be different justifications or bases for ethical evaluations of action, and different justifications given for evaluating an action as right or wrong, but in practice there is ready agreement on very many matters about what it is right or wrong to do. This does not mean that cultural and religious differences are irrelevant in ethics (as we shall see later in this chapter), but despite these differences, there are enough shared values for establishing some basic ethical principles.

Consider the idea, expressed not infrequently in discussions of medical ethics, that 'there are no right or wrong answers in ethics'. Although there are understandable reasons for saying this in some circumstances, it is simply not true as a general rule. If a doctor slapped a patient's face because the patient failed to finish a course of antibiotics, that would clearly be the wrong thing to do. It is not in question; any doctor who took a different view would have the wrong answer. Slapping a patient's face in response to noncompliance with medical treatment is just not ethically justifiable or defensible. This may seem a trivial or ridiculous example, but the point it makes about clear ethical boundaries is crucial. The need to articulate these ethical boundaries or bottom lines is perhaps more evident in relation to financial or sexual exploitation of patients. While some situations in medicine lie in ethical grey areas, in which there is room for reasonable ethical disagreement, many requirements for ethical practice can be clearly set out and are not at all contentious.

3.1 Ethics and law

This chapter is about ethics, rather than law. Subsequent chapters on specific issues refer to both ethical principles and the law, so it is worthwhile to spend a little time on the relationship between law and ethics. The first point to make is that law and ethics are not the same thing, even though there are many matters on which they would endorse or prohibit the same actions. Slapping a patient's face is legally prohibited (as a form of assault), as well as ethically unjustifiable. However, it is possible to have an ethical obligation to act in a certain way (such as treating patients respectfully and not laughing at their concerns), even though there is no clear legal obligation. The law defines some parameters for acceptable practice in medicine and provides some guidance on expected standards, but is not comprehensive. More importantly, in many aspects of medical practice, legal judgements in Australia (and other common-law countries) rely quite heavily on the ethical standards of the profession. In legal cases related to informed consent, to take one example, legal judgements about the type and amount of information that doctors should provide to patients are based on evidence about the accepted ethical standards in the profession. For those interested to know more about this, a good starting point is the chapter on 'Introduction to law' in the Australian text *Ethics and law for the health professions* by Kerridge et al. [5].

When there is a clear legal requirement to act or not act in a certain way, doctors should obey the law. This means that doctors need to know what the relevant laws are in the jurisdiction in which they work. In Australia, laws on some matters vary between states and territories, including, for example, laws about the age at which a young person can consent independently to medical treatment, the circumstances under which an abortion may be performed and whether doctors are permitted to assist terminally ill patients to end their life (voluntary assisted dying). Some jurisdictions have laws enforcing protections for human rights; others don't. Laws also change over time, as all three of the previously mentioned laws have done. There may be change in legislation and changes in common-law principles, as new rulings establish new interpretations and new precedents. So, knowledge of the laws related to medical practice is important for doctors, so that they work within the broad boundaries set by the law. However, the law will frequently not provide a clear-cut answer about what a doctor should do in a particular situation. Understanding of ethical principles and ethical decision making is crucial, and in many instances, judges will be looking to doctors to provide the ethical rationale for their actions.

3.2 Ethics and emotions

Ethical conduct does not mean being unemotional. In fact, the ethical principles of benefit, non-harm and respect for autonomy can only really be put into practice when doctors care about their patients as people, and care about doing the right thing by them. When things get complicated, when a patient's health and wellbeing is at risk and the way forward is not clear, strong emotional reactions are to be expected. There is nothing wrong with this—indeed, it would be ethically problematic if a doctor did not experience any emotions in such a situation. But ethical decision making does require stepping back from gut feelings, instincts and immediate emotional reactions. These can all be signs that something ethically important is at stake. And it may turn out that the immediate emotional reactions to a situation line up with considered ethical decisions about it. But this will not always be the case. When faced with an ethically challenging situation, it is crucial to look past one's immediate feelings and think things through, referring to ethical principles and using an ordered process for ethical decision making, such as the one described below.

3.3 Elements of ethical practice

The focus in the rest of this chapter is on ethical decision making—a systematic cognitive process that involves taking into account the particular facts of a situation and general ethical principles. Ethical decision making is a skill doctors need to have, although it is important to note that they are not expected to make complex ethical decisions alone. Where time allows (and it usually does), such decisions are best discussed with colleagues, including members of the multidisciplinary care team. This will help to ensure all relevant information is at hand, and a range of different perspectives can be brought to bear in the process of interpreting how general ethical principles apply in this particular situation.

Box 3.1 Elements of ethical practice

- Ethical decision-making skills
- Professional integrity (commitment to professional ethical values)
- Ethical motivation and character
- Ethical awareness

Nevertheless, there is more to ethical practice than ethical decision making. The foundation is commitment to the patient-centred values and ethos of the medical profession, as described in Chapter 2, On being a good doctor: the changing face of medical professionalism. In committing to these values, doctors are, to some extent at least, stepping outside their own personal sense of morality and the values of their cultural and religious groups. The values of the medical profession may align quite closely with a doctor's own values, or there may be some divergence. Either way, ethical practice in medicine requires commitment to professional values. Identifying with these values, a process that continues over a whole career, provides internal motivation to act ethically, out of a sense of professional integrity. Motivation is significant because taking the ethically best path is not necessarily easy. It may take more time, demand more self-reflection and greater willingness to think critically rather than act on first impressions. Sometimes it requires courage—to have difficult conversations, or to push back against organisational culture or practices. The theory of virtue ethics (or Aristotelian ethics) delves deeply into the idea of ethical motivation and ethical character traits. For those who would like to read more about this, Beauchamp and Childress [4] provide a good chapter-length discussion, as does Walker [6].

Lastly, although arguably this should come first, is ethical awareness, which is the capacity to recognise when there is something ethically important at stake in a situation. Without ethical awareness, commitment to professional values and ethical decision-making skills alone will not get a doctor very far along the road towards ethical best practice in medicine. Ethical awareness is a capacity that grows over time, with practice. It is founded on the willingness and ability to look at all of medical practice through an ethical lens, to be always open to the question of whether the usual response is really best ethical practice in a clinical situation. Ethical awareness also involves taking seriously the gut feeling that something is not right. While this sense of being uncomfortable is not a sure sign that there is an ethical problem, it can be a warning sign, so more thought and reflection is always warranted when the feeling surfaces.

3.4 Types of ethical issues in medicine

One helpful first step in developing an overall understanding of medical ethics is to recognise the broad types of ethical issues or challenges that arise in medical practice.

Box 3.2 Types of ethical issues in medicine

1. The ethical principle is clear, but the challenge is to put it into practice.
2. Different ethical principles point in different directions.
3. The ethics are contentious because standard ethical principles are disputed or their relevance is questioned.

The first type of issue, by far the most encountered, is where the right thing to do is straightforward based on accepted principles, but the challenge is to put it into practice in a busy, high-stress work environment. One good example of this is the ethical requirement for informed consent (described in more detail below and discussed at length in Chapter 7, Consent and informed decision making). When time is short, the medical diagnosis and treatment are complex, and there are barriers to communicating with the patient (such as language differences or low health literacy), it can be challenging to work out a way to achieve informed consent. The structure and processes of the healthcare system may present additional challenges. But there is no question that it is ethically required. What is needed here is to develop skills and strategies to manage these situations as well as possible, rather than giving up and saying that informed consent is not possible. Some degree of informed consent is preferable to none.

A second type of ethically challenging situation occurs when the standard principles of ethical practice point in different directions. A common example is when a patient does not agree to the treatment that is needed for their medical condition. Taking care of the patient's health points one way, but respecting their wishes points another way—and both are integral to good medical practice [3]. In these situations, doctors need two things: knowledge of the standard resolutions for some of these situations and ethical decision-making skills for the grey areas. For refusal of treatment, there is a standard resolution: if a well-informed patient who has decision-making capacity refuses medical treatment, their wishes should be respected, even if the result will be permanent damage to their health or death. However, an assessment must be made about whether the patient does have decision-making capacity, and whether they have received sufficient information, explained carefully in a way that is understandable. Another standard resolution relates to privacy. Patients can have medical conditions which put others at a significant risk of specific harm (e.g. a patient with poorly controlled epilepsy who works as a bus driver). In these situations, if the patient refuses to allow information about their medical condition to be passed on to others, it is ethically appropriate for the doctor to breach confidentiality and notify those who need to know. But again, professional judgement and ethical decision making is needed to determine the level of risk posed to others, whether it is possible to remove that risk without disclosing the patient's medical information, and whether it would be reasonable to wait a while to give the patient time to reflect and perhaps change their mind, before disclosing the information against their wishes.

There are not always standard resolutions when ethical principles point in different directions. These must be approached entirely on a case-by-case basis, using a systematic framework for ethical decision making, such as the one described below. The idea mentioned earlier that there are no right or wrong answers in ethics has some relevance here. Different doctors, each having the same information and with a good understanding of ethics, could come to a different ethical decision about what to do in these situations. These different decisions might be based on different assessments of how likely it is that the patient or others will be harmed by a particular course of action, or whether the likely benefits of a particular treatment outweigh the potential risks. There are no objective facts that can prove one assessment correct and the others incorrect. However, this does not show that there are no wrong answers in ethics. Instead, it indicates ethical decision making is not fully determinative—there may be more than one ethically justified course of action, or it may not be possible to be sure which course of action is ethically best. This is one among a number of types of uncertainty in medicine which doctors need to accept and work with.

A third type of ethically complex or challenging situation is where even the basic ethical principles or values in medical ethics seem to be in dispute, or insufficient on their own to guide ethical thinking. These are genuinely ethically contentious areas of medical practice. Current examples might include hormone and surgical treatment for transgender adolescents, donation of organs after cardiac death (as distinct from brain death) and voluntary assisted dying (euthanasia). Abortion would have been on this list in the not-too-distant past, but over time, this practice, or at least its legal availability, has become more widely accepted within the medical profession in Australia. Voluntary assisted dying is also arguably moving in the same direction (this is covered in more depth in Chapter 19, Advance care planning and end-of-life care). In both cases, of course, there are doctors with strong ethical objections.

In relation to these highly contested matters, where there are genuine, strongly held value positions diametrically opposed to each other, it might again be said that there are no right or wrong answers. Those who regard voluntary assisted dying as ethically acceptable typically hold the view that continued life is not always beneficial to a person, and that directly causing the death of that person at their request is not a wrong thing to do. Those opposed to voluntary assisted dying may believe either that continued life is always better than death, no matter the quality of that life, or that even if death would not be a bad thing for the person, it is always wrong for a doctor to intentionally cause death. There is no agreed objective standard to adjudicate between these value positions. However, there is an agreed ethical way of managing this value difference, and that is to accept that individual doctors may exercise a conscientious objection to being involved in procedures which they believe to be wrong. This comes with the obligation to inform patients of the doctor's ethical value position (which might be based on religious or secular ethical considerations) and refer patients to another medical practitioner or service. Conscientious objection is ethically permissible only on contested matters such as those discussed here. On fundamentals such as informed consent and the right of competent patients to refuse treatment, there is no scope for conscientious objection.

3.5 Ethical principles for medical practice

The importance of a systematic, analytical approach to ethical decision making in medicine has already been highlighted. Relying solely on intuition or gut instinct is not enough; and good intentions do not necessarily lead to sound ethical practice. The standard systematic approach is to base ethical decisions on a set of fundamental ethical principles. As noted above, these principles are well established, widely accepted and used in codes of medical ethics.

Box 3.3 Ethical principles in medicine

- Beneficence—provide help, produce benefit, do good
- Non-maleficence—do not cause harm, protect people from harm
- Autonomy—respect patients' wishes and values, provide information and choice
- Justice—do not discriminate, allocate limited resources fairly [4]

It is easy enough to say that ethical practice in medicine is based on following the four principles in Box 3.3, but actually using ethical principles to make ethical decisions is a complex task. This is because principles are not rules. They tell us what to think about when deciding on what is the right or ethically appropriate thing to do, but none of them constitute absolute rules which must be followed. There are two reasons for this. Firstly, principles need to be understood and interpreted—in relation to both the ideas behind the principles, and how they apply to each particular situation, with its own unique set of facts. Secondly, the individual principles do not always point in the same direction, as we have already seen—there can be tensions or clashes between principles, which means there are competing ethical considerations to consider. It is simply not always possible to completely fulfil all four ethical principles. These ethical principles are 'prima facie' or 'defeasible', meaning that each one should be taken seriously and followed unless there is a compelling ethical reason not to. That compelling ethical reason would typically refer to another from this group of principles. When principles clash, the competing ethical considerations have to be weighed up and balanced against each other. The principles do not come in a neat order of priority, so their relative weight in each individual situation has to be assessed. This is not an exact science, and there is no algorithm to apply to produce the right answer. The next section will provide some guidance on the balancing and weighing, but first, let's move to a deeper understanding of what each of these principles means—what ideas and values lie behind these terms, and how they may be applied to an example case.

Box 3.4 Case example

Mr X is a 73-year-old man with end-stage renal failure. His doctor has explained to him that his kidney function is now so poor that he will need to go on haemodialysis. Mr X listens carefully to the doctor's explanation of what dialysis will involve, what will happen if he doesn't start dialysis, and what benefits dialysis will offer him (extending his life by several years and preventing his health deteriorating further), even though it is not a cure for his kidney failure. The doctor also explains the potential risks and side effects, gives the recommendation that Mr X is a good candidate for dialysis, and should do well on it. Mr X asks some questions, which his doctor answers, and then says that he wants to go home and talk with his wife before deciding. At his follow-up appointment a few days later, Mr X tells his doctor that he has decided not to go on dialysis.

3.6 Beneficence

It sounds simple and obvious to say that doctors have an obligation of beneficence, to do good for patients and promote their wellbeing, but it becomes more complex the more you think about it. Here are some of the key things to consider in unpacking the meaning and implications of the principle of beneficence.

3.6.1 What counts as benefiting someone?

There are different types or domains of benefit—physical, psychological, emotional, social and spiritual/existential. All are relevant in the ethical practice of medicine, and all need to be considered—an idea that is familiar from the biopsychosocial model of medicine. Medicine is not purely about physical health. Doctors and patients may have different ideas about whether some treatment or outcome would be beneficial, based on the different relative weights they attribute to the different aspects of wellbeing. In Box 3.4's case example, Mr X, the patient who refused dialysis, may have placed less importance on physical health or longevity than his doctor, and more importance on emotional wellbeing—feeling safe and calm at home, in a familiar and much-loved place with the constant company and support of his wife. This preference for the security of being at home over living longer might seem strange, even irrational, to others. They are certainly different types of benefits: increased length of life is a matter of objective fact, visible and measurable from the outside, and essentially the same thing for every patient, whereas feeling secure is entirely subjective, varying greatly between individuals in terms of what produces that feeling and how much it matters.

3.6.2 Who should decide what is beneficial for a patient?

Benefits, then, are partly objective (and broadly the same for different people) and partly subjective, dependent on the particular individual and perhaps varying greatly between people. Doctors have knowledge about the objective physiological benefits of a treatment, but only patients are in a position to know whether or to what extent undertaking the treatment will help them to feel better overall. So, should it be the doctor or patient who makes the call on what will be beneficial for a patient? The standard ethical position is that subjective benefits matter at least as much as the objective (and arguably more). This suggests that patients should be the ones to decide for themselves what will be beneficial to them. The principle of respect for autonomy supports this interpretation. Respecting a person's autonomy is partly about respecting their values, their sense of self and their own understanding of what makes their life go well—even if this results in them making decisions that look unwise or even detrimental from the doctor's perspective.

This understanding of what counts as beneficial and who should decide is quite the opposite of a paternalistic approach to benefit. Paternalism involves doctors making unilateral decisions about what is best for a patient, on the basis of their interpretation of the objective facts, without placing weight on the patient's values and views. Paternalism is ethically problematic because of this narrow understanding of the concept of benefit, in addition to the implicit assumption that patients are not able to cope with or understand medical information well enough to know what is in their own best interests. This assumption takes away or bypasses a person's opportunity to make their own decisions and act on their own behalf.

The subjective aspect of benefit makes for complexity in decision making when a patient is not able to say what they would see as beneficial due to illness, impaired cognitive capacity, inability to communicate and so on. Someone must make that assessment on their behalf. Who should this be? In principle, this sort of assessment should be made by the person or people who know the patient best because they will have greatest insight into the patient's views and values. In these situations, doctors should turn first to family, friends and appointed proxy decision makers, rather than simply acting on their own ideas about the patient's best interests.

3.6.3 Non-maleficence

Harm, like benefit, is partly subjective, so all the considerations above about interpreting what counts as beneficial also apply to interpreting what counts as harmful. One difference between harm and benefit in medicine is that while benefits to patients are typically intended, harms are not. The principle of non-maleficence is a broad injunction to avoid harm coming to patients—certainly by refraining from intentionally causing harm, but also by taking care not to cause unintended but foreseeable harms, and beyond that, by not allowing patients to come to avoidable harm through the doctor's inaction. It is worth noting here a misunderstanding, or perhaps misstatement, about ethical responsibility for the outcomes of inactions (i.e. medical interventions not done, which could have been done). In the end-of-life context, it is not uncommon to hear the idea that when medical interventions (such as drug therapy or ventilation) are not initiated, or are discontinued, this is 'allowing nature to take its course', and the patient will die from their disease.

While this is a reasonable way of understanding the situation, it is not the full picture. What makes this course of action ethically appropriate is not that doctors have refrained from intervening and so are not responsible for the outcome. Doctors are ethically responsible for the consequences of their inaction (omissions), as well as their actions. In other contexts, this is so obvious that it is hardly noticed. A doctor working in an emergency department could not stand by and allow an injured patient to bleed to death, then claim that this was not their responsibility because they did not do anything to cause it. They have an obligation based on non-maleficence to act to protect patients from harm, as well as not doing things that cause harm. In the end-of-life context, what makes withdrawal or withholding of treatment ethically appropriate is the ethical reason, not that it can be seen as omission rather than action. The ethical rationale comes from the assessment that the treatment is overall doing more harm than good (or that the patient has refused the treatment). A better way to think about this issue is to think about the consequences of the decision (the plan for medical management), regardless of whether that plan involves providing medical interventions or not providing them.

The Hippocratic maxim, 'first do no harm', is often cited in relation to the principle of non-maleficence or non-harm. But this is not necessarily helpful, and should not be taken too literally. Taken as stated, it seems to mean that doctors should not perform any intervention unless they are sure it won't do any harm to a patient. However, virtually all medical interventions carry some degree of risk. Following this maxim literally would mean almost never intervening for fear of the possibility of causing some form of harm. That makes no sense because patients would miss out on the great benefits that medical treatment can bring. It makes much more sense to think of harm as an overall or summative concept. Overall harm occurs when the bad effects of an intervention outweigh the good effects—that is when intervention would not be ethically appropriate. In short, we always have to consider benefits when thinking about harm. If an intervention has possible harms associated with it, this is not in itself an overriding reason not to do it. On the other hand, even when an intervention has a high probability of being beneficial overall, the principle of non-maleficence creates an obligation on doctors to reduce and mitigate any harms that might be done to the patient. Benefits should be maximised; harms should be minimised.

3.6.4 Respect for autonomy

The principle of respect for autonomy points to the fundamental ethical importance of respecting patients' capacity and right to make their own decisions about their own lives, based on their own values. Respect for autonomy is put into practice in a number of different ways: informed consent, shared decision making, right to refuse and confidentiality (respect for patients' wishes regarding who knows what information about them). Informed consent is a fundamental ethical requirement in medical practice. Doctors must obtain the patient's informed consent before performing any sort of medical intervention, invasive or not. This includes history taking, physical examination and investigations, as well as treatment. Shared decision making is the precursor to informed consent: a process in which doctor and patient communicate with each other about the medical situation, the options and what matters to the patient, aiming to come to a decision together about what form of treatment or management to proceed with. The outcome is informed consent.

Informed consent is described in more detail in Chapter 7, Consent and informed decision making, but the key idea at the heart of informed consent is that the decision is ultimately the patient's, not the doctor's. The decision-making process is shared, but in the end, the patient makes their own decision for their own reasons. Patients may base their decision on what their doctor recommends—this is still valid informed consent, provided that it is the patient's own idea to reach a decision in this way. Similarly, patients may base their decision on considerations related to their family, rather than thinking of only their own interests. This may have been what was motivating Mr X's decision not to have dialysis. This is entirely in keeping with respect for his autonomy, provided it is what he genuinely wants. It is a patient's right to take into account whatever matters to them (whether for personal, family, cultural or religious reasons, or more likely a complex mix of these) when making decisions about their own medical care.

Refusal of recommended treatment

The flip side of the ethical obligation for doctors to obtain patients' informed consent is that patients who are mentally competent and adequately informed have a right to refuse (or, to use a less emotionally laden term, decline) treatment that has been recommended by their doctor. This is so even if the patient will die or be permanently incapacitated or harmed without treatment. Doctors should seek to understand why a patient is refusing, what their reasons, concerns and motivations are, and then explain any misunderstandings and provide any additional information. It is also ethically appropriate to encourage patients to think again, to try to see the benefits of proceeding with the recommended treatment. But in the end, it is for the patient to decide based on their own sense of what will be beneficial to them, in light of their own values. There are ethical limits to encouraging and persuading patients; it is not ethically justifiable to hector, manipulate, trick or bully patients. Nor should patients be considered as incompetent (lacking decision-making capacity), solely because they decline recommended treatment. This is one of the hardest parts of ethical practice—accepting and witnessing patients like Mr X dying earlier than they could have or suffering harm that could be avoided because respect for patient autonomy in these situations carries the greater ethical weight.

Requests for unrecommended treatment

Patients may sometimes request a specific form of treatment or investigation. A patient with COVID-19 may ask their GP for ivermectin or antibiotics. A patient may present to the emergency department with a headache and insist on a brain MRI. As part of respect for patient autonomy, doctors should take these requests seriously and discuss them with patients in an open-minded and respectful way. Ultimately, though, patient autonomy does not trump all other considerations. In particular, it does not mean that patients have a right to any form of treatment or investigation that they want. Respect for autonomy protects patients against unwanted intrusions on their body, even when they will suffer harm as a result, but it does not compel doctors to take whatever actions a patient wants. If a doctor judges that the investigation or procedure wanted by a patient would cause harm to them, or would not produce any benefit, or would be an inappropriate use of healthcare resources (see section 3.6.5 for more on this), it is ethically justified for the doctor not to provide what the patient is asking for. When declining, doctors should explain their reasons, and in some instances, it may be appropriate to offer the option of a second opinion.

When patients lack capacity to make their own decisions

Where a patient does not have capacity to make their own decisions, temporarily or permanently, shared decision making and informed consent are done with the patient's proxy decision maker (next of kin, substitute decision maker, person responsible, medical decision maker—there are lots of terms for this, but all are essentially referring to the same idea). Proxy decision makers, whether they have been formally appointed using a legal document or are next of kin, have a specific ethical role. For patients who have previously been competent, the job of the proxy is to make the decision that the patient themselves would have made if they were able. That is, the proxy's aim should be to use their knowledge of the patient's previously expressed wishes and known and implied values, goals, hopes and fears to make a decision about medical treatment. It is ethically appropriate for doctors to assist proxy decision makers to understand and carry out this role, but not to direct or take over from them. For patients who have never been competent (such as children or adults with an intellectual disability), the job of the proxy is to make decisions in the best interests of the patient, which is a somewhat different task. If parents or guardians of a never-competent patient make decisions that are clearly harmful to the patient, there are legal avenues by which doctors may challenge these decisions. The decision to challenge is an ethical decision and requires careful ethical consideration.

Referring to patients who have or lack capacity to make their own decisions makes capacity (competence) sound like an all-or-nothing matter. In reality, though, working out whether a patient is sufficiently able to understand and has sufficient insight into their own authentic preferences and values can be very difficult, and is always partly a matter of judgement, not just of fact. Even when patients obviously do not have capacity to make the final decision, they may well have some understanding of the situation and views on what they want to happen. It is ethical best practice to involve non-competent patients, such as children and adults with cognitive impairment, in discussions about their medical treatment to the extent that they are able, to seek their views, offer them opportunities to ask questions and so on. Some of the legal aspects of decision making for people with mental illness is discussed in Chapter 18, People with mental illness and the law.

3.6.5 Justice, including equity, fairness and non-discrimination

The ethical principle of justice must not be confused with criminal justice; it has nothing to do with crime and punishment (and certainly should not be taken as meaning that doctors have any ethical role in enforcement of criminal law). Justice as an ethical principle has two key aspects: non-discrimination against individuals and the fair allocation of scarce resources (distributive justice). The underlying concept here is treating all individuals as having equal worth. It may seem unnecessary to say that doctors should not discriminate against individual patients, for example, by providing a lower standard of care to someone just because of their gender, religion, social class, language, sexual orientation or ethnicity. This is obviously unethical practice. However, such discrimination most commonly happens subconsciously, as a result of implicit bias or unnoticed personal assumptions about patients, rather than as a deliberate decision [7]. So the ethical obligation for doctors is to become aware of their own implicit biases (which everyone has—this is not a moral failing of doctors alone) and actively work to treat all patients fairly, as moral equals. Of course, this does not mean treating all patients the same; it means treating each as an individual, according to who they are as a person, but all worth equal moral regard.

Fair allocation of limited resources is a much more obvious ethical issue in medicine, and a more contentious one. The reality that resources in health care are limited cannot be avoided. The most fundamental implication of the ethical principle of distributive justice is that considered ethical decisions should be made about which patients get access to which medical services, instead of allowing things to simply play out by chance or market forces. These decisions are hard, but they must be made if there is to be any chance of real fairness in health care. Resource allocation is discussed more fully in Chapter 24, Resource allocation and rationing in health care, but as a prelude to that discussion, it is helpful to understand why these decisions are so difficult. Firstly, the ethical principle of distributive justice can be interpreted in a number of different ways, all of which have merit. Severity of medical condition, capacity to benefit from medical treatment (which can be at odds with severity of condition) and equal opportunity to access care all have validity as ethical criteria for allocating resources. Secondly, making decisions about patient care based on fair allocation of resources just feels bad. It can result in patients not getting treatment that could benefit them (because access is limited and other patients could be benefit more), and not getting the treatment that they want (because respect for individual autonomy does not carry as much ethical weight as distributive justice when resources are limited). This is the bitter ethical pill of resource allocation—decisions can be ethically justifiable, even ethically necessary, but *feel wrong*.

3.7 A process for ethical decision making

Ethical decision making in medical practice, when done well, is a systematic process which involves careful consideration of both the facts of a particular situation and the general ethical principles described above. Ethical decision making is complicated by lack of certainty. Often, there is no certainty about how things will turn out; foreseeable good and bad outcomes are only probable, not guaranteed. This is an unavoidable feature of decision making in medicine. After reasonable efforts have been made to gather the needed information, ethical decisions just have to be made taking this uncertainty into account, rather than waiting endlessly for it to go away or be resolved by some new fact.

Box 3.5 Process for ethical decision making

1. Formulate the ethical concern or issue.
2. Gather relevant information.
3. Identify possible options—ways forward or pathways from here.
4. Identify ethical pros and cons of each option (based on ethical principles).
5. Ethically evaluate options and choose the most ethically justified one.

A systematic process is set out in Box 3.5 as a series of steps. The steps are tasks that need to be completed to reach an ethical decision. They are presented in the order of the logic that leads from one to the next. However, in practice it is often the case that each step is not fully completed before the next is embarked on. The formulation of the ethical issue is provisional—as you gather more information and consider possible ways forward, you may develop a different understanding of the nature of the issue or realise that there are actually two separate ethical issues that need to be addressed. The process of identifying ethical pros and cons of the possible options often results in new possibilities being identified. Circling back to previous steps is perfectly fine. As long as you are clear about what you are doing, you are still being systematic and probably also being more thorough than if you worked through from step 1 to step 5 in a straight line.

Let's consider the sort of thinking that each step requires.

3.7.1 Formulating the ethical issue

The formulation of any ethical issue requires identifying what is ethically puzzling, troubling or problematic in the situation. One way of doing this is to consider the ethical principles and get a broad-brush first impression of what each seems to require or point to in the situation. It may be fairly obvious that there is a tension or clash between principles. Or the problem might be uncertainty about how to interpret or put a principle into practice (e.g. uncertainty about whether a form of treatment would actually be beneficial for this particular patient or uncertainty about whether a patient is making an informed decision about treatment).

Some ethically challenging situations arise out of disagreement, typically between the patient (or family) and doctors, but sometimes between different members of the healthcare team involved in the care of the patient. Where there is conflict or disagreement, it is always important to work out the source (or sources) of the conflict to see if they can be addressed. Disagreement does not always mean there is an underlying ethical dilemma—but sometimes it does.

Box 3.6 Questions to ask yourself to uncover addressable sources of disagreement

1. Have I communicated clearly and fully with the patient and/or family? Have I used euphemisms or medical jargon or made unwarranted assumptions about what the patient and family know or want?
2. Have I asked the patient/family what their goals for treatment of the medical condition are?
3. Has the patient/family received mixed messages or conflicting information from other healthcare providers?
5. Does the patient/family mistrust me (or the healthcare system)?

Adapted from Jonsen et al. [8].

3.7.2 Gathering relevant information

The step to gather relevant information is obviously crucial. The information that is needed relates not only to the patient's medical condition and treatment options, but also to the patient as a person and to the context in which the decision is being made. Having a system for seeking this information (from a range of sources, including patient and family members) and organising it, especially in complex situations, is helpful. One well-established guide for doing this is the 'four boxes' or 'four quadrants' method first described by Jonsen and Siegler and recently updated in the ninth edition of their well-known text [8]. Remember, the assembly of relevant information probably won't be completed in one go. The steps of identifying and ethically evaluating possible options will often indicate the need for more information.

3.7.3 Identifying possible options

There are always at least two options—to do X (e.g. to prescribe medication that a patient wants) or not to do X (e.g. not to prescribe it). But almost always there are also other options, intermediate between the two opposites (such as offering an alternative medication that would give some of the effects the patient is seeking but with fewer side effects). An option might include several steps (e.g. agreeing to seek more information about the medication that a patient wants or referring them for a second opinion, before seeing them again to make a final decision—which could be to offer a time-limited trial of the medication). The step of identifying possible options is assisted by experience, creative thinking and the input of others.

3.7.4 Identifying the ethical pros and cons of each option

Identifying ethical pros and cons involves systematic consideration of what each of the ethical principles means in this particular situation. This consideration must take into account the nuances discussed above in relation to each of the principles. Poor ethical decision making often results from superficial understanding of ethical principles or unwillingness to engage with the complexities of interpretation and application. A good rule of thumb is to resist simple answers at this stage.

3.7.5 Ethically evaluating the options

Evaluation will often come down to trying to resolve clashes or tensions between principles. In essence, this is the process of balancing or weighing up competing ethical considerations. This is not a matter of precise calculation, but rather a considered exploration of how much each ethical principle is preserved or lost in each of the possible options that have been identified, leading to a holistic, overall or all-things-considered assessment of which possible pathway is the most ethically appropriate. The most ethically appropriate course of action is the one that provides the best fit overall for the set of ethical principles in comparison to other possible courses of action. Sometimes all options look bad, in which case the most ethically appropriate will be the least-worst option. Other times, as noted earlier, there may not be one option that is clearly a better fit overall than the others. Some options might be identified as ethically poor, but others remain on the table as roughly equally ethically appropriate. While this may feel inconclusive, working out what not to do is a big step forward, and it would be reasonable to proceed with any of the remaining options.

Summary

Ethical decision making requires reasoning. Making an ethical decision based on a gut feeling alone is not sufficient and would not be regarded as acceptable in any forum where a doctor needed to demonstrate accountability for their actions and decisions. The reasons on which an ethical decision is based should be able to be stated explicitly. A doctor should be able to explain why they chose one course of action over the others that were possible in that situation. Being aware of other options and consciously choosing one over others is a hallmark of good ethical decision making. This again emphasises the importance of making time for ethical decisions, seeking advice and input of colleagues and consulting with a clinical ethics committee or service if one is available.

References

1. Blendon RJ, Benson JM, Hero JO. Public trust in physicians—US medicine in international perspective. *N Engl J Med* 2014; 371: 1570–1572.
2. World Medical Association. Declaration of Geneva. 2017. https://www.wma.net/policies-post/wma-declaration-of-geneva/ (accessed May 2025).
3. Medical Board of Australia. Good medical practice: a code of conduct for doctors in Australia. 2020. https://www.medicalboard.gov.au/codes-guidelines-policies/code-of-conduct.aspx (accessed May 2025).
4. Beauchamp TL, Childress JF. Principles of biomedical ethics. 8th ed. Oxford: Oxford University Press, 2019.
5. Kerridge I, Lowe, M, Stewart C. Ethics and law for the health professions. Sydney: Federation Press, 2013.
6. Walker RL. Virtue ethics and medicine. In: Besser-Jones L, Slote M, editors. The Routledge companion to virtue ethics. New York: Routledge, 2015: 515–528.
7. Chadwick AJ, Baruah R. Gender disparity and implicit gender bias amongst doctors in intensive care medicine: a 'disease' we need to recognise and treat. *J Intensive Care Soc* 2020; 21: 12–17.
8. Jonsen AR, Siegler M, Winslade WJ. Clinical ethics: a practical approach to ethical decisions in clinical medicine. 9th ed. New York: McGraw-Hill, 2022.

04 Ethical and legal responsibilities of medical students

Brendan Crotty AM

Introduction

The central role of professionalism in medical practice is a key component of Australian medical programs [1–3]. Modern curricula are designed to support medical students to grow their understanding and the development of professionalism as they progress through their program and take increasing responsibility as members of the healthcare team.

While some of the legal requirements discussed elsewhere in this book do not directly apply to medical students, it is essential that students graduate with a good understanding of the regulatory framework and their legal responsibilities after graduation.

All medical students must understand and incorporate in their day-to-day work fundamental underlying principles of medical practice discussed elsewhere in this book:

- universal human rights
- respect for all individuals, irrespective of age, beliefs, ethnicity, gender or sexuality
- patient autonomy
- privacy and confidentiality
- the limits of an individual practitioner's knowledge and skills
- the roles of all members of the healthcare team
- the impact of an individual practitioner's health and emotional state on the quality and safety of care.

Students should be familiar with the Medical Board of Australia's *Good medical practice: a code of conduct for doctors in Australia* [4] and should observe the Australian Medical Students' Association code of ethics (see Box 4.1) [5].

As students develop their knowledge, clinical skills and professionalism, they will also develop an understanding of:

- the social determinants of health, differing views of the healthcare system and the social accountability of the medical profession
- the limits and challenges of the Australian healthcare system, including the inevitability of error and the responsibility of health practitioners to contribute to systems of quality improvement.

This chapter deals with the ethical and legal responsibilities that apply to medical students while students and after graduation, and summarises the ethical responsibilities of those practitioners who teach medical students.

Box 4.1 Principles of the Australian Medical Students' Association code of ethics

1. Medical students should respect the dignity, beliefs, values and culture of every patient they encounter during their training.
2. Medical students should never exploit patients or their families.
3. Medical students should hold clinical information in confidence.
4. Medical students should obtain informed consent from patients before involving them in any aspect of training.
5. Medical students should appreciate the limits of their role in the clinical setting and in the community.
6. Medical students should respect the staff who teach and assist them in their clinical training.
7. Medical students should maintain their personal integrity and wellbeing [5].

4.1 Objectives of Australian and New Zealand medical programs

Australian medical programs aim to provide students with the necessary knowledge, skills, professional attitudes and behaviours to enter generalist prevocational training, initially with provisional registration in the intern year (Postgraduate Year 1) and then general registration in Postgraduate Year 2.

Medical education is a continuum from medical school to prevocational training to vocational (specialty) training, and then continuing professional development during independent practice to maintain the standard expected by the community. Medical practice is constantly changing, and one of the most important aims of medical programs is to establish a pattern of lifelong learning.

The Australian Medical Council (AMC) is the national accreditation authority for medicine, appointed to this role by the Medical Board of Australia. It assesses medical programs and the standards of medical education and training across all levels of medical education (medical school, prevocational training, specialty training, and continuing professional development) in Australia and in Aotearoa New Zealand with agreement of the Medical Council of New Zealand.

The AMC undertakes regular accreditation and monitoring of medical schools and programs against a set of accreditation standards, which are designed to ensure that graduating students meet the graduate outcome statements contained in the accreditation standards [6]. There are accreditation standards for each level of the medical training continuum. Each set of outcome statements is grouped into four domains. For the medical school graduate outcome statements, these domains are:

1. clinical practice: the medical graduate as practitioner
2. professionalism and leadership: the medical graduate as a professional and leader
3. health and society: the medical graduate as a health advocate
4. science and scholarship: the medical graduate as a scientist and scholar.

Revised medical school and prevocational training outcome statements and the corresponding accreditation standards have been in place since 2024. All accreditation standards and outcome statements are available on the AMC website [6].

4.2 Registration of medical students

Since the introduction of the Health Practitioner Regulation National Law (the National Law) in 2010, medical schools have been required to provide details of all enrolled students to the Australian Health Practitioner Regulation Agency (Ahpra), which maintains a register of Australian medical students [7]. Medical schools are required to update details of new and existing students twice every year. The register is confidential and is not a public document. There are no initial or renewal registration fees for students.

Under the National Law, medical schools are required to notify Ahpra if they reasonably believe that a student has an impairment due to physical or mental ill health that may place patients at substantial risk of harm [8]. The National Law defines impairment as 'a physical or mental impairment, disability, condition or disorder (including substance abuse or dependence) that detrimentally affects or is likely to detrimentally affect' the student's capacity to carry out clinical training [9]. It should be noted that 'substantial risk of harm' is a high threshold and reporting of medical students is uncommon.

Any person or organisation, including supervising health practitioners, may make a voluntary notification about a student if they believe that the student:

- has been charged with an offence, or has been convicted or found guilty of an offence, that is punishable by 12 months imprisonment or more
- has, or may have, an impairment that they believe may harm the public
- has, or may have, contravened a condition of the student's registration or an undertaking given by the student to their national board.

The Medical Board is not involved in disciplinary provisions for medical student misconduct such as cheating, plagiarism or unprofessional behaviours (including intoxication or sexual misconduct that does not put patients at risk of harm) in clinical settings or online. Disciplinary provisions are managed at a medical school, university or health service level.

Students graduating from Australian and Aotearoa New Zealand medical schools are eligible for provisional registration by the Medical Board of Australia for a year of supervised practice in an accredited intern position (Postgraduate Year 1) [10]. Interns are only permitted to work in accredited intern positions as defined by the Medical Board's general registration standard, which was revised for the 2024 intern year [11]. Provisionally registered interns are not permitted to carry out any clinical work outside of their allocated intern rotations.

Final-year medical students complete an online application form for provisional registration about six weeks before completing their program [12]. The application form requests information to confirm the student's eligibility for practice, including details of any impairments or criminal record. The Medical Board may deny provisional registration if there are concerns that a graduating student has an impairment that may place patients at risk or if the student has been convicted of a serious crime.

4.3 Ethics and professionalism for students

Ethics and professionalism are central to good medical practice and are consequently core topics in all modern medical curricula (see also Chapter 2, On being a good doctor: the changing face of medical professionalism, and Chapter 3, Ethical principles for the medical profession). Most graduating medical students recite a version of the Hippocratic Oath at their graduation ceremonies [13,14] (see Box 4.2).

There is evidence that medical students with documented misconduct, including cheating, plagiarism and poor attendance, during their medical program are more likely to demonstrate unprofessional conduct and poor performance after graduation and to be notified to regulatory bodies [15,16]. Poor relationships with other students, teachers and nursing staff appear to be part of this pattern. Medical schools, health faculties and universities have developed mechanisms to address unprofessional behaviour on campus and at clinical teaching sites [3].

In addition to the specific ethical obligations of medical students in clinical settings described in the following sections, there are ethical requirements that apply to all university courses. These include prohibitions against cheating and plagiarism, research misconduct, discrimination, misuse of social media and generative artificial intelligence, bullying, abusive behaviour, and sexual harassment and assault. These obligations are often included in a student code of conduct. Codes of conduct and the penalties applied to any breaches are published on university websites.

Box 4.2 World Medical Association Declaration of Geneva

This declaration is recited at graduation ceremonies by Australian medical graduates.

AS A MEMBER OF THE MEDICAL PROFESSION:

I SOLEMNLY PLEDGE to dedicate my life to the service of humanity;

THE HEALTH AND WELLBEING OF MY PATIENT will be my first consideration;

I WILL RESPECT the autonomy and dignity of my patient;

I WILL MAINTAIN the utmost respect for human life;

I WILL NOT PERMIT considerations of age, disease or disability, creed, ethnic origin, gender, nationality, political affiliation, race, sexual orientation, social standing or any other factor to intervene between my duty and my patient;

I WILL RESPECT the secrets that are confided in me, even after the patient has died;

I WILL PRACTISE my profession with conscience and dignity and in accordance with good medical practice;

I WILL FOSTER the honour and noble traditions of the medical profession;

I WILL GIVE to my teachers, colleagues, and students the respect and gratitude that is their due;

I WILL SHARE my medical knowledge for the benefit of the patient and the advancement of healthcare;

I WILL ATTEND TO my own health, well-being, and abilities in order to provide care of the highest standard;

I WILL NOT USE my medical knowledge to violate human rights and civil liberties, even under threat;

I MAKE THESE PROMISES solemnly, freely, and upon my honour [14].

4.3.1 Learning from patients

As students progress through their medical program, they have increasing contact with patients and an increasing role in patient care. Students should always be aware that patients' trust in their professionalism and ethical behaviour is a great privilege and must never be taken for granted. Students' learning is only possible because of the generosity, goodwill and cooperation of patients who agree to share confidential personal information and consent to a physical examination or procedure.

Patients are under no obligation to allow students to be involved in their care [4,17]. The patient's treating team or hospital should make it clear that they may be approached by students or their teachers, that they are not obliged to participate in clinical teaching, and that their care will not be affected if they do not. In some health services the charter of healthcare rights includes this information. Patients may be vulnerable because they are unwell, tired, or anxious or distressed about their illness. They (or their parents, family or carers) must always be asked if they are willing to spend time with a student without any element of coercion, and should always be treated with courtesy, consideration and respect. The principles of patient consent apply here (see also Chapter 7, Consent and informed decision making). Most patients welcome contact with students and their teachers for reasons that range from a wish to better understand their health problems to a desire to help to improve medical training and the quality of health care. However, those who are ill, in pain, tired or distressed, or who have already seen many students may decline to participate.

Patients rightly expect health professionals and students to maintain a professional demeanour. This often extends to expectations about dress and grooming, particularly by older patients who comprise a majority of inpatients in general hospitals. Students should adhere to the standards required by the hospital, health centre, medical practice or other institution in which they are undertaking clinical training.

When approaching a patient, medical students should always introduce themselves by name, explain that they are students, and seek consent to take a history or perform a physical examination. This consent must be provided by a parent if the patient is a child, or by a substitute decision maker if the patient does not have capacity to give consent (e.g. next of kin or other person with medical power of attorney). Patients and their families or carers should be asked how they prefer to be addressed (by first name or more formally by title and surname). Students should always show respect for patients' autonomy, ethnicity, culture, religion, sexual identification or orientation, and personal beliefs, and should not question or comment on any of these.

Before proceeding to physical examination of a patient, students should explain what is involved in the examination and confirm the patient's consent to proceed. Students must ensure privacy is maintained when interviewing and examining patients. In some clinical settings, particularly hospitals, this can be difficult. Personal or potentially embarrassing questions and responses should not be audible to other patients or to visitors. It may be appropriate to ask visitors to leave the bedside.

Patients must be given the opportunity to undress and dress in private. A student should only assist a patient to undress or dress if the patient is having difficulty and asks for assistance. The patient should be adequately screened and covered during a physical examination and only the relevant part of the body should be exposed for each phase of the examination. The patient should not be exposed or required to remain undressed for any longer than is needed to complete the examination. Physical examination should cease if there is any verbal or non-verbal indication that consent has been withdrawn. It may be appropriate to have another medical student or health practitioner present who is of the same gender as the patient as a chaperone.

All Australian medical schools have policies about intimate examinations, which state that medical students should never conduct breast, genital or rectal examinations without supervision. The Medical Board of Australia's guidelines on sexual boundaries state that 'an unwarranted physical examination may constitute sexual assault. This includes conducting or allowing others, such as students, to conduct examinations on anaesthetised patients, when the patient has not given explicit consent for the examination' [18]. (See also Chapter 8, Sexual and other professional boundaries: being a doctor in modern society.)

After completing the history and examination, the student should thank the patient for their time and assistance, offer to help the patient dress and return to their bed or chair if they need assistance, ensure that the patient is comfortable and that all the equipment they may need (such as their call bell, TV control, spectacles, mobile phone, books) is within reach, and offer to let visitors know that they can return to the bedside.

4.3.2 Confidentiality

Medical students are bound by the same rules of confidentiality as doctors [4]; see also Chapter 6, Confidentiality, privacy and disclosure. These rules apply to disclosure that an individual has attended or has been admitted to a healthcare facility and to any information obtained from the patient, from family, carers or friends, from the patient's medical record, or from healthcare facility staff. Students must ensure that any notes taken during an interview and examination, or from accessing a patient's medical record, are kept secure and destroyed when no longer needed, including electronic notes (see also Chapter 27, Medical records, reports and certificates). It is essential to obtain the patient's consent for any electronic photographs or videos, and to ensure that these are de-identified, used only for educational purposes and not disseminated (see also Chapter 29, Professional practice, digital technology and artificial intelligence, and Chapter 6, Confidentiality, privacy and disclosure).

Any discussion of a patient's confidential information with teachers, other members of the healthcare team or other students must be conducted in private, and the patient should be de-identified wherever possible. Students must take particular care that conversations about patients are not overheard by staff who are not directly involved in the patient's care or in teaching (e.g. in hospital cafeterias), or by members of the public, including the patient's family and friends. As discussed later in this chapter, they should also take great care with online communication, particularly through social media, where there is a significant risk that information will eventually be transmitted to the patient or to someone who knows the patient.

4.3.3 Recognising limits of knowledge and authority

Medical students must recognise that their knowledge and experience is limited, and that they are not authorised to provide medical advice to patients. Students should be careful that their answers to patients' questions do not include advice on diagnosis, treatment or prognosis, particularly if these are still uncertain. In these situations, students should politely explain their role and its limitations and suggest that the questions be addressed to one of the patient's healthcare team. Students should not offer alternative diagnoses or management plans and should never criticise or appear to agree with criticism of a patient's care when the patient may hear them.

Students spend a lot of time with some patients and may establish a degree of rapport that leads to a patient revealing information that may be important to diagnosis or management of their illness. If this occurs, the student should encourage the patient to discuss the new information with one of their healthcare team. In some instances, the patient may ask the student to pass on the information; this is appropriate if it is clear that consent has been given. However, it is usually inappropriate for students to assume a role of patient advocate, confidante or adviser. Students should politely decline requests for assistance unrelated to health care (such as for transport, money, cigarettes or the like).

As students' knowledge and experience grows, they are asked to take a more active role in patient care and are given opportunities to perform or assist with history taking, physical examinations, ordering investigations and performing procedures under supervision. Multilingual students are sometimes asked to act as interpreters for patients. This can be ethically complex, depending on the student's language proficiency and the nature of the clinical interaction. Students should not agree to interpret if they feel it is not appropriate in the circumstances. Most medical courses include a pre-internship term in the final year, where students work with interns, registrars, senior doctors and other members of a healthcare team, and often undertake simple procedures under supervision. It is essential that the consent of the patient or carer is obtained for students to be involved in these activities [4]. The degree of supervision will vary according to the nature of the patient's problem, the student's experience and skills, the procedure, and any relevant regulations of the healthcare facility. Students should not perform any procedure for which they feel they have not been appropriately trained or if they believe that the level of supervision is inadequate. All students can be assured that they are covered by their university's indemnity insurance for any adverse outcomes arising from their involvement in patient care.

4.3.4 Infection prevention and control

To reduce risks to patients, healthcare workers and students, medical schools have developed infection control policies covering vaccination and other infection prevention and control measures. Students are also required to adhere to the infection control policies of each clinical placement site they attend. The requirements of medical school policies are explained before enrolment, and advice and counselling are offered to students as appropriate.

In line with the recommendations of the *Australian immunisation handbook*, medical students must be immunised against (or be immune through past exposure to) a range of infectious diseases including hepatitis B, diphtheria, tetanus, polio, pertussis, measles, mumps, rubella, varicella, influenza and COVID-19 [19]. Many medical schools also require students to be vaccinated against hepatitis A. Students who are at risk of exposure to drug-resistant cases of tuberculosis may be offered the BCG vaccine. Annual influenza vaccination is offered by most medical schools and is usually compulsory in hospital and aged care settings.

Medical schools also require students to assess their risk of infection with bloodborne viruses (hepatitis B, hepatitis C and HIV), and assist students to consult an independent infectious diseases physician where needed. Students are required to demonstrate their immune status on entry to the medical program, in line with the recommendations of the Australian national guidelines for healthcare workers with bloodborne viruses [20]. People infected with HIV, hepatitis B or hepatitis C are not excluded from Australian medical programs. However, they are required to avoid exposure-prone procedures, and must seek counselling and advice about restrictions on training and career opportunities and on measures to prevent transmission to patients or healthcare staff. Graduating medical students who are infected with a bloodborne virus are required to sign a commitment that they will comply with the Australian national guidelines as part of their application for provisional registration by the Medical Board of Australia [21].

Australian and overseas experience shows that many medical students experience needlestick and other injuries that place them at risk of being infected by bloodborne viruses, and that these incidents are under-reported [22]. All Australian medical schools and healthcare facilities have protocols in place for follow-up of needlestick injuries or similar incidents, and students are required to report the incidents immediately and to observe the local protocol.

Medical students undertaking clinical placements must be instructed in and adhere to all of the host healthcare facility's infection control measures, for their own protection and the protection of patients, other students and staff. These measures include hand hygiene, respiratory hygiene and cough etiquette, not working when infectious, contact (gloves, mask and gown) and isolation precautions for infected and immunocompromised patients, and aseptic technique for procedures. There is good evidence that poor hand hygiene techniques play a major role in spreading infection in hospitals and that medical staff have the lowest rates of adherence to hand hygiene protocols [23]. One of the best ways of addressing this problem is for students to establish good habits of hand hygiene before and after each patient contact. More information is available from the *Australian guidelines for the prevention and control of infection in healthcare* [24].

The COVID-19 pandemic has been accompanied by a constantly evolving set of regulations to prevent the spread of the responsible virus in healthcare settings, including mandatory vaccination, not attending a clinical, disability or aged care facility with any respiratory symptoms or after contact with an individual with COVID-19, and mask and gown requirements [25]. There have been frequent changes to these regulations and to recommendations about how long infected individuals and contacts should stay home. In some locations, medical students' clinical placements were restricted during the early phase of the pandemic but these restrictions have been lifted. It is likely that the regulations and recommendations on COVID-19 prevention and control will continue to evolve, and medical students should be aware of and observe the current restrictions for the sites where they undertake clinical training.

4.3.5 Sexual boundaries

One of the most important principles of medical practice is that doctors should not exploit the trust of a patient to establish a sexual relationship. This is an abuse of the inherent power imbalance in the doctor–patient relationship, which can cause significant harm to patients and undermine the trust that patients and the community have in the medical profession.

Doctors and medical students must not engage in any behaviours designed to provide their own sexual gratification through patients in their care. These behaviours form a continuum from inappropriate remarks about a patient's appearance or the use of sexually suggestive language, to performing an unnecessary physical examination, to establishing or attempting to establish an improper emotional relationship or sexual relationship, to sexual harassment, to sexual assault and rape. The risks and consequences of breaching sexual boundaries are greater for more vulnerable patients, particularly patients dealing with mental health problems.

This subject is discussed more fully in Chapter 8, Sexual and other professional boundaries: being a doctor in modern society, and in the Medical Board of Australia's *Sexual boundaries in the doctor–patient relationship* guideline [18].

4.3.6 Social media and other digital communication

Social media and other forms of digital communication are ubiquitous in daily life. Online curriculum delivery and feedback are essential components of modern medical programs. Digital communication is a core component of modern medical practice through electronic health records, digital prescribing, telehealth and the use of My Health Record, and a bewildering array of mobile phone–based health applications. In 2017 Australia adopted a National Digital Health Strategy, which has been updated periodically since [26]. It is likely that generative artificial intelligence will play a role in clinical practice in the future. See also Chapter 29, Professional practice, digital technology and artificial intelligence.

Medical students need to master these digital tools during their training. Most of the features of professionalism described in this chapter and the rest of this book—confidentiality and maintaining privacy (Chapter 6, Confidentiality, privacy and disclosure); maintenance of sexual and professional boundaries (Chapter 8, Sexual and other professional boundaries: being a doctor in modern society); and respect for teachers, colleagues and members of the healthcare team (Chapter 11, The doctor and interprofessional relationships)—apply to communication online. Hospitals and other health providers are developing codes of practice for digital health activities, which students must observe. There is considerable ongoing investment in cybersecurity to protect patient privacy.

Students should be acutely aware of two characteristics of online communication that pose particular challenges: the ongoing accessibility of virtually every piece of information, image, video or comment that is posted online; and the capacity for this information, image, video or comment to be transmitted to a much broader audience than initially intended.

As Australian universities have expanded the use of online delivery and communication, there has been an unfortunate increase in inappropriate online behaviour, which has led to the development of policies on acceptable use of information technology. These policies are often included in student codes of conduct, which are available from university websites. Under these policies, students may face disciplinary action for online communication with other students, teachers, and other academic or professional staff that is abusive, discriminatory or racist, or contains any comments that would be interpreted as sexual harassment or bullying. Online communication with teaching staff should always be respectful, and expectations about the timing of responses should be realistic, particularly to inquiries sent out of normal working hours. Medical schools and clinical placement sites may also take disciplinary action for any online breaches of professionalism in clinical settings, such as compromising patient privacy. Developing the skills of professional online communication with teachers and other students is an important step towards developing the skills that are required in clinical learning and practice.

It is important to recognise that professionalism requirements may also apply to the private use of social media that does not identify the user as a medical student or doctor. Even with the most stringent online privacy settings, it is relatively easy for others to link private online activities to a professional role. There are significant risks to personal privacy; to the privacy of patients; to relationships with colleagues, supervisors and teachers; and potentially to future employment. A good general rule is to assume that anything posted online can be seen by everyone and that it will never be possible to remove it.

Posting clinical photographs or videos without the patient's consent is a breach of privacy legislation. Students should also take great care about posting photographs or videos of themselves or their colleagues in clinical settings as they may contain details that could disclose personal information about a patient or healthcare worker. It is advisable to avoid online relationships with patients because of the relatively high risk of breaching professional or even sexual boundaries.

More information is available from the Medical Board of Australia's guideline on technology-based communication and a guide to online professionalism published by the Australian Medical Association, which has been endorsed by the Australian and Aotearoa New Zealand medical student associations [27,28].

4.4 The student and the healthcare team

The role of the doctor is continually changing in response to patient and community expectations, growing therapeutic complexity, and the acquisition and development of specific skills by other healthcare professionals. In contemporary medical practice, the highest standard of care is generally delivered by collaborative multidisciplinary teams, whose members recognise the skills and roles of all members of the team, including some who have not trained as health professionals, such as peer support workers, pastoral care workers and chaplains. The roles of all these practitioners are described in more detail in Chapter 11, The doctor and interprofessional relationships.

Quality of care depends on mutual respect for the skills and roles of other professionals in the healthcare team and on good communication between team members. While doctors generally lead multidisciplinary teams and retain primary responsibility for patient care, optimal outcomes are not achieved without effective collaboration with all the health professionals contributing to that care [29]. Changes to models of healthcare delivery have been challenging for some doctors, but traditional hierarchical views of the role of the doctor are increasingly recognised as a barrier to high-quality care, depriving patients of many significant benefits available through other healthcare disciplines.

Modern medical programs are designed to support students to develop a good understanding of the roles of all health professionals and of the importance of teamwork in patient care. AMC accreditation standards require that medical programs include interprofessional learning activities, where medical students study or work under supervision with students of other health professions in multi-profession group-learning activities [30]. An understanding of the role of nursing and allied health practitioners is particularly important for hospital practice in the early years after graduation, and medical students should carefully observe and learn from well-functioning multidisciplinary teams during clinical placements to prepare for internship.

4.5 Student health

Doctors are required to ensure that their own physical or mental ill health does not affect the quality of care they provide to their patients [4]. The more limited role of medical students in most clinical settings means that their health problems are less likely to adversely affect patient care. However, many of the poor habits that have characterised some members of the medical profession have their origins in the student years. It is increasingly clear that medical students experience a range of psychological challenges as they progress through their courses. Doctors' health is discussed in more detail in Chapter 12, Personal health of the doctor: illness and impairment.

4.5.1 Maintaining good health

Medicine is a demanding course. The volume of learning, the pressure of exams, navigating complex and hierarchical health services, the emotional toll of dealing with confronting clinical presentations, managing family and peer expectations, and anxiety about caring for patients after graduation are all challenges to students' health and wellbeing. University study is often accompanied by financial stress, and personal and relationship challenges. Avoiding self-diagnosis and treatment is critical to maintaining good health, and it is essential that every medical student has their own general practitioner (GP).

As discussed earlier in this chapter, it is important to be mindful of the risks of infectious diseases to elderly or immunocompromised patients, including spread through the staff and students caring for them. Students should keep their vaccinations up to date and should not attend clinical sites if they are infectious.

4.5.2 Stress and mental illness

Many, if not most, medical students find their course stressful, and there is considerable evidence that the prevalence of psychological distress and mental illness is higher in medical students and doctors (especially recent graduates) than in the general population [31,32]. A meta-analysis of studies from 43 countries reported depression or depressive symptoms in 27% of medical students [31]. Only 15% of those with these symptoms had sought psychiatric treatment. In the same report, suicidal ideation was reported by 11% of medical students from 15 countries. In 2013, Beyond Blue surveyed Australian doctors and medical students and found that just over 40% of the 1811 students who responded had symptoms consistent with a minor psychiatric disorder (depression or anxiety) [32].

A range of factors are thought to contribute to the high prevalence of psychological distress and mental health problems in medical students and to their reluctance to seek help. These factors include academic pressures, exposure to bullying and harassment, the stigma associated with mental health diagnoses, concerns about career progression, and underlying personality characteristics. The Australian Medical Students' Association has published a policy document that discusses these issues and recommends a number of strategies to improve student wellbeing [33].

Medical schools strongly encourage students to discuss any mental health concerns with their GP, a student counsellor or a member of staff. Students should encourage any peers who appear to be struggling with stress or mental health concerns to take up these opportunities. Many medical schools have identified individual academic or professional staff members, who are not involved in assessment, to provide confidential advice to students about managing stress or other psychological symptoms. Some Australian medical schools have developed programs to promote student wellbeing [34,35].

The overwhelming majority of these problems are resolved by a discussion with sympathetic staff or a GP. A few students require a brief period of counselling, and a small minority benefit from contacting or being referred to their state or territory doctors' health service [36]. For some students, more serious mental health problems can commence during medical school study, but these students are usually able to complete their course and make the transition to practice with appropriate support from medical school staff and their healthcare professionals. Notifications of students to Ahpra because of substantial risk to patient safety are very uncommon.

4.5.3 Alcohol and other drugs

Studies from the US and the UK report a higher consumption of alcohol and other drugs by medical students than by young people in the general population [37,38]. A survey of 855 medical students from 49 US medical schools found that 91% had consumed alcohol in the previous year, a third had consumed five or more drinks in one sitting in the previous two weeks, and 26% had used marijuana in the previous year [37]. The 2013 Beyond Blue survey reported moderate-risk drinking among 21% of Australian medical students and high-risk drinking among 4%, which was lower than the rate for the overall university student population (8%). Use of other drugs, mostly cannabis, was similar to the general population: 10% of students used another drug 2–3 times a month, and 0.5% 1–6 times a week [32].

As discussed elsewhere in this book (Chapter 12, Personal health of the doctor: illness and impairment), some doctors become impaired and are a risk to patients because of excessive alcohol consumption or drug use. Although there is a lack of data, it seems very likely that patterns of alcohol and drug use established as a student will continue after graduation, particularly in response to stressful working conditions or life events.

4.5.4 Students with a disability

Medical schools seek to be inclusive and do not discriminate against students with disabilities if they meet admission or selection criteria and are able to satisfactorily complete the essential components of the course. Until recently, medical schools' admissions policies were based on an approach that required students and doctors with a disability to be able to complete all routine clinical tasks undertaken by an intern working in an Australian health service. However, Medical Deans Australia and New Zealand has recently recommended a more inclusive approach for considering otherwise qualified applicants with a disability. This approach emphasises the benefits of an inclusive culture, and of adjustments and supports that allow students with a disability to successfully complete their course, be registered by the Medical Board of Australia and practise as a doctor [39,40].

4.5.5 Work–life balance

As discussed elsewhere in this book (Chapter 12, Personal health of the doctor: illness and impairment), there are increasing reports of burnout among practising doctors [41–43]. There are several possible contributors to this phenomenon, including excessive working hours, lack of control over work processes, limited support and social interaction at work, and a perception that one's work is not worthwhile or valued. Burnout can lead to poor physical and mental health, increased alcohol or other drug consumption, and failed relationships or family problems [41,44]. While many of the underlying causes of burnout relate to workplace conditions rather than individuals, there is evidence that maintaining work–life balance through a broad range of social contacts and maintenance of interests outside medicine, as well as realistic expectations and capacity for self-reflection, all contribute to wellbeing and reduce the likelihood of burnout [45].

The demands and pressures of a medical program lead some medical students to neglect rest, exercise, outside interests and friendships. Unfortunately, students are sometimes taught or supervised by senior clinicians who are poor role models. One of the professionalism goals during a medical program is to learn to recognise the value of balancing professional and personal life. Striking a reasonable balance as medical students will establish good habits that can be carried over to achieving a balance between professional, family and personal needs after graduation. The Australian Medical Students' Association has produced a valuable health and wellbeing guide for medical students [46].

4.6 Responsibilities of, and professional ethics for, medical teachers and supervisors

There is a very long history of codes of medical ethics addressing the importance of teaching and the relationship between learners and their teachers. The Hippocratic Oath includes the following:

> To hold him who taught me this art equally dear to me as my parents, to be a partner in life with him, and to fulfill his needs when required; to look upon his offspring as equals to my own siblings, and to teach them this art, if they shall wish to learn it, without fee or contract; and that by the set rules, lectures, and every other mode of instruction, I will impart a knowledge of the art to my own sons, and those of my teachers, and to students bound by this contract and having sworn this Oath to the law of medicine, but to no others [13].

As noted in Box 4.2, the modern World Medical Association version of this oath, often recited by new doctors at graduation ceremonies, states: 'I will give to my teachers, colleagues, and students the respect and gratitude that is their due' [14].

The Australian Medical Association code of ethics clause on clinical teaching includes the following requirements for clinical teachers:

- Honour your obligation to pass on your professional knowledge and skills to colleagues and students, where appropriate.
- Before conducting clinical teaching involving patients, ensure that the patient is fully informed and has consented to participate.
- Respect the patient's right to refuse or withdraw from participating in clinical teaching at any time without compromising the doctor–patient relationship or appropriate treatment and care.
- Avoid compromising patient care in any teaching exercise. Ensure that the patient is managed according to the best-proven diagnostic and therapeutic methods and that the patient's comfort and dignity are maintained at all times [47].

University codes of conduct for teaching staff prohibit bullying, racism and other forms of discrimination, and sexual harassment of or sexual relationships with students. Clinicians and other teachers engaged by medical schools are bound by these rules as well as by the ethical codes of the medical profession.

4.6.1 Unethical or unprofessional conduct by teachers

While most doctors are grateful to their past teachers and are enthusiastic in their desire to assist medical students, there is considerable evidence that some medical teachers breach professional codes of conduct and abuse the power imbalance inherent in the student–teacher relationship. Responses to student surveys report verbal abuse, teaching by humiliation and belittlement, sexism, racism and lack of cultural safety, and sexual harassment [48–50]. The Medical Board of Australia's national medical training survey reports similar results in postgraduate training programs [51]. Some doctors are poor role models for medical students, demonstrating a paternalistic or discriminatory attitude to patients, lacking respect for patient autonomy or privacy, making critical remarks about other health professionals, or lacking communication skills. These abuses and failings contribute to 'the hidden curriculum', a set of implicit messages about values, norms and attitudes, that undermines teaching about ethical practice and professionalism [52,53].

Experiencing or observing these behaviours can be very confronting and creates real dilemmas for medical students [48]. Students may be unsure whether the observed behaviour is appropriate, particularly if the teacher holds a senior role or has highly regarded skills in their area of practice. Even when it is clear that the behaviour is inappropriate, there is an understandable reluctance among students to discuss their concerns with the teacher or report the behaviour. There is no easy answer to these dilemmas [54]. Discussing concerns with fellow students, a student counsellor or a senior academic such as the clinical dean may help to clarify the most appropriate response. Universities and health services have mechanisms for reporting and responding to discrimination, racism and sexual harassment. Medical Deans Australia and New Zealand has produced a guide—*Preventing and managing bullying, discrimination and harassment, a guide for medical schools*—to assist medical schools to address the specific challenges in addressing these behaviours [55].

Summary

Ethics, professionalism and an understanding of a doctor's legal responsibilities are key components of Australian medical programs. Students graduating with a good understanding of the ethical principles and regulatory framework that underpin modern medical practice and their legal responsibilities after graduation will be well prepared for internship and the years that follow.

References

1. Braunack-Mayer AJ, Gillam LH, Vance EF, et al. An ethics core curriculum for Australasian medical schools. *Med J Aust* 2001; 175: 205–210.
2. Torda A, Mangos JG. Medical ethics education in Australian and New Zealand (ANZ) medical schools: a mixed methods study to review how medical ethics is taught in ANZ medical programs. *Int J Ethics Educ* 2020; 5: 211–224.
3. Medical Deans Australia and New Zealand Professionalism Working Group. Professionalism and professional identity of our future doctors. 2021. https://medicaldeans.org.au/md/2021/02/Professionalism-and-professional-identity-of-our-future-doctors-2021-FEB.pdf (accessed Sep 2024).
4. Medical Board of Australia. Good medical practice: a code of conduct for doctors in Australia. 2020. https://www.medicalboard.gov.au/codes-guidelines-policies/code-of-conduct.aspx (accessed Sep 2024).
5. Australian Medical Students' Association. Code of ethics. 2015. https://www.scribd.com/document/423841067/AMSA-Code-of-Ethics-2015-pdf (accessed Sep 2024).
6. Australian Medical Council. Accreditation standards and procedures. https://www.amc.org.au/accredited-organisations/accreditation-standards-and-procedures/ (accessed Sep 2025).
7. Medical Board of Australia. Student registration. 2013. https://www.medicalboard.gov.au/Registration/Types/Student-Registration.aspx (accessed Sep 2024).
8. Medical Board of Australia. Student registration: fact sheet for education providers. 2019. https://www.ahpra.gov.au/registration/student-registrations/fact-sheet-for-education-providers.aspx (accessed Sep 2024).
9. Medical Board of Australia. Guidelines for mandatory notifications. 2020. https://www.medicalboard.gov.au/Codes-Guidelines-Policies/Guidelines-for-mandatory-notifications.aspx (accessed May 2025).
10. Medical Board of Australia. Provisional registration. 2018. https://www.medicalboard.gov.au/Registration/Types/Provisional-Registration.aspx (accessed Sep 2024).
11. Medical Board of Australia. Registration standards. 2024. https://www.medicalboard.gov.au/Registration-Standards.aspx (accessed Sep 2024).
12. Medical Board of Australia. Forms. 2024. https://www.medicalboard.gov.au/Registration/Forms.aspx (accessed Sep 2024).
13. National Institutes of Health, National Library of Medicine, History of Medicine Division. Translation of the Hippocratic Oath [translated by Michael North]. 2002. https://www.nlm.nih.gov/hmd/greek/greek_oath.html (accessed Sep 2024).
14. World Medical Association. WMA Declaration of Geneva. 2017. https://www.wma.net/policies-post/wma-declaration-of-geneva (accessed Sep 2024).
15. Papadakis MA, Teherani A, Banach MA, et al. Disciplinary action by medical boards and prior behaviour in medical school. *N Engl J Med* 2005; 353: 2637–2682.
16. Krupat E, Dienstag JL, PadrinoSL, et al. Do professionalism lapses in medical school predict problems in residency and clinical practice? *Acad Med* 2020; 95: 888–895.
17. Better Health Channel. Patient and carer rights in hospital: Patient rights in hospital. 2015. https://www.betterhealth.vic.gov.au/health/servicesandsupport/patient-and-carer-rights-in-hospital#patient-rights-in-hospital (accessed Sep 2024).
18. Medical Board of Australia. Guidelines: Sexual boundaries in the doctor–patient relationship. 2018. https://www.medicalboard.gov.au/codes-guidelines-policies/sexual-boundaries-guidelines.aspx (accessed Sep 2024).
19. Australian Technical Advisory Group on Immunisation (ATAGI). Australian immunisation handbook. 2024. https://immunisationhandbook.health.gov.au (accessed Sep 2024).
20. Communicable Diseases Network Australia. Australian national guidelines for the management of healthcare workers living with blood borne viruses and healthcare workers who perform exposure prone procedures at risk of exposure to blood borne viruses. 2019. https://www.health.gov.au/resources/publications/cdna-national-guidelines-healthcare-workers-living-with-blood-borne-viruses-perform-exposure-prone-procedures-at-risk-of-exposure-to-blood-borne-viruses (accessed May 2025).

21. Medical Board of Australia. Application for provisional registration as a medical practitioner—Australian and New Zealand medical school graduates. 2024. https://www.medicalboard.gov.au/Registration/Forms.aspx (accessed Sep 2024).
22. Sharma GK, Gilson MM, Nathan H, Makary MA. Needlestick injuries among medical students: incidence and implications. *Acad Med* 2009; 84: 1815–1821.
23. Gilbert GL. One moment doctor! Have you forgotten hand hygiene? *Med J Aust* 2014; 200: 508–509.
24. National Health and Medical Research Council. Australian guidelines for the prevention and control of infection in healthcare. 2019. https://www.nhmrc.gov.au/about-us/publications/australian-guidelines-prevention-and-control-infection-healthcare-2019 (accessed Sep 2024).
25. Australian Government Department of Health. Coronavirus (COVID-19) resources for health professionals, including aged care providers, pathology providers and health care managers: Personal protective equipment (PPE) for the health workforce. 2022. https://www.health.gov.au/resources/collections/coronavirus-covid-19-resources-for-health-professionals-including-aged-care-providers-pathology-providers-and-health-care-managers#personal-protective-equipment-ppe-for-the-health-workforce (accessed Sep 2024).
26. Australian Digital Health Agency. National Digital Health Strategy. https://www.digitalhealth.gov.au/about-us/strategies-and-plans/national-digital-health-strategy-and-framework-for-action (accessed Sep 2024).
27. Medical Board of Australia. Guidelines: Telehealth consultations with patients. 2023. https://www.medicalboard.gov.au/Codes-Guidelines-Policies/Technology-based-consultation-guidelines.aspx (accessed Sep 2024).
28. Australian Medical Association. A guide to social media and medical professionalism: the tips and traps every doctor and medical student should know. 2020. https://www.ama.com.au/articles/guide-social-media-and-medial-professionalism (accessed Sep 2024).
29. Royal Australasian College of Physicians. Integrated care: physicians supporting better patient outcomes [discussion paper]. 2018. https://www.racp.edu.au/docs/default-source/advocacy-library/integrated-care-physicians-supporting-better-patient-outcomes-discussion-paper.pdf (accessed Sep 2024).
30. Bogossian F, Craven D. A review of the requirements for interprofessional education and interprofessional collaboration in accreditation and practice standards for health professionals in Australia. *J Interprof Care* 2021; 35: 691–700.
31. Rotenstein LS, Ramos MA, Torre M, et al. Prevalence of depression, depressive symptoms, and suicidal ideation among medical students: a systematic review and meta-analysis. *JAMA* 2016; 316: 2214–2236.
32. BeyondBlue. National mental health survey of doctors and medical students. 2013. https://medicine.uq.edu.au/files/42088/Beyondblue%20Doctors%20Mental%20health.pdf (accessed May 2025).
33. Australian Medical Students' Association. Policy document: mental health and wellbeing. 2022. https://amsa.org.au/wp-content/uploads/2023/10/Mental-Health-and-Wellbeing-2022.pdf (accessed Sep 2024).
34. Sloan H, Clayman D. 'Just what the doctor ordered': promoting wellbeing with medical students. *J Aust N Z Stud Serv Assoc* 2018; 26: 51–59.
35. Sugumar D, Fleming O, Ogden K. A mental health programme for medical students. *Clin Teach* 2019; 16: 352–355.
36. Doctors' Health Services. Drs4Drs. https://www.drs4drs.com.au/getting-help#doctors-health-services (accessed May 2025).
37. Ayala EE, Roseman D, Winseman JS, Mason HRC. Prevalence, perceptions, and consequences of substance use in medical students. *Med Educ Online* 2017; 22: 1392824.
38. Bogowicz P, Ferguson J, Gilvarry E, et al. Alcohol and other substance use among medical and law students at a UK university: a cross-sectional questionnaire survey. *Postgrad Med J* 2018; 94: 131–136.
39. Medical Deans of Australia and New Zealand. Inclusive medical education: guidance on medical program applicants and students with a disability. 2021. https://medicaldeans.org.au/md/2021/04/Inclusive-Medical-Education-Guidance-on-medical-program-applicants-and-students-with-a-disability-Apr-2021-1.pdf (accessed Sep 2024).
40. Fitzmaurice L, Donald, K, de Wet C, Palipana D. Why we should and how we can increase medical school admissions for persons with disabilities. *Med J Aust* 2021; 215: 249–251.e1.
41. Shanafelt TD, Boone S, Tan L, et al. Burnout and satisfaction with work–life balance among US physicians relative to the general US population. *Arch Intern Med* 2012; 172: 1377–1385.

42. Imo UO. Burnout and psychiatric morbidity among doctors in the UK: a systematic literature review of prevalence and associated factors. *BJPsych Bull* 2017; 41: 197–204.
43. West CP, Dyrbye LN, Shanafelt TD. Physician burnout: contributors, consequences and solutions. *J Intern Med* 2018; 283: 516–529.
44. Maslach C, Leiter MP. New insights into burnout and health care: strategies for improving civility and alleviating burnout. *Med Teach* 2017; 39: 160–163.
45. Zwack J, Schweitzer J. If every fifth physician is affected by burnout, what about the other four? Resilience strategies of experienced physicians. *Acad Med* 2013; 88: 382–389.
46. Australian Medical Students' Association. Keeping your grass greener: a wellbeing guide for medical students. 2014. https://amsa.org.au/resources/mental-health-support (accessed Sep 2024).
47. Australian Medical Association. Code of ethics 2004. Editorially revised 2006. Revised 2016. https://www.ama.com.au/articles/code-ethics-2004-editorially-revised-2006-revised-2016 (accessed Sep 2024).
48. Wilkinson TJ, Gill DJ, Fitzjohn J, et al. The impact on students of adverse experiences during medical school. *Med Teach* 2006; 28: 129–135.
49. Barrett J, Scott, KM. "Constantly ignored and told to disappear": a review of the literature on "teaching by humiliation" in medicine. *Focus Health Prof Educ* 2015; 16: 3–14.
50. Scott KM, Caldwell PH, Barnes EH, Barrett J. "Teaching by humiliation" and mistreatment of medical students in clinical rotations: a pilot study. *Med J Aust* 2015; 203: 185e1–6.
51. Medical Board of Australia. Medical training survey 2023: reports and results. https://medicaltrainingsurvey.gov.au/Results/Reports-and-results (accessed Sep 2024).
52. Hafferty FW, Franks R. The hidden curriculum, ethics teaching, and the structure of medical education. *Acad Med* 1994; 69: 861–871.
53. Mulder H, Ter Braak E, Chen HC, Ten Cate O. Addressing the hidden curriculum in the clinical workplace: a practical tool for trainees and faculty. *Med Teach* 2019; 41: 36–43.
54. Chapter 11. The student in the health-care environment. In: Kerridge I, Lowe M, Stewart C. Ethics and law for the health professions. 4th ed. Sydney: Federation Press, 2013.
55. Medical Deans Australia and New Zealand. Preventing and managing bullying, discrimination and harassment, a guide for medical schools. https://medicaldeans.org.au/md/2024/05/Preventing-and-Managing-BDH-a-guide-for-medical-schools.pdf (accessed Jun 2025).

Further reading

Australian Medical Association. A guide to social media and medical professionalism: the tips and traps every doctor and medical student should know. 2020. https://www.ama.com.au/articles/guide-social-media-and-medial-professionalism

Australian Medical Students' Association. Code of ethics. 2015. https://www.scribd.com/document/423841067/AMSA-Code-of-Ethics-2015-pdf

Medical Board of Australia. Good medical practice: a code of conduct for doctors in Australia. 2020. https://www.medicalboard.gov.au/codes-guidelines-policies/code-of-conduct.aspx

05 Communication in clinical practice

Peter Greenberg OAM, Peter Martin, Emma Warnecke

Introduction

Consistent, high-quality communication is essential for good medical practice. Communication skills are central to all aspects of patient–doctor relationships. Effective communication is vital for the establishment of rapport; gathering information; explaining aspects of physical examination, diagnostic tests and treatments; facilitating informed consent; seeking, learning and appreciating patient preferences and perspectives; and encouraging adherence to treatment through enhanced patient understanding. It is also vital for developing trust and obtaining the current level of patients' understanding about their condition, as well as exploring patients' ideas, expectations, concerns and the impacts of their illness on their life. Communication in clinical practice is much more than an exchange of spoken words between doctors and patients. Non-verbal communication is also an important way to enhance all patient–doctor interactions.

Effective communication decreases the likelihood of complaints [1], and of acrimony and legal action if adverse events occur [2,3]. Effective communication skills alone are not sufficient for professional medical practice and must be accompanied by competence in clinical knowledge and the other clinical skills, respect for patients, empathy, and ethical behaviour underpinned by professional values. Effective communication skills are also required for effective leadership and collaboration in healthcare teams.

Effective communication improves the quality and safety of health care [4,5] and can improve satisfaction with consultations of patients, carers and doctors. Many major adverse events are a consequence of suboptimal communication. Dissatisfied patients criticise their doctor for not listening, for not providing adequate explanations and/or for appearing uninterested. Satisfied patients perceive their doctor to demonstrate humanity, understanding, the ability to listen without hurrying them, and the skill of involving them in decision making [6,7]. There appears to be a strong relationship between a patient's trust in their doctor and their adherence to treatment [8]. Failure of communication underlies most complaints made against doctors (see Chapter 21, Regulation of the medical profession, Chapter 22, Healthcare complaints and complaint systems, and Chapter 25, Negligence and professional liability). Opportunities for patients to exercise autonomy are undermined when doctors are poor communicators or appear to be unapproachable or unwilling to respond to patients' questions and concerns. Complaints related to communication provide opportunities for urgent professional development as there is a very high risk of further complaints regarding the same issue [9].

The traditional perception was that the possession of good communication skills (as a component of a 'good bedside manner') is innate; however, it is now accepted that effective communication is a clinical skill that can and should be taught, enhanced and put into practice [5,10,11]. Role models remain an important influence on students and young doctors, and there is evidence of negative consequences from exposure to poor role models [12]. Although communication skills receive attention in medical student curricula, more needs to be done to reinforce this learning, including after graduation [13]. Enhancement of communication skills, refining the 'art' of communication and learning how to maintain optimal communication in all circumstances, including stressful times for practitioners and/or patients and also in different settings and contexts, are required by all doctors throughout their professional lives [14].

This chapter describes: key skills for effective communication; challenges to communication; advice on working with interpreters; communicating with telemedicine; open disclosure; and how to approach discussions about sensitive topics, such as gender and sexuality. It also covers providing culturally safe and respectful healthcare services and managing challenging doctor–patient encounters. Chapter 27, Medical records, reports and certificates, addresses the importance of good written communication.

5.1 Key skills for effective communication in medical practice

Most doctor–patient interactions occur within face-to-face consultations. Audiovisual consultations are becoming increasingly common and are preferred by some patients in some contexts. Communication within technology-based consultations is discussed in section 5.9.

All of the various skills used during consultations are dependent on effective communication. These skills include:

- gathering information and establishing understanding and rapport
- establishing who this person/patient is, through details of their social history [15,16]
- determining the key issues to be addressed by prioritising an early shared agenda for the consultation; this has been shown to shorten consultations while increasing patient satisfaction [17]
- when relevant, formulating diagnostic hypotheses, estimating their probabilities and pursuing them effectively—this may include 'sharing your thinking' so that the patient can understand your rationale and consider that they might influence it
- explaining diagnoses and options for management, including the seeking of consent (see also Chapter 7, Consent and informed decision making)
- patient education
- effective and rational prescribing, including explanation of likely benefits and possible harms
- providing frequent opportunities for establishing what patients currently understand about their conditions and what additional questions they have
- providing clarity around the immediate next steps in clinical care and using techniques such as teach-back (see section 5.5) to maximise recall and understanding.

All these skills can be learned and improved. They must be accompanied by perceptiveness and by an attitude that conveys respect, sensitivity and empathy towards patients.

5.1.1 Starting consultations: putting patients at ease

The technique used for starting a consultation varies according to the setting and the clinical problem. An essential first step is to properly acknowledge the patient as a unique person, before establishing the clinical issues.

Introductions should make patients feel welcome and as comfortable as possible. All healthcare practitioners and students need to be properly introduced to patients, their family and carers in clinical settings.

Doctors should introduce themselves by name, although this basic human courtesy is often overlooked [18]. In introducing oneself, doctors should be aware of unconscious signals of power imbalance, even at this stage: 'Hello Mary, I'm Dr Smith' sends a different message from 'Hello Mrs Jones, I'm Dr Smith'. Doctors should ask patients how they wish to be addressed and ensure they are pronouncing their preferred name correctly. The 'Hello my name is ...' campaign in the UK (https://www.hellomynameis.org.uk) has gained international recognition and led to the use of name tags with the health professional's preferred name clearly written and visible to patients.

Reading past records before patients enter consultation rooms allows conversations to begin immediately, permits maintenance of eye contact as required, shows respect for patients, and avoids the impression for returning patients that their doctors may have forgotten them. Patients expect doctors to have reminded themselves of the contents of files before consultations and to pay attention to them rather than the computer if they are using electronic records [19]. The same principle applies to referral correspondence, although some doctors explain to their patients that they deliberately elect to assess them before perusing prior information about them to minimise bias.

Helpful 'open-ended' introductory statements include: 'Can you tell me the reason you have come to see me today?', 'How can I help you?', 'What are your expectations of our discussion today?', 'What is the main issue for you today that I may assist you with?' and 'How have things been since we last met?' When meeting a patient for the first time it is often helpful to then say something like 'Before we start to address your issues, as this is our first meeting, perhaps you can tell me about yourself.'

Broad, 'open' initial questions allow patients to choose what they wish to mention first. Responses to these kinds of questions usually provide more information than responses to 'closed' questions, which often lead only to 'yes' or 'no' answers. More direct questions can be considered after these when more specific details are sought. Screening questions such as 'What else have you noticed?' can help clinical reasoning and reduce the risk of premature closure and confirmation bias.

5.1.2 The consultation

Having commenced a consultation, it is important to avoid premature control of the flow of spontaneous information through direct or 'closed' questions [20]. A 2019 study found clinicians often failed to elicit the patient's agenda and interrupted patients after a median of 11 seconds [17]. This study shows the mean time to interruption of the patient's initial statement has been decreasing over time, from 23 seconds in 1999 to 16.5 seconds in 2004. Patients can adequately convey their issues if doctors encourage them to express themselves in an uninterrupted fashion for 90–120 seconds. Attentive listening to patients' responses improves their satisfaction and the quality of communication [21,22]. Premature interruption of this phase of consultations is likely to prevent the expression of patients' real concerns and may lead to doctors focusing on matters of less relevance to this person at this time. In addition, early interruption reduces the chance of establishing optimal rapport and trust. There are, of course, exceptions to these principles, and doctors' approaches may need to be modified, for example, in emergencies.

5.1.3 Active listening and non-verbal communication

Active listeners can learn more than just what is contained in spoken words [21,22]. Maintaining eye contact and asking open questions are important skills; however, it is important to check if eye contact is culturally appropriate and if it fits with the consultation (in some situations, looking to the side can be less confrontational when dealing with sensitive issues). Active listeners are attuned to tone of voice, demeanour, vocabulary, gestures, linguistic patterns and non-verbal messages. It has been estimated that more than half the information communicated in a consultation is by non-verbal means. Body language is a major element of non-verbal communication and is missed in telephone consultations (see section 5.9). Doctors also need to be aware of their own body language (posture, eye contact, fidgeting and other actions). For doctors with computers on their desks, active listening includes taking care that the patient and not the computer screen is the focus of attention. A common pitfall in active listening is to miss key verbal and non-verbal cues from patients by thinking about the next question, instead of truly listening [23].

Active listeners also convey to patients that they are being seen, heard and understood. This may require verbal acknowledgement when distress is apparent (e.g. 'I can see that this is distressing you'). Silence with maintained eye contact or a simple nod of the head can also convey empathy. Limited verbal encouragements such as saying 'Uh-huh' or 'Yes' or 'Anything else?' assures patients that you are both listening and want them to continue. A useful website for strategies for active listening is VitalTalk (https://www.vitaltalk.org/clinicians).

Summarising information back to patients reassures them that you have listened effectively and provides them with opportunities to correct misunderstandings.

5.1.4 Enhancing use of time

Patients are usually, but not always, aware of doctors' time constraints. The duration of consultations alone, however, is seldom the cause for complaint; it is more often the perception of being rushed. Patients perceive consultations as rushed if they are not listened to, are frequently interrupted, or interpret body language to suggest the doctor is anxious to conclude the consultation and/or be elsewhere [22]. Complex problems that clearly require more listening time are best addressed by frank explanations and offers of additional appointments, with sufficient time allocated. Effective communication provides a range of benefits to patients and takes the same amount of time [24]. The key skills that enhance time efficiency without compromising doctor–patient relationships include:

- investing in early rapport
- discovering the patient's agenda for the consultation early, and negotiating with them what you both can reasonably achieve in the time allocated
- identifying and responding to key cues they provide to you throughout consultations.

In hospital consultations, doctors who stand at the end of the bed when talking with patients may send the following message: 'I have no time to sit and listen and want to stay near the door so that I may move off quickly.' Conversely, a doctor sitting on a chair beside the bed sends a warmer message: 'What you have to say is important to me and I will take the time to listen.' This takes no longer but enhances communication. Sitting down has been shown to double the perceived time spent with patients [25].

5.1.5 Handling patients' prior knowledge, including internet-derived information

Patients frequently come to consultations with preconceived ideas about diagnosis, management and other issues. These ideas may be based on their own experiences and those of family and friends, or on information gleaned from media or the internet. As most patients now have internet access, it is wise to assume that information about health complaints will have been searched for online [26]. It has become quite common for patients to refer to, or to bring with them in printed form, information they have gleaned from elsewhere. Where it can often be sensed or seen that such information is unlikely to be accurate or reliable, let alone relevant to the patient's concerns, doctors may make the mistake of dismissing such information out of hand. This is unlikely to strengthen rapport with patients and risks leaving patients feeling demeaned. It is probably wiser to commend patients for seeking information and defer judgement on materials by asking for copies to read later. Further action will depend upon the quality and relevance of materials. Such situations may provide opportunities to advise patients about sources of trustworthy medical information and about the possibility of raising questions at subsequent consultations, following the doctor's review of the information provided.

It is always worth seeking from patients their own views and understanding of their symptoms, illnesses and diseases, as well as, when appropriate, their thoughts about cause and diagnosis [27].

When there is a large discordance between the doctor and the patient regarding expectations of care it is helpful to understand the reasons for this and to explicitly agree on what you are both trying to achieve; for example, optimal treatment for high blood pressure with minimal side effects.

5.2 Challenges to effective communication

Challenges in providing optimal communication may relate to factors in the doctor, factors in the patient and/or factors in the setting or context of medical practice.

5.2.1 Doctor-related factors

Some doctors may have underdeveloped communication skills for reasons that include:

- lack of opportunities to learn communication skills while training and to improve them subsequently
- limited understanding of the evidence base for effective communication
- inadequate role models during training
- underdeveloped self-analysis skills, including a common language or framework to deconstruct difficult consultations
- challenges in adapting their clinical approach to patients with different health literacies
- inadequate reflective practice about communication skills in time-pressured environments
- failure to integrate the three key domains—content (what), process (how to ask) and perception (what you sense)—to maximise clinical reasoning
- misapprehensions or subconscious anxieties (e.g. anxiety about creating patient dependence and discomfort about anticipated inability to cope with information that might arise when patients have the confidence to be frank); unfortunately, such anxieties can translate into curtness and professional detachment or authoritarianism
- lack of attention to emotional and psychosocial domains of consultations

- current (and often temporary) physical and psychological problems
- upbringing and education within cultures that differ from that of the patient, especially when combined with insensitivity to, or lack of awareness of, such cultural differences
- lack of awareness of and/or denial of personal prejudice and bias towards particular patients.

Doctors' emotions can interfere with communication [28], as can the purpose of the consultation (e.g. clinical care as a treating doctor in contrast to medicolegal assessment by a medical assessor). Our own evoked emotions have been shown to impair active listening [29,30].

A common doctor-related reason for communication failure observed by medical boards and health complaints agencies is underdeveloped self-awareness skills; that is, doctors are unaware of the impact of their communication style.

Another reason for perceived communication difficulty is a mismatch between patients' expectations and their doctors' communication styles. Doctors may assume that patients prefer doctors who seem confidently in control of consultations (i.e. paternalistic in style), whereas many patients prefer and anticipate more shared and participatory doctor–patient interactions. Such patients, while respecting doctors for their expert knowledge, also expect doctors to respect their autonomy and right to make their own decisions about their health care. Determining patients' expectations early during consultations can facilitate communication. Judgement in responding appropriately to individual patients' expectations is another key professional skill. The emerging field of shared decision making has given us new frameworks and evidence on how to individualise clinical decision making for each unique context (see section 5.6). Possessing advanced skills that allow flexibility is critical.

5.2.2 Patient-related factors

It is vitally important to provide safe and inclusive spaces for consultations which take patients' diversity into account. Patients' age, sex, gender, sexual orientation, race, culture, religion, language, socioeconomic background, level of education and health literacy are all relevant. Consider individual attitudes and responses to illness as well as emotions such as fear, embarrassment and intimidation in the clinical setting. Patients may be reluctant to ask questions and be concerned about time pressures. Asking questions designed to elicit what patients have understood and taking care to explain, in terms that patients comprehend, the doctor's understanding of the health issue(s) assists with fostering an inclusive and safe environment [31]. The check-back website (https://checkback.org) empowers patients to build skills and confidence in checking understanding of consultations.

5.2.3 Factors in the context and setting of medical practice

The acuity of the illness, the adequacy of the waiting area, the attitude of reception staff and the physical surroundings of the consulting room can all affect communication between patients and doctors. Effective communication can be impeded by failure to ensure comfortable and secure environments that provide privacy. The consulting room should be soundproof, and staff instructed to knock before entering. In hospital and emergency department settings, inadequate privacy compromises communication.

The use of electronic medical records can also be a barrier to effective communication, and consideration should be given as to how these are used during the consultation; for example, engaging with patients by allowing them to see and read what is entered or accessed on computer screens [19]. When patients cannot see computer screens, explanations of what doctors are viewing may substitute. Doctors should consider how computers deemed essential during consultations might best be included, along with optimal strategies for doctors to look directly at their patients. Using clear explicit statements, such as, 'That is important clinical information which I would like to immediately capture in our records; is that okay?', before breaking eye contact, will mean you have 'signposted' (a micro-skill to make consultation structure explicit) what you are about to do and why, to maintain the rapport already developed (see also Chapter 29, Professional practice, digital technology and artificial intelligence).

Interruptions to take essential telephone calls about clinical matters are unavoidable for most doctors, but every attempt should be made to minimise these. When calls are taken, explanations or apologies should be made to patients, and consideration given to moving to another area before continuing.

5.3 Appreciating psychosocial factors in patients seeking medical help

There is increasing evidence that understanding the wider context of patients' psychosocial context not only increases patients' satisfaction but also increases disclosure of useful information and alters the therapeutic options and choices we make in doctor–patient partnerships [32,33].

Often the primary emphasis of the science-driven, disease-based reductionist Western medical consultation is on establishing a diagnosis and/or treating the disorder and/or relieving its symptoms. Illness, however, is accompanied by psychological distress and social consequences. The best way to acknowledge this and the most effective means of helping to relieve patients' distress is by improving communication [14]. This leads to better understanding of patients within their own settings, which may relate to their symptoms. It often helps for doctors to endeavour to imagine how each patient's symptoms, illnesses and diseases are experienced by that patient. Studies show that many doctors avoid engaging in the social and psychological dimensions of patients' problems, but that when they do engage, better outcomes are achieved [34].

Trauma-informed care acknowledges a complete picture of a patient's life experience and understands traumatic experiences are common. It recognises the widespread impact of trauma (events or circumstances experienced by an individual as physically or emotionally harmful or life-threatening) and avoids any triggering of traumatic experiences. Sensitive screening for any past or current trauma is an important step in providing trauma-informed care [35].

5.4 The physical examination

Effective communication is also essential during the physical examination component of consultations. When examinations require patients to undress, the need for this should be explained and doctors should leave the room or direct the patient to a screened area. A gown and/or cover sheet should be provided, depending on the examination to be undertaken. There are certain situations when even greater care must be taken in explaining the need for and nature of the examination, seeking and obtaining consent, and providing for privacy (and sometimes a chaperone). These include intimate examinations (e.g. breast, vaginal, rectal or scrotal examinations), especially when patients are young or may never have experienced such examinations, and for patients met for the first time. Also included are physical examinations of patients from cultural backgrounds which differ from their doctor's (see also Chapter 7, Consent and informed decision making, and Chapter 8, Sexual and other professional boundaries: being a doctor in modern society).

To reduce anxiety experienced by patients during examinations, it may be useful to engage patients in conversation; for example, by obtaining more detail regarding family, past medical or social history. Alertness to non-verbal communication is also a skill to be valued during examinations (e.g. the first evidence that an area of the abdomen is tender when palpated may come from patients' facial expressions, rather than comments or responses to questions).

5.5 Important aspects of patient education, follow-up and concluding consultations

Information needs to be conveyed slowly, clearly, in limited amounts in a single session; using plain language; and in terms that the patient in their context will understand. Doctors should ensure that patients have understood information given; for example, by asking them what they have been told and then listening carefully to their responses. The use of diagrams, illustrations, models, written action plans and handouts is encouraged for enhancing communication. Note-taking and/or the presence of a relative or close friend should be encouraged so that patients can reconsider important points afterwards. Where medical jargon is unavoidable, it needs to be explained, or written, so that patients can confirm the meaning later. Experienced doctors never presume that patients have prior knowledge, even when the patient is a medical practitioner or other health professional (see section 5.17).

Doctors should encourage and be responsive to questions asked by patients and those they have chosen to accompany them. It often helps during consultations, especially towards the end, to enquire 'What else you would like to tell me or ask me about?' This evokes more patient questions than, 'Have you any questions?' Patients usually understand that not every medical question can be answered but should never be given untruthful answers. It is both acceptable and honest to say 'I don't know' when this is the case. Most patients tolerate some degree of uncertainty.

Teach-back (a cycle of patients describing in their own words what they have understood from the consultation until clear understanding is achieved) is a particularly useful technique to improve recall, retention and clarity of understanding [36]. This should be done in a non-shaming way by the doctor taking responsibility for ensuring patient understanding. This may be facilitated by asking, 'I want to check that I explained clearly what you need to do/know, so please tell me in your own words what you will do/know about your condition.' Be specific about a certain area of information and modify the way information is presented if understanding is not reached. Teach-back is a recommended communication strategy for improving patient outcomes [37]. Audio recordings of consultations have also been shown to be valued by patients [38].

It is human nature to be optimistic, but optimism without discernment and honesty is misplaced. Care must be taken not to imply or promise undeliverable outcomes. It helps doctors to try to imagine patients' feelings, as perceived by this patient in their own situation, while avoiding judging or criticising patients' responses based on their own personal standards or beliefs. It is wise to anticipate that patients will not recall or will only selectively recall what they are told, particularly if the information is unexpected or distressing. When information given to patients is critical, taking the trouble to write it down and arranging to see the patient again and/or ensuring that a relative or friend is present is strongly advised. This helps patients assimilate information not processed at the time. Time should be provided for patient education about the key issues and outcomes of their consultation. This can be enhanced by providing handouts, recommending relevant websites, writing action plans and reiterating in follow-up consultations. Information about anticipated illness outcomes and clear arrangements for follow-up should also be provided. If follow-up is not required, this should be clearly communicated.

5.6 Shared decision making

Doctors need to assist patients, always to the extent that they wish to at that particular time, to make decisions about their own clinical care. So, the first step is to articulate that there are choices, the second step is to ascertain how much involvement they want during this consultation in this choice and the final step is to share what the doctor's recommendation is and why. The extent of the sharing in this process may change over time depending on many factors, including the clinical context and the patient's mindset, as well as their trust and relationship with their doctor [39,40].

Overall, the vast majority of patients (approx. 80%) want this to be a clinical partnership [39]. The literature suggests that for approximately 5% of decisions, patients themselves wish to essentially lead this process, while for approximately 15% of decisions, patients prefer to leave clinical decisions to their medical advisers. Irrespective, they almost always want to know what the broad choices are and what has been recommended for them based on their individual circumstances.

Doctors have an obligation, however, to indicate to all patients the risks and the benefits of the range of options, with these expressed in ways that they understand, taking into consideration their values, goals and preferences. This includes ascertaining what patients already know or perceive about the options available, their possible outcomes and the acceptability or otherwise of the various outcomes. This information needs to be gathered before making recommendations. It may be tempting to provide a detailed explanation of the preferred option but it is much more effective to outline all the options, including that of no intervention, and then make a personalised recommendation for the patient to the extent that they wish, based on what is important to them. Patients expect their doctor's recommendations to be based on knowledge, experience and expertise and therefore consider that they can question the rationale for particular recommendations.

Communicating risk clearly is a key requirement, and consideration should be given to the person's health literacy and their understanding of numeracy. Useful tips include keeping the same denominator when conveying numerical risks and benefits, including 'absolute' expressions of the magnitude of risks and benefits (e.g. the number of patients receiving a particular intervention for one patient to benefit or to be harmed in specific ways), and using decision aids before, during or after consultations [41]. Decision aids are particularly useful when the 'trade-offs' are complex; for example, high-risk surgery [42]. A database of decision aids compiled by the Ottawa Hospital Research Institute can be found at https://decisionaid.ohri.ca. An approach which may help is to outline best, worst and most-likely case scenarios [43].

5.7 Working with interpreters

Living in multicultural Australia means that most doctors encounter patients with backgrounds different from their own, some of whom they will not share common languages with. While most patients do not expect doctors to have great knowledge or understanding of their culture and language, doctor–patient relationships are enhanced when doctors clearly demonstrate respect for such differences and actively seek to improve their understanding. This can be shown in small ways, such as by asking questions about the patient's country and their heritage, by indicating knowledge or awareness of their country of origin, and/or by making additional efforts to ensure that patients are fully understood.

In addition, Aboriginal and/or Torres Strait Islander peoples have many traditional languages and English may be a third or fourth language. Interpreters may also be required, especially for rural and remote health services. In addition, finding out the person's language and clan group as well as their home country is an important part of engagement and will assist in determining who can interpret from the community if required.

As medical consultations involve the exchange of complex and subtle information, language barriers need to be minimised by using interpreters [44] (see also Chapter 7, Consent and informed decision making). Ideally, interpreters should be properly qualified and, if requested by patients, of the same gender as them. The risks of family members and/or other hospital staff acting as interpreters should be carefully considered, to ensure both confidentiality and accurate translation. Where in emergency situations this may be unavoidable, a qualified professional interpreter should be sought as soon as practicable after the event, to ensure that accurate information was indeed obtained and conveyed.

The Medical Board of Australia's code of conduct states that good medical practice involves:

> 4.3.7 Taking all practical steps to ensure that arrangements are made to meet patients' specific language, cultural and communication needs, and being aware of how these needs affect patients' understanding.
>
> 4.3.8 Familiarising yourself with, and using whenever necessary, qualified language interpreters to help you to meet patients' communication needs. Government-funded and fee-for-service interpreter services are available [44].

The Australian Government provides a free Interpreting Service for medical practitioners providing Medicare-rebateable services (http://www.tisnational.gov.au; telephone: 131 450). Telehealth video interpreting for medical consultations became available in August 2020. Aboriginal Interpreting WA has provided Aboriginal language interpreters since 2000 (https://aiwaac.org.au).

Doctors have been the subject of complaints to the Medical Board for failure to seek the assistance of interpreters leading to serious harm [45], and surveys have shown that many doctors are unaware of, or have never used, 'free' non-face-to-face (e.g. telephone or audiovisual) interpreter services [46].

Using interpreters appropriately in face-to-face consultations with both patient and interpreter present is a skill that must be learned and which improves with experience. Useful guidelines are available [47]. Medical interpreters undertake formal training, the nature of which doctors should be aware of (see Chapter 11, The doctor and interprofessional relationships). Problems may arise if patients' languages have not been correctly identified, if an interpreter has not been arranged in sufficient time and if the patient considers that a particular interpreter is inappropriate, for whatever reason. It may help to provide the interpreter (with the patient's consent) relevant background information about the patient and the purpose of the consultation. Interpreters should be introduced to patients by name and their roles explained. Patients should be advised that interpreters are professionally bound to maintain confidentiality. When using interpreters, questions and eye contact should be directed to patients, rather than to the interpreter. This is often easier to achieve when interpreters sit slightly behind patients. Doctors should be alert to signals from interpreters that they are being overloaded. It sometimes helps to request patients and interpreters to repeat critical issues, to ensure that no key information is missed. Doctors should also be alert to suggestions that a patient might be uncomfortable with a particular interpreter.

Communication in face-to-face consultations with patients, even with the assistance of an interpreter, is much more difficult when interpreters participate by telephone, because of the absence of interpreters' non-verbal communications with both patients and doctors, and because interpreters cannot see patients' responses to their conversations with doctors. Fortunately, video interpreting is now available. In addition, there are other circumstances where assistance with communication may be required such as for those with impaired hearing and other language barriers or disabilities. Practitioners should know how to access Auslan or deaf interpreters when needed.

5.8 Cultural safety

Cultural safety in health care is vitally important. Providing culturally safe and respectful health care is part of the Medical Board of Australia's code of conduct [44]. The code outlines the following for culturally safe practice:

- Understand how culture, values, attitudes, assumptions and beliefs influence healthcare interactions.
- Acknowledge the social, economic, cultural, historic and behavioural factors influencing the health of individuals, communities and populations.
- Respect diverse cultures, beliefs, gender identities, sexualities and experiences of people.
- Adapt practice as needed to respect diversity and avoid bias, discrimination and racism while still providing safe and appropriate care.
- Support the rights, dignity and safety of others.

Australian health care also needs to respect Indigenous cultural values and protocols, and address inequity. Effective cross-cultural communication assists in developing culturally safe practice and includes a number of cultural considerations, such as greeting protocols and welcome ceremonies; gender and age issues; avoidance relationships in kinship systems; body language; and interview style to name a few. For more information, please refer to Chapter 17, Culturally safe health care for Aboriginal and/or Torres Strait Islander peoples. The Australian Indigenous Doctors' Association website has resources and training in cultural safety (https://aida.org.au/cultural-safety-program).

Since 2004, as a part of the accreditation process of the Australian Medical Council, all Australian medical schools have been required to incorporate an Indigenous health curriculum framework developed by Medical Deans Australia and New Zealand [48]. In its introduction, the document importantly observes:

> The health outcomes of Aboriginal and Torres Strait Islander Peoples are governed more by the historical and social determinants of health, than with inherent Aboriginality. Prior to colonisation, Indigenous Australians were healthy and maintained physical, emotional, mental and spiritual wellness. Thus, the prevalence of illness in today's society cannot easily be attributed only to genetic or even behavioural causes. Rather, as supported by evidence, the preferred view is that current health outcomes result from a range of interrelated historical, environmental, physiological, political and behavioural factors [48].

This topic is discussed in detail in Chapter 17, Culturally safe health care for Aboriginal and/or Torres Strait Islander peoples.

5.9 Communication for technology-based consultations

Technology-based consultations are defined by the Medical Board of Australia as 'consultations that use technology as an alternative to in-person consultations between a patient and a medical practitioner (doctor)' [49]. The use of telemedicine can improve patient access to medical care, especially for patients in remote and relatively underserviced parts of Australia [50]. The COVID-19 pandemic led to the rapid uptake and advancement of telehealth [51] due to the need to maintain the safety of both patients and doctors by minimising spread of infection. In addition, mask wearing in face-to-face consultations meant that technology-based video consultations made it easier to see faces clearly and therefore ensure better communication [52,53].

Because the practice of telemedicine may alter elements of the usual face-to-face doctor–patient interactions during consultations, there are additional considerations for effective communication [54–56].

These include: ensuring telehealth is appropriate for the setting and a direct physical examination is not required; gaining informed consent; ensuring privacy and confidentiality; explaining where necessary about how the technology-based consultation works; keeping good medical records; ensuring effective communication and patient understanding; and ensuring optimal follow-up. As more than one health professional may participate in these consultations, care must be taken to ensure that all involved are identified and acknowledged at the outset. The arrangements and purpose of consultations need to be explained to ensure that patients understand and agree to the process. Interruptions should be avoided [55–57].

Evidence suggests that consultations last no longer but that a new element of technical talk is inserted at the beginning of the consultation to outline technical issues and what to do if sessions end unexpectedly. Significant audio lag seems to be the major issue in making such consultations ineffective and unsatisfactory [58].

Telehealth requires attention to technical details including the location and backdrop for the doctor's camera, the quality of lighting so that faces are clearly visible, and ensuring good sound quality, with telephone backup when problems arise [56]. The Royal Australasian College of Physicians has produced a helpful guide to conducting consultations by telehealth [57]. The Royal Australian College of General Practitioners has developed a telehealth resource website in response to the rapid changes in healthcare delivery associated with the COVID-19 pandemic [59].

5.10 Communicating when things go wrong

Special attention to communication is needed when unexpected or adverse outcomes or events occur in medical practice. Open disclosure is also covered in Chapter 25, Negligence and professional liability.

When things go wrong, it is essential to be open, frank and honest in communicating with patients and their families and carers. This should involve telling the patient as early as possible that an adverse event has occurred. It is important to recognise and acknowledge patients' distress and to express concern and regret, including the words 'I am/we are sorry', without expressing opinions about blame and responsibility [60–62]. Such advice is consistent with the recommendations of indemnity insurers, given that doctors on their own can seldom make judgements about the likelihood of liability and, if liability is confirmed, how and to what or to whom it might be properly attributed, especially at the time of or soon after an adverse event has occurred [63].

When things go wrong, it is usually helpful to engage the whole team involved as well as some independent colleagues, some with relevant expertise, to further consider the event and to determine together what can be learned, as well as what steps might be taken to institute systems which aim to prevent recurrence. It is also advisable to communicate the findings of the review and the future plans to the patient at a well-considered and appropriate time. See Chapter 21, Regulation of the medical profession, and Chapter 22, Healthcare complaints and complaint systems, for more detail on what happens if the situation results in a complaint or inquiry.

5.11 Dealing with strong emotions

One of the most challenging situations, even for experienced doctors, is dealing with patients with strong emotions, especially those angered because their complaints have been ignored or mismanaged. As Niselle wisely wrote, in such situations 'the patient is allowed to be irrational, illogical, emotional and accusatory, but the doctor is meant at all times to be fair, reasonable, dispassionate, measured, and above all, professional' [64]. The core skill that seems to resolve anger is to explicitly show people that you have listened carefully and heard whatever experience(s) led to these feelings.

Many feelings may be driving this anger and it is important to appreciate the diversity of these emotional drivers. Some educators have used simple tools and mnemonics to 'attend to emotions' (see VitalTalk in section 5.1.3).

Key elements in responses include making time available as early as possible to meet with patients, acknowledging their distress, and making genuine attempts to respond positively to complaints (which may include referring the person to relevant agencies, especially if you are unable to conciliate the issues) [64].

It is critical to avoid becoming angry in response and to project this anger to the patient and others. A calm and confident approach is more likely to defuse the situation. Debriefing and peer support for doctors is an important part of dealing with strong emotions.

5.12 Coping with challenging patient–doctor encounters

Not every patient encounter proceeds according to expectations. All doctors experience consultations and doctor–patient relationships that might be deemed 'difficult', to the extent that doctors may be left 'feeling helpless, frustrated, irritated and even angry' [65]. Difficult encounters can arise through factors originating with the doctor (e.g. poor communication skills, lack of experience, overwork [66]), with the patient (e.g. stress and anxiety, mental illness, personality disorder) and with healthcare systems and settings (e.g. lack of continuity of care, lack of time [67]).

It is more constructive to think about an *encounter* as being difficult and to resist labelling a *patient* as difficult. A range of encounters generally regarded as potentially difficult have been identified, including encounters with angry and demanding patients and/or families, overprotective families, dominating partners, patients who resist getting better, patients who offer gifts or otherwise seek special relationships with doctors, patients who are also doctors or other health professionals (see also section 5.17), as well as patients with whom doctors identify and either like or dislike, at times excessively, for whatever reason.

There may be difficulties in consultations when people other than the patient are also present. If additional people are disturbing the interaction between doctor and patient, it may help to offer the other person a pen and notepad and ask them to make notes during the consultation for discussion with the doctor at the end of the patient's interview.

It is essential to at least reflect on encounters when difficulty first becomes apparent. It is often helpful to discuss potential and perceived difficulties with colleagues. There are strategies that can render potentially difficult encounters less stressful and more productive and rewarding for both patients and doctors, although these are rarely taught to young doctors. Faced with such situations, advice should be sought from more experienced doctors and/or relevant publications [68,69].

5.13 Medicolegal examinations

On a proportional basis, more complaints to medical boards and health complaints agencies arise from the medicolegal examination field of practice than from any other. The reasons include the absence of usual patient–doctor relationships, the requirement for doctors to provide detailed reports of their findings and opinions to third parties, and underlying patient concerns that reports may be unfavourable from their perspective. Good communication is vital in achieving good outcomes in this field. This topic is discussed in detail in Chapter 26, Medicolegal examinations and reports, court procedures and expert evidence.

5.14 Consideration of touch as a means of non-verbal support and empathy

Physical contact is another form of human communication. Touching a patient without consent is assault, yet physical contact is a very human means of conveying concern and warmth and is very much part of the healing role of doctors and other health professionals. During physical examinations, touching is permitted because the patient has given consent, usually implied, for the examination to occur (hence the advice in section 5.4 to explain such examinations before conducting them).

However, there are other times during consultations when physical contact may be appropriate and helpful; for example, if a patient is distressed or receiving unexpected news. It is not possible to provide specific advice as to when physical contact—for example, holding a hand or placing an arm around a shoulder—is safe or appropriate. It is more likely to be safe and appropriately interpreted if a third party is present, the patient is unequivocally distressed, the patient is well known to you and if the physical contact is timely yet brief.

Considerations to keep in mind as factors are the age, gender, sexuality, culture and other beliefs of the patient and their family, and how these differ from those of the doctor.

Doctors also need to be alert to patients' reactions to physical contact, especially if these are either negative or inappropriately positive. A very helpful discussion concerning touching as an aspect of communication is given by Myerscough [70].

In addition, sometimes physical contact may be initiated by the patient or their family at times of distress or through gratitude. It is important to acknowledge the situation and limit or avoid physical contact if possible.

5.15 Sensitive topics including talking about sex, gender and sexuality

In general, the more sensitive the topic the more important it is to explicitly ask permission to discuss it. A key pitfall is to ask about discussing a sensitive topic without then pausing and accurately assessing the emotional, verbal or non-verbal responses. Raise topics in a calm and professional manner. Normalise asking about sexuality and gender. Ideally also ask what personal pronouns a patient likes to use. This is most helpfully done at an initial consultation when gathering relevant patient information. This may be done by stating the personal pronouns you prefer and then ask what pronouns the patient prefers to use. Presumption of standard pronouns (e.g. she/he/they) can make patients with other preferences feel disrespected. The Fenway Institute has educational resources to support the health care and wellbeing of lesbian, gay, bisexual, transgender, queer, intersex, asexual and all sexual and gender minority (LGBTQIA+) people (see https://www.lgbtqiahealtheducation.org).

For all patients it is important to be able to competently and confidently discuss health care relating to sexual issues. Although it is neither necessary nor justified to include questions about sexual issues in every medical interview, doctors should be alert to clinical situations where such issues are more likely to be present. These include patients presenting with gynaecological/urological problems, signs or symptoms suggesting sexually transmissible diseases, relationship problems, conditions associated with sexual dysfunction, and after certain types of surgery (e.g. mastectomy, prostatectomy, colostomy and ileostomy). Introducing such questions should not be done until rapport has been established and should always be preceded by a simple explanation as to why the questions are regarded as necessary. This simple explanation prepares the patient and makes it clear that the doctor is comfortable in having such a discussion. The use of relatively open-ended questions such as 'Are there any other issues, including sexual issues, which you'd like to raise?' may provide an opening to this sensitive area.

5.16 Talking about death and dying

Most doctors will at some time in their careers have the task of conveying information about serious illness to patients and their families. Almost all will be involved in the ongoing care of patients with life-limiting illnesses, who represent about one-third of inpatients in our Australian acute care hospitals; about 70% of these patients will have died within three years [71]. The development of oncology and palliative care services and hospice movements may suggest to some that only particular specialists need to be skilled communicators in these areas. However, all doctors in clinical practice should be alert to opportunities and the need to discuss future care plans with patients with serious illnesses early in the course of the illness [71], and should be able to convey information to patients with sensitivity and with awareness of the needs of patients with fatal illnesses [72]. Consideration should also be given to discussing end-of-life issues and advance care planning [73] (see also Chapter 19, Advance care planning and end-of-life care). All doctors need to be able to discern what is of importance to patients and how to integrate these values and goals into discussions about their care. When this is done well it dramatically improves patient outcomes and minimises potentially burdensome unbeneficial treatment [74]. There is a large body of literature showing that prognostic discordance is very common and almost always patients significantly overestimate their curability or life expectancy [75].

An Australian study analysed the ways in which doctors approach the difficult task of breaking bad news (using case scenarios where patients had died suddenly and with actors playing the role of a close relative) [76]. The researchers identified three distinct approaches, which they labelled as blunt (without preamble), forecasting (preparing the person for the bad news) or stalling (avoiding the delivery of the bad news). Of the three, the forecasting approach, used by just over half the doctors, appears to be closest to the approach generally advised [77]. This approach allows the doctor to determine what the relative or patient already knows, increase rapport by demonstrating empathy and concern, forewarn and prepare the individual, and facilitate effective communication [76]. It is also more likely to meet the needs of the person [78].

Providing hope in the setting of advanced disease may require us to reframe and refocus care on key aspects such as quality of life. False hope may help in the very short term but is nearly always crushing in its impact in the medium to long term.

Principles for conveying unexpected news in common clinical situations have already been mentioned in section 5.5, where it was emphasised that adequate time must be made, privacy must be assured, patients should be encouraged to have relatives or friends present and early follow-up appointments offered. On receipt of unexpected news, patients may respond over time with reactions of denial, anger, bargaining, depression and then acceptance [79], a sequence that may vary in its pace of evolution, and with overlap of the reaction phases. Understanding of this classical response has developed in recent times and complicated grief and trauma reactions are now considered part of the spectrum of responses. See Grief Australia (https://www.grief.org.au) for further information and resources. Very rarely, denial dominates the entire final illness [79]. Denial is to be appreciated as an important mechanism whereby patients and others cope with the news of their likely mortality. Doctors who deny their own eventual mortality may have the greatest difficulty in coping effectively with communication in this domain (see Chapter 19, Advance care planning and end-of-life care).

In this clinical setting, doctors must be sensitive to the stage each patient is at and not try to provide information until the patient wants it. Patients expect doctors to tell the truth and never to deceive them, but also prefer to be given optimistic news, making communication of unexpected or unwanted news a challenging task. The Kubler-Ross approach has emphasised the critical importance of always leaving some room for hope [79].

In the aftermath of a patient's death, doctors can play a valuable role in helping relatives of the deceased cope with grief by making themselves available to answer questions about the death. If this opportunity has, as is often the case, not been offered before the patient's death, it may help to contact an appropriate family member about 7 to 10 days after the death, following the initial grieving and memorial services, to enquire about their wellbeing and if they have residual questions. At times, grief is manifested as anger, which may be directed at others, including the doctor (see section 5.11).

5.17 Doctors and other health professionals as patients

Difficulties arise for doctors regarding seeking care for their own health and in caring for other doctors (addressed in Chapter 12, Personal health of the doctor: illness and impairment). It is well recognised that doctors caring for other doctors or other health professionals can make incorrect and potentially dangerous assumptions about such patients' understanding of their illness, proposed investigations, procedures or treatments, and with their compliance. It is wiser not to make any assumptions about knowledge but to impart information at the appropriate level for that patient, having first established their level of understanding and their need for information, as with other patients. Good communication skills ensure that even when such patients are indeed already well informed, no offence will be taken, and patients will have greater confidence in doctors' abilities to provide good care.

Another issue is that relatively inexperienced doctors may feel anxious about caring for more experienced colleagues, which is sometimes resolved by discussing this with the doctor-patient.

5.18 Ending a doctor–patient relationship

Occasions when it is necessary to end doctor–patient relationships may arise. Such occasions may include patients harassing or threatening doctors, patients repeatedly failing to keep appointments or complying with agreed courses of action, 'doctor-shopping' or drug-seeking behaviour, and loss of mutual trust and respect [80]. This is recognised in the Medical Board of Australia's code of conduct:

> In some circumstances, the relationship between a doctor and patient may break down or become compromised (e.g. because of a conflict of interest), and you may need to end it. Good medical practice involves ensuring that the patient is adequately informed of your decision and facilitating arrangements for the continuing care of the patient, including passing on relevant clinical information [44].

While making such decisions is often quite straightforward, conveying them to patients and facilitating appropriate arrangements for ongoing care can be difficult. Consideration needs to be given to whether the patient is informed face to face, by telephone or by letter. Inexperienced doctors should seek advice from their medical indemnity organisation and from senior colleagues before taking any such action. One expert has suggested a style of letter that could be useful in some situations [80]. If a relationship is terminated, staff members need to be informed and supported, as they may be approached for another appointment and become targets of abuse.

5.19 The importance of written communication

Written records need to be clear, to contain all relevant information (including information regarding the patient's knowledge of their illness and their emotional state) and to be signed by the person who wrote them. It is unwise to include critical, judgemental or emotive descriptors, as these can cause substantial embarrassment if, for example, the record is read by the patient or read out in court. Abbreviations should be limited to those used widely throughout the healthcare system. Medical records and reports are discussed in depth in Chapter 27, Medical records, reports and certificates.

Increasingly, the processes by which we curate, integrate and synthesise a variety of electronic health resources is becoming another key skill. This may occur before, during and after clinical consultations.

Much importance is attached to medical students being able to elicit and record systematically the details of the history and the physical examination. In the early postgraduate phase, attention is paid to the adequacy of progress notes and discharge summaries. Later, the emphasis shifts to record keeping for optimal subsequent patient review and management, and for defensive reasons (e.g. 'Would your medical records stand up to the scrutiny of the court?'). While the latter is a powerful incentive to keep clear and contemporaneous records, there are other reasons why written communication in medical records and in letters to doctors and others should be carefully and conscientiously undertaken [16]. These include the unequivocal educational value of correspondence between colleagues and the increasing desirability of sharing correspondence with patients, so that they can see what is stated about them and comment when they wish to.

Good clinical care requires synthesis and integration of all the relevant information available to the clinician and the associated healthcare team. This can range from hard copy professional letters to increasingly diverse digital clinical information systems. The curation of these information repositories is everyone's responsibility and includes capturing key psychosocial information so that we can truly deliver person-centred care. The processes involved are components of professional development, as we learn from them as well as improving care. As these evolving records become not only available to patients but shaped and checked by them, they can add more to the richness and accuracy of their unique narratives.

As factual errors may become incorporated within even the best of written records, however, critical matters should be confirmed by direct communication with patients and from other sources.

5.20 Intra- and interprofessional communication and relationships

The good communication practices outlined in this chapter also apply to communication between doctors and to communication between doctors and other professionals involved in the care of the patient, so that patients receive optimal care. Patient care may be compromised when there is poor communication between health professionals. As medical practice and health care frequently involve cooperative teamwork, and as care has become more specialised and compartmentalised, with multiple professionals involved concurrently or at different times, the risk of communication failure has increased.

Literature regarding the impact of professional incivility shows us that it has impacts on clinical care at the time of the event and beyond [81,82].

Doctors need to be alert to this risk and openly share relevant information with other professionals, with patients being informed and involved as well. This applies especially to information provided in referrals for consultation and in responses to these, to documentation of progress and changes in treatment, and when health care is transferred to other individuals or teams. For example, when many doctors are involved, each with expertise confined to some but not all the body systems, and each with the capacity to change medications, it is essential that all relevant professional colleagues are involved in, or informed of, decisions about proposed changes, before they are implemented.

Providing relevant information for other healthcare providers implies that doctors must understand and respect the potential contributions of others. Chapter 11, The doctor and interprofessional relationships, is devoted to the roles played by other health professionals. Appropriate respect by doctors for these non-medical professional roles is demonstrated by open and effective oral and/or written communication. Unfortunately, doctors often fail in this regard [83].

A closely related issue is the importance of protecting patients from unjustifiable direct or implied criticism by one doctor of another doctor or health professional. One problem is that criticism might be ill informed, especially if based on incomplete information. Apart from being disrespectful to other health professionals and having the potential to destabilise patient confidence, this behaviour can also be a factor leading to unwarranted complaints or civil litigation by patients (see also Chapter 25, Negligence and professional liability). In many clinical instances, robust evidence for specific interventions is lacking, meaning that there are likely to be well-meant and appropriate variations in professional opinions. In such situations, discussion and resolution of differences of opinion by the professionals involved, before options are presented to patients, represents good medical practice.

5.21 Feedback to and from colleagues

Medical practitioners will need to provide and receive feedback to and from their colleagues during their careers. These conversations and the reflections afterwards are often critical for the professional development of those involved; feedback becomes even more complex if there are concerns about clinical performance.

Box 5.1 Key communication skills that maximise the opportunity for learning and development through feedback

Allow the person receiving feedback to self-analyse their own performance first. This gives you key information. For example, colleagues may make major disclosures about stressors within and outside of work which impact on their performance.

Assist their self-analysis by asking open questions and building rapport, as they are unlikely to disclose sensitive or difficult issues until trust is established.

Make the feedback:

- based on direct observation by yourself—second-hand reports make the feedback process much more difficult, especially if there are concerns around performance

Continued over page

- as timely as possible
- as specific and descriptive as possible (e.g. describe the behavioural aspects)—providing global evaluation rather than specific observations may act as a barrier to learning, particularly for some learners who may become defensive and focus on the interpretation of observed behaviours
- balanced, with reference to skills acquired and a small number (e.g. 1–2 maximum) areas to prioritise for development.

Professional development opportunities or resources include:

- small-group experiential workshops
- reading key texts or articles that outline evidence-based frameworks, tools and outcomes of applying recommended skills
- watching role model videos of clinical examples, with examples of skills, approaches and common pitfalls
- observing role models [84]—this requires a common language and an ability to deconstruct what happens, in order to understand the 'microskills' involved
- consideration of audio or video recording of one's own consultations to aid reflective practice and to discuss with supervisors
- being observed by mentors who are skilled in teaching communication skills—this often only requires short periods of observation and may include:
  - information gathering
  - provision of information
  - evaluation during procedures or examinations.

Such conversations can be of great importance in our colleagues' careers and immensely rewarding when undertaken skilfully. Conversely, providing unskilled feedback can inhibit learning and be harmful to the person receiving it.

5.22 Communicating on social media

The use of social media professionally and personally by medical students and doctors has created the potential for new dilemmas in relation to the doctor–patient relationship and the potential risk of harm to a doctor's reputation and standing in the community [85]. Several agencies have provided advice to doctors and medical students about these matters [86] and the Medical Board of Australia has developed guidance [87]. The guidance defines the term 'social media' and emphasises doctors' obligation to adhere to the board's code of conduct and advertising guidelines when using social media.

Patients who use a doctor's social media page to contact the doctor for legitimate medical reasons may be unaware of the ethical restraints placed on doctors in regard to social relationships with patients.

Doctors should always consider how their social media presence may reflect on their reputation as a doctor, regardless of the platform, purpose or intended audience, whether used in their private or professional capacity [88]. The Medical Board of Australia's guidance on social media states:

> Where relevant, National Boards may consider social media use in your private life (even where there is no identifiable link to you as a registered health practitioner) if it raises concerns about your fitness to hold registration.

> While you may think you are engaging in social media in a private capacity because you do not state you are a registered practitioner, it is relatively easy and simple for anyone to check your status through the register, or make connections using available pieces of information [87].

Posting material such as embarrassing photos or thoughtless comments to friends might come back to haunt a doctor. The use of social media also raises possibilities of deliberate or inadvertent crossing of boundaries between patient and doctor; this is discussed in Chapter 8, Sexual and other professional boundaries: being a doctor in modern society.

A separate risk that has evolved is the use of social media by patients and patient groups to informally rank doctors. Such sites are uncontrolled and can post highly critical or even defamatory comments about doctors that can cause great harm to professional reputation, with little chance of redress. It is very important to seek advice from a professional indemnity provider before responding online to these comments.

Summary

Effective, high-quality communication is crucial for good clinical practice and is vital for effective leadership and collaboration in healthcare teams. Good communication improves the quality and safety of health care and decreases the likelihood of complaints and legal action when things go wrong. Communication skills can be taught and learned effectively, and this chapter has discussed some of these key skills, including building rapport with patients, making them feel comfortable, and using open-ended questions to gather information before following up with closed questions to explore details. Active listening, with close attention to non-verbal clues, can be very valuable in both ascertaining the patient's agenda, and ensuring that they feel heard.

Challenges to effective communication include dealing with patients' preconceived ideas about their health care, often derived from the internet; managing the emotional aspects of the interaction; and striking a balance between the patient's autonomy and need for expert opinion and advice. There are also practical aspects—such as provision of adequate time and an appropriate space, maintaining attention on the patient, and checking whether information has been received accurately—that can influence the quality of communication between a doctor and a patient. Effective communication is also crucial during physical examinations, particularly when patients are asked to undress, and when examination of intimate regions of the body is required. All communication with patients needs to take into account diversity, sociocultural factors and linguistic challenges.

Communication with colleagues also needs to be effective to promote optimal patient care, as well as maintaining the health and safety of all practitioners. Communication needs to remain civil at all times, including when there is professional disagreement or when one party is providing feedback to the other.

References

1. Tamblyn R, Abrahamowicz M, Dauphinee D, et al. Physician scores on a national clinical skills examination as predictors of complaints to medical regulatory authorities. *JAMA* 2007; 298: 993–1001.
2. Levinson W, Rotor DL, Mullooly JP, et al. Physician–patient communication. The relationship with malpractice claims among primary care physicians and surgeons. *JAMA* 1997; 277: 553–559.
3. Lussier M, Richard C. Complaints and legal actions: role of doctor-patient communication. *Can Fam Physician* 2005; 51: 37–39.
4. Simpson M, Buckman R, Stewart M, et al. Doctor–patient communication: the Toronto consensus statement. *BMJ* 1991; 303: 1385–1387.
5. Forsey J, Ng S, Rowland P, et al. The basic science of patient-physician communication: a critical scoping review. *Acad Med* 2021; 96: S109–S118.
6. Laidlaw TS, Kaufman DM, Sargeant J, et al. What makes a physician an exemplary communicator with patients. *Patient Educ Couns* 2007; 68: 153–160.
7. Coulter A. Patients' views of the good doctor. *BMJ* 2002; 325: 668–669.
8. Haskard Zolnierek KB, DiMatteo MR. Physician communication and patient adherence to treatment: a meta-analysis. *Med Care* 2009; 47: 826–834.
9. Bismark MM, Spittal MJ, Gurrin LC, et al. Identification of doctors at risk of recurrent complaints: a national study of healthcare complaints in Australia. *BMJ Qual Saf* 2013; 22: 532–540.
10. Smith S, Hanson JL, Tewksbury LR, et al. Teaching patient communication skills to medical students: a review of randomized controlled trials. *Eval Health Prof* 2007; 30: 3–21.
11. Salmon P, Young B. Creativity in clinical communication: from communication skills to skilled communication. *Med Educ* 2011; 45: 217–226.
12. Paice E, Heard S, Moss F. How important are role models in making good doctors? *BMJ* 2002; 325: 707–710.
13. Gillis AE, Morris MC, Ridgway PF. Communication skills assessment in the final postgraduate years to established practice: a systematic review. *Postgrad Med J* 2015; 91: 13–21.
14. Warnecke E. The art of communication. *Aust Fam Physician* 2014; 43: 156–158.
15. Behforouz HL, Drain PK, Rhatigan JJ. Rethinking the social history. *N Engl J Med* 2014; 371: 1277–1279.
16. Mauksch LB, Dugdale DC, Dodson S, Epstein R. Relationship, communication, and efficiency in the medical encounter: creating a clinical model from a literature review. *Arch Intern Med* 2008; 168: 1387–1395.
17. Singh Ospina N, Phillips KA, Rodriguez-Gutierrez R, et al. Eliciting the patient's agenda- secondary analysis of recorded clinical encounters. *J Gen Intern Med* 2019; 34: 36–40.
18. Granger K. Healthcare staff must properly introduce themselves to patients. *BMJ* 2013; 347: f5833.
19. DeAngelis CD. The electronic health record: boon or bust for good patient care? *Milbank Q* 2014; 92: 442–445.
20. Langewitz W, Denz M, Keller A, et al. Spontaneous talking time at the start of consultation in outpatient clinic: cohort study. *BMJ* 2002; 325: 682–683.
21. Boudreau JD, Cassell E, Fuks A. Preparing medical students to become attentive listeners. *Med Teach* 2009; 31: 22–29.
22. Fassaert T, van Dulmen S, Schellevis F, Bensing J. Active listening in medical consultations: development of the active listening observation scale (ALOS-global). *Patient Educ Couns* 2007; 68: 258–264.
23. Levinson W, Gorawara-Bhat R, Lamb J. A study of patient clues and physician responses in primary care and surgical settings. *JAMA* 2000; 284: 1021–1027.
24. Iversen ED, Wolderslund M, Kofoed PE, et al. Communication skills training: a means to promote time-efficient patient-centered communication in clinical practice. J *Patient Cent Res Rev* 2021; 8: 307–314.
25. Strasser F, Palmer JL, Willey J, et al. Impact of physician sitting versus standing during inpatient oncology consultations: patients' preference and perception of compassion and duration. A randomized controlled trial. *J Pain Symptom Manage* 2005; 29: 489–497.
26. Wald HS, Dube CE, Anthony DC. Untangling the web – the impact of internet use on health care and the physician–patient relationship. *Patient Educ Couns* 2007; 68: 218–224.
27. Kurtz S, Silverman J, Benson J, Draper J. Marrying content and process in clinical method teaching: enhancing the Calgary–Cambridge guides. *Acad Med* 2003; 78: 802–809.

28. Buckman R. Communications and emotions. *BMJ* 2002; 325: 672.
29. Luff D, Martin Jr EB, Mills K, et al. Clinicians' strategies for managing their emotions during difficult healthcare conversations. *Patient Educ Couns* 2016; 99: 1461–1466.
30. Martin Jr EB, Mazzola NM, Brandano J, et al. Clinicians' recognition and management of emotions during difficult healthcare conversations. *Patient Educ Couns* 2015; 98: 1248–1254.
31. Shaw A, Ibrahim S, Reid F, et al. Patients' perspectives of the doctor–patient relationship and information giving across a range of literacy levels. *Patient Educ Couns* 2009; 75: 114–120.
32. Binns-Calvey AE, Sharma G, Ashley N, et al. Listening to the patient: a typology of contextual red flags in disease management encounters. *J Patient Cent Res Rev* 2020; 7: 39.
33. Weiner SJ, Schwartz A. Contextual errors in medical decision making: overlooked and understudied. *Acad Med* 2016; 91: 657–662.
34. Street RL, Makoul G, Arora NK, Epstein RM. How does communication heal? Pathways linking clinician-patient communication to health outcomes. *Pat Educ Couns* 2009; 74: 295–301.
35. Reeves E. A synthesis of the literature on trauma-informed care. *Issues Ment Health Nurs* 2015; 36: 698–709.
36. Talevski J, Wong Shee A, Rasmussen B, et al. Teach-back: a systematic review of implementation and impacts. *PLoS One* 2020; 15.
37. Anderson KM, Leister S, De Rego R. The 5Ts for teach back: an operational definition for teach-back training. *Health Lit Res Pract* 2020; 4: e94–e103.
38. Wolderslund M, Kofoed PE, Holst R, et al. Digital audio recordings improve the outcomes of patient consultations: a randomised cluster trial. *Patient Educ Couns* 2017; 100: 242–249.
39. Kriston L, Hahlweg P, Härter M, Scholl I. A skills network approach to physicians' competence in shared decision making. *Health Expect* 2020; 23: 1466–1476.
40. Baghus A, Giroldi E, Muris J, et al. Identifying entrustable professional activities for shared decision making in postgraduate medical education: a national Delphi study. *Acad Med* 2021; 96: 126.
41. Bonner C, Trevena LJ, Gaissmaier W, et al. Current best practice for presenting probabilities in patient decision aids: fundamental principles. *Med Decis Making* 2021; 41: 821–833.
42. Stacey D, Légaré F, Lewis K, et al. Decision aids for people facing health treatment or screening decisions. *Cochrane Database Syst Rev* 2017; 4.
43. Kruser JM, Taylor LJ, Campbell TC, et al. 'Best case/worst case': training surgeons to use a novel communication tool for high-risk acute surgical problems. *J Pain Symptom Manage* 2017; 53: 711–719.
44. Medical Board of Australia. Good medical practice: a code of conduct for doctors in Australia. 2020. https://www.medicalboard.gov.au/Codes-Guidelines-Policies/Code-of-conduct.aspx (accessed Nov 2021).
45. Bird S. Failure to use an interpreter. *Aust Fam Physician* 2010; 39: 241–242.
46. Fung CC, Lagha RR, Henderson P, Gomez AG. Working with interpreters: how student behavior affects quality of patient interaction when using interpreters. *Med Educ Online* 2010; 15.
47. Queensland Health. Working with interpreters: guidelines. 2007. http://www.health.qld.gov.au/multicultural/interpreters/guidelines_int.pdf (accessed Nov 2021).
48. Phillips G. Indigenous health curriculum framework. Sydney: Committee of Deans of Australian Medical Schools, 2004. https://medicaldeans.org.au/md/2018/07/cdams-indig-health-frameworkreport.pdf (accessed Dec 2021).
49. Medical Board of Australia. Telehealth consultations with patients. 2023. https://www.medicalboard.gov.au/Codes-Guidelines-Policies/Telehealth-consultations-with-patients.aspx (accessed May 2025).
50. Thaker DA, Monypenny R, Olver I, Sabesan S. Cost savings from a telemedicine model of care in northern Queensland, Australia. *Med J Aust* 2013; 199: 414–417.
51. Garfan S, Alamoodi AH, Zaidan BB, et al. Telehealth utilization during the Covid-19 pandemic: a systematic review. *Comput Biol Med* 2021; 138: 104878.
52. Marler H, Ditton A. 'I'm smiling back at you': exploring the impact of mask wearing on communication in healthcare. *Int J Lang Commun Disord* 2021; 56: 205–214.
53. Samarasekara K. 'Masking' emotions: doctor–patient communication in the era of COVID-19. *Postgrad Med J* 2021; 97: 406.

54. Allen DT, Caldwell P, Komesaroff PA, et al. Practical aspects of telehealth: set-up and preparation for video consultations. *Intern Med J* 2013; 43: 1133–1136.
55. Greenhalgh T, Vijayaraghavan S, Wherton J, et al. Virtual online consultations: advantages and limitations (VOCAL) study. *BMJ Open* 2016; 6: e009388.
56. Wherton J, Shaw S, Papoutsi C, et al. Guidance on the introduction and use of video consultations during COVID-19: important lessons from qualitative research. *BMJ Leader* 2020; 4: 120–123.
57. Royal Australasian College of Physicians. Telehealth: Guidelines and practical tips. https://www.racp.edu.au/docs/default-source/advocacy-library/telehealth-guidelines-and-practical-tips.pdf (accessed Nov 2021).
58. Seuren LM, Wherton J, Greenhalgh T, Shaw SE. Whose turn is it anyway? Latency and the organization of turn-taking in video-mediated interaction. *J Pragmat* 2021; 172: 63–78.
59. Royal Australian College of General Practitioners. Guide to providing telephone and video consultations in general practice. https://www.racgp.org.au/running-a-practice/technology/clinical-technology/telehealth/guide-to-providing-telephone-and-video-consultatio/introduction (accessed May 2025).
60. Lamb R. Open disclosure: the only approach to medical error. *Qual Saf Health Care* 2004; 13: 3–5.
61. Jacob H, Raine J. Openness and honesty when things go wrong: the professional duty of candour (GMC guideline). *Arch Dis Child Educ Pract Ed* 2016; 101: 243–245.
62. Rathnayake D, Sasame A, Radomska A, et al. What can we learn from patient and family experiences of open disclosure and how they have been evaluated? A systematic review. *BMC Health Serv Res* 2025; 25: 1–22.
63. Avant. Open disclosure: responding when things go wrong. https://avant.org.au/resources/factsheet-open-disclosure-how-to-say-sorry (accessed May 2025).
64. Niselle P. Angered patients and the medical profession. *Med J Aust* 1999; 170: 576–577.
65. Breen KJ, Greenberg P. Difficult physician-patient encounters. *Intern Med J* 2010; 40: 682–688.
66. Krebs EE, Garrett JM, Konrad TR. The difficult doctor? Characteristics of physicians who report frustration with patients: an analysis of survey data. *BMC Health Serv Res* 2006; 6: 128.
67. Haas JL, Leiser JP, Magill MK, Sanyer ON. Management of the difficult patient. *Am Fam Physician* 2005; 72: 2063–2068.
68. Pearce C. The difficult patient. *Aust Fam Physician* 2002; 31: 177–181.
69. Teo AR, Du YB, Escobar JI. How can we better manage difficult patient encounters? *J Fam Pract* 2013; 62: 414–421.
70. Myerscough PR. Talking with patients: a basic clinical skill. Oxford: Oxford University Press, 1989.
71. Boyd K. Why is talking about dying such a challenge? *BMJ* 2014; 348: g3699.
72. Srivastava R. Critical conversations: navigating between hope and truth. *Lancet* 2011; 378: 1213–1214.
73. Silvester W, Detering K. Advance care planning and end-of-life care. *Med J Aust* 2011; 195: 435–436.
74. Ariadne Labs. Serious illness conversation guide. Boston: Harvard School of Public Health, 2023. https://www.ariadnelabs.org/resources/downloads/serious-illness-conversation-guide (accessed Oct 2024).
75. Yennurajalingam S, Rodrigues LF, Shamieh O, et al. Perception of curability among advanced cancer patients: an international collaborative study. *Oncol* 2018; 23: 501–506.
76. Shaw J, Dunn S, Heinrich P. Managing the delivery of bad news: an in-depth analysis of doctors' delivery style. *Patient Educ Couns* 2012; 87: 186–192.
77. Fallowfield L, Jenkins V. Communicating sad, bad and difficult news in medicine. *Lancet* 2004; 363: 312–319.
78. Randall TC, Wearn AM. Receiving bad news: patients with haematological cancer reflect upon their experience. *Palliat Med* 2005; 19: 594–601.
79. Tyrrell P, Harberger S, Schoo C, Siddiqui W. Kubler-Ross stages of dying and subsequent models of grief. Stat Pearls, 2025. https://www.ncbi.nlm.nih.gov/books/NBK507885/ (accessed May 2025).
80. Bird S. Ending the doctor–patient relationship. MDA National, 2015. https://www.mdanational.com.au/advice-and-support/library/articles-and-case-studies/2015/05/end-dr-patient-relationship (accessed May 2025).
81. Riskin A, Erez A, Foulk TA, et al. The impact of rudeness on medical team performance: a randomized trial. *Pediatrics* 2015; 136: 487–495.
82. Gilam G, Horing B, Sivan R, et al. The decline in task performance after witnessing rudeness is moderated by emotional empathy—a pilot study. *Front Psychol* 2020; 11: 1584.

83. Zwarenstein M, Rice K, Gotlib-Conn L, et al. Disengaged: a qualitative study of communication and collaboration between physicians and other professions on general internal medicine wards. *BMC Health Serv Res* 2013; 13: 494.
84. Rosenbaum ME. Dis-integration of communication in healthcare education: Workplace learning challenges and opportunities. *Patient Educ Couns* 2017; 100: 2054–2061.
85. Mansfield SJ, Morrison SG, Stephens HO, et al. Social media and the medical profession. *Med J Aust* 2011; 194: 642–644.
86. Australian Medical Association. Guide to social media and medical professionalism. 2020. https://www.ama.com.au/articles/guide-social-media-and-medical-professionalism (accessed Oct 2024).
87. Medical Board of Australia. Social media: How to meet your obligations under the National Law. 2019. https://www.ahpra.gov.au/Resources/Social-media-guidance.aspx (accessed Oct 2024).
88. Avant. Social media for doctors – keeping it professional. 2021. https://www.avant.org.au/Resources/Public/Social-media-for-doctors-keeping-it-professional/ (accessed Oct 2024).

Further reading

Gawande A. Being mortal: illness, medicine and what matters in the end. London: Profile Books, 2014.

Pendeleton D, Schofield T, Tate P, et al. The new consultation: developing doctor–patient communication. Oxford: Oxford University Press, 2003.

Silverman J, Kurtz S, Draper J. Skills for communicating with patients. 3rd edition. Oxford: Radcliffe Medical Press, 2013.

06 Confidentiality, privacy and disclosure

Georgie Haysom, Michael Isaacs

Introduction

Maintaining confidentiality and protecting the privacy of patient information are fundamental to the doctor–patient relationship and are key legal, ethical and professional requirements. Patients must be willing to trust their doctor, and the basis for this trust is knowing that relevant information they provide will be kept confidential.

The basis of the obligation of confidentiality lies in one of the oldest ethical principles of medical practice, stated in the Hippocratic Oath as:

> Whatsoever I shall see or hear in the course of my profession in my intercourse with men [sic], if it be what should not be published abroad, I will never divulge, holding such things to be holy secrets [1].

This obligation is repeated in the World Medical Association's Declaration of Geneva, as 'I will respect the secrets confided in me, even after the patient has died' [2], and in the Medical Board of Australia's *Good medical practice: a code of conduct for doctors in Australia* [3].

From a legal perspective, privacy law outlines the legal requirements for doctors when collecting, using and disclosing a patient's health information. Because privacy law is the framework within which a patient's health information is handled, this chapter focuses primarily on privacy law.

Australia's complex privacy law includes different legislation, not only at federal and state/territory levels but also between the public and private sectors. However, the key principles are common to all legislation. In some states, privacy law is contained within legislation that covers medical record keeping. Thus, this chapter needs to be read with Chapter 27, Medical records, reports and certificates, in mind.

6.1 Confidentiality distinguished from privacy

Although the words *privacy* and *confidentiality* are at times used interchangeably, they are not the same thing, especially when considering privacy in its legal context.

Confidentiality is a legal, ethical and professional obligation to keep patient information secret. The professional obligation of confidentiality, first stated in the Hippocratic Oath, has been one of the cornerstones of ethical medical practice for more than 2000 years. To provide appropriate care to patients, doctors must be able to obtain information that is often highly personal and sensitive, and patients must be able to trust that doctors will keep this information confidential. The duty of confidentiality 'promot[es] candour in disclosure in the doctor–patient relationship' [4].

Information gained in the course of a professional relationship with a patient must not be disclosed to other parties without the patient's consent. Do not assume that patients consent to the release of information to family members or relatives. A patient may release a doctor from their duty of confidentiality by providing consent for the doctor to share information with a third party. The duty of confidentiality is not absolute and is subject to some exceptions, including where permitted or required by law.

Privacy is a fundamental human right that underpins freedom of association, thought and expression. The concept of privacy is difficult to define because it can include the domains of information privacy, bodily privacy, privacy of communications and territorial privacy. In the context of health care, privacy includes the right to control who can see or use information about an individual, and it relates to how an individual's personal health information is handled ('information privacy').

Privacy law relates to the collection, use and disclosure of 'personal information'; that is, information or an opinion that could identify an individual. Health and genetic information is considered to be 'sensitive information' and has a higher level of privacy protection than other personal information. Privacy law also covers patients' access to their records, security of those records and maintenance of accurate and up-to-date records.

The duty of confidentiality exists alongside privacy obligations, and the duty of confidentiality may affect whether to disclose information under the Australian Privacy Principles (APPs).

In its confidentiality and privacy section, the Medical Board of Australia's *Good medical practice: a code of conduct for doctors in Australia* states:

> Patients have a right to expect that doctors and their staff will hold information about them in confidence, unless release of information is required or permitted by law. Good medical practice involves:
>
> 4.4.1 Treating information about patients as confidential.
>
> 4.4.2 Appropriately sharing information about patients for their health care, consistent with privacy laws and professional guidelines about confidentiality.
>
> 4.4.3 Accessing an individual's medical record only when there is a legitimate need.
>
> 4.4.4 Using consent processes, including forms if required, for the release and exchange of health information.
>
> 4.4.5 Being aware that there are complex issues related to genetic information and seeking appropriate advice about its disclosure.
>
> 4.4.6 Ensuring that your use of digital communications (e.g. email and text messages) and social media is consistent with your ethical and legal obligations to protect patient confidentiality and privacy and the Board's social media guidance [3].

6.2 The legal basis of privacy

Box 6.1 Key points about the legal basis of privacy

- Personal information means information or an opinion about an identified individual, or an individual who is reasonably identifiable, whether true or not.
- Doctors must comply with the 13 Australian Privacy Principles, as outlined in the *Privacy Act 1988* (Cth).
- As a basic requirement, doctors should only collect personal information that is necessary for their functions, ideally directly from the individual to whom it relates, and should make individuals aware of who, why and for whom the information is being collected [5].

Doctors working in private practice are required to comply with the Commonwealth *Privacy Act 1988*, which applies to all private-sector health service providers, including private hospitals and facilities.

Most states and territories have equivalent legislation that applies to public-sector agencies, including public hospitals (see Chapter 32, Legal frameworks: rights, responsibilities and protections). Doctors working in New South Wales, Victoria and the Australian Capital Territory must also comply with jurisdictional health privacy legislation.

Doctors need to be aware of and follow the legislation that applies in their practice context and state or territory [6]. The legislation and the websites of the federal, state and territory information commissioners are given in Table 6.1.

At the time of writing, the Commonwealth Privacy Act is under review, and recommendations for reform have been made [7].

The structure of Australian federal and state/territory privacy legislation is broadly similar. It defines the information to which it applies and the organisations on which obligations about that information are imposed, and it uses principles to describe those obligations. The federal legislation applies to 'APP entities', which are defined as agencies or organisations. Agencies are Commonwealth authorities, whereas organisations include individuals, bodies corporate, partnerships, unincorporated associations and trusts. The Privacy Act does not apply to state or territory government entities. Doctors come under the definition of organisations because of their involvement with health information. There are 13 APPs that apply to APP entities.

The legislation applies to 'personal information', which is defined in subsection 6(1) of the Privacy Act as follows:

> ***personal information*** means information or an opinion about an identified individual, or an individual who is reasonably identifiable: (a) whether the information or opinion is true or not; and (b) whether the information or opinion is recorded in a material form or not.

Within the category of personal information is sensitive information, which includes health information. Health information is also defined in the legislation and includes information about a patient obtained by a doctor during the course of providing a health service, an opinion formed by a doctor about a patient, and genetic information. It also includes the patient's name, address and contact details, medical history, Medicare number and social circumstances, as well as the health service requested or provided and any wishes expressed about future provision of health services.

The basic requirements of the Privacy Act are that:

- organisations must only collect personal information that is necessary for their functions, with the patient's consent and only by lawful and fair means
- if reasonable and practicable, organisations should collect personal information from the individual to whom it relates
- at or before collection, organisations must take steps to ensure individuals are aware of who the organisation is, why the information is being collected and to whom the organisation usually discloses it, any laws that require the collection, that there is access to the information and any consequences of not collecting the information.

Privacy law is complex and technical. Doctors should refer to the Office of the Australian Information Commissioner (OAIC) *Guide to health privacy* for health service providers [8] for more information and seek legal advice if unsure about how privacy laws apply in practice.

Table 6.1 Health privacy and information legislation and websites

Government	Legislation	Information commissioner and website
Commonwealth	*Privacy Act 1988*	Office of the Australian Information Commissioner (http://www.oaic.gov.au)
New South Wales	*Health Records and Information Privacy Act 2002*; *Privacy and Personal Information Protection Act 1998*	Information and Privacy Commission NSW (https://www.ipc.nsw.gov.au)
Victoria	*Health Records Act 2001*	Office of the Victorian Information Commissioner (https://ovic.vic.gov.au)
Australian Capital Territory	*Health Records (Privacy and Access) Act 1997*	ACT Human Rights Commission (http://www.hrc.act.gov.au)
Queensland	*Right to Information Act 2009*; *Information Privacy Act 2009*	Office of the Information Commissioner Queensland (https://www.oic.qld.gov.au)
Western Australia	Does not have specific legislation; some privacy principles included in *Freedom of Information Act 1992*	Office of the Information Commissioner (https://www.oic.wa.gov.au)
South Australia	Code of Fair Information Practice 2020	Privacy Committee of South Australia (https://www.archives.sa.gov.au/privacy-committee/privacy-committee-of-south-australia)
Tasmania	*Personal Information Protection Act 2004*	Ombudsman Tasmania (http://www.ombudsman.tas.gov.au)
Northern Territory	*Information Act 2002*	Information Commissioner Northern Territory (https://infocomm.nt.gov.au)

The OAIC provides a helpful summary of the legislation and oversight of privacy in the states and territories [6].

6.3 The Australian Privacy Principles

What follows is a summary of the relevant APPs and a brief outline of how each principle affects good medical practice [9].

6.3.1 APP 1: Open and transparent management of personal information and APP 5: Notification of the collection of personal information

To comply with these principles, medical practices must notify patients of certain matters regarding how they handle health information, at or before the time of collection (unless it is not reasonable or practicable to do so, such as in an emergency).

Practices must also have an APP privacy policy that contains information about how patients can access and correct information held about them, how they can make a complaint and whether information is disclosed overseas. Generic privacy notices are available from various professional associations that can be adapted for use in private practice (e.g. see the Australian Medical Association's sample privacy policy [10]).

6.3.2 APP 2: Anonymity and pseudonymity

This principle provides that, where it is lawful and practicable, people have the option of not identifying themselves when entering transactions with organisations that have their personal information. The principle does not apply if it is not practical to deal with individuals who have not identified themselves or who have used a pseudonym.

The OAIC points out that:

> While it may often be unlawful or impracticable to provide a health service anonymously or pseudonymously, you should still consider whether there are situations in which you can offer anonymous or pseudonymous healthcare in certain situations and ensure patients are aware of this possibility if applicable. For example, your privacy policy could explain the circumstances in which a patient may deal anonymously or by pseudonym with you, and the procedures for doing so [8].

If a patient does wish to be anonymous or use a pseudonym, it is important to point out to patients the difficulty that anonymity or pseudonymity might create for providing adequate medical care and that the patient would be denied access to Medicare, pharmaceutical benefits and private healthcare benefits.

6.3.3 APP 3: Collection of solicited personal information

APP 3 addresses the collection of information. It provides that sensitive information can generally only be collected with consent and when it is reasonably necessary for one of the entity's functions or activities. Collection of health information is permitted to provide a health service and, if collected in accordance with guidelines, for certain research (section 95 of the Privacy Act).

In a usual patient consultation, consent to take a patient's history can be implied as long as it is clear to the patient what information is being recorded and why. This will be outlined generally in the organisation's privacy notice. However, in certain situations—for example, in regard to sexual health, sexually transmissible infections or suspected domestic violence—more attention should be paid to explaining why certain questions need to be asked and to obtaining consent to record information. In healthcare team situations, it may be necessary to inform patients about how other members of the team will have access to information; this will give the patient the opportunity to request that certain information not be recorded (or used or disclosed to other members of the treatment team if it is not necessary).

Health information may be collected without consent [8]:

- where collection is required or authorised by law (e.g. under legislation or an order of a court or tribunal)
- where collection is necessary to lessen or prevent a serious threat to the life, health or safety of an individual or to public health or safety, and it is unreasonable or impracticable (but not merely inconvenient) to obtain consent
- where collection is necessary for research or statistical activities relevant to public health or public safety, or for the management, funding or monitoring of a health service, and certain other criteria are met
- for other specific purposes, such as taking action relating to suspected unlawful activity or serious misconduct, locating a missing person or where reasonably necessary in relation to a legal claim or confidential alternative dispute resolution process.

6.3.4 APP 4: Dealing with unsolicited personal information

Unsolicited information is information that has not been requested but has been received or come across by accident. This may include health information about a patient offered (but not requested from) the patient's relatives, or information sent to the practice in error or in the absence of a request, such as test results that were not ordered by the practice.

A practice that receives unsolicited health information needs to consider within a reasonable time whether it could have been collected under the Privacy Act (as per the requirements outlined above). If the information could not have been collected, it must be destroyed or de-identified as soon as practicable if it is lawful and reasonable to do so. If the information could have been collected without consent, then it must be handled in the same way as solicited personal information.

6.3.5 APP 6: Use or disclosure of personal information

Health information can be used or disclosed for the primary purpose for which it was collected or for a secondary purpose in certain circumstances. The intent behind the use and disclosure requirements is to ensure that health information is only used and disclosed in ways the patient would expect [8].

In routine medical practice, the primary purpose is for the assessment, diagnosis and treatment of the patient. From the perspective of a treating doctor, this purpose includes not only the care delivered by the doctor, but also usual medical practice elements, such as referral to specialists or referral for investigation, as well as sharing information between members of the broader healthcare team.

Making sure that patients know the purpose of collection and routine disclosure practices (e.g. to specialists) is an obligation that arises under APP 3 when collecting health information. However, consulting or showing X-rays to colleagues for advice, accessing previous test results by computer where the tests were requested by a different doctor, or giving all members of a group practice, including locums, access to patients' health information may not appear, to patients, as clearly falling within that primary purpose [11]. Where patients may have this view and have doubts that their privacy is being protected, it will be important to tell patients that such use and disclosure directly relate to their treatment and are practices that they should reasonably expect. This could be included in a privacy notice or privacy policy, but it is always preferable to obtain the patient's express consent to use and disclose highly sensitive and personal information. Examples include information that might lead to stigmatisation, such as HIV or hepatitis infection, or information about sexual preferences.

A secondary purpose is any purpose other than the primary purpose. Information can be used or disclosed for a secondary purpose:

- with the patient's consent
- if the patient would reasonably expect the use and disclosure of information for that purpose, and the purpose is directly related to the secondary purpose (examples of directly related purposes are billing or debt recovery, quality assurance activities, clinical audit activities, incident monitoring, disclosure to an indemnity insurer or lawyer for the purposes of reporting an adverse incident and legal proceedings or for obtaining legal advice)
- where required or authorised by law or a court or tribunal order (examples include disclosure required under a subpoena or summons, or under legislation, such as mandatory reporting of child abuse, mandatory notification of notifiable conduct under the Health Practitioner Regulation National Law, mandatory notification of communicable diseases under public health legislation, reporting deaths to the coroner, and disclosing information to road traffic authorities about a patient's fitness to drive), legislation indemnities usually protect the doctor against the patient taking legal action for disclosure in accordance with a statutory requirement (see Chapter 15, Family violence, child maltreatment and elder abuse; Chapter 18, People with mental illness and the law; and Chapter 32, Legal frameworks: rights, responsibilities and protections, for examples where legal requirements outweigh privacy)
- where use or disclosure is necessary to lessen or prevent a serious threat to the life, health or safety of any individual or to public health or safety, and it is unreasonable or impracticable (but not merely inconvenient) to obtain consent (an example is where a patient is seriously mentally ill and a danger to themselves, and a crisis assessment team or the police need to be notified—see also Chapter 18, People with mental illness and the law)
- where use or disclosure is necessary for research or statistical activities relevant to public health or public safety, or for the management, funding or monitoring of a health service, and certain other criteria are met
- where use or disclosure of a patient's genetic information is necessary to prevent a serious threat to the life, health or safety of a genetic relative, and certain other conditions are met, as outlined in relevant National Health and Medical Research Council (NHMRC) guidelines [8,12]
- where disclosure to a person responsible for a patient is necessary because a patient lacks capacity or is unable to communicate (a treating doctor may disclose information, provided that the doctor is satisfied that the disclosure is necessary to provide appropriate care or treatment to the individual or for compassionate reasons; the doctor must also be satisfied that the disclosure is not contrary to any wish previously expressed by the patient, and disclosure in such situations must be limited to the extent reasonable and necessary for providing health care)
- where required for enforcement-related activities (there must be a reasonable basis for a belief that disclosure is necessary, and disclosure must be justifiable)
- for other purposes, such as taking action relating to suspected unlawful activity or serious misconduct, locating a missing person or where reasonably necessary in relation to a legal claim or confidential alternative dispute resolution process.

Except for disclosure under legislation pursuant to a court order, the exceptions outlined here permit or allow disclosure, but they do not require it. Doctors need to consider the circumstances carefully to ensure that disclosure outweighs the patient's privacy rights.

An example is disclosure of information to the police for enforcement-related activities (in the absence of a warrant). A doctor may become aware from a patient that a serious criminal offence has been committed. Patients may disclose that their condition has arisen as a result of the crime, or patients may disclose that they have committed a crime. There is generally no duty on a doctor to disclose information to the police about the commission of an offence by their patient or where their patient is a victim. If the consent of the patient to disclose such information is not obtainable, doctors must use their own judgement as to what course to take. APP 6 permits but does not require disclosure, so doctors need to consider whether they have a reasonable belief that disclosure is necessary and justifiable. It would be appropriate for doctors to seek advice before disclosing information in these circumstances.

6.3.6 APP 7: Direct marketing

Direct marketing is directly promoting goods or services to an individual using personal information. Patient information can only be used for direct marketing with the patient's express or implied consent.

An example of direct marketing in the healthcare context is a communication that is not targeted to an individual but is sent to everyone listed in a practice's database [13].

6.3.7 APP 8: Cross-border disclosure of personal information

Cross-border disclosure can occur if health information is held on an overseas server or otherwise sent overseas or shared with an overseas recipient or revealed at an international conference or meeting.

If health information is disclosed overseas, the entity must take reasonable steps to ensure that the recipient does not breach the APPs in relation to that information, and the entity will be accountable for any conduct of the recipient that would breach the APPs [9].

6.3.8 APP 9: Adoption, use or disclosure of government-related identifiers

A patient's government-related identifier (e.g. their Medicare number or Individual Healthcare Identifier) can only be used or disclosed in certain circumstances. This includes where it is reasonably necessary to verify the patient's identity [9].

6.3.9 APP 10: Quality of personal information

This APP provides an obligation to take reasonable steps to ensure that health information is accurate, complete and up to date. Good medical practice that keeps accurate records of all attendances and services provided will ensure compliance.

6.3.10 APP 11: Security of personal information

This APP imposes an obligation to take reasonable steps to ensure that health information is protected from unauthorised access, modification or disclosure and from misuse or loss (see Chapter 27, Medical records, reports and certificates, and Chapter 29, Professional practice, digital technology and artificial intelligence).

Healthcare records are increasingly being targeted in cyber attacks, so it is vital that systems and records are protected. Doctors should ensure that procedures are in place to ensure the cybersecurity of their practice systems. Information and advice are available from the Australian Digital Health Agency and the Australian Cyber Security Centre [14,15].

Care should be taken regarding where records are placed, how computer screens are protected and with conversations in the reception and waiting areas, whether in person or by telephone, which may be overheard by others. All staff must be aware of the requirements for computer access and computer security, including strict use of passwords.

Practices using My Health Record (MHR) are required under the *My Health Records Act 2012* (Cth) and regulations to have, communicate and enforce a written security and access policy to use the MHR system [16].

This principle also applies when transferring and sharing health information electronically, via email or text message and when consulting patients via telehealth. Consider using encryption or password protection when sending health information by email [17]. Ideally, use secure messaging when sharing health information between clinicians [18].

If consulting via telehealth, it is important to ensure that the system is secure from other parties and that any recording or photographs arising from the consultation are also securely held [19–21].

The law that applies to recording consultations is complex [22]. It includes state- and territory-based legislation on surveillance devices, which differs depending on the jurisdiction. Doctors need to be aware of and follow the legislation that applies in their practice context and state or territory.

6.3.11 APP 12: Access to personal information

Patients have a right to access the health information held about them, except in certain circumstances [8]. Medical practices should have a policy on handling patient requests for their records. Access requests should be responded to within 30 days.

Access can be provided in several ways, including allowing the patient to read their record (and take notes), talking the patient through their record or providing a copy of the requested information. Access must be provided in the manner the patient requests unless it is unreasonable or impractical.

Patients cannot be charged for lodging a request for access. However, while there is no legal requirement to charge a fee, fees can be charged, for example, to cover staff costs in searching for the information, photocopying and postage costs.

Patients need to be informed of their options (such as photocopying, as opposed to going through the record with the doctor) and informed ahead of time of the costs likely to be incurred. Where a patient opts to see the doctor to go through the record with them, a consultation fee commensurate with an ordinary consultation of that length may be charged. However, the patient may not claim reimbursement from Medicare, and the account must include GST. Legislation in the ACT and Victoria limits the fee that can be charged for giving access to and for transferring health records.

The Privacy Act contains 10 grounds on which access can be refused. These include where:

- giving access would pose a serious threat to anyone's life or would have an unreasonable impact on someone else's privacy (these exceptions are most likely to apply in the context of health care)
- the information relates to an existing or anticipated legal proceeding, and the information is subject to legal professional privilege
- the request is frivolous or vexatious, or giving access would be unlawful
- access might prejudice an investigation of possible unlawful activity or enforcement-related activities.

6.3.12 APP 13: Correction of personal information

Reasonable steps should be taken to ensure that information held is correct and to correct any information when requested to do so by a patient [8].

6.4 Notifying data breaches

A data breach occurs when there is unauthorised access to or disclosure or loss of personal information held by the practice. This could be an email sent to the wrong person, a lost laptop containing patient information or the practice database being subjected to a cyber attack.

Organisations covered by the Privacy Act are required to notify individuals who are likely to be at risk of serious harm because of a data breach and to notify the OAIC, unless remedial action can be taken to prevent the likelihood of harm [23,24].

Practices using MHR have separate obligations under the My Health Records Act to notify the Australian Digital Health Agency of:

- actual or suspected unauthorised collection, use or disclosure of health information in an individual's MHR
- events or circumstances that have compromised or have the potential to compromise the security or integrity of the MHR system.

6.5 Enforcement and regulatory action

The OAIC has a range of enforcement and regulatory powers. It can investigate a matter in response to a privacy complaint or on its own initiative. Following an investigation, the Commissioner may decide to take enforcement action against an entity. Enforcement powers escalate from less serious to more serious options; the latter include applying to the court for a civil penalty order in the case of serious or repeated interference with privacy [25].

Maximum penalties for serious or repeated interference with privacy under the Privacy Act are $2.5 million for an individual and, for a body corporate, the greater of $50 million or three times the value of the benefit obtained by the corporation that is attributable to the conduct.

Breaches of the privacy provisions of the My Health Records Act are criminal offences punishable by a penalty or imprisonment.

6.6 Specific situations

6.6.1 Differences between the federal and state/territory privacy laws

In Victoria, the *Health Records Act 2001* has additional health privacy principles covering transfer of records, closing of a practice and making information available to another doctor. The Health Records Act extends privacy protection to health information of deceased individuals for 30 years after their death. In Victoria, requests for access are to be in writing, and time limits apply. Where access is denied on the grounds of risk to the patient, arrangements are to be made to provide the information via another doctor.

In NSW, privacy in health matters in both the public and private sectors is covered by the *Health Records and Information Privacy Act 2002*, which became applicable in September 2004. In the ACT, both the *Health Records (Privacy and Access) Act 1997* and the federal Privacy Act apply.

In Queensland, the *Information Privacy Act 2009* applies to the collection, use and disclosure of personal information by government entities. In Tasmania, the *Personal Information Protection Act 2004* applies to the collection, use and disclosure of personal information in the public sector. South Australia and Western Australia do not have state legislation on privacy, but they have standards or codes that apply to public-sector entities and are consistent with the federal legislation.

Doctors need to be aware of and follow the legislation that applies in their practice context and the jurisdiction(s) in which they work [6].

6.6.2 Medicolegal and specialist reports

A medicolegal report is health information about the patient and is generally accessible by the patient under privacy law. However, when a report is an expert report or opinion that has been commissioned from a doctor who is not the treating doctor by a third party, such as a solicitor in legal proceedings, and the report is subject to legal privilege, then access can be denied under the Privacy Act. Always seek advice from the instructing solicitor before responding to a request for records relating to a medicolegal report (see also Chapter 27, Medical records, reports and certificates, and Chapter 26, Medicolegal examinations and reports, court procedures and expert evidence).

Specialists' reports to the referring doctor sometimes contain a proviso about non-release to third parties. Specialist reports are part of the medical record and are 'health information' under privacy legislation. Specialists' letters should be handled in the same way as any other health information, and access to the letter cannot be denied on the basis of any proviso to this effect.

6.6.3 Other reports and certificates

Doctors may be asked to provide reports, records or certificates to third parties, such as employers, insurance companies or solicitors, about their patient's medical conditions. A doctor should only provide records or information if the patient has consented to that information being disclosed.

Such a request should be accompanied by a valid consent from the patient, authorising release of the information. Authorities should be current, signed by the patient and specific enough for the doctor to comply. Only disclose information that the patient has consented to be disclosed, tailoring to their particular circumstance and the purpose of the report or certificate [26].

Providing medical certificates for employers about patients who are employees can create challenges, particularly if the employer asks for more information than the patient is prepared to provide. Ultimately, it is up to the patient to decide how much information they wish the doctor to disclose on the certificate. If a patient requests that the diagnosis not be included, the term 'on medical grounds' or a similar phrase should be used. A general medical certificate should not include the patient's diagnosis, to protect the patient's privacy.

If an employer asks a doctor to confirm details provided in a certificate, a doctor can do so but should not elaborate further without the patient's express consent [27].

Doctors are often asked for reports relating to their patients' workers compensation claims. When a patient who has a work-related illness or injury is seeking compensation or salary maintenance, or is being encouraged to enter a work-based rehabilitation program, it is appropriate, with the patient's consent, to release sufficient information to assist the patient in their claim.

More detail is given in Chapter 26, Medicolegal examinations and reports, court procedures and expert evidence, and Chapter 27, Medical records, reports and certificates.

6.6.4 Disclosure for research

Health information can be used or disclosed for research where the patient has consented or where personal information is necessary (i.e. the research question cannot be answered using de-identified information) and seeking consent is impracticable, in accordance with guidelines issued by the NHMRC and approved by the OAIC (see Chapter 31, Medical research).

6.6.5 Deceased patients

Commonwealth privacy legislation does not cover health information about a deceased patient, so the law relating to the duty of confidentiality applies.

The duty of confidentiality continues after a patient dies. Thus, the right to release a doctor from this duty passes to the legal representative of the deceased, who is usually the executor appointed in the deceased's will or the administrator of the estate of the deceased where there is no will.

In NSW, Victoria and the ACT, health privacy laws continue to protect health information after the patient dies (for 30 years, in NSW and Victoria), and requests for access by others, such as relatives, must be dealt with in accordance with the legislation.

6.6.6 Digital images and messaging apps

Digital images are now often taken in medical practice for legitimate clinical and teaching purposes (e.g. for local referrals or specialist opinion at a distance, such as teledermatology and rural outreach services). Any images taken and stored should be handled as securely as any medical record, as the images are health information and thus a component of the patient's record and covered by privacy legislation [28–31].

It is always preferable to obtain express patient consent to take and use images. Applying the privacy principles, images can only be used for the purpose for which they have been collected, so it is important to explain to a patient why the image is being taken and how it is intended to be used. Specific and express consent should be obtained for non-treatment purposes, such as in education or research, even if identifying information is removed. Digital images for treatment purposes should always be stored in the clinical record.

Using messaging apps, such as WhatsApp, Signal and Messenger, is increasingly common in day-to-day clinical practice. These apps provide a convenient method of coordinating medical teams, integrating text-based communication and enabling quick transfer of images and data. However, they present a multitude of privacy concerns that must be carefully managed. The more convenient and widely used apps tend to have poor or absent encryption for messages, so care should be taken to ensure the app of choice has good security. The apps may also require local storage of messages and images on personal devices, which will need to be regularly reviewed and secured. Information may be uploaded to a server overseas. Finally, the use of group messaging, online pseudonyms or sharing app usage between personal and professional roles runs the risk of inadvertent transmission of private information to unintended recipients. Care should be taken to independently verify the recipients of messages before sharing private information.

Use of digital technology in health care is also explored in Chapter 29, Professional practice, digital technology and artificial intelligence.

6.6.7 Disclosure in court

In common law, there is no privilege that entitles doctors to refuse to answer questions on the grounds of keeping a professional confidence. Courts may compel a doctor to divulge such information in answer to questions, and doctors cannot claim privilege any more than the ordinary citizen. Where information is sought by subpoena, especially the production of documents (such as medical records), the scope of subpoenas must be confined to information relevant to the issues in the court proceedings. Responses to subpoenas are to the court, not to the parties in the proceedings. Submissions can be made to the court that only medical information relevant to the issues be disclosed, thereby protecting other material in a patient's record from disclosure.

Always seek legal advice if there is any doubt about the documents to be provided in answer to a subpoena and if the scope of a subpoena is to be challenged. Failure to comply with a valid subpoena is a contempt of court.

In some jurisdictions, such as NSW, Victoria, Tasmania and the Northern Territory, there are statutory privileges in the relevant evidence legislation that would prevent disclosure of patient information in court. These privileges generally rest with the patient, not the doctor, and are rarely relied upon.

Doctors who fail to attend court to give evidence when properly served with a subpoena, or who, when called as a witness in court, decline to answer questions on the grounds of protecting confidentiality, may be charged with contempt of court.

Summary

Doctors have a legal, ethical and professional duty to keep their patients' information confidential. Doctors are also required to comply with privacy law when handling their patients' health information.

Privacy law is complex and technical, and different legislation applies in different practice contexts and jurisdictions. Doctors need to be aware of and comply with the law and policies that apply in their particular practice context.

The OAIC has detailed privacy guidance for health service providers but, if in doubt, doctors should always seek legal advice.

References

1. Hippocrates; Jones WHS, translator. Hippocrates, Vol.1. Cambridge: Harvard University Press, 1968.
2. World Medical Association. WMA Declaration of Geneva. 2018. https://www.wma.net/policies-post/wma-declaration-of-geneva/ (accessed Oct 2024).
3. Medical Board of Australia. Good medical practice: a code of conduct for doctors in Australia. 2020. https://www.medicalboard.gov.au/Codes-Guidelines-Policies/Code-of-conduct.aspx (accessed Oct 2024).
4. White B, McDonald F, Willmott L, Then S-N. Health law in Australia. 4th ed. Lawbook Co, 2023.
5. Office of the Australian Information Commissioner. What is privacy? https://www.oaic.gov.au/privacy/your-privacy-rights/what-is-privacy (accessed Oct 2024).
6. Office of the Australian Information Commissioner. State and territory privacy legislation. 2024. https://www.oaic.gov.au/privacy/privacy-legislation/state-and-territory-privacy-legislation (accessed May 2025).
7. Attorney-General's Department. Privacy Act review report. https://www.ag.gov.au/integrity/consultations/review-privacy-act-1988 (accessed Oct 2024).
8. Office of the Australian Information Commissioner. Guide to health privacy. https://www.oaic.gov.au/privacy/privacy-guidance-for-organisations-and-government-agencies/health-service-providers/guide-to-health-privacy (accessed Oct 2024).
9. Office of the Australian Information Commissioner. Australian Privacy Principles guidelines. https://www.oaic.gov.au/privacy/australian-privacy-principles/australian-privacy-principles-guidelines (accessed Oct 2024).
10. Australian Medical Association. AMA sample privacy policy. https://ama.com.au/sites/default/files/documents/AMA_Sample_Privacy_Policy_Final.docx (accessed Oct 2024).
11. Braunack-Mayer AJ, Mulligan EC. Sharing patient information between professionals: confidentiality and ethics. *Med J Aust* 2003; 178: 277–279.
12. National Health and Medical Research Council. Use and disclosure of genetic information to a patient's genetic relatives under Section 95AA of the Privacy Act 1988 (Cth): Guidelines for health practitioners in the private sector. https://www.nhmrc.gov.au/about-us/publications/guidelines-approved-under-section-95aa-privacy-act-1988-cth (accessed Oct 2024).
13. Office of the Australian Information Commissioner. Communications with patients. 2017. https://www.oaic.gov.au/privacy/privacy-for-health-service-providers/communications-with-patients (accessed Oct 2024).
14. Australian Digital Health Agency. Cyber security for healthcare providers. 2024. https://www.digitalhealth.gov.au/healthcare-providers/cyber-security-for-healthcare-providers (accessed Oct 2024).
15. Australian Signals Directorate. Australian Cyber Security Centre [website]. https://www.cyber.gov.au (accessed Oct 2024).
16. Office of the Australian Information Commissioner. My Health Record: security and access policies – Rule 42 guidance. 2022. https://www.oaic.gov.au/privacy/guidance-and-advice/my-health-record/security-and-access-policies-rule-42-guidance (accessed Oct 2024).
17. Avant. Email communication with patients: privacy and patient safety. 2024. https://www.avant.org.au/Resources/Public/Email-communication-with-patients-privacy-and-patient-safety/ (accessed Oct 2024).
18. Australian Digital Health Agency. Secure messaging. https://www.digitalhealth.gov.au/healthcare-providers/initiatives-and-programs/secure-messaging (accessed Oct 2024).
19. Australian Digital Health Agency. Using online conferencing technologies securely. 2021. https://www.digitalhealth.gov.au/sites/default/files/2020-11/Online_conferencing_technologies-Connected_secure_consultations.pdf (accessed Oct 2024).
20. Australian Government Department of Health and Aged Care. MBS Online: Privacy checklist for telehealth services. https://www.mbsonline.gov.au/internet/mbsonline/publishing.nsf/Content/Factsheet-TelehealthPrivChecklist (accessed Oct 2024).
21. Burns K, Belton S. Clinicians and their cameras: policy, ethics and practice in an Australian tertiary hospital. *Aust Health Rev* 2013; 37: 437–441.
22. Prictor M, Johnston C, Hyatt A. Overt and covert recordings of health care consultations in Australia: some legal considerations. *Med J Aust* 2021; 214: 119–123.e1.

23. Office of the Australian Information Commissioner. Notifiable data breaches. https://www.oaic.gov.au/privacy/notifiable-data-breaches (accessed Oct 2024).
24. Avant. Responding to a data breach flow chart. https://avant.org.au/resources/responding-to-data-breach (accessed Oct 2024).
25. Office of the Australian Information Commissioner. Guide to privacy regulatory action: Chapter 7: Civil penalties — serious or repeated interference with privacy and other penalty provisions. https://www.oaic.gov.au/about-us/our-regulatory-approach/guide-to-privacy-regulatory-action/chapter-7-civil-penalties (accessed Oct 2024).
26. Avant. Providing medical records to a third party. 2021. https://www.avant.org.au/Resources/Public/providing-medical-records-to-a-third-party/ (accessed Oct 2024).
27. Avant. Medical certificates and your responsibilities. 2019. https://www.avant.org.au/Resources/Public/Medical-certificates-and-your-responsibilities/ (accessed Oct 2024).
28. Office of the Australian Information Commissioner. Taking photos of patients. https://www.oaic.gov.au/privacy/privacy-guidance-for-organisations-and-government-agencies/health-service-providers/taking-photos-of-patients (accessed Oct 2024).
29. Australian Medical Association. Clinical images and the use of personal mobile devices. 2014. https://www.ama.com.au/articles/clinical-images-and-use-personal-mobile-devices (accessed Oct 2024).
30. MacDonald J, Sohn S, Ellis P. Privacy, professionalism and Facebook: a dilemma for young doctors. *Med Educ* 2010; 44: 744–745.
31. Moubarak G, Guiot A, Benhamou Y, et al. Facebook activity of residents and fellows and its impact on the doctor–patient relationship. *J Med Ethics* 2011; 37: 101–104.

Further reading

Australian Digital Health Agency. Information security guide for small healthcare businesses. https://www.digitalhealth.gov.au/sites/default/files/2020-11/Information_security_guide_for_small_healthcare_businesses.pdf

Medical Board of Australia. Guidelines: Telehealth consultations with patients. 2023. https://www.medicalboard.gov.au/Codes-Guidelines-Policies/Telehealth-consultations-with-patients.aspx

Office of the Australian Information Commissioner. Guide to health privacy. https://www.oaic.gov.au/privacy/privacy-guidance-for-organisations-and-government-agencies/health-service-providers/guide-to-health-privacy).

07 Consent and informed decision making

Georgie Haysom

Introduction

Doctors have a legal, ethical and professional obligation to adequately inform patients about proposed examinations, treatments or procedures and to obtain their consent for these. Obtaining consent is more than obtaining a signature on a consent form. The informed consent process involves a discussion with a patient about the risks, benefits and alternatives to a proposed course of action. After this discussion, a patient can decline to provide consent if they do not wish to proceed. The key to an effective informed decision-making process is communication. It involves the doctor and patient coming to a shared understanding about the patient's condition, treatment options and recommendations, taking a patient-centred, shared decision-making approach.

This section does not cover consent for the collection, use and disclosure of a patient's health information under privacy legislation (see Chapter 6, Confidentiality, privacy and disclosure).

7.1 The ethical, legal and professional requirements for consent

7.1.1 Ethical requirement

From an ethical perspective, the requirement to obtain informed consent stems from the Western philosophical principle of autonomy—the right of a person to decide what they wish to do with their own body (ethical principles are discussed in more detail in Chapter 3, Ethical principles for the medical profession). This includes decisions about diagnostic and screening tests, examinations, medications, other treatments and procedures. It also includes the right of a person to make decisions about providing their health information to others.

7.1.2 Legal requirement

The legal requirement for consent stems from two areas of law:

1. The law of trespass to the person: interfering with a person's body integrity without consent is battery or assault [1,2].

   Consent 'has the effect of transforming what would otherwise be unlawful into accepted and therefore acceptable contact' [1]. The consent necessary 'to negate the offence of battery is satisfied by the patient being advised in broad terms of the nature of the procedure to be performed' [3].

2. The law of negligence: it is a breach of a doctor's duty of care to fail to inform a patient of the material risks associated with a treatment or intervention.

   Medical practitioners have a duty to exercise reasonable care and skill in the provision of professional advice and treatment of patients. The duty extends to examination, diagnosis and treatment of the patient and to the provision of information [3].

The doctor's duty to provide advice and information to a patient was articulated by the High Court in *Rogers v Whitaker* as:

> a duty to warn a patient of a material risk inherent in the proposed treatment; a risk is material if, in the circumstances of the particular case, a reasonable person in the patient's position, if warned of the risk, would be likely to attach significance to it or if the medical practitioner is or should reasonably be aware that the particular patient, if warned of the risk, would be likely to attach significance to it [3].

In Queensland and Tasmania, this has been enacted in legislation (*Civil Liability Act 2003* [Qld], section 21, and *Civil Liability Act 2002* [Tas], section 21).

A breach of a doctor's duty of care leaves the doctor open to a claim of negligence.

South Australia and Victoria have legislation that deals with consent for medical treatment generally (*Consent to Medical Treatment and Palliative Care Act 1995* [SA] and *Medical Treatment Planning and Decisions Act 2016* [Vic]). Most states and territories also have legislation dealing with specific issues, such as organ donation and transplantation, substitute decision making and consent for special medical procedures.

It is important for doctors to know and follow the law that applies in the state or territory in which they practise.

7.1.3 Professional requirement

The professional requirement for consent is outlined in the Medical Board of Australia's *Good medical practice: a code of conduct for doctors in Australia* (the code of conduct):

> Informed consent is a person's voluntary decision about medical care that is made with knowledge and understanding of the benefits and risks involved. Good medical practice involves:
>
> 4.5.1 Providing information to patients in a way they can understand before asking for their consent.
>
> 4.5.2 Obtaining informed consent from the patient or where the patient does not have the capacity, from their substitute decision-maker and taking into account any advance care directive (or similar) before you undertake any examination, investigation or provide treatment (except in an emergency), or before involving patients in teaching or research.
>
> 4.5.3 Ensuring that your patients are informed about your fees and charges in a timely manner to enable them to make an informed decision about whether they want to proceed with consultations and treatment.
>
> 4.5.4 When referring a patient for investigation, treatment or a procedure, advising the patient that there may be additional costs, which patients may wish to clarify before proceeding [4].

Failure to comply with the code of conduct leaves a doctor open to regulatory action by the Medical Board (or Medical Council in New South Wales).

Consent is not required for treatment in an emergency, subject to any applicable, valid advance care directive and where there is no available substitute decision maker [5]. Treatment is required in an emergency if it is required to save a person's life or prevent serious injury to the patient's health (see section 7.4.1).

The law recognises the notion of therapeutic privilege as a basis for withholding information from the patient if, in the doctor's opinion, disclosure may harm the patient. This approach was once widely followed but is now regarded as paternalistic and contrary to the principle of respect for patient autonomy. It is rarely used in contemporary clinical practice.

A patient with decision-making capacity can refuse to consent to a treatment, examination or procedure [5] and, if given, can withdraw their consent at any time.

More information about refusal of treatment is covered in Chapter 18, People with mental illness and the law (for people with mental illness), and in Chapter 15, Family violence, child maltreatment and elder abuse, and Chapter 26, Medicolegal examinations and reports, court procedures and expert evidence (when legal requirements can override a patient's wishes).

7.2 Elements of the informed decision-making process

There are several elements relevant to the decision-making process:

- capacity
- voluntariness
- disclosure and discussion
- documentation and form of consent.

7.2.1 Capacity

A patient must have capacity to provide valid consent. At law, a person over the age of 18 years is presumed to have decision-making capacity [5]. This applies in all Australian states and territories except SA, where legislation states that a person is presumed to have medical decision-making capacity once they turn 16 years of age.

As capacity is presumed at law for adults, a doctor is not required to undertake a capacity assessment unless the circumstances or the patient's behaviour suggest that they are unable to make the required decision. Whether a patient has healthcare decision-making capacity is a matter for a doctor's clinical judgement. When required, the treating doctor should conduct a capacity assessment or refer the patient to an appropriate specialist.

The legal test for capacity varies slightly between jurisdictions in Australia. In general, to have capacity, a person must be able to:

- understand the information and consequences relevant to the decision
- retain the information and recall the details for long enough to be able to make the decision
- use and evaluate the information throughout the decision-making process
- communicate their decision and understanding verbally or by other means.

There are differences between the legal test for capacity to make healthcare decisions and the legal test for capacity to make other decisions, such as making a will (testamentary capacity) [6].

Capacity:

- is decision-specific; for example, the capacity required to consent to having a vaccination will be different from the capacity required to consent to a complex surgical procedure
- may fluctuate; a person's capacity may be affected by their medical condition or medication, and a patient may lose capacity temporarily.

The fact that a patient may make a decision that is not, in the view of medical practitioners, in their best interest does not mean that the patient lacks capacity. People with capacity can make decisions that might appear irrational or unwise to others. It is important to assess the patient's decision-making ability, not their decision.

Similarly, a diagnosis of a mental illness does not necessarily mean a patient lacks decision-making capacity.

Table 7.1 outlines an approach to assessing capacity [7].

Table 7.1 An approach to assessing decision-making capacity

Capacity	Questions for clinical assessment
Communicating a choice	• Have you decided whether to follow my advice about treatment? • Can you tell me what your decision is?
Understanding relevant information	• Can you please tell me, in your own words, what I have told you about your health problem; the recommended treatment; the benefits, risks or discomfort of the proposed treatment; any other options; and the risks and benefits of no treatment?
Appreciating the situation and its consequences	• Can you please tell me what you believe is wrong with your health now, whether you believe you need treatment, what the treatment will do for you, and what you think will happen if you have no treatment?
Reasoning about treatment options	• How did you decide to accept or reject the recommended treatment? • What makes this choice better than another option?

Source: Adapted from Grisso T, Applebaum PS. Assessing competence to consent to treatment: a guide for physicians and other health professionals. New York: Oxford University Press, 1998.

There is increasing recognition of the notion of supported decision making, including the role of a supporter in assisting people with disabilities to exercise their autonomy in decision making to the greatest extent possible [8].

If a patient does not have capacity to make a medical decision (including with support), the intervention or treatment is not required for an emergency and the patient does not have an advance care directive, consent should be obtained from the appropriate substitute decision maker (see section 7.3.3).

7.2.2 Voluntariness

A patient's consent must be freely and voluntarily given. It must not be given under duress or undue influence. Undue influence can occur when a third party pressures a patient to consent to or refuse treatment. This can happen, for example, when the patient is in a vulnerable position, such as being elderly and frail or in great pain, so that the patient's will is overborne, and they do not decide for themselves [9]. If a patient feels rushed into agreeing to a procedure, they may also feel they did not consent freely.

7.2.3 Disclosure and discussion

The informed decision-making process involves a doctor having a discussion with a patient about their condition and providing the patient with enough information to allow them to make an informed decision.

Informed decision making is not only relevant to major procedures. It extends to all elements of care, including:

- taking a history, particularly when there is a clinical need to ask sexual or personal questions, and the link between such questions and the patient's reason for attending may not be immediately obvious to the patient
- physical examinations, particularly for any intimate or invasive examination and especially when the patient is young, inexperienced as a patient or there is any reason to anticipate communication difficulties, such as undue anxiety, cultural differences or language barriers
- investigations, particularly where the results could be significant or sensitive, such as HIV testing, genetic screening or cancer screening tests
- procedures, including minor procedures such as certain injections and vaccinations that carry a real risk of serious (although rare) complications
- prescribing medications, especially when prescribing a medication for the first time and where the medication has known serious or predictable side effects
- diagnostic procedures, such as invasive radiology, endoscopy and organ biopsy
- participation in medical research or innovative or experimental treatment
- billing, costs and whether the patient will have any out-of-pocket expenses, including those expected from other specialists (see section 7.5)
- collection and release of patient information (see also Chapter 6, Confidentiality, privacy and disclosure).

The legal test from *Rogers v Whitaker* outlined in section 7.1.2 indicates that the disclosure of information to a patient about a treatment or procedure should be patient-centred [3]. This involves exploring with the patient what is important to them, allowing them to ask questions and coming to a shared view about the proposed intervention or approach.

The key elements that should be disclosed to and discussed with the patient, taking a patient-centred approach, are:

- information about the patient's condition—the possible or likely nature of their illness or condition, including the degree of uncertainty in any diagnosis
- the proposed approach to investigation, diagnosis and treatment, including what these involve and whether they are conventional, experimental or innovative
- who is going to perform the procedure or intervention—if a training doctor is going to perform part of the procedure with the consultant, or under the consultant's supervision, the patient should be advised of this

- timeframes for performing the procedure and possible waiting times if the procedure or treatment is to be performed as a public patient in a public hospital
- the expected benefits—the expected outcome, benefits or improvements, including the degree of uncertainty (if any) about the therapeutic outcome
- known and material risks—the risks the particular patient or a reasonable person in the patient's position would like to know; this involves exploring what is important to the patient and what outcomes they are prepared to live with and should include discussion of the possibility that their condition may not improve, may stay the same or could get worse
- side effects, including common side effects and complications and uncommon side effects of importance to the patient, as well as any potential significant long-term adverse outcomes and expected recovery time if there is a complication
- alternatives to the proposed approach, including the advantages, disadvantages and potential consequences of the available options, surgical versus non-surgical treatment, and the consequences of not choosing or delaying the recommended approach
- costs, including the costs of the procedure and whether there are likely to be any out-of-pocket expenses (see section 7.5)
- follow-up arrangements and recovery time, including where to go and who to contact if the patient experiences any side effects or complications.

Ideally, the doctor undertaking the examination or procedure, recommending the treatment or prescribing the medication should have the informed decision-making discussion with the patient. The discussion can be delegated to, for example, an appropriately trained staff member or, in the hospital context, a more junior doctor. If a doctor wishes to delegate this discussion, they should be confident that their delegate has sufficient knowledge and skill to undertake this process with the patient. If a junior doctor is asked to undertake the discussion, they should feel confident that they have the required background knowledge to describe the procedure fully and answer any questions about it. Junior doctors should not be pressured into having such discussions with patients if they do not have this confidence.

The discussion should also cover who is going to perform the procedure and their level of experience with it. This should cover whether a training doctor will perform some or all of the procedure.

A patient is entitled to decline to consent to a procedure or to prefer an approach that is different from the one that has been recommended.

Box 7.1 Practical tips for informed decision-making discussions

- Avoid using technical words and jargon.
- Use written material, information sheets, diagrams and models to aid patient understanding.
- Ask the patient what is important to them and target the discussion to those aspects.
- Listen to the patient's concerns and give them time to consider the information and to ask questions. A second consultation or a second opinion may be required.
- Test the patient's understanding by asking them to explain in their own words what has been discussed and recommended.

Continued over page

- Where there are language barriers, use an accredited interpreter, not a family member, to facilitate discussion.
- Be alert to any indications that the patient is experiencing pressure to agree to a proposed procedure or being subjected to undue influence; if this is suspected, have a private discussion with the patient.
- Communicate with patients in a culturally safe manner.

7.2.4 Documentation and form of consent

Consent may be given verbally or in writing, or it may be implied.

Consent is implied when the patient indicates by their action that they are willing to undergo a course of action. An example is a patient putting out their arm for blood to be taken or for a blood pressure measurement to be made. Care should be taken in interpreting actions as implied consent (e.g. for consent to an intimate examination), as some patients do not feel empowered to object or to ask questions. It is always advisable to specifically ask for consent in these situations.

Written consent is required under some legislation for certain interventions, such as:

- organ donation and transplantation or removal of gametes after death
- certain mental health treatments
- assisted reproductive treatment.

Hospital or practice policy can also require written consent for certain interventions. Doctors should always follow their hospital or practice policy and obtain written consent when required.

If there is no legislative, hospital or practice requirement to obtain written consent, a good rule of thumb is that the more serious, complex or sensitive the proposed course of action is, the more advisable it is to obtain written consent.

A signed written consent form is evidence that a patient signed the consent form. It is not evidence that an informed decision-making discussion took place or that the patient understood what was discussed with them.

Whether consent is implied or obtained verbally or in writing, it is important in all cases to document the discussion in the patient's medical records. Be as specific as possible and include in the patient's medical record:

- your own notes
- consent forms
- a copy of any written material you have provided
- diagrams or illustrations you have drawn
- correspondence to other practitioners (e.g. referring doctors); consider also sending this correspondence to the patient.

7.3 Specific situations

7.3.1 Consent of children and young people

Unlike adults, capacity is not presumed for young people under the age of 18 years (16 years in SA). However, children and young people under the age of 18 years may have capacity to make healthcare decisions.

There is no age threshold for a child or young person's decision-making capacity, despite the common misconception that there is. This misconception is based on a misunderstanding of the effect of the Medicare rules and of section 49 of the *Minors (Property and Contracts) Act 1970* (NSW). This section provides doctors with a defence to a claim for battery for proceeding with treatment on the basis of consent of a minor over 14 years of age, and protection from liability for assault when a doctor treats a minor under 16 years of age with the consent of a parent or guardian. The provision says nothing about the capacity of a child or young person to consent. Doctors are permitted to bulk-bill Medicare for consultations with patients over the age of 14 years without advising the child's parent.

A child or young person will have capacity to consent where they are 'Gillick competent' or a 'mature minor'. Under the legal principle of Gillick competence (otherwise known as the 'mature minor doctrine'), a child or young person has the capacity to make a specific healthcare decision when they have achieved 'a sufficient understanding and intelligence to enable him or her to understand fully what is proposed' [10]. This principle was adopted in Australia in *Marion's Case* [1].

In SA, doctors can administer medical treatment to a child aged under 16 years if they are of the opinion that the child is capable of understanding the nature, consequences and risks of the treatment; that the treatment is in the best interest of the child's health and wellbeing; and that a second doctor has assessed the child and has concurred in writing (*Consent to Medical Treatment and Palliative Care Act 1995* [SA]).

Whether a child or young person has capacity is a matter for a doctor's clinical judgement.

If a child or young person has capacity to make a healthcare decision, the child or young person's consent is sufficient, and parental consent is not required. If a child or young person has decision-making capacity, it is not permissible to contact their parents to discuss their treatment without the child or young person's permission. In many situations, doctors should encourage children and young people to seek the advice and support of a trusted adult when making healthcare decisions.

If there is a dispute between a child or young person with capacity and their parents, the wishes of the child or young person will prevail.

If a child or young person does *not* have decision-making capacity, the consent of a parent or guardian is required. Parents can generally consent to medical procedures for their children, provided that the proposed procedure is in the child's best interests.

Generally, each parent will have parental responsibility for a child's healthcare decisions, and the consent of either parent is sufficient. The exception is where there is a court order giving parental responsibility to only one parent, or an order giving shared responsibility to both parents. In these cases, doctors should refer to the court order for guidance on who is able to provide consent for the child's healthcare decisions.

If there is a dispute between parents and children, between parents, or between parents and the treatment team about whether a treatment is in the child's best interests, it may be helpful to obtain advice from the institution's clinical ethics service or, as a last resort, approach the court to resolve the dispute. Legal advice should always be obtained before proceeding with an application to the court.

Where a child without decision-making capacity is temporarily in the care of a teacher, babysitter, relative, sports coach or the like, care should be taken to obtain consent from a parent for medical treatment, other than for first aid or in an emergency.

Emergency treatment of children is dealt with in section 7.4.1.

7.3.2 Gender-affirming treatment of children and young people

There have been significant changes in the law during the past decade regarding whether and when consent of the court is required for gender-affirming treatment of children, as well as the consent of parents and the child or young person. The courts have considered:

- whether the child or young person is Gillick competent to consent to treatment, given the irreversible nature of the treatment
- whether the treatment is in the child or young person's best interests
- what to do when there is a dispute or lack of consensus between the child or young person, the parents and the clinicians.

It is important to refer to the current *Australian standards of care and treatment guidelines for trans and gender diverse children and adolescents* [11] and the latest court decisions when considering gender-affirming treatment for children or young people. Legal advice should always be obtained before proceeding with an application to the court or if in any doubt about the legal requirements for consent to gender-affirming treatment.

7.3.3 Substitute decision making

If a patient does not have capacity to make a healthcare decision (with or without support) and there is no advance care directive applying to the situation (see Chapter 19, Advance care planning and end-of-life care), doctors must obtain consent from a substitute decision maker. The exception to this is if emergency treatment is required (see section 7.4.1).

The person identified as the person's 'next of kin' is not necessarily the legally correct substitute decision maker [5]. The law outlining who is the correct substitute decision maker and the terminology used is different in each jurisdiction. In general (with the exception of the Northern Territory, noting that new laws are coming into effect from 2025), there is a legislative hierarchy for identifying the patient's default substitute decision maker. This hierarchy includes a guardian appointed by a court or tribunal, a guardian or attorney appointed by the patient, a spouse, sibling or other relative, or a carer, in various orders of priority. It is important for doctors to know and follow the law that applies in the state or territory in which they practise [12].

When communicating with substitute decision makers, doctors should discuss the information outlined in section 7.2.3.

If a doctor is concerned that the substitute decision maker is not making decisions that are in the best interests of the patient, they can approach the relevant guardianship tribunal for an order that an alternative substitute decision maker be appointed.

If there is a dispute between the substitute decision maker and clinicians about a treatment decision, it may be helpful to obtain advice from the institution's clinical ethics service or, as a last resort, approach the court or tribunal to resolve the dispute. Legal advice must always be obtained before proceeding with an application to the court.

7.3.4 Special medical procedures where patients lack capacity

In most jurisdictions, there are legislative provisions covering consent for sterilisation, termination of pregnancy and other procedures termed 'special' or 'prescribed' medical treatment, where a person lacks decision-making capacity for these procedures. The focus is generally on procedures that lead to infertility but may include other medical or surgical treatments and clinical research. Only a court or tribunal can provide consent for these procedures where the patient lacks capacity.

An example is the NSW legislation, which includes sterilisation, termination of pregnancy (see also Chapter 14, Termination of pregnancy and related issues), treatment using an aversive stimulus and new treatments not yet supported by a substantial number of doctors. These procedures can only be authorised by the NSW Civil and Administrative Tribunal [13].

There are differences in the definitions and requirements in each jurisdiction, so it is important for doctors to know and follow the law that applies in the state or territory in which they practise. Gender-affirming treatment of children is dealt with in section 7.3.2.

7.4 Treatment without consent

7.4.1 Emergencies when the patient is unable to consent

In general, treatment can be provided without consent in an emergency, if immediate treatment is necessary to save the patient's life or prevent serious damage to their health, where there is no advance care directive indicating that the patient does not consent to the treatment and no substitute decision maker is immediately available to provide consent.

There is legislation in all Australian jurisdictions, except the Australian Capital Territory, that deals specifically with treatment in an emergency. There are differences in the legislation in each jurisdiction, so it is important for doctors to know and follow the law that applies in the state or territory in which they practise. For example, the legislation in SA and the NT requires the supportive opinion of a second medical practitioner. In the ACT, the same principles apply, based on the common law rather than specific legislation.

The general principle also applies to treatment of children in an emergency. In NSW, there is specific legislation relating to the treatment of children and young people in an emergency. In addition, legislation in Victoria, Queensland, Western Australia, Tasmania and the ACT permits blood transfusions to be given to children in a life-threatening emergency without the consent of their parents.

7.4.2 Other treatment without consent

In NSW and Queensland, minor treatment can be carried out on a patient without capacity to consent if necessary to promote the patient's health and wellbeing, where there is no substitute decision maker and the patient does not object. This must be certified in writing in the patient's medical record. In Tasmania, any treatment (other than special treatment) can be carried out in these circumstances, and where there is no advance care directive.

If there is any doubt about whether a treatment or procedure can be provided without consent, doctors should seek the advice of their institution, state or territory guardianship office, or medical indemnity provider.

7.4.3 Consent and patients with mental illness

A diagnosis of a mental illness does not necessarily mean a patient lacks decision-making capacity. Capacity is decision-specific, and it is important to assess the patient's capacity to make the specific decision at the relevant point in time.

Mental health legislation in all states and territories outlines the circumstances in which patients can be involuntarily admitted and treated without their consent.

Mental health legislation in all states and territories except Tasmania also contains provisions relating to consent for treatments such as electroconvulsive therapy and psychosurgery.

The legislation in each state and territory is different, and it is important for doctors to know and follow the law that applies in the state or territory in which they practise.

Chapter 18, People with mental illness and the law, covers this in more detail.

7.5 Informed financial consent

One of the components of informed decision making is ensuring that patients are advised of, understand and accept the likely costs associated with a procedure or treatment, before the procedure or treatment is provided. This includes providing patients with information about:

- the total cost of the procedure or treatment, including the costs of any implant, prosthesis or other device
- any Medicare benefit available
- any private health insurance benefits available
- expected out-of-pocket costs for the patient
- whether there will be fees for other practitioners, such as surgical assistants or anaesthetists, and how to obtain more information about these costs.

Ideally, doctors should provide written information to patients about the likely costs.

Summary

The key to an effective informed decision-making process is good, patient-centred communication. Doctors should explore with patients (or, where they lack capacity, their substitute decision makers) what is important to them and target their discussions accordingly. The aim is to have a shared understanding and expectations of the likely outcomes of proposed treatment and of the costs associated with the treatment, particularly if there will be any out-of-pocket expenses for the patient. A patient can decline to provide consent if, after this discussion, they do not wish to proceed.

Doctors should be aware of and follow the legal requirements in the state or territory in which they practise and the requirements of the institutions in which they work.

If there is any doubt about whether a treatment or procedure can be provided without consent, doctors should seek the advice of their institution, state or territory guardianship office, or medical indemnity provider.

References

1. *Secretary, Department of Health and Community Services v JWB (Marion's Case)* [1992] HCA 15; 175 CLR 218.
2. *Dean v Phung* [2012] NSWCA 223.
3. *Rogers v Whitaker* [1992] HCA 58; 175 CLR 479.
4. Medical Board of Australia. Good medical practice: a code of conduct for doctors in Australia. 2020. https://www.medicalboard.gov.au/Codes-Guidelines-Policies/Code-of-conduct.aspx (accessed Oct 2024).
5. *Hunter New England Area Health Service v A* (2009) 63 NSWLR 22, NSWSC 761.
6. Avant. Determining testamentary capacity. https://avant.org.au/resources/determining-testamentary-capacity (accessed Jun 2025).
7. Grisso T, Applebaum PS. Assessing competence to consent to treatment: a guide for physicians and other health professionals. New York: Oxford University Press, 1998.
8. Office of the Public Advocate. Supported decision-making in Victoria. 2020. https://www.publicadvocate.vic.gov.au/resource/file?id=31 (accessed Oct 2024).
9. Stewart C, Lynch A. Undue influence, consent and medical treatment. *J R Soc Med* 2003; 96: 598–601.
10. *Gillick v West Norfolk AHA* (1986) AC 112.
11. Telfer MM, Tollit MA, Pace CC, Pang KC. Australian standards of care and treatment guidelines for trans and gender diverse children and adolescents. Melbourne: The Royal Children's Hospital, 2020. https://www.rch.org.au/uploadedFiles/Main/Content/adolescent-medicine/australian-standards-of-care-and-treatment-guidelines-for-trans-and-gender-diverse-children-and-adolescents.pdf (accessed Oct 2024).
12. Avant. Substitute decision makers. 2020. https://www.avant.org.au/Resources/Public/Substitute-decision-makers/ (accessed Oct 2024).
13. NSW Civil and Administrative Tribunal. Special medical treatment guidelines. 2016. https://www.ncat.nsw.gov.au/documents/factsheets/gd_factsheet_special_medical_treatment_guidelines.pdf (accessed Oct 2024).

Further reading

Australian Commission on Safety and Quality in Health Care. Informed consent - fact sheet for clinicians. 2020. https://www.safetyandquality.gov.au/publications-and-resources/resource-library/informed-consent-fact-sheet-clinicians

Australian Medical Association. AMA guide to informed financial consent. 2024. https://www.ama.com.au/articles/informed-financial-consent

Avant. Children and consent. 2019. https://avant.org.au/resources/children-and-consent

End of Life Directions for Aged Care (ELDAC). Substitute decision-making [factsheet]. https://www.eldac.com.au/Toolkits/End-of-Life-Law/Substitute-Decision-Making/Factsheet

Royal Australian and New Zealand College of Psychiatrists. Mental health legislation Australia and Aotearoa New Zealand. 2023. https://www.ranzcp.org/clinical-guidelines-publications/in-focus-topics/mental-health-legislation

White B, McDonald F, Willmott L, Then S-N. Health law in Australia. 4th ed. Lawbook Co, 2023.

08 Sexual and other professional boundaries: being a doctor in modern society

Anne Tonkin AO, Christine Gee AM

Introduction

> Respectful relationships with medical colleagues, other healthcare professionals, team members and patients are essential for patient care. ... Professional boundaries in medicine are the limits that define the relationship between a doctor and their patient. Professional boundaries are integral to a good doctor–patient relationship. They promote good care for patients and protect both parties [1].

Entering the medical profession is a significant moment in every doctor's life. Society generally holds the profession in high regard, and the impact of recognition as a doctor usually extends beyond an individual's workplace and permeates almost every aspect of their life. With the title comes privilege, but also great responsibility, and doctors are required to meet the ethical standards expected by the communities they serve (see section 2.1.2 of Chapter 2, On being a good doctor: the changing face of medical professionalism).

The interface between an individual's personal and professional life is not always very clear to doctors or to their patients. It is at these boundaries that great care is required to ensure that these standards are upheld, to prevent harm to individuals and to maintain the reputation of the profession as a whole. In particular, the relationship of trust between patient and doctor must never be abused by the establishment of any inappropriate or exploitative relationships, including intimate personal and sexual relationships.

This principle has been recognised since the time of Hippocrates, and has been restated in the Medical Board of Australia's *Good medical practice: a code of conduct for doctors in Australia* [1] and in the associated *Guidelines on sexual boundaries in the doctor–patient relationship* [2]. The code of conduct includes the following statement:

> Good medical practice involves:
>
> Never using your professional position to establish or pursue a sexual, exploitative or other inappropriate relationship with anybody under your care. This includes those close to the patient, such as their carer, guardian, spouse or the parent of a child patient [1].

The Guidelines expand on this further as follows:

> Patients need to trust that their doctor will act in their best interests, treat them professionally, not breach their privacy and never take advantage of them. Exploitation of the doctor–patient relationship undermines the trust that patients have in their doctors and the community has in the profession. It can cause profound psychological harm to patients and compromise their medical care [2].

This chapter covers the concept of professional boundaries, the principles underpinning them and their application in current medical practice. Understanding the principles can assist doctors to identify feelings or behaviours that may threaten the boundary between a professional role and a personal role in the doctor–patient relationship. It also describes the management by the Australian regulatory system of alleged boundary breaches.

8.1 The role of the doctor in today's society and the importance of professional boundaries

> In professional life, doctors must display a standard of behaviour that warrants the trust and respect of the community. This includes observing and practising the principles of ethical conduct [1].

The role of a doctor in society carries with it significant privilege and authority, and with that comes an essential requirement for a sense of responsibility and trustworthiness. Patients frequently entrust their doctor with very private information and allow them access to their bodies in ways that would otherwise be restricted to their most intimate personal relationships. It is crucial that doctors do not betray that trust because it can lead to serious harm to patients individually and to the community's trust in the profession overall.

The doctor–patient relationship has embedded within it an imbalance of power that leads to the potential for exploitation. This arises from an imbalance in knowledge and experience, together with the power vested in doctors to facilitate access to diagnostic tests or treatments that would not be available to the patient acting alone. Patients rely on the knowledge and experience of doctors when seeking help for medical issues, and often need the support of their doctor to access social supports. For example, doctors can certify illness or disability, facilitate time off work, and control access to driving licences and financial support. Patients need to be able to trust that their doctor is always acting in their best interests and is not being motivated by self-interest or self-gratification (see Chapter 3, Ethical principles for the medical profession).

The power imbalance inherent in the doctor–patient relationship opens it to the potential for exploitation or abuse, which may take many forms, including social, financial and, most seriously, sexual. Avoiding exploitation requires the doctor to set boundaries between themselves and their patients, while at the same time behaving with empathy and compassion. The boundaries of the relationship need to make it absolutely clear that the relationship exists for a professional purpose only and is not a precursor to a friendship or romantic interaction. Such boundaries are essential to ensure that patients can have confidence in the professional relationship and doctors can maintain the critical component of objectivity necessary to ensure safe practice. It is crucial to recognise that the responsibility for a boundary violation lies entirely with the doctor, regardless of which party initiates the change in the nature of the relationship. Clear professional boundaries can thus provide safety for the practitioner as well as for the patient. Despite this recognition, sexual misconduct by doctors continues to be an issue, including in Australia [3,4].

8.2 Types of boundary breaches with patients

While all doctors should know about the need to avoid breaching sexual boundaries with patients, some may not be fully aware of other types of boundary breaches. Professional boundaries ensure that there is an appropriate psychological and social distance between a health professional and patient, protecting the objectivity of medical decision making and promoting the safety of patients within the professional relationship [5]. There is some controversy about which types of relationships and caring acts are acceptable and which cross boundaries and represent a potential risk. A recent survey of primary care physicians in the US revealed that about a third had engaged in acts such as providing a ride home and paying for medicines, and 10% had gone to dinner with a patient [6].

8.2.1 Social boundaries

Ideally, doctors should not enter into social relationships with people who are also patients, and conversely should not accept as a patient someone who is already a friend or relative. While this can be a difficult balancing act for doctors in rural and remote settings, it is important to separate as much as possible the professional relationship from the personal. Some doctors avoid dual relationships entirely (arguably the safest option where feasible) while others compartmentalise the different parts of their lives by making it clear to patients what is acceptable behaviour within and outside the clinical setting [7]. A professional indemnity organisation advises that, where there is no alternative but to treat someone you otherwise have a personal relationship with (e.g. towns with only one doctor, or one specialist in a particular field), it is important to discuss the situation and document that discussion so both doctor and patient understand the boundaries. In addition, doctors should ensure that all professional interactions occur in a formal setting, such as the consultation room, and are well documented [8].

By extension of this principle, doctors should not be involved in the medical care of members of their family, close friends or colleagues, including providing referrals or prescriptions [9]. Several cases have been managed by the Medical Board of Australia over recent years in which such behaviour has been deemed to be professional misconduct by tribunals [10]. This principle is difficult for some practitioners to accept; however, it is now very well established and is specifically listed in the Medical Board's code of conduct [1]. The reasons include a loss of objectivity, poor continuity of care, inadequate record keeping and poor communication with other treating practitioners, leading to a risk of poor patient outcomes [9].

8.2.2 Financial boundaries

There are doctors who misuse their relationship with patients for financial gain, and there have been examples of doctors being made a patient's major beneficiary in their will, while continuing to treat the patient. The Medical Board and tribunals agree that this behaviour constitutes professional misconduct. One example involved a general practitioner (GP) who formed a close relationship with an elderly patient, assisting her with shopping, household maintenance and inviting her to share family events. He continued to be her treating GP. Over time, she started giving him expensive gifts, and eventually made him the major beneficiary of her will. While awaiting the tribunal hearing, the patient died and the GP inherited her substantial estate. The tribunal ruled that this was professional misconduct and imposed a reprimand and a significant fine.

Other forms of financial exploitation may occur when a practitioner uses their position of trust to encourage patients to purchase devices or substances, with significant profits accruing to the practitioner. A recent example is encouragement to buy ozone-generating devices, supplied by the practitioner, for use in the treatment of COVID-19.

Conflicts of interest are dealt with in the Medical Board's code of conduct (sections 10.12 and 10.13) where it is made clear that potential conflicts of interest must be recognised and appropriately managed, including being transparent in financial and commercial matters and declaring to patients any professional and financial interest in any product sold from a doctor's practice [1]. (See also Chapter 9, Doctors, industry and conflicts of interest.)

8.2.3 Sexual boundaries

Breaches of sexual boundaries span a wide spectrum of inappropriate activity [2], from verbal sexual harassment (such as sexually themed jokes; comments about appearance, sexuality or relationships; and inappropriate sexual comments during a consultation or procedure) through written harassment (including text messages or emails with sexual content) to physical sexual touching and sexual assault, sometimes under the guise of a medical examination or procedure. Some doctors may not recognise that sexualised comments can be a source of great distress for patients, and that these can be regarded as professional misconduct. An example of this was a practitioner who, being about to conduct a clinically indicated vaginal examination, paused and said words to the effect that he had not even had to take the patient dancing first. This comment sexualised the procedure and made the patient feel violated and very distressed. The tribunal ruled that this behaviour constituted professional misconduct and the practitioner's registration was suspended.

Intimate physical examinations without adequate prior explanation and the obtaining of informed consent may also be regarded as a breach of sexual boundaries [2]. Many reports of alleged sexual boundary violations to the Medical Board arise from a lack of informed consent processes (see Chapter 7, Consent and informed decision making) and inadequate communication by the practitioner, potentially causing the patient to feel shocked, violated and exploited during the physical examination because they did not know what to expect (see Chapter 5, Communication in clinical practice). Less commonly, a doctor may use the clinical setting to make contact with a patient for their own sexual gratification, such as performing intimate examinations when they are not clinically indicated or required [10].

It is never appropriate for a doctor to pursue a sexual or improper emotional relationship with a patient or someone close to a patient. Given the power imbalance, it is now generally recognised that there is no such thing as a 'consensual' sexual relationship between a doctor and patient, or a person close to a patient (e.g. parent, partner or child). It is always the doctor's responsibility to ensure that a sexual relationship does not occur, and doctors should be aware of the warning signs that may indicate a risk that boundaries may be crossed. These include social invitations; patients requesting non-urgent appointments at unusual hours or locations, especially when other staff are not present; and patients using sexually explicit language, being overly affectionate or attempting to give substantial gifts. In these circumstances, the doctor should generally transfer the care of the patient to another doctor [2].

There is a consensus view that, while there are a few doctors who engage in deliberately predatory sexual behaviour, the majority of damaging boundary violations start with minor, non-exploitative boundary crossings [11], such as disclosure of personal details of the doctor's life, acceptance of gifts or making a particular effort to accommodate a patient in terms of timing of appointments, provision of transport or other minor departures from usual practice. Such behaviour may start the practitioner on a 'slippery slope' towards more serious boundary breaches, including sexual exploitation of the patient [11].

It is clear that sexual exploitation of a patient, or a person close to a patient (e.g. parent, partner or child) can have very destructive effects [3], including intense shame, guilt, depression, post-traumatic stress disorder, misuse of alcohol or drugs, break-up of other relationships, and suicidal thoughts or actions, including completed suicide.

Forming a sexual relationship with a former patient may also be regarded as unprofessional if this breaches the trust the patient placed in the doctor, or if the power imbalance in the doctor–patient relationship continues after the professional relationship has ended. In some specialties, such as psychiatry, intimate relationships with former patients are prohibited regardless of the timeframe [12]. If the Medical Board is notified about such a relationship in other areas of medicine, it will assess each situation individually, taking several factors into account, including the duration, frequency and type of care provided; the vulnerability of the patient; and the time elapsed since the end of the professional relationship. Further details are provided in the Medical Board's *Guidelines on sexual boundaries* [2].

Clearly, any practitioner who is convicted of sexual assault or rape is very likely to be referred to the tribunal by the Medical Board, and tribunals have imposed disqualification periods of up to 15 years in recent cases, potentially ending the practitioner's career in medicine.

It is also important to recognise that sexual boundaries exist between colleagues in the workplace, and it has been established by several tribunal decisions over recent years that inappropriate comments or unwanted sexual touching of a colleague (medical or non-medical) by a doctor can be determined to be professional misconduct and lead to serious sanctions. This extends to supervisors of trainees. There have been several recent cases in which the tribunal has judged such unwanted sexual advances to be professional misconduct, leading to suspension or cancellation of registration [10]. This topic is discussed further in section 8.4.

Finally, conduct online has led individual practitioners to be severely sanctioned by boards and tribunals. In particular, offences involving accessing and/or possessing child exploitation materials (child pornography) are regarded as professional misconduct and have led to cancellations of registration for 10 years or more.

8.3 Risk factors for boundary breaches

8.3.1 Isolation

Doctors who are isolated, whether professionally (solo practitioners), geographically or culturally, are at higher risk of boundary breaches, and need to take particular care to avoid them. Isolation can make it very difficult to ensure there is a clear distinction between professional and personal roles. Geographical isolation from other practitioners, particularly where the doctor is the only one in a rural or remote location, can make it particularly difficult to maintain a professional relationship that is kept separate from other social interactions. Research in the US suggests that the smaller the population of the area, the less choice a doctor has about whether or not to interact with patients in social or community settings, or conversely, about whether or not to accept people with whom they have social relationships as patients [6,7]. In this scenario, there needs to be a discussion about the situation up front, careful separation of the clinical from the social relationship, and full documentation of all clinical interactions [8,13].

8.3.2 Demographic factors

A very clear majority (about 90%) of practitioners who are notified to the Medical Board for professional boundary issues are male [3,10]. Some age groups appear to be more at risk, particularly between 40 and 60 years (Australian Health Practitioner Regulation Agency [Ahpra]; unpublished information). Over recent years, several cases related to inappropriate use of social media by practitioners in their twenties or thirties have been notified to the board; this is an area of potential risk [14] that needs to be understood by all doctors, but particularly those younger practitioners who are more likely to use social media. Guidance is provided both in the Medical Board's code of conduct and in specific social media guidelines on the Ahpra website [15].

8.3.3 Specialty areas of practice

Although there are few objective data, it appears that GPs, psychiatrists, and obstetricians and gynaecologists are at particular risk of being notified for breaching boundaries [3,10]. The development of long-term clinical relationships with patients is more common for GPs and psychiatrists, and this is likely to represent a potential area of risk for inappropriate relationships to develop. Similar long-term relationships develop in other specialties, such as renal medicine [16], and practitioners need to exercise particular care to ensure that these relationships remain professional and trusting. Obstetricians and gynaecologists are required to ask personal questions and conduct intimate examinations that may give rise to allegations of sexual harassment or assault. Excellent communication skills and informed consent processes that ensure that patients are aware of what is going to be done and the reasons for it help to reduce this risk.

8.3.4 Illness and impairment

In some cases of boundary breaches, the practitioner has been found to be unwell, particularly with a psychiatric disorder that may impair their judgement or self-control (see also Chapter 12, Personal health of the doctor: illness and impairment). In many instances, the background issue may be exacerbated by an additional life crisis, such as relationship breakdown, work-related stress or burnout [4].

8.4 Relationships with colleagues and trainees

Any interaction between individuals occurs within the context of the relationship between them, which may be of varying complexity but almost always involves some differential in the relative power of the participants, which overarches all the other aspects of the relationship. Interactions between healthcare colleagues are also subject to these complex factors, and unprofessional behaviours between staff are common and can lead to poorer outcomes for patients [17,18]. A staff survey carried out in seven Australian hospitals [18] showed that about 90% of respondents reported experiencing at least one instance of unprofessional behaviour over the preceding year, including 39% who reported these experiences occurring at least weekly.

Experiencing unprofessional behaviour is more common for younger staff members and for nurses (about twice the rate as for doctors). The Medical Training Survey, an annual survey of doctors in training in Australia, now has six years of data (2019 to 2024 inclusive) which consistently show that about one-third of respondents experienced and/or witnessed bullying, harassment, discrimination and/or racism over the preceding year. In the 2023 survey, nearly half of the perpetrators of these behaviours were senior doctors [19]. While the survey has not included specific questions related to sexual boundary breaches with colleagues as yet, there have been several high-profile cases where senior male practitioners have been found to have assaulted younger, female colleagues [20] and it is likely that such incidents are under-reported.

A UK survey of the experiences of the surgical workforce [21] show that 63% of women and 24% of men had experienced sexual harassment and 30% of women and 7% of men had been sexually assaulted by colleagues, including such behaviours as unwanted touching and forced physical contact in exchange for career opportunities. Similar behaviours have been reported across professions and directed towards support staff, including receptionists in private practices. Regulators, including the Medical Board, are taking reports of such unacceptable behaviour very seriously because of the moral imperative as well as its well-documented negative impacts on the wellbeing of victims and the safety of patients [21].

Clearly, well-functioning healthcare teams require all participants, whatever their position is in the medical hierarchy or in other professions, to interact with each other with respect and civility, and to avoid breaching professional boundaries (see Chapter 11, The doctor and interprofessional relationships). The same principles apply to teaching, supervising and mentoring roles, where there is a clear power imbalance and the potential for inappropriate behaviour.

8.5 Social media and digital communication

Doctors from all areas of medicine are increasingly using digital technologies, including internet and social media, in their practice. While there are many positive aspects of the professional and appropriate use of social media, it also raises ethical issues related to the use of social networking sites as well as various forms of digital communications such as emails, texts and online chats. Ethical issues include the management of clinical boundaries in a digital setting, maintaining privacy and confidentiality in the face of unprecedented availability of personal information online (see Chapter 6, Confidentiality, privacy and disclosure), establishing realistic expectations for digital communication, and establishing a definition of digital professionalism [14,22]. While the COVID-19 pandemic acted as a catalyst for further adoption of digital forms of communication to support medical practice, clear and consistent guidelines and processes to support these have been slower to emerge.

The use of social and digital media by doctors can be problematic in several ways (see Chapter 29, Professional practice, digital technology and artificial intelligence). It provides avenues for patients to attempt to connect outside of the professional relationship, thus blurring professional and personal identities. 'Friending' a patient on a social media platform is a potential boundary crossing that may start a 'slippery slope' towards a harmful boundary violation. On the other hand, refusing a friend request can make a patient feel rejected [14]. Practitioners may self-disclose on their social media accounts and reveal more personal information than would usually be available to patients. Some posts by medical students or practitioners may be inconsistent with professional standards (e.g. depicting intoxication, profanity or sexual innuendo). Both patients and practitioners may use search engines to find out more about each other, and some of the information may not be relevant to the therapeutic relationship [22]. This can sometimes lead to inappropriate online interactions between patients and practitioners, which can become personal and sometimes overtly sexual in nature. It is very clear that this type of interaction is inappropriate and sometimes constitutes professional misconduct.

Additionally, there are risks to patient safety where clinical information and advice is provided via digital communication and not recorded within the contemporaneous medical record, which may also lead to medicolegal issues for the doctor.

Guidance on the appropriate use of social media is provided by the Medical Board in its code of conduct [1], Ahpra in its social media guidelines [23] and by many of the professional indemnity providers (e.g. Avant [24]).

8.6 Regulatory aspects of boundary breaches

8.6.1 Obligation to report

Under the Health Practitioner Regulation National Law (the National Law), all registered health practitioners must make mandatory notifications in some circumstances, including serious impairment affecting the ability to practise safely, intoxication while practising, significant departure from accepted professional standards and sexual misconduct (see Chapter 21, Regulation of the medical profession).

In Western Australia, a doctor treating an impaired practitioner is exempt from this requirement but may still make a voluntary notification if they are concerned that the public is being put at serious risk of harm. Details on the obligation to report are available in Ahpra's *Guidelines for mandatory notifications* [25].

8.6.2 Management of notifications

Notifications of concern about possible boundary breaches are reported to Ahpra in most states and territories of Australia, and to the Office of the Health Ombudsman in Queensland and the Health Care Complaints Commission in New South Wales (see Chapter 22, Healthcare complaints and complaint systems). Similar processes occur in all jurisdictions. The cases managed by Ahpra are allocated to a team of specifically trained regulatory advisers and are reviewed clinically by a medical practitioner at an early stage. If the risk to the public is assessed as being high, the matter may be considered for immediate action to restrict the practitioner's practice (usually by suspension of registration or imposition of conditions, such as gender-based restrictions or supervision) until a full investigation can be completed. The decision to take immediate action and the final decision at the end of the investigation are made by a specialised delegated committee on behalf of the Medical Board. If the committee forms a reasonable belief that the reported behaviour constitutes professional misconduct, the matter will be referred to the relevant tribunal for a formal hearing and determination (see Chapter 21, Regulation of the medical profession). Matters not meeting the threshold of professional misconduct but requiring regulatory action may be managed by the committee through the imposition of conditions on the practitioner's registration; for example, education, mentoring or audits of practice.

8.6.3 Outcomes of notifications

Australian reviews of notifications to the health practitioner regulator (Ahpra) showed that the risk of regulatory action restricting the doctor's practice was significantly higher in cases of boundary breaches than concerns about clinical care [3,10]. A review of tribunal cases occurring during the first seven years of the Australian national regulatory system [10] showed that doctors were more likely to be involved than other health professionals, and the large majority were male practitioners. Outcomes were more severe for sexual misconduct compared with poor clinical care, with 79% of doctors involved in sexual misconduct being removed from practice, at least temporarily (48% deregistered and 31% suspended from the register) [10].

Tribunal findings are made public in all jurisdictions, and there is therefore also a risk of reputational harm to individual practitioners who are found to have engaged in professional misconduct.

Summary

The maintenance of professional boundaries in the doctor–patient relationship is vital to good medical care, and breaches of these boundaries can lead to great harm to patients (and those close to them) and serious outcomes for practitioners. Doctors need to be vigilant about the way they communicate with patients, and need to ensure they have appropriate informed consent processes, particularly when required to undertake intimate examinations. It is also very important to be aware of the warning signs that a relationship with a patient may be becoming personal rather than remaining professional (including in online communications) and to take steps very early in the process to prevent any further development, usually by ceasing contact and referring the patient on to a colleague. Useful guides to avoiding the risk of boundary violations are provided by professional indemnity providers [13,26,27] and in the Medical Board of Australia's codes and guidelines [1,2,25].

Non-sexual boundaries also need to be respected, and doctors should avoid providing formal or informal consultations, prescriptions or referrals to family members, friends or colleagues, and should develop strategies for dealing with these requests [9].

Good medical practice requires a doctor–patient relationship grounded in trust, in which the sole motivation for both parties is the health and welfare of the patient. Such relationships, grounded in professionalism, can be rewarding for the practitioner and therapeutic for the patient, and are key to achieving the best possible outcomes for patients and maintaining the community's trust in the medical profession.

References

1. Medical Board of Australia. Good medical practice: a code of conduct for doctors in Australia. 2020. https://www.medicalboard.gov.au/Codes-Guidelines-Policies/Code-of-conduct.aspx (accessed Nov 2024).
2. Medical Board of Australia. Sexual boundaries in the doctor–patient relationship. 2018. https://www.medicalboard.gov.au/Codes-Guidelines-Policies/Sexual-boundaries-guidelines.aspx (accessed Nov 2024).
3. Bismark MM, Studdert DM, Morton K, et al. Sexual misconduct by health professional in Australia, 2011–2016: a retrospective analysis of notifications to health regulators. *Med J Aust* 2020; 213: 218–225.
4. Galletly CA. Sexual misconduct by doctors: a problem that has not gone away. *Med J Aust* 2020; 213: 216–217.
5. Lampe L, Hitching R, Hammond TE, et al. Being a 'good' doctor: understanding and managing professional boundaries is challenging and can lead to stress and burnout. *Australas Psychiatry* 2023; 31: 764–767.
6. Nieva HR, Ruan E, Schiff GD. Professional–patient boundaries: a national survey of primary care physicians' attitudes and practices. *J Gen Intern Med* 2020; 35: 457–464.
7. Brooks KD, Eley DS, Pratt R, Zink T. Management of professional boundaries in rural practice. *Acad Med* 2012; 87: 1091–1096.
8. Avant. Treating family members, friends or staff. 2023. https://avant.org.au/resources/treating-family-members-friends-or-staff (accessed Nov 2024).
9. Smyth C. Treating family, friends and colleagues: why and how to say 'no'. Adelaide: Medical Insurance Group Australia, 2023. https://www.miga.com.au/Bulletin/treating-family-friends-and-colleagues (accessed Mar 2024).
10. Millbank J. Serious misconduct of health professionals in disciplinary tribunals under the National Law 2010–17. *Aust Health Rev* 2020; 44: 190–199.
11. Galletly CA. Crossing professional boundaries in medicine: the slippery slope to patient sexual exploitation. *Med J Aust* 2004; 181: 380–383.
12. Royal Australian and New Zealand College of Psychiatrists. Zero tolerance policy on proven sexual boundary violations. 2024. https://www.ranzcp.org/clinical-guidelines-publications/clinical-guidelines-publications-library/zero-tolerance-policy-on-proven-sexual-boundary-violations (accessed Nov 2024).
13. Watson-Kyme C. Beware boundary violations. MDA National, 2020. https://www.mdanational.com.au/advice-and-support/library/articles-and-case-studies/2020/06/beware-boundary-violations (accessed Nov 2024).
14. Rukavina TV, Viskić J, Poplašen LM, et al. Dangers and benefits of social media on e-professionalism of health care professionals: scoping review. *J Med Internet Res* 2021; 23: e25770.
15. Australian Health Practitioner Regulation Agency. Social media: How to meet your obligations under the National Law. 2019. https://www.ahpra.gov.au/Resources/Social-media-guidance (accessed Nov 2024).
16. Cousins M, Bradshaw J, Bonner A. Professional relationships between nephrology clinicians and patients: a systematic review. *J Ren Care* 2020; 46: 206–215.
17. Aunger JA, Maben J, Abrams R, et al. Drivers of unprofessional behaviour between staff in acute care hospitals: a realist review. *BMC Health Serv Rev* 2023; 23: 1326.
18. Westbrook J, Sunderland N, Li L, et al. The prevalence and impact of unprofessional behaviour among hospital workers: a survey in seven Australian hospitals. *Med J Aust* 2021; 214: 31–36.

19. Australian Health Practitioner Regulation Agency. Medical Training Survey. https://medicaltrainingsurvey.gov.au (accessed Mar 2024).
20. Davey M. 'The system teaches you to be quiet': doctor indecently assaulted by senior colleague identifies herself. The Guardian, Sep 2023. https://www.theguardian.com/australia-news/2023/sep/24/the-system-teaches-you-to-be-quiet-doctor-indecently-assaulted-by-senior-colleague-identifies-herself (accessed Mar 2024).
21. Begeny CT, Arshad H, Cuming T, et al. Sexual harassment, sexual assault and rape by colleagues in the surgical workforce, and how women and men are living different realities: observational study using NHS population-derived weights. *Br J Surg* 2023; 110: 1518–1526.
22. Sabin JE, Harland JC. Professional ethics for digital age psychiatry: boundaries, privacy, and communication. *Curr Psychiatry Rep* 2017; 19: 55.
23. Australian Health Practitioner Regulation Agency. Social media: How to meet your obligations under the National Law. https://www.ahpra.gov.au/Resources/Social-media-guidance.aspx# (accessed Nov 2024).
24. Avant. Social media for doctors—keeping it professional. 2021. https://avant.org.au/resources/social-media-for-doctors-keeping-it-professional (accessed Nov 2024).
25. Australian Health Practitioner Regulation Agency. Guidelines for mandatory notifications. 2020. https://www.medicalboard.gov.au/Codes-Guidelines-Policies/Guidelines-for-mandatory-notifications.aspx (accessed Mar 2024).
26. Avant. Boundary issues. 2020. https://avant.org.au/resources/boundary-issues (accessed Nov 2024).
27. Parisi C. How close is too close? Adelaide: Medical Insurance Group Australia, 2022. https://www.miga.com.au/Bulletin/how-close-is-too-close (accessed Nov 2024).

09 Doctors, industry and conflicts of interest

Ian Kerridge, Wendy Lipworth

Introduction

Despite an increasing emphasis on patient autonomy and choice, and the ease with which patients can obtain information about illnesses and treatments, patients still place considerable trust in their doctors, and rely upon their independence and trustworthiness. This trust is underpinned by the ethical principle that doctors should act in the best interests of their patients. In this regard, the Medical Board of Australia's *Good medical practice: a code of conduct for doctors in Australia* reads as follows: 'Doctors have a professional responsibility to be familiar with *Good medical practice* [the code of conduct] and to apply the guidance it contains' [1].

In recent decades there has been enormous growth in collaborations between the medical profession and health-related industries, including pharmaceutical, device and diagnostic industries. Collaborations between the medical profession and these industries has undoubtedly generated the bulk of evidence to support the registration and translation of new drugs, devices and diagnostic technologies, with the vast majority of clinical trials (more than 70%) worldwide being sponsored by manufacturers [2].

At the same time, these industries have been the subject of considerable criticism for behaviours including misleading marketing, deliberate concealment of clinical trial data, including serious adverse effects, ghost-writing of manuscripts that overestimate benefits and under-report risks of new treatments, exaggeration of the cost of developing new drugs, and conducting low-quality clinical trials as a form of marketing. The industry has also been accused of 'disease mongering'—medicalising normal human experiences and overstating the need for drug treatment for relatively minor conditions solely for the purpose of creating markets or increasing product sales [3]. As a result, collaborations with pharmaceutical and device industries have raised questions about the trustworthiness of the medical profession and the extent to which clinical practice, research, health policy and education are inappropriately influenced by commercial interests [3]. While these collaborations are beneficial for the collaborators, their extent, nature and consequences have been the subject of ongoing concern.

Many patients, research participants and the public are likely to be unaware that medical professionals engage with industry. Others might be aware of this but assume that self-reflection would nevertheless guide the doctor towards the best interests of the patient, research participant or public [4]. It is therefore crucial for the medical profession and for individual medical practitioners to take the lead in managing industry interactions.

9.1 How industry interacts with doctors

9.1.1 Product promotion

Manufacturers use a wide range of promotional strategies to sell their products. For doctors in clinical practice, one of the most common forms of interaction with the pharmaceutical and medical device industries is engagement with company representatives seeking to influence the behaviour of doctors. These representatives use a variety of techniques to influence doctors, including creation of a personal relationship, giving of gifts, drug samples, invitations and literature, educational resources and quoting of authority figures ('key opinion leaders') [5,6].

Companies have also been known to offer gifts to medical students, although this is increasingly precluded by medical school policies [7]. Advertising of products also occurs through product displays at conferences, direct-to-consumer advertising, disease awareness campaigns and advertisements in medical journals [8].

9.1.2 Industry-funded education

Doctors are also likely to interact with industry by attending educational events conducted or sponsored by industry. The pharmaceutical industry has contributed large amounts of funding to continuing medical education (CME). Some authorities have called for a ban on such support, and disengagement is slowly occurring [9–11]. The Australian Medical Association's guidelines, *Doctors' relationships with industry*, remain quite permissive in some aspects:

> It is acceptable for industry to support meetings that contribute to doctors' education and continuing professional development (CPD); however, such support should be untied, fully disclosed, at arms-length to the organisation of the meeting [12].

In the US, medical schools have also been criticised for accepting support for educational initiatives from the pharmaceutical industry [13] (see Chapter 10, Continuing professional development).

9.1.3 Key opinion leaders and peer networks

Some clinicians, particularly interventional physicians (e.g. cardiologists), surgeons and those who prescribe medicines to large populations (e.g. psychiatrists) or medicines that are high cost (e.g. oncologists) might have more extensive interactions with industry. The benefits derived are likely to be both tangible and intangible. They might, for example, be invited to speakers' bureaus, be named as key opinion leaders, and be appointed (paid or unpaid) to companies' medical advisory boards [14,15]. These doctors are often asked to speak as experts at conferences in Australia and overseas and serve on industry advisory boards. Key opinion leaders often benefit from such roles through enhanced access to support for their clinical research and access to cutting-edge information. Acting in this role also enables them to shape the research and innovation agenda. Key opinion leaders are also unavoidably influenced by the relationships they form and they, in turn, have considerable influence over their peer networks and the profession more generally [14].

9.1.4 Clinician involvement in research

In Australia as in other industrialised nations, the majority (>60–70%) of clinical trials are funded by industry [16]. This means that the research agendas, research questions, study designs and the interpretation and reporting of results are largely determined by industry interests. Clinicians can be involved in industry-funded research in a number of ways, including participating in study design, recruiting participants, promoting the trial and the product being tested to their patients and colleagues, assisting with interpretation of findings and authoring manuscripts and presenting findings at conferences, seminars and clinical meetings. Hospitals and departments are always paid to conduct industry-sponsored studies, and clinician researchers might also be remunerated for other trial-related activities (see Chapter 31, Medical research).

9.1.5 Indirect modes of influence

Doctors' practices might also be shaped by industry in indirect ways because the clinical trials they rely on are sponsored by industry, the professional bodies they belong to are supported by industry, the clinical guidelines they follow are drafted by experts with ties to industry, and even the definitions of the diseases they diagnose are shaped by commercial imperatives [17,18]. Industry also has a major effect on the treatments that doctors are able to prescribe, not only because companies decide what products to produce, but also because they design research and decide what results to publish, and lobby (often with the assistance of patient groups and key opinion leaders) for specific products to be publicly subsidised on the Pharmaceutical Benefits Scheme (for medicines) or the Medicare Benefits Schedule (for devices) [17]. Industry also shapes prescribing by influencing the information that is available to patients. While there is currently a ban in Australia on direct advertising of prescription medicines to the public, industry funding of patient advocacy organisations provides an indirect mechanism for providing information to patients which, in turn, shapes the doctor–patient interaction when patients request specific products [19].

9.1.6 Measuring industry interactions

The extent of the interactions between doctors and the pharmaceutical industry is difficult to quantify, although this has been made easier by regulations that mandate disclosure by both industry and physicians. The Medicines Australia *Code of conduct* now requires companies to publicly report exchanges of value to health professionals [20,21]. This system has, however, been criticised for not collecting all relevant information, for the way it reports this information, and for being difficult to search [22]. Interactions can be measured in several ways. These include: the proportion of doctors who regularly agree to see company representatives; the estimated amount of money spent by industry per doctor per year; and the number of doctors who accept benefits by attending educational events and conferences supported or conducted by industry. Data from the US has demonstrated that in 2016, health-related companies spent almost US$30 billion on medical marketing. Of this, around 68% (or about US$20 billion) was spent on persuading doctors and other health professionals of the benefits of specific prescription drugs [8]. In Australia, between October 2011 and September 2015, 42 companies sponsored 116,845 events for health professionals. Oncology, surgery and endocrinology were the most frequent clinical areas of focus. Most events (64%) were held in a clinical setting. The mean cost per event was A$2449 and over 90% included food and beverages [23].

9.2 Influence and conflict of interest

Interactions with industry can influence practice in positive ways. Industry funding can make it possible for clinicians to conduct research. Industry-sponsored clinical trials can also be of high quality and provide important evidence regarding new medicines, diagnostics or devices. Similarly, information provided by industry can alert clinicians to important advances in science and medical practice.

At the same time, industry activities serve the interests of companies in generating profits for their shareholders and are not always aligned with those of patients and health systems. This creates a situation in which conflicts of interest may arise.

There is no single agreed definition of what constitutes a conflict of interest. According to the Medical Board of Australia [1],

> [a] conflict of interest in medical practice arises when a doctor, entrusted with acting in the interests of a patient, also has financial, professional or personal interests, or relationships with third parties, which may affect their care of the patient.

The *Australian code for the responsible conduct of research* [24] states that:

> a conflict of interest exists in a situation where an independent observer might reasonably conclude that the professional actions of a person are or may be unduly influenced by other interests.

The guide that supports the code [25] emphasises that:

> the perception that a conflict of interest exists is a serious matter and can raise concerns about the integrity of individuals or the management practices of the institution, potentially undermining community trust in research.

It is important to recognise that a conflict of interest is an objective situation rather than an internal mental state. A conflict of interest also needs to be distinguished from any behaviour that might be the result of the conflict. For this reason, a doctor cannot simply deny the existence of a conflict of interest by asserting that their behaviour has not been affected by it or that they do not believe they have a conflict [26].

While most attention has been paid to financial conflicts of interest (where the relevant interest is a monetary or in-kind gain), non-financial interests related to personal, career, family, religious and other obligations or commitments may also create a conflict of interest. Importantly, although these might be less obvious than financial interests, they are often stronger drivers of behaviour [27–30].

When doctors interact with industry, conflicts of interest arise primarily as a result of the loyalty or sense of reciprocity that doctors develop towards companies, their employees or their products. This might stem from the creation of close relationships between doctors and drug representatives or the companies for which they consult (whether or not this is paid) or from which they receive funding for research or education. The sense of reciprocity arises as a result of what social psychologists refer to as the 'gift relationship' [31,32]. It is human nature to accept gifts (other than from people one does not like), to feel that the donor is likely to be offended if a gift is refused, and to want to reciprocate for gifts.

In the context of doctors' interactions with industry, information, food and sponsored education or research are all types of gifts, and doctors can meet the obligation of reciprocity by, for example, using the company's product, providing access to patients or their data; providing access to educational forums and students; agreeing to collaborate on research and author papers; agreeing to act as a consultant or adviser, and speaking positively about the company's product at conferences, seminars, departmental meetings and the like.

Interestingly, small gifts can be more influential than large ones and it can be more difficult to refuse a small gift than a large, disproportionate gift. Importantly, social science research shows that recipients of gifts are often unaware of these dynamics, which could be why some doctors deny or rationalise the effects of gifts. There is also evidence that some doctors might be unaware of, or deny, the influence that industry might have over their attitudes and actions [33–35].

Socialisation also plays an important role in facilitating interactions with industry, and in generating interests and conflicts of interest. Medical students and specialist trainees observe their seniors interacting with companies, which normalises and can even give status to such practice. Companies also seek to form relationships with medical students and trainees as early as possible in their career development [36,37]. Studies have shown pharmaceutical company contact with students is widespread and some students believe that they are immune to any influence from this contact. Some medical schools and student societies in Australia and internationally have developed policies to limit students' interactions with industry [13,38].

There is now considerable evidence that marketing, funding support, and sponsorship by the pharmaceutical and device industries may adversely affect how doctors practise medicine, prescribe drugs, treat patients, conduct and publish research, participate in CME, conduct peer review and contribute to the development of clinical practice guidelines.

9.2.1 Effects on prescribing

Multiple studies from different countries and different healthcare systems have demonstrated how readily doctors' prescribing patterns can be influenced. Studies have shown that there is an association between interacting with industry and prescribing the company's product. While it cannot be assumed that all such prescribing is inappropriate, there is a moderate association between industry interaction and the use of more expensive or less clinically appropriate products [39,40] (see also Chapter 30, Prescribing and administering medicines).

9.2.2 Effects on requests to hospital pharmacies

Not only do industry methods alter prescribing practices, but they also impact on hospital pharmacies. Studies have shown that after interactions with industry, doctors are more likely to request that their hospital pharmacy stock new drugs linked to those companies with which they have interacted [41,42].

9.2.3 Effects on research

Much adverse publicity received by the pharmaceutical industry in recent years has related to its influence on research. Industry practices that have received criticism have included distorting the research agenda (e.g. producing profitable 'me too' drugs and neglecting rare diseases or those associated with poverty), deficient study design (e.g. choosing a comparator drug or dose likely to favour the new drug), delay or failure to publish results of clinical trials, publication of positive studies only (publication bias), and incomplete or selective reporting (omitting or minimising adverse effects). Pharmaceutical companies have also been criticised for not allowing clinical investigators to have full access to data from clinical trials they have conducted and for employing ghost writers to draft reports for publication [17,43–45].

Interestingly, industry-funded studies are less likely than investigator-initiated studies to be found to be affected by outright scientific misconduct (e.g. falsification, fabrication or plagiarism). Rather, the influences are subtle and systemic and fit within the bounds of what is generally considered good scientific practice. In Australia and internationally, compulsory registration of all clinical trials has been introduced to circumvent some of these problems. Nevertheless, an Australian survey revealed that a small proportion of medical specialists admitted to involvement in questionable research practices (e.g. premature discontinuation of clinical trials, delayed publication of trial findings or concealment of data from publication) on the part of industry [46] (see Chapter 31, Medical research).

9.2.4 Effects on clinical guidelines

Until quite recently, little attention has been paid to the conflicts of interest that clinical experts might bring to the panel discussions involved in drafting guidelines. If conflicts of interest are not adequately addressed, there are risks that patient care may be compromised, healthcare expenditure skewed, and doctors' trust in guidelines diminished. In response to these concerns, Australia's National Health and Medical Research Council (NHMRC) has promulgated guidelines that cover possible conflicts of interest on the part of guideline panel members [47]. This is also an issue internationally [48]. The most recent edition of the *Diagnostic and statistical manual of mental disorders* [49] issued by the American Psychiatric Association (APA) and used extensively throughout the world for clinical and medicolegal purposes, has been criticised because the APA receives 20% of its funding from industry, and many of those who worked on the new edition had financial conflicts of interest [50].

9.2.5 Effects on patient trust

To date, revelations about the impact of interactions between doctors and industry have not seriously undermined the trust Australian patients have in their doctors. This might reflect lack of awareness of the extent of these interactions. Studies have shown that, when informed about interactions with industry, patients are less likely to trust their doctors [51]. At the same time, the public may have permissive attitudes towards gifts, (particularly if they are small) and may respond positively to disclosure [52,53].

9.3 Response to public concerns

Medicines Australia is the major pharmaceutical industry association in Australia. Its code of conduct [20] has been progressively modified in response to public opinion particularly in relation to a ban on providing entertainment, a ban on paying delegates to attend meetings, and seeking to reduce any appearance of extravagance regarding venues and catering. While the code is voluntary, members can be reported for alleged breaches of the code and investigated by the association. Breaches found to be proven are published on the association website.

The Medical Technology Association of Australia also has a code of practice for its members. Members are primarily companies that develop and market medical and surgical devices and companies providing in-vitro diagnostics. In relation to interaction with the medical profession, the code covers issues around gifts and possible inducements, as well as guidelines for support for conferences, education and training [54].

While companies have curtailed some behaviours, they still maintain the position that interactions with health professionals are mutually beneficial. In the UK, for example, the Association of the British Pharmaceutical Industry supported and promoted a position statement on the topic [55], although this was met with some criticism [56,57]. The position that medicine and industry should collaborate continues to be supported not only by industry itself, but also by medical research associations, universities and government departments [58,59]. It is therefore important for all health professionals to be aware of both the benefits and risks of doing so, and of how to manage the resulting influence and conflict of interest.

9.4 Management of influence and conflicts of interest

9.4.1 Managing conflicts of interest

In response to concerns about industry influence and conflicts of interest, medical professional organisations, health services, universities, research institutes and government bodies have developed codes of conduct. The codes cover the relationships between doctors and the pharmaceutical and medical devices industries and how these relationships may result in a breach of a doctor's ethical duty. They articulate the risks of industry engagement and suggest ethical frameworks for identifying and managing them.

Disclosure and transparency

The first step in managing conflict of interest is to identify and disclose it. Here, it is important to bear in mind that it is *interests*, not *conflicts of interest*, that need to be declared [26]. This is important because it is not solely up to the individual to decide whether they have a conflict of interest, but also those receiving the declaration [26]. In this regard it is noteworthy that common legal tests for conflict of interest state that a conflict of interest exists if a 'reasonable member of the public properly informed would conclude that a conflict exists.'

Instructions for disclosing financial interests are usually quite clear (e.g. industry payments greater than $500 in the past 3 years). While it can be more difficult to determine what non-financial interests to declare, the existence of an intangible benefit (such as one that is likely to confer status among peers) might be considered more influential and therefore riskier in ethical terms. Although it is often useful to consider what a 'reasonable observer' might perceive to be a relevant interest and whether they believe a conflict of interest exists, from an ethical perspective this is insufficient. Komesaroff et al. [26] offer some useful additional guiding principles for determining whether an interest should be declared, arguing that an interest should be declared if it is:

- pertinent—applicable to the issue being considered
- substantial—generating substantive outcomes in the specific context
- immutable—not readily susceptible to change as a result of conversation, dialogue or reflective deliberation.

Many countries have 'sunshine policies' (including in Australia, the US, France, Portugal, Latvia, Slovenia, Turkey and Japan) that aim to make the ties (particularly financial ones) between individual health professionals and health-related industries publicly transparent. Policies vary in terms of what is reported and whether they are legislated or not. In the US, the Physician Payments Sunshine Act is federal legislation that requires manufacturers of drugs, medical devices, biologicals and medical supplies covered by federal health insurance programs to disclose a broad range of payments to physicians and teaching hospitals if valued at over US$10 or totalling more than US$100 in one calendar year. It excludes product samples and educational materials that are intended to directly benefit the patient.

Australia was one of the first countries to introduce transparency policies related to pharmaceutical company payments to health professionals in 2007. The most recent (19th) edition of the Medicines Australia *Code of conduct* requires reporting of payments for consulting or advisory board membership, sponsorship to attend an educational event including travel, and speaker honoraria and travel support. Companies are not, however, required to disclose the provision of food and beverages, or payments for research [20].

There are, however, a number of points to bear in mind when thinking about disclosure of interests. First, it is not obvious that the requirement to disclose alters the practices of those who are disclosing. The biases associated with industry interaction might arise long before any disclosure occurs. For example, in research, biases might occur at the point at which a study question is chosen, or a study is designed. Second, it is not clear what effect disclosure has on the recipients, who may come to incorrect conclusions about the trustworthiness, or otherwise, of the discloser. Patients and research participants who are told about industry relationships might interpret these both as evidence of greater and lesser trustworthiness. This point is acknowledged by the NHMRC code [24]. Third, those making disclosures might believe that this is all that needs to be done to manage conflicts of interest—so-called 'moral licensing'. Finally, if a large number of declarations are made simply to satisfy bureaucratic requirements, this can create 'noise' that obscures the significance of the more substantial declarations [60–63]. For all of these reasons, disclosure 'does not expunge or exonerate bias' [64] and is not an end in itself, but rather a way of facilitating more active management.

Management

If a conflict is identified, it is then necessary to determine how it should be managed. If a conflict is determined to be of minor significance, then it may be sufficient for it simply to be taken into account by those receiving the information. More significant conflicts might need more active management. For example, a person with a conflict of interest might need to abstain from voting on a committee or withdraw from a committee altogether. A clinical researcher who is researching their own patients may have to hand over the role of recruitment to an independent third party; or a researcher investigating their own discovery in a clinical trial may have to hand data analysis over to a third party; and a researcher who has ties to industry may not be allowed by journals to write editorials or review articles. The NHMRC has detailed guidelines on the management of conflicts of interest on guideline panels. The emphasis is on transparency in disclosure, independent NHMRC consideration of the significance of any disclosures, and having a working party chair who has no conflicts of interest [47].

Importantly, as Komesaroff et al. note:

> Whatever the chosen course of action, it is important that the assessments and decisions are recognised as ethical judgments made by relevant groups of stakeholders engaging in reflective dialogues about the social consequences of values [26].

Prevention

Critics of industry have argued that even the most stringent management strategies are not sufficient, and that conflicts of interest should be prevented or eliminated entirely by disengaging from industry. Strategies for doing so are discussed in the next section.

9.4.2 Other approaches to managing industry influence

Research and publication

A number of strategies have been instituted to try to minimise undue industry influence over research. These include expanded government and NGO funding for research (such as the Drugs for Neglected Diseases initiative—DNDi [65]), formation of public–private partnerships [66], taxing industry to create research funds [67], registration of all clinical trials (in part so that publication bias can be detected) [68], prohibiting the use of ghost writers (industry authors who are not listed or acknowledged) and 'guest authors' (academics who put their names to papers without having contributed significantly to research) [69], ensuring unrestricted access to data [70], and having data analysed and manuscripts prepared by independent academics [71].

Independent medical education and clinical practice

A relatively straightforward step for practitioners to reduce the influence of product promotion (and also conflict of interest) is to simply choose not to see pharmaceutical representatives or participate in industry-funded CME. However, the educational benefit of CPD conducted by industry and representative visits can be valuable to maintain currency, and as a practical matter it is relied on by many practitioners. In this regard, it is important to note that there are independent sources of information available. For example, the Cochrane Collaboration database is a highly regarded and readily available source of evidence-based reviews of treatments for many common medical conditions (https://www.cochrane.org).

Numerous policies have been generated by industry, professional organisations, or clinical or educational institutions that restrict interactions between clinicians and industry. These include rules about drug representatives, distribution of industry-created materials, gifts, samples, off-label promotion, sponsorship of educational programs, contact with students and trainee doctors, and so on. There are also grassroots initiatives aimed at limiting industry interactions, such as the No Advertising Please initiative [72].

9.4.3 Education about industry influence and conflicts of interest

Education of medical students and early-career doctors about the marketing techniques of industry and their influence (especially their unconscious influence) is essential to facilitate early identification of potentially difficult ethical situations and reflection and judgement on methods to manage conflicts when they arise. Education in its broadest sense includes much more than lectures; it should encompass good role modelling, including limiting and disclosing interactions. The Australian Medical Students' Association [38] states that all doctors should 'be open and transparent with members and medical students about all sponsorship received' and that medical schools are responsible for 'educating medical students about issues around industry interaction including the role of pharmaceutical companies in Australia, laws and guidelines on industry interaction, and the influence of marketing strategies.'

Professional colleges, such as the Royal Australasian College of Physicians, have also developed educational resources to help trainees and members understand the implications of industry interactions and manage them [73].

Summary

Interactions between health professionals and health-related industries are a reality of contemporary medical practice and may generate positive outcomes for patients and health systems. However, these interactions may have both benefits and risks, and clinicians need to be alert to these, and make informed decisions about how they will conduct themselves. Rules and policies provide some constraints, but there will always be a need for reflection and judgement. Ultimately, clinicians need to manage interactions in a manner that preserves public trust, protects the integrity of the profession and scientific endeavour, ensures the best interests of patients and promotes public wellbeing.

References

1. Medical Board of Australia. Good medical practice: a code of conduct for doctors in Australia. 2020. https://www.medicalboard.gov.au/codes-guidelines-policies/code-of-conduct.aspx (accessed May 2025).
2. MTPConnect, Australia's Clinical Trials Sector. 2021. https://www.mtpconnect.org.au/images/MTPConnect_2021_AustraliasClinicalTrialsSectorReport.pdf (accessed May 2025).
3. Elliott C. White coat, black hat: adventures on the dark side of medicine. Boston: Beacon Press 2010.
4. Dubois J, Kraus EM, Mikulec AA, et al. A humble task: restoring virtue in an age of conflicted interests. *Acad Med* 2013; 88: 924–928.
5. Somerset M, Weiss M, Fahey T, et al. Dramaturgical study of meetings between general practitioners and representatives of pharmaceutical companies. *BMJ* 2001; 323: 1481–1484.
6. Roughhead EE, Harvey KJ, Gilbert AL. Commercial detailing techniques used by pharmaceutical representatives to influence prescribing. *Aust N Z J Med* 1998; 28: 306–310.
7. Kesselheim AS. Drug company gifts to medical students: the hidden curriculum. *BMJ* 2013; 346: f1113.
8. Schwartz LM, Woloshin S. Medical marketing in the United States, 1997–2016. *JAMA* 2019; 321: 80–96.
9. Korn D, Carlat D. Conflicts of interest in medical education. Recommendation from the Pew Task Force on medical conflicts of interest. *JAMA* 2013; 310: 2397–2398.
10. Fugh-Berman A. Industry-funded medical education is always promotion—an essay by Adriane Fugh-Berman. *BMJ* 2021; 373: n1273.
11. Kerridge I. Pharmaceutical industry support for continuing medical education: is it time to disengage? *J Paediatr Child Health*. 2011; 47: 690–692.
12. Australian Medical Association. Doctors' relationships with industry. 2018. https://www.ama.com.au/position-statement/doctors-relationships-industry-2018 (accessed May 2025).
13. American Medical Student Association. Evidence and recommendations for a model pharmfree curriculum. https://amsa.org/wp-content/uploads/2015/03/ModelPharmFreeCurriculum.pdf (accessed May 2025).
14. Price SM, O'Donoghue AC, Rizzo R, et al. What influences healthcare providers' prescribing decisions: results from a national survey. *Res Social Adm Pharm*. 2021; 17: 1770–1779.
15. Donohue JM et al. Influence of peer networks on physician adoption of new drugs. *PLoS ONE* 2018; 13: e0204826.
16. Moses H, Matheson DHM, Cairns-Smith S, et al. The anatomy of medical research: US and international comparisons. *JAMA* 2015; 313: 174–189.
17. Moynihan R, Bero L, Hill S, et al. Pathways to independence: towards producing and using trustworthy evidence. *BMJ* 2019; 367: i6576.
18. Akl EA, Khamis AM. The intersections of industry with the health research enterprise. *Health Res Policy Syst* 2019; 17: 53.
19. Fabbri A, Parker L, Colombo C, et al. Industry funding of patient and health consumer organisations: systematic review with meta-analysis. *BMJ* 2020; 368: i6925.
20. Medicines Australia. Code of conduct. Edition 19. https://www.medicinesaustralia.com.au/code/about-the-code/code-of-conduct-current-edition (accessed May 2025).
21. Medicines Australia. Disclosure Australia database. https://www.disclosureaustralia.com.au (accessed May 2025).
22. Parker L, Karanges EA, Bero L. Changes in the type and amount of spending disclosed by Australian pharmaceutical companies: an observational study. *BMJ Open* 2019; 9: e024928.
23. Fabbri A, Grundy Q, Mintzes B, et al. A cross-sectional analysis of pharmaceutical industry-funded events for health professionals in Australia. BMJ Open 2017; 7: e016701.
24. National Health and Medical Research Council, Australian Research Council, Universities Australia. Australian code for the responsible conduct of research. 2018. https://www.nhmrc.gov.au/research-policy/research-integrity/2018-Australian-Code-Responsible-Conduct-Research (accessed May 2025).
25. National Health and Medical Research Council. Disclosure of interests and management of conflicts of interest: a guide supporting the *Australian Code for the Responsible Conduct of Research*. 2019. https://www.nhmrc.gov.au/file/14503/download?token=YtUTSjW4 (accessed May 2025).
26. Komesaroff PA, Kerridge I, Lipworth W. Conflicts of interest: new thinking, new processes. *Intern Med J* 2019; 49: 574–577.

27. Ghinea N, Wiersma M, Kerridge I, et al. Are my religious beliefs anyone's business? a framework for declarations in health and biomedicine. *J Med Ethics* 2020; 47: 803–806.
28. Wiersma M, Kerridge I, Lipworth W. Status, respect and stigma: a qualitative study of non-financial interests in medicine. *J Bioethic Inq 2020*; 17: 203–216.
29. Wiersma M, Kerridge I, Lipworth W. Dangers of neglecting non-financial conflicts of interest in health and medicine. *J Med Ethics* 2018; 44: 319–322.
30. Wiersma M, Kerridge I, Lipworth W, et al. Should we try to manage non-financial interests? *BMJ* 2018; 361: k1240.
31. Mauss, M. The gift: the form and reason for exchange in archaic societies. London: Routledge, 2002 (first published 1925).
32. Titmuss R. The gift relationship: from human blood to social policy. London: Allen and Unwin, 1970.
33. Dana J, Lowenstein G. A social science perspective on gifts to physicians from industry. *JAMA* 2003; 290: 252–255.
34. MacNeill PM, Kerridge IH, Henry DA, et al. Giving and receiving of gifts between pharmaceutical companies and medical specialists in Australia. *Intern Med J* 2006; 36: 571–578.
35. Sah S, Loewenstein G. Effect of reminders of personal sacrifice and suggested rationalisations on residents' self-reported willingness to accept gifts. *JAMA* 2010; 304: 1204–1211.
36. Keys T, Ryan MH, Dobie S et al. Premedical student exposure to pharmaceutical marketing: too much too soon? *Fam Med* 2019; 51: 722–727.
37. Brown SR and Fugh-Berman A. Changing pharmaceutical industry interaction in US Family Medicine Residencies: a CERA study. *J Am Board Fam Med* 2021; 34: 105–112.
38. Australian Medical Students' Association. Pharmaceutical financing and relationship with industry policy. 2022. https://amsa.org.au/wp-content/uploads/2023/10/Pharmaceutical-Financing-and-Relationship-with-Industry-2022.pdf (accessed May 2025).
39. Fickweiler F, Fickweiler W, Urbach E. Interactions between physicians and the pharmaceutical industry generally, and sales representatives specifically and their association with physicians' attitudes and prescribing habits: a systematic review. *BMJ Open* 2017; 7: e016408.
40. Brax H, Fadlallah R, Al-Khaled L, et al. Association between physicians' interactions with pharmaceutical companies and their clinical practices: a systematic review and meta-analysis. *PLoS ONE* 2017; 12: e0175493.
41. Spurling GK, Mansfield PR, Montgomery BD, et al. Information from pharmaceutical companies and the quality, quantity and cost of physicians' prescribing: a systematic review. *PLoS Medicine* 2010; 7: e1000352.
42. Mitchell AP, Trivedi NU, Gennarelli RL, et al. Are financial payments from the pharmaceutical industry associated with physician prescribing? A systematic review. *Ann Intern Med* 2021; 174: 353–61.
43. Lundh A, Lexchin J, Mintzes B, et al. Industry sponsorship and research outcome. *Cochrane Database Syst Rev* 2017; 2: MR000033.
44. Fabbri A, Lai A, Grundy Q, et al. The influence of industry sponsorship on the research agenda: a scoping review. *Am J Public Health* 2018; 108: e9–e16.
45. Ahn R, Woodbridge A, Abraham A, et al. Financial ties of principal investigators and randomised controlled trial outcomes: cross sectional study. *BMJ* 2017; 356: i6770.
46. Henry DA, Hill SR, Doran E, et al. Medical specialists and pharmaceutical industry-sponsored research: a survey of the Australian experience. *Med J Aust* 2005; 182: 557–560.
47. National Health and Medical Research Council. Identifying and managing conflicts of interest. In Guidelines for guidelines handbook. 2018. https://www.nhmrc.gov.au/guidelinesforguidelines/plan/identifying-and-managing-conflicts-interest#toc__69 (accessed May 2025).
48. Nejstgaard CH, Bero L, Hróbjartsson A, et al. Association between conflicts of interest and favourable recommendations in clinical guidelines, advisory committee reports, opinion pieces, and narrative reviews: systematic review *BMJ* 2020; 371: m4234.
49. American Psychiatric Association. Diagnostic and statistical manual of mental disorders.5th ed. Arlington, VA: American Psychiatric Publishing, 2013.
50. Cosgrove L, Wheeler EE. Industry's colonization of psychiatry: ethical and practical implications of financial conflicts of interest in the DSM-5. *Fem Psychol* 2013; 23: 93–106.
51. Kanter GP. US nationwide disclosure of industry payments and public trust in physicians. *JAMA Netw Open* 2019; 2: e191947.

52. Macneill PU, Kerridge IH, Newby D, et al. Attitudes of physicians and public to pharmaceutical industry 'gifts'. *Intern Med J* 2010; 40: 335–341.
53. Green MJ, Masters R, James B, et al. Do gifts from the pharmaceutical industry affect trust in physicians? *Fam Med* 2012; 44: 325–331.
54. Medical Technology Association of Australia. Medical technology industry code of practice. Edition 13. 2023. https://www.mtaa.org.au/sites/default/files/uploaded-content/field_f_content_file/medical_technology_industry_code_of_practice_edition_13_2023.pdf (accessed May 2025).
55. Association of the British Pharmaceutical Industry. Ethical Standards in Health & Life Sciences Group. Healthcare community agree on principles for working together to improve patient health. 2012.
56. Hawkes N. Lancet withdraws support of document on collaboration between doctors and drug industry. *BMJ* 2013; 346: f770.
57. Rogers W, Zutlevics T, Raven M, et al. Guidance offers little in the way of ethics or transparency. *BMJ* 2012; 344: e2910.
58. Universities Australia. Clever collaborations: the strong business case for partnering with universities. 2019. https://www.universitiesaustralia.edu.au/wp-content/uploads/2019/06/Clever-Collaborations-FINAL.pdf (accessed May 2025).
59. Austrade. Australia: a go-to destination for clinical trials. 2022.http://www.austrade.gov.au/ArticleDocuments/2814/Clincal-Trials-Capability-Report.pdf.aspx (accessed May 2025).
60. Smith E. Toward a postmodernist view of conflict of interest. *J Bioeth Inq* 2012; 9: 223–224.
61. Rifkind AB. Competing interests: expanding rapidly. *Nature* 2012; 488: 590–591.
62. Loewenstein G, Sah S, Cain DM. The unintended consequences of conflict of interest disclosure. *JAMA* 2012; 307: 669–670;
63. Komesaroff P. Disclosure forms: what is revealed about the Emperor's clothes? *Intern Med J* 2011; 41: 297–298.
64. Isaacs D. Conflict of interest: no such thing as a free lunch. *J Paediatr Child Health* 2011; 47: 679–680.
65. Drugs for neglected diseases initiative. https://dndina.org/about/ (accessed May 2025).
66. Aerts C, Sunyoto T, Tediosi F, Sicuri E. Are public-private partnerships the solution to tackle neglected tropical diseases? a systematic review of the literature. *Health Pol* 2017;121: 745–754.
67. The Italian Medicines Agency Research and Development Working group. Feasibility and challenges of independent research on drugs: the Italian Medicines Agency (AIFA) experience. *Eur J Clin Invest* 2010; 40: 69–86.
68. Australian Clinical Trials. https://www.australianclinicaltrials.gov.au (accessed May 2025).
69. Ghost, guest, or gift authorship in a submitted manuscript. https://publicationethics.org/resources/flowcharts/ghost-guest-gift-authorship-submitted-manuscript (accessed May 2025).
70. Packer M. Data sharing in medical research *BMJ* 2018; 360: k510.
71. Fisher MR, Roecker EB, DeMets EL. The role of an independent statistical analysis center in the industry-modified National Institutes of Health model. *Ther Innov Regul Sci* 2001; 35: 115–129.
72. Coopes A. Australian campaign aims to stop visits from drug representatives. *BMJ* 2014; 349: g6183.
73. Royal Australasian College of Physicians. Guidelines for ethical relationships between health professionals and industry. 2018. https://www.racp.edu.au/fellows/ethical-guidelines (accessed May 2025).

Further reading

Carl E. White coat black hat: adventures on the dark side of medicine. Boston: Beacon Press, 2010.

Komesaroff PA, Kerridge I, Lipworth W. Conflicts of interest: new thinking, new processes. *Intern Med J* 2019; 49: 574–577.

Lo B, Field MJ, editors. Conflict of interest in medical research, education, and practice. Washington, DC: National Academies Press, 2009.

Royal Australasian College of Physicians. Guidelines for ethical relationships between health professionals and industry. 4th edition. 2018. https://www.racp.edu.au/fellows/ethical-guidelines.

10 Continuing professional development

Richard Doherty

Introduction

The concepts underpinning continuing professional development (CPD) are familiar to virtually every medical practitioner. It is very evident that knowledge and practice changes over time and that some form of continuous learning and evolution of practice is a fundamental part of medical practice and a key professional responsibility for medical practitioners (see Chapter 2, On being a good doctor: the changing face of medical professionalism). Despite this, the role and place of CPD remain somewhat contested, particularly among some practitioners who have watched it appear and change in Australia over the last few decades. The profession remains uncertain about the necessary or desirable elements of CPD and sceptical about the effectiveness of various activities. This chapter provides an introduction to the requirements for CPD that must be completed each year for ongoing registration as a medical practitioner. It also summarises the key evidence underlying the effectiveness of CPD, both within the medical profession and in other professions, and the activities that provide the most benefit for maintaining professional competence.

10.1 Continuing professional development requirements for ongoing registration as a medical practitioner

As with virtually all other professions, participation in a formal CPD program has become a formal requirement for renewal of registration in all Western medical regulatory systems. Since 2010, Australian medical practitioners have been required to confirm their participation in CPD at the time of each annual renewal of registration. The Medical Board of Australia has set a CPD standard which was revised in 2022 for implementation partially in 2023 and fully in 2024 [1]. Chapter 21, Regulation of the medical profession, provides a summary of the regulatory role of the board in section 21.2.1.

The activities currently included in CPD have evolved over the last few decades. The most notable change has been a shift in focus from continuing medical education (CME), which tends to be passive and involves 'being taught' by reading journals or attending traditional lectures, often sponsored by industry (see Chapter 9, Doctors, industry and conflicts of interest), to a broader, more active concept of professional development. In addition, the range of activities considered appropriate to be included in CPD has widened to include more active learning, review of performance and issues such as cultural safety (see Chapter 17, Culturally safe health care for Aboriginal and/or Torres Strait Islander peoples) as well as individual medical specialist knowledge. At the same time, evidence has been collected to demonstrate the effectiveness of CPD at several levels [2], although possibly not yet demonstrating an effect on individual clinical outcomes or community-wide indicators.

Formal and informal surveys of Australian medical practitioners suggest that accessibility and convenience are strong factors in determining the choice of professional learning activity with lectures, seminars and conferences all rated highly. There has traditionally been a bias towards individual activity rather than learning in teams or social groups, and favoured activities often tend to require only passive engagement of the practitioner. Unless mandated, reviews of performance or measurement of outcomes do not form a prominent part of the CPD activities of most Australian medical practitioners. It is also relevant to note, however, that many practitioners see CPD as an imposed requirement which is separate from their normal professional role and do not recognise that many of the activities they perform in their ordinary work contribute strongly to learning and professional development [3] and are bona fide elements of CPD.

The challenge now for regulators is to develop models for CPD which engage practitioners so that they plan and undertake CPD activities which are integrated into their professional roles, that use learning methods that are more likely to be effective and which they may already be doing, rather than discrete additional requirements. The CPD program needs to encourage practitioners to use various forms of data and information to reflect on their performance in their role and the outcomes of their work, and to develop further knowledge, skills and behaviours in a planned fashion. It is central to this challenge that any effective model allows practitioners to feel that their CPD activity is authentic in both content and type of activity and results in benefit to their professional role.

10.2 Professional development outside the medical profession

The most comprehensive body of research into professional development addresses its role in the teaching profession and the effectiveness of professional development in teachers. Garet et al. [4] drew attention to the features of professional development which were perceived by teachers to be effective, including the role of active learning and coherence with other learning activities. The authors concluded that '(a) the form of the activity (e.g. workshop vs study group); (b) collective participation of teachers from the same school, grade, or subject; and (c) the duration of the activity' significantly affected teacher learning.

This issue has been reviewed comprehensively by Webster-Wright, who challenged the traditional view that any learning must have an element of supervision or external direction associated with it [5]. In contrast, the concept of continuous professional learning as the self-directed and targeted learning of practising professionals is a more appropriate way to describe effective learning behaviour. This provides a way to avoid a false dichotomy between learning situated within practice and the formal events conducted outside normal work which are more typical of traditional views of CPD. It also allows explicitly for inclusion of a wide range of activities in the learning portfolio of a practising professional [5]. Furthermore, it addresses a criticism of CPD requirements linked to professional registration of educators which is also often raised in the medical profession: 'few states award credit for the types of professional development educators most value—job-embedded, team-based, and collaborative learning' [6].

10.3 Professional development within the medical profession

10.3.1 The terminology of continued learning and professional development

Continuing education and professional development of medical practitioners around the world occurs in many forms. The terms used can be confusing, and they are not defined consistently between jurisdictions.

CME was probably the earliest term used and most commonly refers to development activities focused on expanding the knowledge base of a doctor's scope of practice. In its simplest form, this can be passive, without reflection on deficiencies in knowledge or on the impact of any educational activity. Many ongoing professional learning programs in medicine were introduced as CME in both name and format, and the term is often still used generically long after program requirements have evolved to include other components. Despite all subsequent developments, adequate and current content knowledge remains a key part of medical competence or fitness to practise and contemporary CPD programs generally provide for a substantial amount of this in a CPD portfolio.

Recognition that a practitioner's overall performance involves components additional to content knowledge led to the emergence of the concept of CPD [2]. While a multitude of individual (and sometimes idiosyncratic) definitions for CPD have been published, the registration of Australian health practitioners involves adherence to a formal standard which provides a clear articulation of the dimensions of CPD which are additional to traditional CME: 'CPD is how health practitioners maintain, improve and broaden their knowledge, expertise and competence, and develop the personal and professional qualities required throughout their professional lives' [7].

10.3.2 Evidence of effectiveness of continuing professional development

Studies evaluating the effectiveness of continuing education in the professions have been reported since 1977 and are well reviewed in several reports including some updated systematic reviews [2,8]. These have evaluated the evidence for the effectiveness of continuing education in a range of healthcare settings, mostly in primary care medicine but also in dental and nursing practice. Despite the (acknowledged) variability in the educational activities involved in the studies reviewed, the authors concluded that CME was at least moderately effective in improving both the performance of practitioners and patient outcomes. In 2015, Cervero and Gaines noted that the effect on practitioner performance was more positive than the effect on patient outcomes [2]. They concluded also that:

> the eight systematic reviews support previous research showing CME activities that are more interactive, use more methods, involve multiple exposures, are longer, and are focused on outcomes that are considered important by physicians lead to more positive outcomes [2].

The impact of the format of the educational activity has been investigated in a wide range of studies. Much of the available literature examines the acceptability to practitioners of individual activities rather than the elements which together comprise an effective CPD program. It seems entirely logical that optimal activities to be included in a CPD portfolio will differ between specialty groups, although the elements of traditional CME, such as lectures, may show little difference between groups. Programs in a range of health professions have traditionally focused on tallying hours spent in activity or used a points system to record inputs, but are increasingly moving towards requiring documentation of outputs such as completion of learning plans, quality improvement activities and audits [9]. Introducing elements which require active participation and reflection will assist programs develop a focus on outcomes. Cervero and Gaines note that a wide range of CPD activities were included in the studies reviewed and that there was little consistency between studies in this respect. This did not change their eventual conclusion regarding the overall effectiveness of CPD [2].

Some newer approaches to professional learning may be effective as part of CPD programs. These include competency-based medical education, which is based on outcomes of practitioner proficiency, and entrustable professional activities (EPAs), which frame learning around components of work. These newer techniques are being implemented at multiple levels of medical education. They have been proposed as possible components of CPD programs because they are likely to conform to the model of an optimal continuing professional learning activity. Sargeant et al. envisaged competency-based CPD placing 'health needs and patient outcomes at the centre of a CPD system that will be guided by a set of competencies to enhance the quality of practice and the safety of the health system' [10]. In developing an agenda for ongoing research into the role and effectiveness of EPAs in medical education, Ten Cate et al. discuss how EPAs 'could serve as the framework to support continuing learning and skill development to achieve higher levels of proficiency and mastery' [11]. They postulate a role for them for practitioners at the early stage of independent practice as well as for mid- and late-career practitioners, who need to show maintenance of existing skills as well as learning new skills [11].

EPAs as a means of demonstrating competence at any level of practice offer considerable face validity and are clearly set within the workplace, easily aligned to scope of practice and focused on development or maintenance of key skills and attributes. On the other hand, one underlying feature of EPAs is that they typically involve formal assessment through observation of performance, an aspect which might limit acceptability in many CPD settings.

A number of Australasian specialty colleges (e.g. Australian and New Zealand College of Anaesthetists and Royal Australian College of General Practitioners [RACGP]) already include competency-based elements in their CPD programs as a means of ensuring ongoing competence in emergency responses [12] or basic life support [13].

10.3.3 Continuing professional development in international settings

Depending on the regulatory setting, CPD as a term is used to describe programs which are limited to content knowledge as well as to others which involve specific requirements of planning, review and data collection. In some jurisdictions, more complex programs have been developed in which strictly defined CME or CPD becomes just one component. These are commonly known by other terms, such as revalidation, recertification and maintenance of competence (MOC).

In 2011, the UK's General Medical Council released a comprehensive review of international CPD systems [14]. The review assessed the CPD programs of some 30 countries across Europe, Asia, North America and Australasia and provides an interesting perspective on the wide variation in regulatory requirements across these regions. One key observation is that CPD and related programs everywhere undergo continuous change with evolution, revision and adaptation as constant features. It was noted that programs are voluntary in some settings but compulsory in others and that the activity required ranges from a few hours of typical CME to more comprehensive programs with multiple components. The model in which a national or regional regulator sets the standards for CPD while specialist colleges and professional associations provide supporting advice and templates for their members is acknowledged, but many variants exist.

The Medical Council of New Zealand's CPD program is integral to its process for annual re-registration of doctors, termed 'recertification' by the Council. In its updated form, the Council provides explicit guidance for doctors depending on their registration status [15]. One of the central features of the program for doctors registered in a general scope of practice (i.e. not recognised as specialists or in prevocational or training programs) is the requirement for regular practice review (RPR) by peers. This involves pre- and post-visit activity as well as observation of practice and review of records and clinical reasoning among other things. A long-term evaluation of the practice review program was completed in 2019 [16] and included qualitative feedback from the reviewed doctors. It concluded that RPR helped many doctors to identify and act on areas of practice that could be improved. The evaluation also concluded that RPR was likely to be improving the quality of care, although data on patient outcomes were not available. A peer review program based on practice visits has also been implemented in Aotearoa New Zealand for some specialists (most notably orthopaedic surgeons). Recertification as implemented in Aotearoa New Zealand describes a very different model compared to the one in place in the US [17].

The approach to renewal of certification, professional development and demonstration of currency of knowledge and skills has evolved significantly in the US over the past 50 years. In the early 1990s, the American Board of Medical Specialties (ABMS) widened a program previously only required of family medicine practitioners. As a result, all medical graduates who were board certified from 1990 onwards in one of the specialties under the ABMS banner now need to pass a comprehensive test of their contemporary knowledge of their specialty at set intervals after their initial certification [18]. For example, in internal medicine this is now an eight-hour multiple choice examination which must be taken every 10 years. This process of recertification by periodic examination was expanded further by the introduction of requirements for the documentation of patient outcomes and provision of evidence from peer assessment and patient satisfaction surveys. These additional requirements are known as MOC requirements [18]. While not usually required for registration with state regulatory boards, recertification is normally required for renewal of hospital appointments and thus has effectively become compulsory. To complicate matters, state medical boards usually have separate CME requirements for registrants which require additional activity and documentation.

Widespread dissatisfaction with the ABMS recertification requirements (based on cost, allegations of conflict of interest and lack of evidence of efficacy) led to the emergence of an alternative group, the American Board of Physician Specialties (ABPS), which offers recertification programs at reduced cost and without the MOC requirement [19]. In response to criticism of its complex program, the ABMS has recently introduced a series of revisions to its MOC recertification program, including removal of some of the requirements for review of physician performance and the introduction of a more interactive longitudinal assessment process. This longitudinal knowledge assessment program is delivered over two years every five years as an alternative to the 10-year recertification exam. It nevertheless remains a test of currency of medical knowledge rather than an assessment of performance in practice. Both ABMS and ABPS programs allow little room for practitioners to focus their professional learning on their actual scopes of practice but rather emphasise currency with the broad contemporary knowledge base relevant to each specialty.

In the UK, a much more comprehensive program to ensure fitness and currency of doctors has been implemented under the banner of revalidation [20]. In 2012, the UK General Medical Council (GMC) introduced a formal program of revalidation for medical practitioners seeking to renew or retain their practising certificate. This came after a very long period of gestation and was at least partly in response to significant events such as the conviction of Harold Shipman for murdering patients and the conclusion of a GMC investigation into the Paediatric Cardiac Surgery Unit at Bristol Royal Infirmary. In its 2019 online advice to doctors, the GMC describes revalidation as 'an evaluation of your fitness to practise' and specifies that the process supports doctors to develop or improve, 'gives patients confidence that doctors are up to date with their practice' and 'promotes improved quality of care' [20].

Two key features of the British medical system inform this process: the separation of being listed on the medical register from being licensed to practice and the overarching role of the National Health Service (NHS) in providing governance and the necessary infrastructure to support the program.

The GMC requires doctors to undergo revalidation every five years and makes revalidation decisions in the great majority of cases on the basis of the recommendation by each practitioner's responsible officer (usually a service medical director or similar senior doctor). The central activity of revalidation is an annual appraisal at which each practitioner provides details of their practice to their responsible officer. These include:

- details of all practice activities as well as voluntary clinical work and nonclinical activity
- involvement in significant events
- whether complaints have been made
- whether there have been concerns about fitness to practise
- whether practice has been restricted by the GMC or employer.

In addition, doctors are expected to collect and reflect on a range of supporting information including CPD activity, quality improvement activity, feedback from patients and colleagues and details of complaints and compliments. Online portfolios to assist doctors preparing for revalidation are provided to members of specialty colleges and allow easy collection of the information needed for the formal revalidation exercise every five years. The support of the colleges and the structure of the NHS in supporting the appraisal process are essential elements of the implementation of the UK's program. Tazzyman and colleagues assessed the implementation of the GMC's revalidation program and found that initial scepticism about the purpose and value of revalidation lessened over time as 'participants recognised the benefits it brought to their practice' [3]. This finding was tempered by recognition that not all doctors saw that revalidation was a legitimate part of their role.

In one way, the GMC's revalidation program can be seen as a highly developed form of CPD with its set formal requirements. But its own documents specify that CPD is actually only one part of the supporting information practitioners need to provide in their appraisal and revalidation process. Apart from requiring the formation of a personal development plan and reflection on outcomes of CPD activity undertaken (as opposed to documentation of activity conducted) the GMC's guidance to doctors on CPD provides only limited detail as to the nature of acceptable CPD and does not specify an amount of time which should be devoted to CPD in each appraisal cycle.

10.4 Elements of effective continuing professional development for doctors

10.4.1 Planning and reflection in effective continuing professional development

Virtually all contemporary literature on CPD supports the use of reflection and planning in a cyclical process, and regulators such as the Medical Board of Australia explicitly require doctors to participate in a reflective CPD program [1]. The original concepts of reflective practice are attributed primarily to Donald Schön, who proposed a model of intuitive 'reflection in action' [21], and John Dewey, whose 1933 model involved a more methodologically rigorous and systematic process of consideration of all possible options [22]. The inclusion of reflection and reflective practice in professional learning programs has become so widely accepted as to be essentially ubiquitous.

Despite critical examination of the concepts of reflective models (e.g. Hébert [23]), the idea that a medical practitioner should think carefully about where they might or should direct their efforts in continuing professional learning makes sense at the simplest level, and the term 'reflection' fits this activity well in the ordinary sense of the word. The Medical Board of Australia has stipulated the preparation of an annual professional development plan for which most specialty colleges have provided templates or guidance for participants. At a practical level, the 'plan' and 'study' stages of a traditional quality cycle can be used to provide a framework for reflection and offer the additional benefit of providing for inclusion of clinical experience, practice data, feedback or other information in the process. The use of plan-do-study-act (PDSA) cycles in CPD has been considered by a number of authors as a fundamental tool in quality improvement exercises. Picarillo [24] offers an overview of the model for improvement developed by the Institute for Health Improvement (IHI), in which a range of tools and methods have been adopted from manufacturing [25]. The IHI model uses a process of analysis and planning to feed into a PDSA cycle, which in turn further informs the assessment of outcomes achieved.

10.4.2 What is considered a continuing professional development activity?

One of the consistent themes which emerged from the Medical Board of Australia's 2021 public consultation on its proposed changes to the CPD standard for Australian doctors was the view expressed that CPD (often termed CME by respondents) was something distinct from normal practice, opportunistic rather than planned in terms of the topic, usually done after hours and thus intrusive of personal time and incurring a cost to the practitioner. Conversely, effective CPD is increasingly understood to be embedded in practice, to involve interaction rather than passive attendance and to be directed deliberately towards improved quality of care.

The Medical Board of Australia has introduced the concept of CPD 'homes' into the CPD standard which became fully implemented on 1 January 2024 [1]. In this model, the homes stipulate the formal requirements of a CPD program which complies with the board's new standard and provide the means by which participants can document compliance. The requirements must meet 'high level' minimum standards set by the accredited training college for each specialty. Although most homes are postgraduate medical colleges, the initiative provides for other organisations to offer CPD programs, and at the time of writing, five non-college CPD homes have been accredited. The extent to which homes offer CPD content in addition to providing the structure of the program is expected to vary considerably. Colleges have provided guidance to fellows via comprehensive CPD handbooks which detail the types of activities which meet program requirements (the CPD handbooks and frameworks published by Australasian colleges are available electronically; examples include Australian College of Rural and Remote Medicine [ACRRM] [26], Royal Australasian College of Physicians [27] and RACGP [28]).

Although it is unsurprising that recognised activities vary widely between specialties or scopes of practice even within a single college, common elements include the provision of templates for developing personal development plans, conducting audits, seeking patient feedback and undertaking peer review. At the same time, dividing CPD activities into specific categories is a common technique in both regulatory and member organisation–based programs. This allows recognition of a very wide range of activities, from attendance at international conferences to conduct of planned quality improvement projects and participation in formal degree courses, to peer group case discussions. Further, segregating activities on the basis of levels of engagement and interactivity allows organisations to allocate higher value to some activities. This obviously requires a framework which tallies more than hours of participation. The Medical Board of Australia's framework for implementation in 2024 requires that practitioners distribute activity over three categories: educational activities, measuring performance and measuring outcomes, and has set minimum time requirements for activity in each of the three categories [1].

Simulation activities have been incorporated into CPD programs in a number of ways (e.g. in competency-focused activities described above) and can be seen as an exemplar of CPD activity because of the active engagement, skill development, opportunity for feedback and collegial approach involved. Dort et al. reported the evolution of a formal simulation-based training program in surgery in response to the COVID-19 pandemic among other things [29]. In their model, telementoring allows participants to learn new surgical techniques in a high-fidelity setting over one day or less. The process of training the mentors and faculty involved in the exercise would of course be an effective form of professional development for those practitioners.

The Royal College of Physicians and Surgeons of Canada (RCPSC) administers a CPD program, which is referred to as a MOC program. Participation in the MOC program is required for renewal of Fellowship of the college. College guidelines include explicit details of compliant activities and the credit associated with each activity [30]. Fellows are required to log activity from each of three categories: group learning, self-learning and assessment. This latter category includes both knowledge and performance assessment options and a wide range of acceptable activities are listed in each of the three categories. Fellows have access to an ePortfolio which standardises documentation of activity. As noted below, a number of organisations have been accredited by the RCPSC to provide simulation-based CPD programs.

Chorley et al. reported their experience with redesigning the CPD offering for emergency medicine physicians in Hamilton, Ontario, following falling participation rates in a traditional rounds- and conference-based program [31]. They used a formal design thinking method in association with a prior analysis of the needs and experiences of the region's emergency doctors and generated five key pillars of a program for further development. These were:

1. simulation/procedural learning
2. asynchronous learning (including online and podcast resources)
3. synchronous learning (with emphasis on small group discussion)
4. community connections (within the craft group)
5. individual experiences such as coaching and mentorship.

In essence, this redeveloped program plan incorporates desirable elements by being collegial, team focused and embedded in practice, and offering review and feedback on performance. Additionally, it recognises the opportunities presented by technology and social media through use of online services such as podcasts and private messaging platforms. Although their model is still to be implemented, it is worth noting that the reflection and planning involved had been conducted at the program level. The model would also be highly amenable to planning of activities at both team and individual levels at the point of delivery.

Practitioners in nonclinical scopes of practice such as public health, medical administration or medical research have expressed concern about how their needs can be met by CPD programs that focus on elements such as practice outcomes and feedback from patients. In the Australian setting, nonclinical fields of practice which are recognised as specialties by the Medical Board of Australia have been able to use the resources of their respective colleges to develop appropriate guidelines and materials. The situation is perhaps less clear for a medical researcher who wishes to retain registration and, for example, the right to prescribe. The board's revised standard requires such practitioners to nominate a CPD home appropriate for the field of practice in which they seek registration. Given that the outcomes of research inevitably involve rigorous peer review at several levels, it seems logical that at least some work-embedded CPD could be acknowledged.

10.4.3 Accreditation and approval in continuing professional development

Accreditation processes appear at two levels in the development and delivery of CPD programs: first, in accreditation of the objectives, structure and processes of a program; and second, in the accreditation of specific providers or activities being made available to participants in those programs. Both examples are evident in the Australian CPD environment and both work to ensure that the CPD programs and activities offered to participants are fit for purpose.

Specialist medical colleges are accredited by the Medical Board of Australia for the purpose of training practitioners who are then permitted to use the specialist title matching the training program completed. The CPD program for each college is reviewed as part of the periodic accreditation review conducted by the assigned accreditation agency, the Australian Medical Council (AMC) [32]. This level of accreditation ensures that each college offers its fellows a CPD program which complies with the Medical Board of Australia's registration standard. With the introduction of CPD homes into the Australian regulatory model, the AMC has been assigned responsibility for accreditation of these organisations as well. A consistent standard for both college homes and non-college CPD homes has been developed by the AMC. As noted previously, the Medical Council of New Zealand maintains its own standard for recertification [15] and similarly accredits CPD programs offered by Australasian colleges with transnational membership.

Accreditation of CPD resources or activities is a well-established model for ensuring quality of offerings. Canada's RCPSC publishes on its website the standards for accreditation as a CPD provider [33]. These require a level of institutional governance, program maturity and resourcing which are assessed formally. Successful accreditation allows the provider to develop resources and to offer these to RCPSC fellows. The accredited providers are largely either medical school offices of CME or national medical specialty organisations.

In the US, the Accreditation Council for Continuing Medical Education (ACCME) is a not-for-profit organisation founded in 1981 whose members represent the spectrum of medical education and training, medical practice, specialty certification and medical regulation. The ACCME offers standards-based accreditation of providers with a stated aim of realising their 'shared vision of leveraging the power of education to improve the quality of care for the patients and communities we serve' [34]. The US Federation of State Medical Boards is one of the ACCME's member organisations and, as noted previously, the state boards often have CME or CPD requirements which are additional to the specialty recertification requirements of the ABMS or ABPS.

In Australia, both the RACGP and ACRRM offer providers accreditation of specific activities and have published guidelines for their respective processes on their websites. Both colleges adjudicate suitability of the resources offered internally. The RACGP has recently streamlined its accreditation process [35] but does charge fees to providers seeking accreditation, albeit with an exception for resources addressing cultural safety and cultural awareness.

Continuing professional development as a group or team activity, a role for organisations and institutions?

Embedding CPD in the work setting is a key step in improving its effectiveness and authenticity [2,5]. There are many activities which are both part of normal practice and appropriate for recognition in expanded or strengthened CPD programs. These include team meetings that involve discussion of cases, audits of unit activity, formal morbidity and mortality meetings as well as informal discussion and mentoring. In all of these examples, professional learning may not be the primary outcome for which the events are convened, but learning and changes to practice are an inevitable secondary outcome of these activities. The learning which arises is effective because the discussions are directly relevant to the scope of practice of the individual or team and can stimulate reflection or identify deficiencies in knowledge or skills.

Use of practice or other clinical data in workplace-based quality activities such as these is widely accepted and usually afforded some degree of legal privilege. As a result, active engagement of organisations through providing access to patient data and service profiles should be seen as a key part of a future CPD environment. Such use of patient data raises issues of security, confidentiality and privacy, and the obligations of individual doctors to protect these are unchanged by their CPD requirements. Contemporary developments in health care such as electronic health records and datasets for practice analysis are likely to assist with both access to data and assurance of its security.

Summary

Synthesis of learnings from CPD research outside the medical profession and an understanding of the format and processes of modern medical care suggest that an optimal CPD program for medical practitioners should feature a series of key components. It should:

- include mechanisms where practitioners are helped to identify their blind spots or areas where their competence differs from their self-assessment
- encompass a practitioner's actual scope of practice rather than permit a focus on preferred topics
- be planned in a cycle using conclusions from reflection on previous activities, analysis of needs and using evidence gathered from that practice to inform the next plan
- address more than the knowledge and technical aspects of practice and include attention to outcomes, the use of clinical benchmarks such as practice guidelines and markers of professionalism
- be integrated into practice as much as possible to minimise the logistic impact of the activity and recognise the professional learning which is inextricably linked to practice
- accommodate the formats of contemporary practice such as unit-based or shared-care models and include, where appropriate, involvement of practitioners from other health professions
- include formal review processes such as clinical audits, quality improvement activity or case reviews, with appropriate attention to confidentiality
- attribute enhanced value to components that require active participation and include a range of different types of activity
- be collaborative and collegial
- feel authentic, relevant and of value to the practitioner and contribute to an overall improvement in the quality of care provided.

It is clear that developing a program that has these features and can be incorporated into a regulatory framework is a considerable challenge. The effort involved in documentation of activity to satisfy regulatory requirements can become a significant burden and discourage participation in a range of activities. Further, the activities that can be documented most easily, such as lectures and seminars, are usually those that do not require active engagement of participants. Achieving the cultural change that will be needed to gain wide acceptance of CPD activities which involve observation, review, assessment or receipt of feedback will also be a significant challenge to implementation of ideal models in CPD. Finding the lightest effective regulatory touch in formal requirements while encouraging CPD activity which is compliant, authentic and valued stands is a worthy goal.

References

1. Medical Board of Australia. Registration standard: continuing professional development. 2023. https://www.medicalboard.gov.au/Registration-Standards.aspx (accessed May 2025).
2. Cervero RM, Gaines JK. The impact of CME on physician performance and patient health outcomes: an updated synthesis of systematic reviews. *J Contin Educ Health Prof* 2015; 35: 131–138.
3. Tazzyman A, Ferguson J Hillier C, et al. The implementation of medical revalidation: an assessment using normalisation process theory. *BMC Health Serv Res* 2017; 17: 749.
4. Garet MS, Porter AC, Desimone L, et al. What makes professional development effective? results from a national sample of teachers. *Am Ed Res J* 2001; 38: 915–945.
5. Webster-Wright A, Reframing professional development through understanding authentic professional learning. *Rev Educ Res* 2009; 79: 702–739.
6. Procopio M. Reconsidering teacher recertification in Maryland. *The Abell Report* 2021; 34: 1–20.
7. Australian Health Practitioner Regulation Agency and National Boards. Continuing professional development. 2024. https://www.ahpra.gov.au/Registration/Registration-Standards/CPD.aspx (accessed May 2025).
8. Forsetlund L, O'Brien MA, Forsén L, et al. Continuing education meetings and workshops: effects on professional practice and healthcare outcomes. *Cochrane Database Syst Rev* 2021; 9: CD003030.
9. Bullock A, Kavadella A, Cowpe J, et al. Tackling the challenge of the impact of continuing education: an evidence synthesis charting a global, cross-professional shift away from counting hours. *Eur J Dent Educ* 2020; 24: 390–397.
10. Sargeant J, Wong BM, Campbell CM. CPD of the future: a partnership between quality improvement and competency-based education. *Med Educ* 2018; 52: 125–135.
11. Ten Cate O, Carraccio C, Damodaran A, et al. Entrustment decision making: extending Miller's pyramid. *Acad Med* 2021; 96: 199–204.
12. Australian and New Zealand College of Anaesthetists. Continuing professional development activity guide. 2024. https://www.anzca.edu.au/getContentAsset/6403fd59-f3a2-439c-81b8-510a854447ea/80feb437-d24d-46b8-a858-4a2a28b9b970/CPD-activity-guide_2025.pdf?language=en (accessed May 2025).
13. Royal Australian College of General Practitioners. CPD handbook: RACGP – your CPD home. 2022. https://www.racgp.org.au/FSDEDEV/media/documents/Handbook.pdf (accessed May 2025).
14. Murgatroyd GB, Continuing professional development: the international perspective. 2011. https://www.gmc-uk.org/-/media/documents/cpd---the-international-perspective-jul-11_pdf-44810902.pdf (accessed May 2025).
15. Medical Council of New Zealand. Recertification and professional development. https://www.mcnz.org.nz/registration/maintain-or-renew-registration/recertification-and-professional-development/ (accessed May 2025).
16. Malatest International. Evaluation of Regular Practice Review Programme: final evaluation report. 2019. https://www.mcnz.org.nz/assets/Publications/Reports/a185d7b752/Evaluation-of-RPR-final-report-August-2019.pdf (accessed May 2025).
17. Norcini J. Recertification in the United States. *BMJ* 1999; 319: 1183.
18. American Board of Medical Specialties. Why become board certified? https://www.abms.org/board-certification/getting-board-certified/ (accessed May 2025).
19. American Board of Physician Specialties. Physician Board recertification standards. www.abpsus.org/physician-board-recertification-standards/ (accessed May 2025).
20. General Medical Council. Revalidation. www.gmc-uk.org/registration-and-licensing/managing-your-registration/revalidation (accessed May 2025).
21. Schön DA, The reflective practitioner: how professionals think in action. New York: Basic Books, 1983.
22. Dewey J. How we think: a restatement of the relation of reflective thinking to the educative process. Chicago: Henry Regnery, 1933.
23. Hébert C, Knowing and/or experiencing: a critical examination of the reflective models of John Dewey and Donald Schön. *Reflective Pract* 2015; 16: 361–371.
24. Picarillo AP. Introduction to quality improvement tools for the clinician. *J Perinatol* 2018; 38: 929–935.

25. Institute for Healthcare Improvement. How to improve: model for improvement. https://www.ihi.org/resources/how-improve-model-improvement (accessed May 2025).
26. Australian College of Rural and Remote Medicine. ACRRM CPD framework. https://www.acrrm.org.au/CPDHome/cpd-framework (accessed May 2025).
27. Royal Australasian College of Physicians. My CPD framework. 2025. https://www.racp.edu.au/fellows/continuing-professional-development/2025-cpd-framework (accessed May 2025).
28. Royal Australian College of General Practitioners. CPD at the RACGP. www.racgp.org.au/education/professional-development/cpd (accessed May 2025).
29. Dort J, Paige J, Qureshi A, et al. SAGES Reimagining Education & Learning (REAL) project. *Surg Endosc* 2022; 36: 1699–1708.
30. Royal College of Physicians and Surgeons of Canada. The MOC framework. https://www.royalcollege.ca/en/cpd/moc-program/moc-framework (accessed May 2025).
31. Chorley A, Azzam K, Chan TM. Redesigning continuing professional development: harnessing design thinking to go from needs assessment to mandate. *Perspect Med Educ* 2022; 11: 121–126.
32. Australian Medical Council. Accreditation standards and procedures. https://www.amc.org.au/accredited-organisations/accreditation-standards-and-procedures/ (accessed May 2025).
33. Royal College of Physicians and Surgeons of Canada. About CPD accreditation. https://www.royalcollege.ca/en/standards-and-accreditation/cpd-accreditation.html (accessed May 2025).
34. Accreditation Council for Continuing Medical Education. https://accme.org/about-accme/mission-responsibilities/ (accessed May 2025).
35. Royal Australian College of General Practitioners. CPD program provider handbook. https://www.racgp.org.au/getattachment/bacb2f9e-0762-4c73-bad8-24bb063f06e1/Continuing-Professional-Development-CPD-Program.aspx (accessed May 2025).

11 The doctor and interprofessional relationships

Gary Rogers

Introduction

Healthcare is team work. Doctors enhance patient outcomes by working with other health practitioners to provide constructive, collaborative care and to support patients and their families to navigate the healthcare system.

This chapter outlines principles of interprofessional collaboration, the healthcare professions working in clinical settings in Australia, and some of the regulations pertinent to their practice.

Recent decades have seen an increase in both the complexity and chronicity of the most prominent health problems affecting communities in Australia, as the population ages and multimorbidity becomes more common [1]. Over the same period, the importance of the social [2] and environmental [3] determinants of health and disease has increasingly been recognised. Since the turn of the present century, the per capita cost of the Australian healthcare system, in real terms, has risen at an average rate of 2.7% annually [4], underlining the importance of optimising the effectiveness of health service delivery.

Taken together, these effects point to the growing need for a wide range of healthcare and health-promotion professional capabilities in order to continue to impact positively on the health of Australians into the future. Successful practice in this environment requires workers from multiple different health professions, doctors included, to use their full scopes of practice and collaborate effectively with each other to meet the needs of the patients, clients and communities they serve. Multiple inquiries into instances of healthcare misadventure [5–8] have also pointed to faulty interactions between health professionals as a major source of serious adverse outcomes for patients, underlining the importance of successful collaboration. (See also Chapter 23, Patient safety.)

Interprofessional collaborative practice has been defined as:

> Health and community service professionals working together using complementary knowledge and skills, to provide care to patients, clients and communities, based on trust, respect and an understanding of each others' expertise [9].

For this kind of practice to be effective, doctors and other health professionals need to develop particular capabilities that enable productive collaboration, in addition to those required for the practice of their own professions. The metaphor of the orchestra has been suggested [10] to illustrate this concept. In this context, it is easy to see that musicians need to develop particular skills and techniques, in addition to virtuosity in playing their own instrument, in order to work effectively with colleagues to perform an orchestral work. These capabilities cannot be learned in solitude; they can only be developed through interactive learning with musicians who play other instruments, a process known in health practice as interprofessional education.

The metaphor has other elements that also symbolise collaborative health practice well. It emphasises the within-team collaboration for a shared, noble purpose that characterises both good health practice and fine orchestral performance, without allusions to between-team competition that follow from the more common comparison between healthcare teams and sporting teams. It also provides insight into the optimal timing for interprofessional educational activities in the training of health workers. Musicians can only benefit from playing together after they have developed at least some rudimentary capabilities on their own instruments, but from the very beginning they need to know how the other instruments work and roughly what they sound like. In health professional education, this kind of understanding—of the history, philosophy, expertise and scope of practice of each profession, including the learner's own—has been dubbed 'health professions literacy' [11]. Similarly, musicians can be part of multiple different performing groups at different times, just as health workers may move between different teams for different aspects of their professional work. Perhaps most significantly, in an orchestra there is no particular instrument whose player is always the conductor—conductors may be violinists, but they may equally be trumpeters or timpanists. In health, the metaphor reminds us that no particular profession will, or should, always be the leader of a care team. Rather, which profession leads the collaboration will depend on the purpose and nature of the care being provided [10].

Multiple frameworks have been proposed to describe the capabilities that health workers need in order to collaborate effectively with colleagues from other professions. A 2017 synthesis by O'Keefe et al. [12] derived a common set of interprofessional collaborative 'competencies':

- Explain interprofessional practice to patients, clients, families and other professionals
- Describe the areas of practice of other health professions
- Express professional opinions competently, confidently, and respectfully avoiding discipline specific language
- Plan patient/client care goals and priorities with involvement of other health professionals
- Recognise and resolve disagreements in relation to patient care that arise from different disciplinary perspectives
- Critically evaluate protocols and practices in relation to interprofessional practice
- Give timely, sensitive, instructive feedback to colleagues from other professions, and respond respectfully to feedback from these colleagues [12].

The aim of this chapter is primarily to support doctors and medical students to develop the first two of these capabilities as a foundation for the development of the others, assisted by other chapters in this book. It will provide an overview of the training, skills, philosophies and ethical imperatives of the wide range of health and other professionals (including interpreters, librarians, pastoral care workers, lawyers and police) with whom they will work throughout their careers.

Nursing and pharmacy are discussed first, as these are the two professions with which doctors most frequently interact. Other clinical professions are then considered alphabetically, with the exception of chiropractic, osteopathy and Chinese medicine, which are described under the heading of complementary medicine.

The chapter also provides guidance on the relationships that are expected between doctors and lawyers acting on behalf of patients, attends to the spiritual dimension that is important in the care of some patients, and discusses some of the ethical and professional issues related to complementary medicine.

11.1 The legal and ethical context

Health professionals, including doctors, share common ideals related to helping people to prevent or overcome illness, relieving suffering and maintaining good quality of life. They share similar codes of ethics, being bound to respect patients, maintain their confidentiality, be honest and behave with integrity. Many are subject to regulation, some through the same scheme as applies to medical practitioners, the National Registration and Accreditation Scheme, and some through state-based or profession-managed processes, with mechanisms for dealing with professional misconduct and with practitioners whose health or performance is impaired to the extent that the public is at risk. Rules and, in some cases, legislation define the scope of each profession's practice (see also Chapter 21, Regulation of the medical profession). Recent and ongoing reviews that focus on healthcare reform, scope of practice and the benefits of enabling health professionals to work at the top of their scope are likely to result in expansion of activities such as prescribing to additional professions.

11.2 Nurses and midwives

In their training, doctors work alongside nurses and may well feel they are familiar with their training and the scope of their responsibilities. However, Australian and US studies indicate that doctors do not have a clear understanding of the philosophy of nursing practice; the regulations governing it; the development of specialisation in nursing, including the role of the nurse practitioner; or changes in nursing education [13–15]. Doctors are probably unaware of how the medical and nursing professions view each other's roles. In an American survey, two-thirds of each profession indicated general satisfaction with working relationships but observed that, when problems arose, the professions sought to solve them competitively rather than collaboratively [16]. Doctors valued nurses for their capacity to communicate with doctors, their willingness to help and their competence, whereas nurses valued doctors who demonstrated trust and respect for nurses [16]. Other studies have found considerable discordance between nurses' and doctors' views on the health of their interprofessional relationship, with doctors being more positive than nurses [13–15].

In the nurse–doctor working relationship when caring for patients, there are responsibilities that are clearly those of nurses, clearly those of doctors, and responsibilities that may be shared. Even when it is clear where a particular responsibility lies, there are overriding responsibilities for both professions to act always in the best interests of the patient. Nurses who recognise a situation of potential or actual harm to a patient must take steps to prevent it. This may lead to a nurse intervening as a patient advocate to argue for a different course of action or refusing to follow a treatment order. Failure to take such action could be for the nurse a serious abrogation of responsibility to the patient and a breach of codes of ethics. Nurses, like doctors, are accountable in law primarily to patients and must take personal responsibility for their own professional actions. Misunderstandings about responsibilities will be prevented if there is a collaborative partnership role based on mutual respect and appreciation of the training, philosophies, skills and expertise that each profession brings to patient care. Where differences arise, as they frequently will in the complexity of hospital practice and health care, open respectful discussion achieves the best for the patient, while allowing each profession to support the other and providing checks and balances when needed. It is well established that a highly functioning care team achieves better care for patients as well as better job satisfaction for members of both professions [10]. In addition, most new medical graduates can learn a lot from nursing staff, particularly in specialised areas such as the emergency department or coronary care unit.

11.2.1 Philosophy

Nursing and midwifery courses contain significant components of science and clinical practice and have elements in common with medicine. Although nurses and midwives generally share the care of patients with doctors, they are accountable for their own actions. They act as the patient's advocate and particularly consider the social and psychological dimensions of being ill. Through longer time spent with patients, nurses and midwives may have greater insight into their real concerns and those of their families.

Nursing philosophy focuses on partnership with patients and sharing their goals. Consistent with this philosophy, nurses seek a collaborative working relationship with doctors. Their role in clinical care is complementary to that of doctors and it is important that they are respected, listened to and worked with positively in a genuine team approach.

Midwifery focuses on providing evidence-based health care to women and their babies across 'pregnancy, birth, the postnatal period and transition to parenting' [17].

11.2.2 Education and registration

The Nursing and Midwifery Board of Australia (NMBA) registers two main categories of nurses: enrolled nurses (ENs) and registered nurses (RNs). It also registers midwives, who may or may not also be RNs. All three of these titles (together with 'nurse', 'nurse practitioner' [see section 11.2.3] and 'midwife practitioner') are protected titles under the Health Practitioner Regulation National Law (the National Law), as in force in each state and territory, and it is illegal for persons who do not hold appropriate registration with the NMBA to use them. ENs complete diploma-level courses at institutes of technical and further education or with private providers, typically lasting 18 months full time. They usually work under the direct supervision of an RN. The basic qualification for work as an RN is a three- to four-year full-time bachelor degree, provided by more than 30 universities and a small number of other approved providers throughout Australia. These courses include multiple supervised clinical placements in hospitals and other healthcare settings.

Some midwives complete a standalone three-year bachelor degree and register only in midwifery. Others complete a longer double degree and gain qualification in both nursing and midwifery. Another pathway to midwifery qualification is for existing RNs to undertake an approved postgraduate program of study at graduate diploma or master level. At the completion of their degrees, new graduates are eligible for registration with the NMBA as an RN, a registered midwife or both depending on their qualification. Many Australian jurisdictions offer 'graduate nurse' or 'transition-to-practice' programs for RNs and midwives in their first year of practice but these are not a mandatory prerequisite for full registration in the way that the intern year is for medical practitioners.

11.2.3 Post-registration training and career paths

Many RNs choose to specialise in particular areas of practice such as critical care, emergency nursing, mental health nursing, diabetes education, oncology, sexual health, child and maternal health, primary care nursing or stomal therapy. These specialisations are achieved through practice experience, with or without formal postgraduate qualifications. Some nurses function as consultants in relation to their specialties to other nurses and healthcare teams. Some nurses and midwives move into leadership roles within their profession or more broadly in health services and prepare for this through postgraduate degrees in nursing or general management and leadership. Others pursue careers in nursing education and research. Most nursing faculties offer postgraduate research master and doctoral courses.

Nurse practitioners are RNs who have undertaken approved additional qualifications at master level and gained appropriate endorsement of their registration by the NMBA to practise in an expanded nursing role. They can work in a diverse range of clinical settings—from acute hospitals to rural health centres, sexual health clinics, aged care, public health and other community services. Their role can include aspects of care that were previously provided by doctors, such as diagnosing some medical conditions, referring patients, prescribing some medicines and requesting and interpreting investigations.

11.2.4 Ethical and legal responsibilities

In law, nurses and midwives are regarded as members of the healthcare team, taking professional responsibility for their role. They have been sued personally for negligence, have been apportioned responsibility for the deaths of patients by coroners and are subject to disciplinary action by the NMBA for unprofessional conduct. Weighing heavily on the minds of nurses are situations where their duty of care will not be fulfilled if they follow a doctor's treatment decision; for example, where a nurse genuinely believes a proposed treatment plan is not in the patient's best interests. Good communication between doctor and nurse should minimise the risk of such situations arising. Where they do occur, the nursing profession's strong view is that their ultimate responsibility is to the patient; this needs to be understood by doctors and respected as a legitimate exercise of professional judgement.

11.2.5 Codes of ethics and conduct

The nursing and midwifery professions, like the medical profession, have developed codes of ethics at international and national levels. First issued in 1953, the preamble to the 2021 edition of the International Council of Nurses code of ethics for nurses states that:

> [N]urses have consistently recognised four fundamental nursing responsibilities: to promote health, to prevent illness, to restore health, and to alleviate suffering and promote a dignified death. The need for nursing is universal.
>
> Inherent in nursing is respect for human rights, including cultural rights, the right to life and choice, the right to dignity and to be treated with respect. Nursing care is respectful of and unrestricted by considerations of age, colour, culture, ethnicity, disability or illness, gender, sexual orientation, nationality, politics, language, race, religious or spiritual beliefs, legal, economic or social status.
>
> Nurses are valued and respected for their contributions to improving the health of individuals, families, communities and populations locally, nationally and globally. They coordinate services with those of other health care professionals and related groups [18].

The International Confederation of Midwives has produced a corresponding code for that profession [19]. At the national level, the NMBA has developed Australian codes that are complementary to the international documents [20].

11.2.6 Mutual expectations and responsibilities

Several medical responsibilities cannot be delegated to registered or enrolled nurses, including making a medical diagnosis by history and physical examination, prescribing drugs, requesting tests, anaesthetising patients and performing surgery. There is currently a move towards providing appropriately trained nurses with limited prescribing rights. As noted in section 11.2.3, nurse practitioners have a broader scope of practice that can include diagnosis, referral and prescribing in specific circumstances. In specialised areas such as coronary care and intensive care, nurses are trained and expected to be skilled in resuscitation including defibrillation. Although there are minor differences between Australian jurisdictions, nurses share with doctors responsibilities such as giving intramuscular or intravenous injections, as well as storage of and recording the use of drugs of dependence. Nurses make nursing diagnoses (clinical judgements about patient, family or community experiences and responses to health problems, based on information obtained from a nursing assessment) and such diagnoses are frequently the basis for medical intervention. Nurses and other health professionals are currently able to undergo training to perform several other procedural tasks, such as gastrointestinal endoscopy [21], although introduction of nurse endoscopists remains controversial.

In all Australian jurisdictions, qualified midwives are legally able to conduct antenatal care in relation to uncomplicated pregnancies and deliver babies without the supervision of doctors. The NMBA's *Midwife standards for practice* [22] identify that they are responsible and accountable for 'promoting normal physiological childbirth and identifying complications for the woman and her baby' then, where necessary, for 'consultation with and referral to medical care ... and implementing emergency measures'. They go on to require that midwives engage in professional relationships with other health practitioners that are conducted within a context of collaboration, mutual trust, respect and cultural safety. The safety and wellbeing of women and babies requires that medical practitioners demonstrate reciprocal respect from their side of these relationships.

11.3 Pharmacists

Doctors and pharmacists have distinct and joint responsibilities to ensure that patients can benefit from pharmaceutical treatments safely and effectively. The commonest problem that arises between doctors and pharmacists relates to communication, usually due to a failure on the part of the doctor. Much less frequently, interprofessional tensions arise when doctors seek to dispense and sell medicines or when doctors misunderstand the role pharmacists legitimately play in giving advice and recommending medicines. Pharmacists, through their training and experience, recognise common ailments by their symptoms and, if necessary and appropriate, can recommend treatment with medicines that may be legally sold without prescription. Where this is not appropriate, the pharmacist will advise that medical attention be sought, although at the time of writing there have been trials of prescribing by pharmacists and this may become more general. In 2006, following amendment to the *Workplace Relations Act 1996* (Cth), pharmacists were provided with the authority to certify illness causing unfitness for work.

In dispensing a prescription, a pharmacist must exercise an independent judgement to ensure that the medicine is safe and appropriate for the patient, and that it conforms to the prescriber's intentions. If there is any doubt, the prescriber is to be contacted [23]. See also Chapter 30, Prescribing and administering medicines.

New medical graduates usually develop an understanding of the role and expertise of pharmacists while working in hospitals, where hospital pharmacists play an important role in supporting safe and effective prescribing. Most doctors thus appreciate the central role of pharmacists in the healthcare team in dispensing drugs and contributing to their safe and effective use through providing advice to prescribers on medication choice, side effects and drug interactions. The basic means of communication between doctor and pharmacist is the prescription itself, so doctors must ensure prescriptions are legible and precise (see section 11.3.5).

The education and training of pharmacists covers the following responsibilities:

- dispensing prescriptions
- providing general information and drug administration instructions to patients
- counselling patients with regard to minor ailments, the use of over-the-counter drugs and the need to see a doctor
- conducting medication reviews of patients taking multiple medications to inform optimisation of their treatment regimens
- keeping up to date with the laws and regulations about drugs
- keeping up to date with knowledge about drugs, their effects, side effects and potential interactions, as well as being able to access specialised information about them when required
- recognising the nature of common drug side effects
- recognising and resolving problems related to a patient's drug therapy, such as incorrect dosing, in collaboration with the prescriber where necessary.

Pharmacists seek to work collaboratively with doctors. They wish to be respected for their particular skills and knowledge and want, by collaboration with doctors, to ensure that patients benefit maximally from the skills of both professions. In providing advice, pharmacists direct many people to their family doctor and are sensitive to the judgement required to avoid unnecessary or late referrals.

11.3.1 Education and registration

Most pharmacy students undertake a four-year undergraduate degree based on science, pharmacology and pharmacy practice. Another training pathway is the completion of a two-year master-level qualification after an undergraduate degree, typically in biomedical science. These courses are accredited by the Australian Pharmacy Council and approved by the Pharmacy Board of Australia. They include practical training supervised by pharmacists in various settings. On completion of their approved qualification, pharmacy graduates are required to complete a year of supervised practical intern training then successfully complete written and oral examinations to be eligible for full registration.

To practise as pharmacists, practitioners must be registered with the Pharmacy Board of Australia. The requirements for registration, composition of the board and its disciplinary processes are similar to those of the Medical Board of Australia. Pharmacists are also bound by state and territory laws relating to drugs of dependence (see Chapter 30, Prescribing and administering medicines) and Commonwealth laws relating to the Pharmaceutical Benefits Scheme (PBS) (see Chapter 20, The Australian healthcare system). Pharmacists must be approved by Medicare before they can participate in the PBS and dispense PBS prescriptions. In addition, state or territory legislation may cover matters such as the qualifications required to be able to prescribe, and administrative requirements for owning and running pharmacies. The legal and ethical implications of these strict regulations are detailed in section 11.3.3.

11.3.2 Post-registration training and career paths

The Pharmaceutical Society of Australia, the Pharmacy Guild of Australia and Advanced Pharmacy Australia (AdPha; formerly the Society of Hospital Pharmacists of Australia) conduct national and state-based continuing professional development programs similar to those undertaken by medical practitioners. The Pharmacy Board of Australia requires registered pharmacists to undertake a specified amount of professional development each year, involving a range of activities such as attendance at conferences and workshops and participation in online learning.

The largest proportion of pharmacists work in community pharmacies either as proprietors or employees. Other career opportunities exist in hospital pharmacies, regulatory authorities, the pharmaceutical industry, research and teaching. There are no formally recognised pharmacy specialties or specialist qualifications within Australia, but AdPha has developed 'specialty practice streams' for its members in a wide range of areas such as geriatric medicine, infectious diseases, oncology, mental health, and rural and remote pharmacy [24]. Some pharmacists engage in research or pharmacy education and undertake research degrees at a master or doctoral level.

11.3.3 Ethical and legal responsibilities

Pharmacists must conform to the regulatory framework discussed previously or risk legal sanction by the federal department responsible for Medicare or state or territory authorities regulating the handling of drugs and poisons. They are also bound to act in accordance with professional standards by the Pharmacy Board of Australia. To prevent harm to patients, a pharmacist is required to dispense a prescription only if it is consistent with patient safety. Thus, pharmacists must not dispense prescriptions if the prescription is not clearly legible or if the dose is thought to be dangerously incorrect. This ethical and legal duty must be understood and respected by doctors. Pharmacists have at times been joined with doctors in actions for damages where both parties should and could have collaborated to resolve a medication safety issue. Pharmacists also have an obligation to ensure patients are instructed in the use of medications and their side effects, including provision of consumer product information leaflets relating to prescribed drugs where required. Doctors need to appreciate this obligation and inform the pharmacist when a prescription has been written with unusual directions or for a purpose for which it has not been formally approved, as the consumer product information leaflet may not be fully relevant in such situations. If satisfied of the therapeutic need, pharmacists may supply certain drugs, including Schedule 3 drugs, directly to patients, keeping records as required by legislation, but currently may only dispense Schedule 4 and 8 drugs on receipt of a written prescription from a doctor or other approved prescriber such as a nurse practitioner (see also Chapter 30, Prescribing and administering medicines). Pharmacists are subject to disciplinary action if they are found guilty of misconduct by the Pharmacy Board. They may be sued for negligence and have been subject to adverse findings by the coroner for dispensing errors.

11.3.4 Codes of ethics and conduct

The Pharmacy Board of Australia shares a *Code of conduct* [25], which applies to registered health practitioners in 12 professions and has much in common with the code issued for doctors by the Medical Board. The Australian Health Practitioner Regulation Agency (Ahpra) also advises practitioners that they 'have a responsibility to be familiar with and apply their relevant code' [25]. The Pharmaceutical Society of Australia's *Code of ethics for pharmacists* [26] and AdPha's *Code of ethics* [27] are also appropriate guides. The Pharmaceutical Society's code includes the following principles:

- A pharmacist makes the health and wellbeing of the patient their first priority.
- A pharmacist practises and promotes patient-centred care.

- A pharmacist exercises professional judgement in the interests of the patient and wider community.
- A pharmacist acts with honesty and integrity to maintain public trust and confidence in the profession.
- A pharmacist only practises under conditions which uphold the professional independence, judgement and integrity of themselves and others.
- A pharmacist demonstrates a commitment to the continual development of self and the profession to enhance pharmacy practice.
- A pharmacist works collaboratively with others to deliver patient-centred care and optimise health outcomes [26].

11.3.5 Mutual expectations and responsibilities

Pharmacists expect and rely on doctors to write legible prescriptions with clear instructions as to how the medication is to be taken. Pharmacists are obliged to adhere to *Guidelines for dispensing of medicines* [23] issued by the Pharmacy Board. By law, pharmacists cannot dispense a prescription unless the pharmacist is certain of which drug is being prescribed and what directions have been given for its administration. Doctors expect pharmacists to dispense the medication prescribed accurately and to attend to labelling and record-keeping requirements. Doctors can create problems for pharmacists and their joint patients when they:

- write illegible prescriptions or prescriptions with unhelpful or unclear instructions about dispensing requirements, strength or quantity
- fail to provide on the prescription a telephone number for contact and the address of the doctor, information that is legally required
- fail to include directions for use of prescribed drugs
- refuse to accept a telephone call or behave discourteously when asked by a pharmacist to clarify details of a prescription
- ignore the obligations of pharmacists to be concerned for patient safety and to ensure that patients understand what a medication is for and how it is to be used
- make comments that can be interpreted as denigrating pharmacists or undermining their legitimate professional role.

Doctors who fail to meet their professional responsibilities in their dealings with pharmacists are open to disciplinary action by the Medical Board of Australia. Complaints in this area often relate to rudeness and abruptness. They are important because of their potential impact on patient care and because they reflect poorly on the doctor's approach to professional communication.

The medical profession in Australia has not involved itself in stocking, dispensing and selling medicines for profit. This approach of differentiating between the professional roles of pharmacists and doctors has developed with the best interests of patients in mind. This differentiation of roles:

- provides a system of checks and balances, whereby pharmacists contribute to patient safety by monitoring their use of medications and by drawing the attention of doctors to possible prescribing errors
- reduces conflict of interest in doctors' prescribing and distances doctors from direct incentives to prescribe a sponsor's products

- ensures that medicines are dispensed in a regulated framework, where pharmacists are subject to regulations covering record keeping, labelling and dispensing
- maintains records of all items dispensed
- for PBS prescriptions, ensures that patients have full access to the benefits of this system, including its safety net provisions.

There are some exceptions to this separation of roles. They include the use of drugs from a doctor's emergency bag, the provision of drugs in remote areas or where a pharmacy is not immediately available, and the supply of 'starter' packs. Doctors who dispense drugs in these situations are obliged to meet all the regulatory requirements facing pharmacists, including recording, labelling and adequately instructing patients about the medication's purpose and side effects. On the other hand, it is possible that limited prescribing rights may become available to appropriately trained pharmacists over the next few years.

Apart from their professional accountabilities to patients and their responsibility to collaborate with medical practitioners, pharmacists have additional obligations. For example, pharmacists are expected to play a key role in ensuring that residents in care facilities, low-level aged care hostels and special accommodation have appropriately supervised and supported pharmacy services to support the safe use of medicines in these settings.

11.4 Aboriginal and/or Torres Strait Islander health workers and practitioners

Aboriginal and/or Torres Strait Islander health worker and health practitioner roles developed from a need to provide culturally safe primary healthcare services to Indigenous Australians whose health needs were not being met by mainstream services. Aboriginal and/or Torres Strait Islander *health workers* are Indigenous Australians who have gained a Certificate II or higher qualification in Aboriginal and/or Torres Strait Islander Primary Health Care [28]. Aboriginal and/or Torres Strait Islander *health practitioners* are Indigenous Australians who have completed an approved 'Certificate IV' or equivalent program (under the Australian Qualifications Framework) in Aboriginal and Torres Strait Islander Primary Health Care Practice and gained registration with the Aboriginal and Torres Strait Islander Health Practice Board. This board, like the Medical Board of Australia, is supported by Ahpra.

Aboriginal and/or Torres Strait Islander health workers and practitioners work in a wide range of urban, regional, rural and remote settings, including Aboriginal community controlled health organisations, government health services and private medical practices. They work as part of healthcare teams or autonomously, with scopes of practice determined by their qualifications, experience and community needs. They use their knowledge of Indigenous culture and communities to promote good health. Aboriginal and/or Torres Strait Islander health workers and practitioners occupy a broad range of roles within the Australian healthcare system. Examples include generalist clinician within a multidisciplinary care team, specialist (e.g. dental, diabetes, renal, mental health, cardiology, aged care, disability, addiction, infant and maternal, sexually transmitted infections, bloodborne viruses, emergency department, justice and youth justice health), on-call generalist, healthcare promoter and educator, trainer, researcher, and roles in executive leadership and management [29]. They are also trained to act as the first contact point in health services, as well as to facilitate the care given by doctors, nurses and other health professionals. Their focus includes encouraging and empowering Indigenous Australians to manage their own health. They take on additional responsibilities including immunisation, health screening, counselling, interpreting, maintaining medical records and having input into the development and delivery of community health programs (see Chapter 17, Culturally safe health care for Aboriginal and/or Torres Strait Islander peoples).

As of 2023–24, the national board registered 972 Aboriginal and/or Torres Strait Islander health practitioners, of whom about one-quarter, worked in New South Wales and one-fifth in the Northern Territory [30].

The Aboriginal and Torres Strait Islander Health Practice Board has adopted the shared *Code of conduct* for registered practitioners [25], which has much in common with the code issued by the Medical Board of Australia for doctors.

11.5 Audiologists

Audiologists are allied health professionals who 'promote healthy hearing, communication competency, and quality of life for persons of all ages through the prevention, identification, assessment, and rehabilitation of hearing, auditory function, balance, and other related systems' [31]. They work autonomously and in close collaboration with doctors, particularly ear, nose and throat surgeons. Audiologists provide detailed assessment of hearing and vestibular function using sophisticated equipment including electrophysiological methods. They are also involved in the prescription and fitting of hearing aids and other assistive devices, as well as providing patients with education in their effective use.

Audiology is not a regulated profession under the National Law but Audiology Australia certifies individuals as accredited audiologists. This certification signifies that practitioners have undertaken an approved course of study followed by a one-year clinical internship. Practitioners are bound by a *Code of conduct* [32] that is used by Audiology Australia and the Australian College of Audiology, as well as being required to undertake appropriate continuing professional development. Approved qualifications comprise a two-year, graduate-entry master degree and include practical placement. A limited range of the activities undertaken by accredited audiologists can also be performed by members of a related occupation known as audiometrists, who have undertaken a two-year program of vocational education.

11.6 Dental practitioners

The Dental Board of Australia registers and regulates multiple professions that contribute to oral health, including dentists, dental specialists, dental therapists, dental hygienists, oral health therapists and dental prosthetists. Dentistry is 'the science and art of preventing, diagnosing and treating diseases, injuries, developmental and acquired defects of the teeth, oral cavity and associated structures within the context of general health' [33]. A primary qualification in dentistry was traditionally a five-year full-time undergraduate degree but some institutions now offer a combination of bachelor and master degrees or allow graduate entry to their programs. Entry requirements and competition for entry are very similar to those for medicine. Most dentists work in general private dental practice and are eligible to do so immediately upon graduation with their primary qualification, unlike in medicine where specialised post-registration training is required for all areas, including general practice. Some dentists undertake additional training, often in the form of an approved doctoral degree, in one of 13 specialties, including orthodontics, periodontics, endodontics, prosthodontics, paediatric dentistry and public health dentistry. Some undertake oral and maxillofacial surgery, which involves also obtaining a medical degree.

Other practitioners registered by the Dental Board include dental hygienists, dental prosthetists, dental therapists and oral health therapists, each with different but overlapping scopes of practice [34]. Dental practitioners are often supported in their work by dental assistants and technicians who have vocational qualifications but are not registered practitioners.

The Dental Board of Australia has adopted the shared *Code of conduct* [25], which has much in common with the code issued by the Medical Board of Australia for doctors. The Australian Dental Association also publishes codes of ethics, which are developed by its state and territory branches [35].

Interactions between dental practitioners and doctors occur reasonably commonly, especially in relation to patients who are on anticoagulants, who have serious chronic illness or who might require prophylactic antibiotics to reduce the risk of bacterial endocarditis. Some medical treatments may also have significant impacts on oral health. Thus, it is important that doctors make themselves accessible to dental practitioners who are seeking information or advice about shared patients.

11.7 Dietitians and nutritionists

Dietitians are professionals 'who appl[y] the science of food and nutrition to promote health, prevent and treat disease to optimise the health of individuals, groups, communities and populations' [36]. As the knowledge of dietary factors in health and disease has grown, doctors have increasingly come to collaborate with dietitians, who are skilled in eliciting detailed dietary histories, making nutritional assessments and providing specific counselling about dietary modifications. For diseases where dietary therapy is the primary or major mode of therapy, doctors who do not possess adequate knowledge and skills to undertake these tasks have an ethical obligation to refer patients to dietitians.

Dietitians undertake an approved program of study, typically as a specialised four-year bachelor degree or a postgraduate master program. Their education covers biochemical, physiological and psychological factors relating to human nutrition as well as the principles of communication, education and health promotion. Dietetics is not covered by the National Law that regulates many health professions through Ahpra, but rather has a profession-led recognition program operated by Dietitians Australia. This organisation approves programs of study and awards the title of Accredited Practising Dietitian, with attendant requirements to adhere to its *Code of conduct*, practise within their areas of expertise and undertake continuing professional development. Neither 'dietitian' nor 'nutritionist' are protected titles in Australia, and people practising under the latter title may have a wide range of qualifications and experience. Typically, nutritionists tend to provide education to groups rather than assessment and advice for individuals, but this is not formally regulated. The Nutrition Society of Australia has established a voluntary registration scheme for nutritionists [37].

Accredited Practising Dietitians work predominantly in hospitals, community health centres and private practice, but may also work in food service management in hospitals, government, industry, or education and research. Dietitians value, but do not necessarily require, letters of referral from doctors. However, doctors should consider providing a letter in every instance, to improve communication and enhance the value of the dietitian's contribution to the care of the patient. In return, dietitians undertake to provide written communication to the referring doctor, outlining assessment and treatment plans.

11.8 Exercise physiologists

Exercise physiologists 'design, deliver and evaluate safe and effective exercise interventions for people with acute, sub-acute or chronic medical conditions, injuries or disabilities' [38]. They can work autonomously but also accept referrals from doctors or other health professionals and often work in interprofessional teams. They work in private and public healthcare settings, rehabilitation centres and aged care facilities, as well as in fitness centres and in private practice.

Exercise physiology is not a regulated profession under the National Law but Exercise and Sports Science Australia recognises individuals as Accredited Exercise Physiologists. This certification signifies that practitioners have undertaken an approved course of study and are bound by the organisation's *Code of professional conduct and ethical practice* [39], as well as undertaking appropriate continuing professional development and maintaining professional indemnity insurance. Approved qualifications usually comprise a four-year undergraduate degree, often with an additional graduate diploma, and include practical placement. Exercise and Sports Science Australia also accredits professionals who have undertaken an approved three-year bachelor degree to undertake a narrower range of activities as Accredited Exercise Scientists.

11.9 Medical radiation practitioners

Medical radiation practitioners are health professionals registered with the Medical Radiation Practice Board of Australia, supported by Ahpra. The profession has three divisions: diagnostic radiographer, nuclear medicine technologist and radiation therapist. Each requires training with an approved specialised four-year bachelor degree that includes extensive clinical placement. Medical radiation practitioners collaborate very closely with medical practitioners in their field of practice. Diagnostic radiographers use medical imaging technologies such as X-rays, computerised tomography and magnetic resonance imaging to obtain high-quality diagnostic images and then collaborate with medical radiologists to interpret those images. They also support radiologists when they undertake interventional radiological procedures such as arterial stenting. Nuclear medicine technologists prepare the radiopharmaceuticals and operate the equipment used to obtain images through nuclear medicine techniques. They collaborate closely with nuclear medicine physicians and may also be involved in the preparation of radioactive materials used for therapeutic purposes. Radiation therapists work closely with medical radiation oncologists to plan and deliver radiation therapy, primarily in the treatment of cancer.

The Medical Radiation Board of Australia, which is supported by Ahpra, has adopted the shared *Code of conduct* in relation to the profession [25].

11.10 Occupational therapists

Occupational therapists 'use a whole person perspective to work with individuals, groups and communities to achieve optimal health and wellbeing through participation in the occupations of life' [40]. Their focus on 'occupation' refers not only to formal employment but also to supporting all of the activities that people find meaningful, including the activities of daily living and providing care to others, as well as participating in hobbies and social events. They undertake capability assessments and devise individual therapy programs that may include retraining of skills, provision of adaptive equipment, home assessment and worksite visits.

Occupational therapists undertake an approved program of study that is typically a four-year university undergraduate course but may be a combination bachelor/master pathway or a standalone graduate-entry master qualification. Studies are undertaken in anatomy, physiology, neurosciences, psychology, human development, ergonomics, medical sciences, psychosocial assessment and intervention, design and development, experiential studies and research. Practical training takes place in teaching hospitals, rehabilitation centres and community-based organisations. Graduates most frequently work with patients in hospitals, rehabilitation centres, community health centres, special education services or aged care facilities. Specialised fields include workplace safety and ergonomics, hand therapy, and motor vehicle driving assessment and support.

Occupational therapists are registered by the Occupational Therapy Board of Australia, which is supported by Ahpra and has adopted the shared *Code of conduct* in relation to the profession [25].

Many occupational therapists work very closely with doctors and value referrals that provide sufficient information regarding medical diagnosis and prognosis to enable them to work effectively with the patient. They have a professional responsibility to make their own assessment of the problem and advise on its appropriate treatment.

11.11 Optometrists

Optometrists are primary care practitioners who focus on eye health. They are trained to diagnose and manage a range of ocular conditions including dry eye, allergies and infections, as well as refractive errors, for which they prescribe and dispense spectacles and contact lenses. Their training is typically an approved five-year program comprising a bachelor and a master degree. Their studies resemble basic medical training and include ocular and orbital anatomy, ocular physiology, pathology and optics, as well as clinical skills, eye-related public health, ethics and professionalism. Most current optometry programs also include the training required to obtain endorsement from the Optometry Board of Australia (which regulates the profession and is supported by Ahpra) to prescribe a range of scheduled medicines for common eye conditions. Optometrists are trained to conduct comprehensive ocular assessment including examination and imaging of the ocular fundus in order to screen for and monitor retinal pathology. They are also able to prescribe a limited range of treatments for ocular conditions. Optometrists can refer patients with more complex ocular and orbital conditions directly to ophthalmologists (medical specialists in diseases of the eye) with whom they often collaborate in the management of ongoing disorders.

11.12 Orthotists/prosthetists

Orthotists/prosthetists provide treatment to people with physical and functional disabilities through the prescription, design, fitting and monitoring of orthoses (externally applied devices fitted to the body to correct deformity or support joints) and prostheses (artificial devices attached or applied to the body to replace a missing part). They draw on knowledge of biomechanics and materials to design devices intended to promote mobility and independent function. Orthotic management is provided to people with a wide variety of problems, including paediatric disorders such as congenital hip dislocation; post-trauma care such as fracture management or devices for people with spinal cord injuries; and degenerative disorders such as arthritis. Prosthetic management is provided to people undergoing amputation of a limb from immediate and early postoperative care through rehabilitation to long-term care. Training involves a four-year bachelor degree that includes theoretical and practical work and clinical placement within orthotic/prosthetic services. Studies are taken in anatomy, physiology, biomechanics, materials technology, pathology, neurology, prosthetics and orthotics.

Orthotics/prosthetics is not a regulated profession under the National Law. The Australian Orthotic Prosthetic Association awards certification to appropriately trained and experienced practitioners; certified members of the association are required to adhere to its *Ethical principles and code of professional conduct* [41]. Orthotists/prosthetists work within the public hospital system, in private practice and to a more limited extent in research and education. They expect health professionals who refer patients for treatment to provide sufficient information regarding diagnosis and suggested functional outcome to facilitate their assessment of the condition. They ensure that the prosthetic or orthotic design is appropriate for the individual patient's disability, provide prostheses and orthoses that are structurally sound, and educate the patient about appropriate use of the devices.

11.13 Paramedics

On 1 December 2018, 'paramedic' became a protected title in Australia and the occupation became a regulated profession overseen by the Paramedicine Board of Australia, which has adopted the shared *Code of conduct* in relation to the profession [25] and is supported by Ahpra. Paramedics provide 'emergency or unscheduled care to acutely ill or injured persons, predominantly in an out of hospital or primary care environment' [42]. Particularly in urban areas, they are the major source of immediate care for people who have been involved in serious accidents; who have collapsed, are unconscious or have had a cardiac arrest; and those with urgent medical symptoms such as chest pain. Entry to practice as a paramedic now requires completion of an approved program of study, which is typically a three-year bachelor-level university degree. Some universities offer four-year double degrees in paramedicine and nursing. Different Australian jurisdictions have different classifications for more senior members of the profession, such as 'intensive care paramedics', who have acquired higher-level capabilities and will sometimes be dispatched separately to assist paramedic teams to provide higher-level assessment and treatment at an accident scene or where a patient is gravely ill. In 2019, the Australian Institute of Paramedic Practitioners was formed to promote and regulate the development of senior registered paramedics to provide primary care and health promotion services in settings such as remote communities, independently or in collaboration with doctors and nurse practitioners [43]. A small number of Australian universities now offer master or professional doctoral qualifications at paramedic practitioner level, though this specialisation within the profession had not yet been formally recognised by the Paramedicine Board of Australia at the time of writing.

Paramedics make a very important contribution in providing crucial information to doctors and nurses working in emergency departments, as they have often been witness to the earliest phases of rapidly evolving illnesses. Information gleaned from direct conversation or from the report that accompanies the patient can be very valuable in establishing a diagnosis and guiding early management. Paramedics are trained to observe and record vital signs and other observations. This information is handed over verbally and in writing to emergency department nurses and doctors, who value it highly [44].

Ambulance services are a valuable resource that must be used with due consideration. Apart from patient- or doctor-initiated services in a genuine emergency, all other requests for paramedic attendance and ambulance transport should involve the doctor considering whether cheaper transport alternatives are available, within reasonable bounds of patient safety. In some cities, alternative and less expensive transport for elective procedures and ambulatory consultations is available and should be used where appropriate.

With the introduction of computer-aided dispatch technology to ambulance communications in Australia, the detail of information doctors provide to the call takers is vital in determining the level of response, namely whether that be a standard paramedic team or a mobile intensive-care crew and whether that resource is sent 'lights and sirens' or under normal driving conditions.

In emergency situations, the person who is with the patient is in the best position to call for an ambulance because that person can answer the call taker's questions accurately with up-to-date details of the patient's condition. As ambulance communications systems vary within and between states, doctors should familiarise themselves with their local service protocols to elicit the appropriate ambulance response for their patients.

11.14 Physiotherapists

Physiotherapists are 'experts in the structure of the human body and its movement' [45]. Through the use of physical modalities of treatment, physiotherapists aim to facilitate recovery or to retrain function that has been lost through disorders or injuries, particularly of the musculoskeletal, neurological and cardiorespiratory systems. They undertake an approved program of study, which is generally a four-year bachelor degree, a two-year postgraduate master or a three-year extended master qualification course involving theoretical and practical learning with clinical placements. Studies typically include anatomy, physiology, psychology and physiotherapy practice. Physiotherapists must be registered with the Physiotherapy Board of Australia, supported by Ahpra. They are subject to disciplinary and impairment provisions similar to those applying to doctors.

Physiotherapists work predominantly in hospital or independent private practice, but also may be employed in rehabilitation centres, sports medicine centres, community health services, schools, industry, research and education. The Australian College of Physiotherapists also provides formal specialisation leading to fellowship [46], though specialist recognition is not regulated by the board or Ahpra in this profession, as it is in medicine. Physiotherapy specialties include musculoskeletal, neurological, cardiorespiratory and paediatric. The Physiotherapy Board has adopted the shared Code of conduct [25] and the Australian Physiotherapy Association also has its own complementary Code of conduct, which describes the profession's ethical principles and outlines its values [47].

Physiotherapists have traditionally worked very closely with doctors but also accept patients without referral. They expect doctors who refer patients to provide sufficient information regarding the patient's history and medical diagnosis, as it gives context for their own assessment of the problem and its appropriate management. Only a small proportion of doctors claim expertise in and provide treatment by manipulation or by such methods as transcutaneous electrical nerve stimulation or ultrasound. The vast majority will refer patients who may benefit from such treatments to physiotherapists.

11.15 Podiatrists

Podiatrists are primary contact practitioners who deal with the prevention, diagnosis, treatment and rehabilitation of medical and surgical conditions of the feet and lower limbs. They are able to administer local anaesthesia and perform procedures on the foot such as ingrown toenail removal. They may also refer patients for appropriate imaging studies of the foot and ankle. The profession is regulated by the Podiatry Board of Australia, supported by Ahpra. The board has adopted the shared *Code of conduct* [25]. The board can also provide suitably qualified podiatrists with endorsement to prescribe certain drugs related to their work. The profession has one registered specialty: podiatric surgery. Podiatrists must complete an accredited post-registration podiatric surgery program of study approved by the Podiatry Board of Australia in order to perform more major surgical procedures on the foot and ankle, usually in private hospitals or day-surgery centres under regional or general anaesthesia administered by medical anaesthetists [48].

Many podiatrists are in private practice, while others work in community health centres and hospitals. Primary training in podiatry typically involves a four-year bachelor degree or a two-year graduate-entry master qualification.

11.16 Psychologists

Psychologists 'study individuals and groups to better understand how people, communities and societies function, and devise ways to empower them and help them thrive ... through [an] understanding of mental and biological functions that drive behaviour' [49]. 'Psychologist' is a protected title under the National Law and in order to practise, psychologists must be registered with the Psychology Board of Australia, supported by Ahpra. To qualify for general registration, they must complete either a six-year sequence comprising a bachelor as well as a master or doctoral degree, or a five-year university qualification followed by a year of supervised practice as a psychological intern. Formerly, a four-year honours degree followed by a two-year internship pathway was available, but this was retired by the board in mid-2022. At the time of writing, the board required registered psychologists to adhere to the Australian Psychological Society's *Code of ethics* [50], which will be in effect until the board's own code of conduct takes effect in December 2025.

In addition to general registration, psychologists can undertake additional training and supervised practice as a registrar to obtain endorsement of their registration by the board in one or more of nine specialty practice areas, including clinical psychology, clinical neuropsychology and health psychology. Psychologists are equipped to treat social, emotional and behavioural problems in children, adults and families and are thus a critical component of the healthcare system. They use diagnostic categorisation systems (such as the *Diagnostic and statistical manual of mental disorders* or International Classification of Diseases systems) in common with the medical specialty of psychiatry, with which they often collaborate in interprofessional teams. Thus, they share a common language with doctors. Psychologists can accept referrals from doctors or clients may refer themselves.

11.17 Social workers

'Social work is a practice-based profession and an academic discipline that promotes social change and development, social cohesion, and the empowerment and liberation of people' [51]. It is founded on the principles of social justice, human rights, collective responsibility and respect for diversities [51]. Social workers have a dual focus on both helping individuals and families cope with personal or social problems and addressing systemic or structural issues that may impact on wellbeing through inequality, injustice or discrimination. As much of the distress that presents to doctors is triggered by social problems, and as serious illness or hospitalisation can be associated with social and financial difficulties, close cooperation between doctors and social workers has great value. Social workers have a broad knowledge of the service system, which enables them to access resources on behalf of patients and families. Social workers are trained to work as members of interprofessional teams.

Social work is not a regulated profession under the National Law, but the Australian Association of Social Workers accredits individuals to use its registered trademarks designating Accredited Social Workers and Accredited Mental Health Social Workers. This accreditation signifies that practitioners have undertaken an approved course of study, are bound by the association's Code of ethics [52] and undertake appropriate continuing professional development. Approved qualifications usually comprise a four-year bachelor degree or a two-year graduate-entry master qualification and include practical placement with qualified social workers. Social workers are extensively employed in community services, public hospitals, justice agencies, voluntary organisations and government departments.

Social workers in hospital settings appreciate early identification where possible of social concerns by doctors and others in the healthcare team as assessment, and more particularly the harnessing of resources prior to the patient's discharge, can take considerable time. Timely intervention can mitigate the effects of crisis situations. The assistance of social workers to patients will be enhanced by doctors providing a clear outline of the patient's condition, including diagnosis, prognosis, psychological state and medical plan of management.

11.18 Speech pathologists

Speech pathologists are trained to diagnose and treat patients with communication disorders including problems with the use of language and the use of voice. Their work includes teaching compensatory strategies to assist communication. Speech pathologists also assess and manage patients with pharyngeal swallowing disorders and, with the healthcare team, assist patients to return to oral intake as safely and quickly as possible following conditions such as stroke or traumatic brain injury [53]. Speech pathologists typically undertake either an approved four-year bachelor degree or a two-year graduate-entry master qualification. Studies include a wide range of theoretical and practical subjects including linguistics, speech and language development and disorders, psychology, anatomy and physiology, and audiology. The course also includes clinical training, which is carried out in a variety of settings including hospitals, schools and community health centres.

Speech pathology is not a regulated profession under the National Law, but Speech Pathology Australia accredits individuals who have completed appropriate training as Certified Practising Speech Pathologists. These practitioners work in a variety of settings within the school system, community health centres, hospitals, special institutions, rehabilitation centres and education and research centres. Speech pathologists also work in independent private practice throughout Australia. They have different referral expectations dependent on the work setting. Speech pathologists working in hospitals accept patients on referral from a doctor. They expect the doctor who refers the patient to provide sufficient information in regard to the patient's medical history to provide context for their diagnosis and assessment. The speech pathologist liaises closely with the doctor in regard to results of assessment and patient management.

11.19 Chaplains and spiritual care practitioners

Patients who are seriously ill, in hospital or facing major surgery frequently avail themselves of support offered by spiritual or pastoral care practitioners. This may include patients who have not claimed adherence to a religion or who have declared themselves to be agnostic. This is consistent with the common experience, even in a secular society, that there is a spiritual component or deeper meaning to life, or an awareness of an inner being or soul, especially when reminded of one's mortality [54].

These feelings are not always shared or even recognised by younger people, including young doctors who have not themselves faced serious illness. Doctors should recognise the important role played by spiritual care practitioners and hospital chaplains in the overall care of many patients and regard them as members of the care team who are committed to a holistic approach to healing. Pastoral care departments have long existed in hospitals founded by Christian religious orders and, more recently, an organisation called Spiritual Care Australia has been formed as the professional association of practitioners in spiritual care, pastoral care and chaplaincy [55]. The organisation seeks to unify, consolidate, support, promote and encourage the development of spiritual care within contemporary multi-faith, multicultural Australia [55]. It accredits practitioners at Certified Member and Certified Advanced Member levels based on a primary bachelor or master degree in an appropriate field, followed by completion of training in clinical pastoral education provided by one of the state-based members of the Australian and New Zealand Association for Clinical Pastoral Education [56]. This training includes minimum requirements for supervised practice in pastoral care, and Spiritual Care Australia's practice standards include a requirement to collaborate effectively with other members of an individual's care team [57].

On admission to hospital, patients frequently experience a sense of depersonalisation or of being lost. They may struggle to cope with the threat of illness and its physical and emotional effects, as well as the confusion created by separation from family and friends and by receiving care from many members of a complex team. It is of great value to many patients to have access to a pastoral care practitioner who is an independent advocate yet part of the healthcare team and who can respond to their non-medical, non-physical needs. This support, and the deeper spiritual needs of some patients, should be recognised and respected by clinicians. The pastoral care practitioner's role is to address the spiritual and other affective needs of patients, which may involve religious issues. This is achieved by visiting patients, listening to their stories, accompanying them on their journey through their illness and offering support and counselling to them and their families.

In many areas, pastoral care practitioners can play important additional roles. They can be critically valuable in anticipating grief and in grief counselling, especially in fields such as organ donation and transplantation. They can also assist hospital staff by facilitating debriefing sessions when patients have died in distressing situations. They can help staff recognise distress, burnout and associated depersonalisation. In addition, they can assist staff by sharing the emotional burden of caring for seriously ill and dying patients and their families, both while the patient is in hospital and in the weeks and months that follow deaths in hospital.

11.20 Interpreters

Interpreting is '[t]he process of first fully understanding, analyzing, and processing a spoken or signed message and then faithfully rendering it into another spoken or signed language' [58]. It involves a different set of skills from the translation of written language and is critically important to the effective provision of health care to people whose first language is different from those of their health providers. The interpreting profession is regulated in Australia by the National Accreditation Authority for Interpreters and Translators, which is a not-for-profit company owned jointly by the Commonwealth and state and territory governments [59]. The authority assesses and verifies individuals' capabilities for a variety of interpreting roles, such as Certified Specialist Health Interpreter, in particular language combinations based on formal qualifications and practice experience.

The Royal Australian College of General Practitioners–endorsed *Guide for clinicians working with interpreters in healthcare settings* points to the importance of using professional interpreters where required:

> As a matter of good practice, clinicians should ensure the person understands the discussion that takes place and the proposed care plan, engaging an interpreter if necessary. Failure to determine the need for, and engage, an interpreter in consultations with people with limited English proficiency or Deaf people may be considered to be a breach in duty of care. From a medico-legal perspective, engaging interpreters helps clinicians to ensure that they have adequately assured informed consent, and that a person understands complex instructions and is competent to make decisions. These all underpin informed decision-making [60].

Doctors should also be aware that bilingual staff or students, unless appropriately accredited, should not be presumed to have the necessary skills to act as interpreters. Australian health practitioners have ready access to very high-quality professional interpreting services through the Commonwealth's Translating and Interpreting Service (TIS National), which offers the Free Interpreting Service when doctors are providing care claimable under Medicare. This includes 24-hour access to immediate phone interpreting, pre-booked telephone interpreting for planned appointments, in-person interpreting for more complex matters and a telehealth video interpreting service. Doctors need to register to access the full range of services by phone or online (1300 575 847; https://tisonline.

tisnational.gov.au/RegisterAgency). If an unqualified interpreter such as a family member has been used—for example, in an extreme emergency—a qualified interpreter should be introduced as soon as possible to ensure the patient has understood what has taken place.

Interpreters expect to be recognised for their professional capabilities and to work as part of a team. Their code of ethics [61] demands that they interpret accurately and honestly, maintain confidentiality and act impartially and objectively.

11.21 Lawyers

The role of the law in medical practice has been noted in several chapters of this book. The expectations upon doctors when providing medicolegal reports, responding to subpoenas and appearing in court are described in Chapter 26, Medicolegal examinations and reports, court procedures and expert evidence. Doctors, however, may come into contact with lawyers in other ways, and it is important that in such contact, both parties adopt a cooperative stance where each party understands the professional role of the other. Where difficulties do arise, this can often be traced to an uncooperative, defensive or ill-informed attitude of a doctor or an aggressive, confrontational and equally ill-informed attitude of a lawyer. In most jurisdictions, there are formal mechanisms for regular discussions between representatives of the two professions to develop better understanding and to prepare protocols to guide each profession [62]. These are clearly helpful but unlikely to be at hand to guide a doctor responding to a telephone call from a lawyer. As it is rare that an instantaneous response is required of the doctor, the doctor who is uncertain of the approach to be taken should seek advice, usually from their medical indemnity organisation, before responding. Contact by lawyers with doctors usually occurs by way of:

- referral for medicolegal assessment
- request for access to records or a report on care previously given to a patient
- request for an independent opinion on medicolegal reports prepared by other doctors
- a subpoena to produce records or to appear in court to give evidence.

The appropriate responses to these types of contact are described in Chapters 26, Medicolegal examinations and reports, court procedures and expert evidence, and 27, Medical records, reports and certificates. In responding, doctors must keep in mind the need to act professionally at all times, to respect patient confidentiality (see also Chapter 6, Confidentiality, privacy and disclosure) unless the patient has given express permission to waive this right or unless directed by a court, and to respect the powers that the community has granted to the courts and their officers.

11.22 Health librarians

As the information explosion continues, and as the means of accessing that information expands, librarians are becoming increasingly important as guides for health professionals to obtain the best-quality information to guide clinical care quickly and efficiently. The Australian Library and Information Association accredits bachelor, postgraduate diploma and master courses that lead to eligibility for professional membership of the organisation, with an attendant requirement to engage in continuing professional development. Within the association, a special interest group known as Health Libraries Australia has developed a set of competencies and a process for recognition as a Certified Health Specialisation Professional [63].

Medical librarians expect doctors to be aware of the complexity and diversity of information resources and to recognise and use the expertise of librarians in managing and retrieving information. This includes learning information management skills from librarians. Librarians are assisted when doctors communicate their requirements clearly, working directly with the librarian and not through an intermediary. Doctors need to appreciate that high-quality information retrieval is labour intensive and that, for other than genuinely urgent needs, sufficient time should be allowed for processing requests. Library regulations must be observed and librarians appreciate feedback from users on the library's resources and services.

11.23 Police

As the police play a key role in the protection of the community, it is highly desirable that doctors work cooperatively with them. Conflicts occasionally arise, as in the following situations:

- Doctors believe that the illness or injury is such that its treatment needs to take precedence over the duties of the police to investigate a crime, take statements or obtain blood and tissue samples.
- Police misunderstand the ethical responsibilities of doctors, especially in regard to patient confidentiality.
- Doctors misunderstand the responsibilities of police under the law.

Interacting with patients in circumstances where police have an interest (e.g. in cases of physical or sexual assault, or where the wellbeing of a person held in custody or where the fitness of a person to be interviewed is in question) requires knowledge and experience. If the doctor has any uncertainty about how to proceed, they should seek advice from their medical defence organisation. Difficulties and conflict can be avoided by approaching these situations with courtesy and consideration and by spending time making sure that the views of both sides are understood. Should an impasse remain, higher authority should be consulted both by the doctors and the police.

Doctors have a responsibility, as does any citizen, to assist the police in the investigation of serious crime. Release of confidential information regarding a patient in this situation may be justified in the public interest but should be done with forethought and appropriate advice (see also Chapters 6, Confidentiality, privacy and disclosure, 26, Medicolegal examinations and reports, court procedures and expert evidence, and 27, Medical records, reports and certificates).

11.24 Complementary medicine practitioners

Alternative or complementary medicine may create educational, philosophical and ethical issues for the medical profession, leading at times to ambivalent or contradictory stances taken by segments of the profession. The World Health Organization notes that 'the terms "complementary medicine" and "alternative medicine" refer to a broad set of health care practices that are not part of that country's own tradition or conventional medicine and are not fully integrated into the dominant health-care system' [64]. Although the two terms are often used interchangeably, they differ subtly in their meaning in that 'complementary' normally refers to the use of one or more 'non-mainstream approach ... *together with* conventional medicine', while 'alternative' is the use of such approaches '*in place of* conventional medicine' [65]. The Australian Medical Association uses the term 'complementary medicine', which it defines as 'a wide range of products and treatments with therapeutic claims that are not presently considered to be part of conventional medicine' [66]. It considers 'complementary medicines' to include 'herbal medicines, some vitamin and mineral supplements, other nutritional supplements, homeopathic formulations, and traditional medicines such as Ayurvedic medicines and traditional Chinese medicines', while 'complementary therapies' include 'acupuncture, chiropractic, osteopathy, naturopathy, homeopathy and meditation' [66].

In 1991, the US Government established an Office of Alternative Medicine within the prestigious National Institutes of Health, and this has since developed into the National Center for Complementary and Integrative Health [65]. With an annual budget of over $170 million, the Center's mission is 'to determine, through rigorous scientific investigation, the fundamental science, usefulness, and safety of complementary and integrative health approaches and their roles in improving health and health care' [67]. In Australia, since 2006, the National Health and Medical Research Council (NHMRC) has also supported research and conducted evidence evaluations in relation to complementary medicine [68]. This work was used by the Australian Government in 2019 when it excluded 16 complementary therapies from eligibility for private health insurance coverage under Australian law. The NHMRC has also prepared a valuable resource for clinicians titled *Talking with your patients about complementary medicine* [69].

The international network Cochrane (formerly Cochrane Collaboration), which aims to ensure that decisions about health and care globally are informed by high-quality evidence, has undertaken a very large number of systematic reviews of the available evidence related to the use of a wide range of complementary treatments and therapies for many common conditions [70]. Its website provides plain language summaries, often supported by audio podcasts, that are very useful for supporting conversations between doctors and their patients about their interest in the use of complementary approaches.

It is probably fair to comment that complementary medicine practitioners tend to be ambivalent about their professional place in the healthcare system—some would like to be recognised via registration processes and sit alongside mainstream medicine [71], while others fear that such recognition might reduce the mystique of complementary medicine and affect its popularity with the general public. In terms of regulation, there is currently something of a paradox in Australia in that chiropractors, osteopaths and Chinese medicine practitioners are regulated under the national health registration scheme (and discussed specifically below), with protected titles under the National Law, while the remainder of individuals offering complementary treatments and therapies are either self-regulated or unregulated. This might be taken by the public to imply governmental endorsement of these three professions relative to the others when, in fact, the inclusion of particular complementary (or indeed 'conventional') health professions or not in the national scheme appears to have been more an accident of history than anything intentional on the part of legislators. Each of the national boards for the three regulated professions emphasises the importance of 'evidence-based practice' in its practice standards and practitioner capability documents, but the evidence summarised in the Cochrane database does not appear to support the contention that the practice of these three professions is, in fact, more evidence based than that of self-regulated 'Western herbalists', for example [70].

In relation to self-regulated and unregulated complementary medicine practitioners, several state/territory governments have enacted legislation that empowers their health complaints authorities to receive and act upon complaints in relation to any 'health services' provided in their jurisdiction. The Victorian *Health Complaints Act 2016*, for example, includes a definition of 'health service' that is inclusive of all activities 'intended or claimed (expressly or otherwise)' to 'assess, predict, maintain or improve' a person's physical or mental health [72]. It also prescribes a code of conduct for the unregistered providers of such services and empowers the state's Health Complaints Commissioner to investigate and resolve alleged breaches of the code through conciliation or the issuing of prohibition orders on practitioners.

The medical profession has been reluctant to oppose complementary medicine completely. From time to time, remedies arising from alternative approaches find their way into mainstream medical practice; the risk of harm is usually low and doctors recognise that some elements of orthodox medical practice represent art rather than science. Many doctors are highly critical of the quantity and, especially, the quality of empirical scientific evidence concerning the efficacy, safety and cost of complementary interventions in comparison to mainstream medical practice. Additional concerns relate to the real, but at times unknown, potential for adverse events as a consequence of interactions between orthodox and less orthodox therapies, as well as the problems of sharing patient care with providers whose ethical principles may not always be explicit. Some doctors undertake additional training in acupuncture and their registration can be endorsed for acupuncture practice.

It is important that opinions and attitudes concerning complementary medicine are conveyed to patients in a responsible manner. Doctors have a professional duty to advise patients about the benefits and risks of conventional and less conventional therapeutic and investigational interventions, and about what is known and not known about them. The reality is that some patients seek access to complementary therapies out of frustration that orthodox medicine is not helping them, out of distress and, in some instances, out of the desire to have more sense of control over their own health care. Wise doctors will be alert to these possibilities and seek to work uncritically and positively with such patients in a spirit of partnership, with a focus on the minimisation of harm.

11.24.1 Chiropractors

The Australian Chiropractors Association defines chiropractic practice as being 'concerned with the diagnosis, management and prevention of mechanical disorders of the musculoskeletal system (spine); this includes the effects of these disorders on the function of the nervous system and general health' [73]. It points out what it sees as a 'common misconception' that chiropractic practice involves the single technique of spinal manipulation, arguing that it 'incorporates a range of manual therapies which may include spinal adjustment, but also includes mobilisation, muscle and soft tissue techniques along with electrotherapies, exercise prescription, rehabilitation, nutritional recommendations and lifestyle advice' [74].

Becoming a chiropractor in Australia requires completion of an approved five-year program of study at one of five Australian higher education providers, configured as either a bachelor–master sequence or two bachelor degrees. 'Chiropractor' is a protected title and may only be used by individuals who are registered with the Chiropractic Board of Australia, supported by Ahpra. Registered chiropractors are required to adhere to the shared *Code of conduct* [25] and meet registration standards related to indemnity insurance, recency of practice and continuing professional development. They may refer patients for X-rays of the spine or pelvis and are also entitled to perform these investigations themselves, subject to state/territory-based regulations and where clinically indicated.

11.24.2 Osteopaths

Osteopathy originated in the US in the 1870s. Osteopaths believe that the human body has all of the necessary elements to attain, and maintain, optimal health, and an in-built repair system that enables people to recover from injury and disease. Via techniques believed to promote blood flow, osteopaths claim to maintain optimal function of the internal organs, which in turn promotes and maintains the body's balanced production of natural chemicals. In the US and a few other countries, some accredited medical schools incorporate osteopathic principles in addition to orthodox medicine and graduate 'osteopathic physicians' who are licensed to practise medicine and train in the full range of medical specialties. In most parts of world, including Australia, practitioners are known as osteopaths and have a narrower scope of practice that is considered a form of complementary therapy. The principal technique employed is osteopathic manipulative therapy, which includes soft tissue massage, muscle stretching, passive range of motion and gentle joint manipulation. The majority of people treated present with acute musculoskeletal complaints [75]. Osteopaths also consider the roles of appropriate exercise programs, a healthy diet and nutrition, and emotional wellbeing (through techniques such as stress reduction exercises and strategies) as important factors in treatment.

Training in Australia involves an approved four- to five-year program of study at one of three universities, configured as two bachelor degrees or a bachelor–master sequence. Osteopaths must be registered with the Osteopathy Board of Australia, which is supported by Ahpra.

11.24.3 Chinese medicine practitioners

Chinese medicine became a regulated profession under the National Law in Australia in 2012. It comprises two major divisions, 'acupuncturist' and 'Chinese herbal medicine practitioner', with most individuals practising in one or both areas, while some work only as 'Chinese herbal dispensers', providing therapies prescribed by other practitioners within the profession. Chinese medicine has a very long history dating back 5000 years. As a system, its emphasis is on bodily functions and balance of opposing factors rather than on anatomy and physiology. Practitioners focus on the interplay between body and mind, with therapeutic interventions including acupuncture, moxibustion (a technique in which dried plant leaves are burned close to the skin), massage, dietary therapy and the prescription of traditional herbal preparations. Many of these herbal agents are potentially toxic and the Chinese Medicine Board of Australia has produced detailed *Guidelines for safe practice of Chinese herbal medicine* [76]. Some preparations may interact significantly with conventional pharmacotherapeutics and it is very important for doctors to inquire about the use of Chinese (and other) herbal medicines when taking a medication history prior to prescribing.

In order to qualify for registration as Chinese medicine practitioners, candidates need to complete an approved program of study at bachelor or master level at one of two Australian universities or several private education providers. Practitioners are registered with the Chinese Medicine Board of Australia, supported by Ahpra, and are required to adhere to the shared *Code of conduct* [25] and meet registration standards related to indemnity insurance, recency of practice and continuing professional development.

Summary

To work collaboratively, doctors should understand and respect the contributions of other healthcare professionals and actively include them in care planning. This chapter has outlined the particular knowledge, skills and attributes such health professionals bring to patient care and has outlined some principles of collaborative care. The key principles to bring to any interaction with other professions involved in the care of patients are understanding of and respect for their role, and good communication skills.

It is very important to recognise that a patient's care may require multiple healthcare professionals to support patients to understand and access other services. Equally, patients have the right to choose health care that is broader than the medical approach alone, and an open-minded conversation about such choices is likely to provide the best outcomes.

References

1. Australian Institute of Health and Welfare. Chronic condition multimorbidity. Canberra: AIHW, 2021. https://www.aihw.gov.au/reports/chronic-disease/chronic-condition-multimorbidity (accessed Sep 2021).
2. Australian Institute of Health and Welfare. Australia's health 2020: Social determinants of health. Canberra: AIHW, 2021. https://www.aihw.gov.au/reports/australias-health/social-determinants-of-health (accessed Sep 2021).
3. Australian Institute of Health and Welfare. Australia's health 2020: Natural environment and health. Canberra: AIHW, 2021. https://www.aihw.gov.au/reports/australias-health/natural-environment-and-health (accessed Sep 2021).
4. Australian Institute of Health and Welfare. Australia's health 2020: Health expenditure. Canberra: AIHW, 2021. https://www.aihw.gov.au/reports/australias-health/health-expenditure (accessed Sep 2021).
5. Kohn LT, Corrigan JM, Donaldson MS, editors. To err is human: Building a safer health system. Washington DC: National Academy Press, 2000. https://www.nap.edu/catalog/9728/ to-err-is-human-building-a-safer-health-system (accessed Oct 2021).
6. Bristol Royal Infirmary Inquiry. Learning from Bristol: The report of the public inquiry into children's heart surgery at the Bristol Royal Infirmary 1984–1995. London: Stationery Office, 2002. https://psnet.ahrq.gov/issue/learning-bristol-report-public-inquiry-childrens-heart-surgery-bristol-royal-infirmary-1984 (accessed Oct 2021).
7. Garling P. Final report of the special commission of inquiry: Acute care in NSW public hospitals. 2008. https://www.dpc.nsw.gov.au/publications/special-commissions-of-inquiry/special-commission-of-inquiry-into-acute-care-services-in-new-south-wales-public-hospitals/ (accessed Oct 2021).
8. Francis R. Report of the Mid Staffordshire NHS Foundation Trust Public Inquiry. London: National Archives, 2013. https://www.gov.uk/government/publications/report-of-the-mid-staffordshire-nhs-foundation-trust-public-inquiry (accessed Oct 2021).
9. Rogers GD, Thistlethwaite JE, Anderson ES, et al. International consensus statement on the assessment of interprofessional learning outcomes. *Med Teach* 2017; 39: 347–359.
10. Rogers GD, Chesters JE. An orchestral metaphor for interprofessional learning and collaborative practice? *Clin Teach* 2014; 11: 317–318.
11. Teodorczuk A, Khoo TK, Morrissey S, Rogers GD. Developing interprofessional education: Putting theory into practice. *Clin Teach* 2016; 13: 7–12.
12. O'Keefe M, Henderson A, Chick R. Defining a set of common interprofessional learning competencies for health profession students. *Med Teach* 2017; 39: 463–468.
13. Ebert L, Hoffman K, Levett-Jones T, Gilligan C. 'They have no idea of what we do or what we know': Australian graduates' perceptions of working in a health care team. Nurse Educ Pract 2014; 14: 544–550.
14. Rosenstein AH. Nurse–physician relationships: impact on nurse satisfaction and retention. Am J Nurs 2002; 102: 26–34.
15. Greenfield LJ. Doctors and nurses: a troubled partnership. *Ann Surg* 1999; 230: 279–288.
16. Nelson GA, King ML, Brodine S. Nurse–physician collaboration on medical-surgical units. *Medsurg Nurs* 2008; 17: 35–40.
17. Nursing and Midwifery Board of Australia. Midwife standards for practice. Ahpra, 2018. https://www.nursingmidwiferyboard.gov.au/Codes-Guidelines-Statements/Professional-standards/Midwife-standards-for-practice.aspx (accessed Nov 2021).
18. International Council of Nurses. Code of ethics for nurses. 2021. https://www.icn.ch/resources/publications-and-reports/icn-code-ethics-nurses (accessed Nov 2021).
19. International Confederation of Midwives. International code of ethics for midwives. 2014. https://internationalmidwives.org/resources/international-code-of-ethics-for-midwives (accessed Nov 2021).
20. Nursing and Midwifery Board of Australia. Professional standards. Ahpra, 2023. https://www.nursingmidwiferyboard.gov.au/Codes-Guidelines-Statements/Professional-standards.aspx (accessed Jan 2025).
21. Austin Health. State endoscopy training centre. 2021. https://www.austin.org.au/StateEndoscopyTrainingCentre/ (accessed Nov 2021).

22. Nursing and Midwifery Board of Australia. Midwife standards for practice. Ahpra, 2018. https://www.nursingmidwiferyboard.gov.au/Codes-Guidelines-Statements/Professional-standards/Midwife-standards-for-practice.aspx (accessed Nov 2021).
23. Pharmacy Board of Australia. Guidelines for dispensing of medicines. Ahpra, 2024. http://www.pharmacyboard.gov.au/Codes-Guidelines.aspx (accessed Jan 2025).
24. Advanced Pharmacy Australia. Specialty practice. 2025. https://adpha.au/workforce-research/specialty-practice (accessed Jan 2025).
25. Australian Health Practitioner Regulation Agency. Shared code of conduct. Ahpra & National Boards, 2022. https://www.ahpra.gov.au/Resources/Code-of-conduct/Shared-Code-of-conduct.aspx (accessed Jan 2025).
26. Pharmaceutical Society of Australia. Code of ethics for pharmacists. 2017. http://www.psa.org.au/membership/ethics (accessed Nov 2021).
27. Advanced Pharmacy Australia. SHPA Code of ethics. 2016. https://adpha.au/publicassets/0835179a-de53-ec11-80dd-005056be03d0/6._shpa_code_of_ethics.pdf (accessed Nov 2021).
28. National Association of Aboriginal and Torres Strait Islander Health Workers and Practitioners. Who we are and what we do. 2021. https://www.naatsihwp.org.au/who-we-are-and-what-we-do (accessed Nov 2021).
29. National Association of Aboriginal and Torres Strait Islander Health Workers and Practitioners. Professional Scopes of Practice Project: Achieving greater national consistency for the Aboriginal and/or Torres Strait Islander Health Worker and Health Practitioner professions. 2025. https://www.naatsihwp.org.au/storage/naatsihwp_report_web_250211.pdf (accessed Aug 2025).
30. Aboriginal and Torres Strait Islander Health Practice Board. Annual report 2023/24. 2025. https://www.atsihealthpracticeboard.gov.au/News/Annual-report.aspx (accessed May 2025).
31. University of Nebraska–Lincoln. Definition of an audiologist. 2021. https://cehs.unl.edu/secd/aud-student-handbook/definition-audiologist/ (accessed Dec 2021).
32. Hearing Professional Conduct and Complaints Body. Code of conduct for audiologists and audiometrists. 2024. https://hpccb.org.au/code-of-conduct/ (accessed Jan 2025).
33. Australian Dental Association. Policy Statement 3.2 – Dentists. 2021. https://ada.org.au/policy-statement-3-2-dentists (accessed Dec 2021).
34. Dental Board of Australia. Guidelines for scope of practice. Ahpra, 2020. https://www.dentalboard.gov.au/Codes-Guidelines/Policies-Codes-Guidelines/Guidelines-Scope-of-practice.aspx (accessed Dec 2021).
35. Australian Dental Association, NSW Branch. Code of Ethics. 2022. https://www.adansw.com.au/wp-content/uploads/ADA-NSW-Code-of-Ethics-2022.pdf (accessed Jun 2025).
36. International Confederation of Dietetic Associations. Standards: definition of dietitian-nutritionist. 2014. https://internationaldietetics.org/standards/ (accessed Dec 2021).
37. Nutrition Society of Australia. About the registration scheme. 2021. https://www.nsa.asn.au/nsa-registration/registration/about-the-registration-scheme/ (accessed Dec 2021).
38. Exercise and Sports Science Australia. What is an Accredited Exercise Physiologist (AEP)? 2021. https://www.essa.org.au/Public/Consumer_Information/What_is_an_Accredited_Exercise_Physiologist_.aspx (accessed Dec 2021).
39. Exercise and Sports Science Australia. Code of professional conduct and ethical practice. 2024. https://www.essa.org.au/Web/Resources/Standards/code-of-professional-conduct-and-ethical-practice.aspx (accessed Jan 2025).
40. World Federation of Occupational Therapists. About occupational therapy. 2021. https://wfot.org/member-organisations/australia-occupational-therapy-australia (accessed Jun 2025).
41. Australian Orthotic Prosthetic Association. Ethical Principles and Code of Professional Conduct. 2018. https://www.aopa.org.au/documents/item/473 (accessed Dec 2021).
42. Paramedicine Board of Australia. Fact sheet: What is a registered paramedic. 2022. https://www.paramedicineboard.gov.au/Registration.aspx (accessed Mar 2025).
43. Australian Institute of Paramedic Practitioners. About AIPP. 2021. https://www.acpp.net.au/about-aipp (accessed Mar 2025).
44. Yong G, Dent AW, Weiland TJ. Handover from paramedics: observations and emergency department clinician perceptions. *Emerg Med Australas* 2008; 20: 149–155.

45. Allied Health Professions Australia. Physiotherapy. 2021. https://www.ahpa.com.au/physiotherapy (accessed Dec 2021).
46. Australian Physiotherapy Association. Australian College of Physiotherapists. 2021. https://australian.physio/pd/australian-college-physiotherapists (accessed Dec 2021).
47. Australian Physiotherapy Association. Code of conduct. 2023. https://australian.physio/sites/default/files/APA_CODE_OF_CONDUCT_2023.pdf (accessed Mar 2025).
48. Podiatry Board of Australia. Registration Standards. https://www.podiatryboard.gov.au/Registration-Standards.aspx (accessed Aug 2025).
49. Australian Psychological Society. How can psychology help me? 2021. https://psychology.org.au/psychology/about-psychology/what-is-psychology (accessed Dec 2021).
50. Australian Psychological Society. APS code of ethics. 2007. https://psychology.org.au/about-us/what-we-do/ethics-and-practice-standards/aps-code-of-ethics (accessed Dec 2021).
51. International Federation of Social Workers. Global definition of social work. 2014. https://www.ifsw.org/what-is-social-work/global-definition-of-social-work/ (accessed Dec 2021).
52. Australian Association of Social Workers. Code of ethics. 2020. https://www.aasw.asn.au/about-aasw/ethics-standards/code-of-ethics/ (accessed Dec 2021).
53. Speech Pathology Australia. What is a speech pathologist? 2024. https://www.speechpathologyaustralia.org.au/Public/Public/services/About-speech-pathologists/What-speech-pathologists-do.aspx (accessed Mar 2025).
54. Grant L, Murray SA, Sheikh A. Spiritual dimensions of dying in pluralist societies. *BMJ* 2010; 341: 659–662.
55. Spiritual Care Australia. Strategic plan 2021-2025 [v2.1 July 2024]. 2021. https://www.spiritualcareaustralia.org.au/about-us/sca-strategic-plan/ (accessed Mar 2025).
56. Australian and New Zealand Association for Clinical Pastoral Education. ANZACPE Member Associations. 2022. https://www.anzacpe.org.au/member-associations/ (accessed Jan 2022).
57. Spiritual Care Australia. Standards of practice. 2013. https://www.spiritualcareaustralia.org.au/public/103/files/SCA_Standards_of_Practice_Document-1.pdf (accessed Jan 2022).
58. Cross-Cultural Communications. Definition of interpreting. 2022. https://www.thecommunityinterpreter.com/what-is-interpreting (accessed Jan 2022).
59. National Accreditation Authority for Interpreters and Translators. About us. 2022. https://www.naati.com.au/about-us/ (accessed Jan 2022).
60. Migrant and Refugee Women's Health Partnership. Guide for clinicians working with interpreters in healthcare settings. 2019. https://culturaldiversityhealth.org.au/wp-content/uploads/2019/10/Guide-for-clinicians-working-with-interpreters-in-healthcare-settings-Jan2019.pdf (accessed Jan 2022).
61. Australian Institute of Interpreters and Translators. AUSIT code of ethics. 2012. https://ausit.org/code-of-ethics/ (accessed Aug 2025).
62. Australian Medical Association (Vic Branch); the Law Institute of Victoria. Guidelines for co-operation between doctors and lawyers. Melbourne: LIV, 2008. http://civilforensicpsychiatry.com.au/wp-content/uploads/2014/05/Guidelines-for-Doctors-and-Lawyers.pdf (accessed Jan 2022).
63. Australian Library and Information Association. HLA Health Professional Development Scheme. 2022. https://hla.alia.org.au/professional-development-education-and-training/ (accessed Jan 2022).
64. World Health Organization. Traditional, complementary and integrative medicine. 2022. https://www.who.int/health-topics/traditional-complementary-and-integrative-medicine#tab=tab_1 (accessed Jan 2022).
65. National Center for Complementary and Integrative Health. Complementary, alternative, or integrative health: what's in a name? 2021. https://www.nccih.nih.gov/health/complementary-alternative-or-integrative-health-whats-in-a-name (accessed Jan 2022).
66. Australian Medical Association. AMA position statement—complementary medicine—2018. https://www.ama.com.au/position-statement/ama-position-statement-complementary-medicine-2018 (accessed Jan 2022).
67. National Center for Complementary and Integrative Health. About NCCIH. https://www.nccih.nih.gov/about (accessed Jun 2025).
68. National Health and Medical Research Council. Complementary medicines. 2022. https://www.nhmrc.gov.au/health-advice/all-topics/complementary-medicines (accessed Jan 2022).

69. National Health and Medical Research Council. Talking with your patients about complementary medicine – a resource for clinicians. 2014. https://www.nhmrc.gov.au/about-us/publications/talking-your-patients-about-complementary-medicine-resource-clinicians (accessed Jan 2022).
70. Cochrane Complementary Medicine. Cochrane reviews related to complementary medicine. 2022. https://cam.cochrane.org/cochrane-reviews-related-complementary-medicine (accessed Jan 2022).
71. Naturopaths and Herbalists Association of Australia. Welcome to the Naturopaths & Herbalists Association of Australia. 2022. https://nhaa.org.au/ (accessed Jan 2022).
72. *Health Complaints Act 2016* (Vic), Pt 1, s 3.
73. Australian Chiropractors Association. Chiropractic and you. 2022. https://www.chiro.org.au/about-chiropractic/chiropractic-and-you/ (accessed Jan 2022).
74. Australian Chiropractors Association. FAQs. 2022. https://www.chiro.org.au/about-chiropractic/faq/ (accessed Jan 2022).
75. Burke SR, Myers R, Zhang AL. A profile of osteopathic practice in Australia 2010–2011: a cross sectional survey. *BMC Musculoskelet Disord* 2013; 14: 227.
76. Chinese Medicine Board of Australia. Guidelines for safe practice of Chinese herbal medicine. 2024. https://www.chinesemedicineboard.gov.au/Codes-Guidelines/Guidelines-for-safe-practice.aspx (accessed Mar 2025).

Further reading

Day J. Interprofessional working: An essential guide for health and social care professionals. Melbourne: Cengage Learning, 2013.

Slusser M, Garcia LI, Reed C-R, McGinnis PQ. Foundations of interprofessional collaborative practice in health care. Maryland Heights: Mosby, 2018.

12 Personal health of the doctor: illness and impairment

Kathryn Hutt, Margaret Kay AM

Introduction

Doctors' health is a vital element in good medical practice.

Over a century ago, Sir William Osler paraphrased Shakespeare, stating that 'the doctor who doctors himself has a fool for a patient' [1]. Today, we recognise that doctors looking after their own health are not fools but have a personal and professional responsibility to do so. There are, however, specific challenges for doctors seeking to maximise their own physical and mental health and wellbeing. It is essential that all doctors recognise appropriate limits for self-diagnosis and treatment and are able to access professional support when needed.

A healthy doctor provides improved care for patients and supports the overall wellbeing of communities. Maintaining doctors' health remains a fundamental issue for the medical profession today—not only for each individual doctor but for the profession as a whole (see Chapter 2, On being a good doctor: the changing face of medical professionalism, section 2.1.1).

The importance of doctors' health is well recognised internationally and has been integrated within the World Medical Association's Declaration of Geneva (the 'Modern Hippocratic Oath') and International Code of Medical Ethics:

> I WILL ATTEND TO my own health, well-being, and abilities in order to provide care of the highest standard
>
> World Medical Association Declaration of Geneva [2]

> In order to provide care of the highest standards, physicians must attend to their own health, well-being, and abilities. This includes seeking appropriate care to ensure that they are able to practise safely.
>
> World Medical Association International Code of Medical Ethics [3]

This chapter outlines multiple facets of doctors' health, including health issues experienced by doctors, understanding how doctors' health intersects with the delivery of health care, impacts of the medical profession on doctors' health, how doctors should care for themselves, and strategies to help doctors access health care. The concept of 'impairment'—an important issue for all doctors and their communities—is discussed, along with key points on how to care for the doctor-patient.

12.1 Defining doctors' health

Understanding the broad range of factors, including cultural, environmental and spiritual elements, that make up doctors' health is essential to enable doctors to maintain and support their personal health and the health of their colleagues.

The World Health Organization defines health as a state of complete physical, mental and social wellbeing and not merely the absence of disease or infirmity [4]. Because of their professional focus on disease or infirmity, doctors often narrow their understanding of their own personal health to focus on the absence of disease. There is much to learn about health and wellbeing from First Nations communities, who recognise the importance of connection to culture, community, environment and history [5]. This broad definition of health also applies to doctors.

As with the general community, many doctors have physical or mental health issues, and acute issues can often complicate chronic health problems. Managing doctors' health includes preventive health care, as well as specific types of health care at various stages of life, such as maternal health care. Understanding doctors' health only through the lens of impairment restricts the profession's understanding of the breadth and complexity of doctors' health issues. The concept of impairment is addressed in section 12.11.

Proactively addressing wellbeing can assist doctors to flourish in medicine. This includes incorporating preventive activities to maintain doctors' physical health, such as wearing protective gear and receiving appropriate vaccinations. For doctors' mental health, preventive activities might include peer support and allowing time for reflection. Connectedness facilitates social health.

12.1.1 Physical health

Physical health issues are part of the shared human experience, and the prevalence of these in doctors often mirrors that in the general population [6]. Doctors do experience a lower mortality rate, which has much to do with their health literacy, education and other social determinants of health. This is not, however, a nuanced measure of health or wellbeing for any population, and more research investigating the physical health of doctors is required [6].

More than 40% of doctors are managing chronic physical health issues [6]. Doctors remain vulnerable to infectious disease, as highlighted during the COVID-19 pandemic. The profession must remain mindful of the need to consider doctors' physical health issues, understanding how acute illness can interrupt their short- and long-term career plans and how physical health issues affect their career and life decisions.

Infections with bloodborne viruses, including hepatitis B, hepatitis C and HIV, have specific regulatory requirements. All doctors should be aware of whether they are working in defined exposure-prone activities. If so, appropriate monitoring for bloodborne viruses is required. Doctors who test positive for a bloodborne virus need to follow the relevant guidelines to maintain their health and reduce public risk [7].

12.1.2 Mental health

Mental health issues in doctors, such as stress, anxiety and depression, have been well documented in the literature [8]. Most studies that describe the prevalence of mental health issues in doctors report on mental health screening tools, rather than diagnoses, which allows useful comparisons between populations.

A Beyond Blue study, published in 2013, was the first national investigation of the mental health of doctors and medical students in Australia [8]. This study found that 9% of doctors reported a current diagnosis of anxiety. Depression is not uncommon in doctors and can be under-recognised, with stigma contributing to late presentations. Eating disorders are increasingly being recognised as an issue for doctors, particularly for younger doctors.

Suicide is often discussed as a mental health issue, but doctor suicide is complex (see section 12.5).

12.1.3 Social health

Social health is an important aspect of wellbeing, and lack of social support has been associated with poor outcomes for doctors with mental health issues, including suicide. Peer support became an important consideration throughout the COVID-19 pandemic, although previous research had already identified the association between doctors attending continuing medical education activities and their improved wellbeing (see section 12.7).

Throughout their medical careers, doctors will experience a variety of health issues and stressors. New health issues are to be expected at different stages of life. Doctors have a responsibility to regularly self-reflect on their health issues and to anticipate or recognise when their physical or mental health may be more fragile. Proactive reflection should include a review of their current workload and the quality of care they are delivering, as well as time available to address their health issues. Ensuring regular independent review with a general practitioner (GP) allows objective feedback to support these personal self-reflections.

12.2 Doctors' health and the delivery of health care

Addressing all aspects of doctors' health enables the delivery of quality care.

The personal health of doctors cannot be separated from the quality of care they give their patients. Across the medical literature, many doctors have attested to how their own experience as a patient has enhanced the care they provide. The philosopher Plato recognised that doctors could benefit from personally experiencing significant health issues:

> It is true enough of doctors that the ablest might prove to be men who, from childhood up, besides mastering their profession, had been in contact with the largest number of the worst cases, and moreover were not of a robust constitution and had themselves suffered from every malady [1].

Personal illness can enable doctors to deliver care with empathy and with a deeper understanding of the patient's perspective and expectations [11]. From an organisational perspective, doctors' health is acknowledged as a key quality indicator for the delivery of quality health care [12,13]. It is therefore an organisational responsibility to maximise doctors' health and wellbeing [14], which also makes sound business sense [15].

Doctors' wellbeing requires a positive and supportive workplace culture. Medical professional organisations, including medical colleges, medical associations, training organisations, universities and hospitals, have important roles in supporting the health and wellbeing of doctors and medical students [14,16,17].

Many doctors hold leadership roles within such organisations. Ideally, all doctors should proactively support the health of their colleagues, and those in leadership roles have a clear professional responsibility to do so, as well as to ensure that the workplace is mentally and physically safe [18].

All doctors need to develop a personal awareness of how their actions and words influence the wellbeing of colleagues, peers and those they educate. Doctor-leaders can support doctor wellbeing by identifying and supporting workplace interventions that foster a positive culture, as well as identifying emerging concerns and addressing these effectively [14,19,20].

12.3 Impacts of the medical profession on doctors' health

The health and wellbeing of every doctor is fundamentally affected, both positively and negatively, by their medical training and ongoing professional role.

Doctors working in Australia come from a wide range of backgrounds. Each person brings to the profession a unique set of personal characteristics, strengths, vulnerabilities and life stories. These variables can all have positive and negative impacts on a doctor's personal health and wellbeing. It is clear, however, that the act of training to be a doctor, and subsequently working as a member of the profession, has a profound impact on each doctor's health and wellbeing, including on their ability to seek care when required.

There are many reasons why medical training can improve the personal health of a doctor. Doctors frequently enjoy reasonably good socioeconomic status and quality of life and may thrive on their sense of accomplishment and high level of job satisfaction. Increased health literacy may result in healthier life choices and early recognition of disease indicators. Doctors might have enhanced knowledge of services or treatments available for their health condition. An understanding of the local health system can improve access to care for a doctor or their family members.

However, becoming a member of the profession can also have a negative impact on the health and wellbeing of the individual. Many doctors experience significant barriers when accessing health care [21]. Doctors can often provide timely and effective self-care and may not recognise the need to seek professional support until their illness has progressed. Some doctors find they are uncomfortable accepting the role of a patient and may feel they are burdening a colleague by doing so [22].

Doctors are often expected to work long hours, handle high levels of stress and perform physically demanding tasks, which can take a toll on their health and wellbeing. The pressure to make life-and-death decisions, the emotional toll of caring for patients, working in an often hierarchical system and the stress of dealing with administrative tasks can lead to burnout, depression and anxiety.

There are many factors and potential hazards in training or working as a doctor that may have a negative impact on health and wellbeing. Identifying aspects of the profession with the potential to have a negative impact on a doctor's health is the first step in developing strategies to mitigate these risks. Personal reflection on each of these factors can assist individual doctors to proactively identify relevant barriers and recognise solutions that will enhance their personal health and wellbeing.

12.3.1 Working hours (extended hours and shiftwork)

The often long working hours, shiftwork and lack of time for self-care that doctors experience can contribute to their mental load. There is strong evidence that shiftwork can have a negative impact on physical and mental health [23].

12.3.2 Physical requirements of the job

Physical strain may have an impact on health. Doctors often experience physical pain from the repetitive motions they perform, such as bending over patients, performing surgeries and procedures, and being on their feet for extended periods [24]. Doctors also run the risk of exposure to infectious diseases and hazardous materials that can negatively affect their health [25].

12.3.3 Occupational hazards

Doctors face many occupational hazards, which vary according to their role. It is important that individuals familiarise themselves with any hazards particular to their workplace, such as exposure to sharp objects, radiation or toxic agents, or aggressive members of the public. They may need to take special precautions to protect their safety [26].

12.3.4 Other workplace stressors

Doctors often face stressful work environments, sometimes involving non-collaborative relationships with colleagues or other staff. This can lead to feelings of isolation and lack of support, accompanied by increased stress levels. See section 33.8 of Chapter 33, Entering and leaving practice and practice management, for more information on managing the work environment.

The healthcare system is often bureaucratic, leading to significant rules, regulations and administrative tasks that can be time consuming and take doctors away from direct patient care, which may detract from their job satisfaction.

12.3.5 Professional culture

Doctors often work within a culture of norms regarding their behaviour and performance. These expectations, relating to performing well academically, may have been in place for many years. Medical culture often prioritises technical expertise and scientific knowledge over emotional intelligence and empathy. Additionally, there may be expectations around 'getting things right 100% of the time' and the amount of time dedicated to the job, as well as a focus on individual achievement over teamwork.

These cultural expectations can have a significant impact on the wellbeing of doctors and can contribute to issues such as burnout, stress, lack of self-care and lack of attention to other aspects of their personal lives.

To promote the health and wellbeing of doctors, it is important to examine and challenge these cultural expectations, improve work conditions and find ways to create a more supportive and inclusive culture among doctors.

12.3.6 Vicarious trauma

Doctors are vulnerable to the impact of recurrent exposure to traumatic events [27]. Individual personal responses vary but can include acute anxiety, depression and post-traumatic stress disorder. Vicarious trauma is more common when the situation resonates with a doctor's personal experience, such as their own previous trauma history or the age of an unwell patient in relation to a member of their own family.

12.3.7 Moral injury

Moral injury can occur when a doctor feels powerless to act, or has failed to respond, in a manner in which they feel they should [28]. Structural and hierarchical issues are often involved, altering a doctor's ability to respond. When this is beyond the doctor's personal control, feelings of distress can result. Being able to identify when a moral injury occurs can be key to ameliorating the distress [29].

12.3.8 Impostor syndrome

The 'impostor syndrome' is a common experience for those practising medicine. Individuals who are extremely capable can feel like impostors and become fearful that others will 'discover' their lack of knowledge or inadequate skill, despite being very capable in their work [30].

For doctors, particularly for those early in their careers, feeling like an impostor can cause distress, potentially eroding self-esteem. This feeling can be paralysing and reduce the doctor's efficiency and confidence in delivering care. There is a risk that when a doctor feels this way, they will be less likely to request support from colleagues about a case they are managing, as they fear that no-one else would need help in the same situation.

Identifying and managing these fears with appropriate strategies can result in safer medical care. Strategies could include ensuring adequate peer support to enable camaraderie and normalisation of the experiences associated with the practice of medicine. An environment that promotes non-threatening, safe conversations between peers and between doctors-in-training and their supervisors is essential for normalising feelings of uncertainty and enhancing opportunities for collegial support.

12.3.9 Burnout

Burnout is an occupational phenomenon that can cause psychological distress [31]. It is important to understand the role of the healthcare organisation in the development of burnout in an individual [18].

Doctors experience high levels of burnout compared with the general population [32]. Burnout in doctors has a negative impact on their personal health and the quality of patient care they provide. Doctors experiencing burnout are more likely to self-report medical errors and to demonstrate reduced empathy for patients, increased unprofessional behaviour and reduced altruism [33]. Burnout increases the rate of intention to leave medicine and impacts on mental health among doctors [33,34]. There is evidence of burnout occurring in doctors across the career spectrum, including medical students, as well as across the many specialties in both clinical practice and academia.

Australian doctors have similar rates of burnout to those reported internationally [8]. Since the COVID-19 pandemic, rates of burnout have increased, with a recent study reporting the prevalence of burnout in frontline workers to be 70.9% [34].

12.3.10 Bullying, discrimination and harassment

Bullying, discrimination and harassment (including sexual harassment) in the workplace deserve special consideration. They are harmful to individuals and have no place in the profession of medicine, or in broader society, yet doctors report that these issues persist in the health workforce [35,36].

Embedded cultural issues that are established early in a doctor's medical career foster these behaviours [37]. Discrimination (including discrimination related to race or gender) is prevalent in medicine and is associated with burnout and suicidal ideation [36].

These behaviours are unacceptable, and it is the responsibility of every doctor to identify and address them. All doctors should be aware of the definition of bullying in the workplace, understanding how this differs from standard feedback given during clinical training and performance management. When doctors are bystanders (witnesses of these behaviours), they often feel powerless, yet their role can be crucial [38]. Daring to maintain a presence, being a witness and maintaining a record of the event (time, date and place) can help reduce such behaviour. Ensuring that the colleague subjected to the bullying feels supported after such an event is also important. Validating the reality of the experience can help reduce the ongoing impact of these experiences. At times, bystanders can experience moral injury (see section 12.3.7) when exposed to this behaviour. Senior personnel have an important role in supporting their junior colleagues who are experiencing such behaviours and in supporting the expectation of a safe workplace for all [39].

Reporting of bullying, discrimination or harassment by those experiencing or witnessing it can be difficult because of the cultural issues noted above and associated stigma. However, one of the common reasons given for not reporting it is simply not knowing the pathway for doing so. It is the responsibility of individuals, team leaders and healthcare organisations to ensure that all doctors are aware of the appropriate pathways for such reporting [39]. The federal *Sex Discrimination and Fair Work (Respect at Work) Amendment Act 2021* and *Anti-Discrimination and Human Rights Legislation Amendment (Respect at Work) Act 2022* highlight the responsibilities of employers and provide the Australian Human Rights Commission with greater powers to support best practice in these areas. Although employers, including healthcare organisations, may have policies and procedures for managing any concerns about these behaviours in the workplace, simply having such policies is not enough, as employers now need to demonstrate how these policies are enacted.

Many postgraduate colleges have developed educational modules to ensure that supervisors know how to deliver training in an appropriate manner [37]. The entire profession will benefit from doctors proactively working together with their various professional organisations to ensure effective implementation of these strategies for addressing bullying, discrimination and harassment in medicine. As individuals, all doctors should be aware of their professional and personal supports in case they are personally affected or need to support a colleague.

12.4 How personal attributes and the medical career intersect

When wearing the mantle of the white coat, it is important that doctors maintain their sense of self.

Self-knowledge and the capacity for honest self-reflection are essential elements in maintaining personal health and wellbeing. Doctors are individuals, with a range of personal values, vulnerabilities and motivators. Developing self-understanding and practising self-compassion can assist each individual to recognise their role as a doctor as distinct from their personal identity [40]. This can be protective when dealing with workplace difficulties or when things go wrong at work.

12.4.1 Resilience

Resilience is a personal quality often identified as a requirement for a medical role, in which long hours and difficult decisions are required.

The process of medical education can involve fear-based learning, with mobbing and bullying being regularly reported [35], which can erode self-confidence and make individuals feel devalued.

Supporting the resilience of individuals in the profession includes teaching and supporting the practice of self-care skills and modelling positive self-care behaviours, as well as a collective responsibility to ensure collegiate support [41].

12.4.2 Dealing with adversity

Examinations and assessments are frequent during medical training, and these are significant contributors to stress. In addition, complaints about professional performance can occur at any time in a medical career.

Medical students and doctors who are unsuccessful in an assessment can find themselves confronted with failure for the first time. The stakes can be high, and it is important for individuals to understand the options and supports available to them when things go wrong.

Although managing clinical care always has challenges, there are some moments, such as breaking bad news, delivering palliative care, managing severe trauma and coping with the death of a patient, that can be more stressful.

Adverse clinical events and medicolegal difficulties bring a different layer of anxiety, with concerns that these could be career-ending for the doctor and adding to the concerns for the patient [42]. Shame and stigma can complicate access to support.

12.4.3 Life beyond the professional role

Many doctors and medical students wrestle with aspects of life beyond their medical careers, such as their relationships, making decisions about financial matters or having children. These can be significant stressors, even when they are positive or expected life events [43]. Personal illness or injury can be life changing, as well as having an impact on the doctor's medical career.

As doctors progress along their professional pathway, the changes and decisions that all individuals face at different life stages can bring unexpected challenges [43]. Maintaining adequate flexibility and time to address these challenges among work commitments is important and often requires planning.

Adequate income protection insurance, supportive personal connections and strong peer networks can provide some safety netting. Most importantly, however, ensuring adequate time for processing, reflection and personal decision making is essential throughout a doctor's medical career.

12.5 A reflection on suicide

12.5.1 Suicidal ideation

Suicidal ideation is common among doctors, who need strategies for both supporting their colleagues and managing their own thoughts of suicide [44]. High levels of burnout and stress are associated with suicidal thoughts [45]. Although the prevalence of suicidal ideation is high, its relationship to suicide among doctors is complex. Doctor suicide has been a serious concern for the profession for more than a century [46]. Doctor suicide has immense repercussions for the doctor's family, colleagues and community. Figures vary, but it is generally recognised that the rate of suicide among doctors is about twice as high as that in the general community [9,47], with the rate being higher for female doctors than for male doctors. Both physical and mental health issues have been associated with increased risk of suicide in doctors, as has substance use [9]. There is a clear association between regulatory investigation and doctor suicide [48,49].

12.5.2 Seeking help

All doctors need to have robust personal and professional supports in place for their own health care. Stigma surrounding mental health and help seeking may be a barrier for doctors who are struggling with mental health challenges, stress or burnout [50]. Doctors who report having stigmatising attitudes towards mental disorders are less likely to seek help for their own mental health challenges [51].

All doctors have a role in preventing doctor suicide. Supporting colleagues to seek help, reducing stigma about health issues and providing robust peer support when colleagues are dealing with hospital or other regulatory investigations are important steps. Proactive support involves more than reminding a doctor that all doctors should have a GP. Having robust strategies for responding to colleagues in distress can improve engagement with appropriate health services [52]. Prioritising empathy, active listening and collaboration can reduce stigma related to help seeking.

When a treating doctor identifies that a doctor-patient is experiencing suicidal ideation, this needs to be taken seriously, while remembering that thoughts of suicide are common [9,45,53]. Appropriate steps to ensure the safety and wellbeing of the doctor-patient should be taken, maintaining their connectedness to care [54]. Referral to specialist services may be required.

12.5.3 The impact on a doctor after someone dies by suicide

When discussing suicide, it is important to acknowledge the impact of a patient's suicide on a doctor. This impact can be significant and multifaceted, resulting in a range of emotions, such as sadness, anger, guilt or confusion [55–57]. The impact can vary depending on factors such as the doctor's level of experience, the relationship they had with the patient and the support they receive from colleagues and from their organisation.

Similarly, when a medical colleague dies by suicide, doctors can feel intense emotional distress, including grief, guilt or regret. While experiencing feelings of loss, doctors may also be confronted by professional expectations to increase their workload to address a gap in service, which can reduce the time available for the normal processing of grief. Similarly, other colleagues may look to the doctors in the healthcare team for leadership in responding to a doctor suicide, yet these doctors may feel unqualified to provide such leadership and too overwhelmed to step into this role.

12.5.4 Postvention

Postvention refers to the provision of support and intervention after a traumatic event, particularly a suicide, to help those affected cope with their experience and to reduce the risk of further harm. Postvention focuses on the survivors, families and communities left behind, rather than the individual who died. Postvention is an organisational responsibility [58]. All organisations (e.g. hospitals, medical schools and private practices) should have a postvention process that is regularly reviewed with input from all levels of medical staff and, where appropriate, medical students.

Postvention can help by providing emotional support, information and resources to help individuals understand and cope with their feelings and reduce their risk of harm. Linkage to appropriate specialised postvention community services can help, although these services may have limited expertise in providing specific support for doctors [59]. Resources provided should include education about pathways to care. For doctors and medical students, ensuring an awareness of the range of pathways to care is important, given the barriers they may experience in accessing health care. Understanding the role of the local doctors' health service, as well as being aware of other services, is vital (see section 12.13).

12.6 The medical student and doctor-in-training experience

It is vital that doctors-in-training and medical students are supported throughout their early career.

The medical education process supports the formation of an individual's identity as a 'doctor' [60]. The medical training environment is highly competitive, and this often reduces collaboration between individuals. Trainees can feel isolated and unable to demonstrate vulnerability and be unwilling to access support.

Competition to get into medicine is fierce, and this rivalry can continue for many years, particularly when hospital placements and training positions are in limited supply. Individuals often conceal distress from their peers and supervisors in an attempt to maintain a façade of perfection and invulnerability. This can result in increased stress and have a negative impact on their mental health [61].

12.6.1 Career transitions

There are many transitions throughout the medical career, each of which can be a stress point. It is common for students and doctors-in-training to have to move regularly to continue their training and, each time this happens, they are likely to be uprooted from their family, social supports and personal healthcare team.

When things do not go as planned, such as failure in an examination, some individuals aim to keep going down the same pathway, but for others this is a time of reflection about alternative career opportunities. Supportive mentoring and career coaching can assist individuals to make informed and considered decisions [62].

12.6.2 The 'hidden curriculum'

It is common for doctors to adopt the behaviours they witness—the normative behaviours of the profession. As the formal medical teaching unfolds, there is also a well-described 'hidden curriculum' that contributes significantly to professional identity formation over time [63]. The cultural understandings of how doctors perceive expectations about their behaviour are internalised as a subtext to their clinical learning.

In this hidden curriculum, resilience is applauded, with little space provided for being open about vulnerability. Bravado regularly goes unquestioned, and honest discussions about error are rare. Doctors learn early in their training that there is an expectation in the profession that doctors should be perceived as healthy [64]. This professional expectation is compounded by the general community's expectation of 'physician, heal thyself'.

In many aspects of practice, the doctor is called upon to maintain equanimity, no matter what unfolds during the patient narrative or how the operation unfolds. The doctor is to remain invulnerable, and, for many, the taking up of the mantle of the white coat (actual or figurative) symbolises acceptance of this narrative.

The formative years of training as a medical student and doctor-in-training are important ones for establishing positive strategies for supporting health and wellbeing [65]. Positive messaging about doctors' health throughout these early years needs to be included as part of the overt curriculum and integrated with the hidden curriculum. It is therefore the responsibility of all doctors to support appropriate messages about doctors' health in their daily work (see also Chapter 4, Ethical and legal responsibilities of medical students).

12.7 Peer support and social connectedness

Medicine is best practised with collegial support, and social connection is an enabler of doctors' wellbeing.

The medical profession has always thrived on collegial support systems. The medical culture, with its own linguistic nuances, humour and behaviour, provides a sense of belonging for many doctors that transcends other cultural differences. Although problems can emerge from like-minded thinking and clique-like behaviours, there are also benefits related to this collegial support.

12.7.1 Professional interaction

Most doctors benefit from contact with mentors as they move forward in their careers [66]. For many doctors, regular engagement with continuing medical education helps them maintain a relationship with their peers as they share case discussions and workplace experiences. Collegial support is often found at professional meetings, including educational evenings and conferences. Regular participation in educational events is associated with better maintenance of personal wellbeing, as well as lower risk of medicolegal problems [67]. Building relationships with experienced clinicians can support the development of clinical skills and provide a depth of understanding of the culture and practice of medicine that adds to clinical knowledge. Role modelling is a recognised part of these professional interactions. These relationships can provide doctors with a safe place to discuss their clinical concerns about a case, in an environment of empathy and support rather than judgement and competition.

12.7.2 Peer support

Existing relationships with medical peers can enable support to be found during difficult times. All doctors will struggle at some time during their careers, such as when managing a difficult case or making important career or life decisions. At these times, knowing where there is a safe space to talk can be important [10]. Although the doctor's family may be supportive, the medical lens and understanding of the nuances of medical work that peers offer can be helpful when needing to debrief. For some doctors, specific doctors' health services or peer support programs can provide a safe space for these discussions (see section 12.13).

However, the practice of medicine has an element of competitiveness that can affect the development of peer support. Starting even before students have secured their place in medical school, and continuing throughout training, there is a degree of intellectual competitiveness on which many doctors thrive. Even after completing their training, many specialist doctors may continue to feel that they are competing with their colleagues [68]. As they step up to face the challenges before them, the thrill of competition can add a layer of excitement.

The danger of prolonged immersion in a highly competitive environment is that there is potential for individuals to feel isolated from their peers, who would otherwise be a natural source of support. This highly competitive aspect of medicine results in doctors often feeling unable to communicate any fallibility or vulnerability. It becomes more difficult to feel safe enough to share personal narratives of error or feelings that may be perceived as weakness, fearing judgement or negative consequences for their career or reputation. This reduces access to authentic peer support. Yet, the need to acknowledge fallibility and humanity is inherent in all individuals [69]. The reality is that mistakes and failures occur throughout the professional life of every clinician.

It is an important task for all doctors to identify peer support options that provide a safe space for open dialogue. These peer relationships may begin during medical training but need to be proactively fostered and maintained throughout the doctor's career.

12.7.3 Peer pressure

Interaction with medical peers can sometimes be detrimental to a doctor's wellbeing, potentially increasing distress or unhealthy behaviour. There may be strong collegial bonds, particularly in smaller craft groups, in which unhealthy behaviours, such as heavy drinking or presenteeism, may be normalised. There may be codes of behaviour that are accepted by the group, and may even be seen to be expected, which do not accord with an individual's values. It is important that doctors are alert to these instances of potentially harmful peer pressure and feel empowered to maintain their own personal and professional standards.

12.7.4 Isolation

The risk of isolation can be magnified for some doctors at different times during their careers. The social lives of doctors are frequently disrupted during their training. International medical graduates can find themselves disconnected from important cultural supports when they arrive in Australia, particularly if they are practising in a small Australian town. Cultural isolation can be magnified when connectedness with family and friends is lost [70].

Connectedness can be enhanced through online conversations, which break through geographic borders. Social media offers other opportunities for connectedness, but understanding professional ethical engagement with these platforms is vital [71].

12.7.5 Social connection beyond the professional role

Although there are advantages to peer support, it is also important for doctors to connect with their community beyond the medical profession. Individual choices of activities and social connections will vary greatly, but all doctors need to cultivate this broader engagement so that their professional identity is not their sole identity. Integrating work and non-work will support doctor wellbeing [72].

12.8 Caring for yourself as a doctor

Self-care is an important starting point for doctors' wellbeing, and recognising the barriers and boundaries to self-care is integral to professional practice.

Doctors have a responsibility to be proactive in maximising their health and wellbeing. Wellbeing may depend on managing the physical, mental, social, workplace, spiritual, cultural, financial and medicolegal dimensions of health [73]. Optimising doctors' health and wellbeing also benefits their patients, family and colleagues.

Doctors' personal self-care and help-seeking behaviours are established during medical school training [64]. In taking up medical professional culture, some doctors find themselves adopting attitudes that can negatively affect their personal health. They may be more likely to minimise their own health issues while prioritising care for their patients, and they may be more reluctant to seek independent health care [74]. Much of this cultural learning occurs through the hidden curriculum—through observation and assumed expectations, implicitly taught by example.

Doctors can be effective in their self-care because of their extensive health literacy [22]. Once a doctor identifies a health issue, they often know how it should be treated. Many doctors self-treat appropriately, and the health issue may quickly resolve. Sometimes the only treatment required is observation or a simple remedy. Self-care is a normal part of health care in the community and is no less relevant for doctors.

There are, however, limits to appropriate self-care. Doctors have the potential to self-prescribe medications and self-refer for investigations or specialist review. It is important that doctors are aware of specific guidance to avoid these practices from the Medical Board of Australia (in section 11.2 of *Good medical practice: a code of conduct for doctors in Australia*) [75] and any relevant restrictions in their local jurisdictions or workplaces.

Self-care requirements change over time but usually include healthy eating, adequate sleep and regular exercise. Regular engagement with mindfulness or other activities that support mental health can also be essential. Having an established pathway to formal health care reduces a doctor's risk of continuing inappropriate self-care.

12.9 Seeking independent care as a doctor-patient

All doctors need access to independent formal health care, and understanding the pathways to care can reduce the barriers to help-seeking.

12.9.1 Seeking formal health care

Despite their knowledge, doctors may not prioritise their own health or may neglect their personal health needs when they are busy caring for their patients. Routine preventive health is frequently deferred. The cultural crafting of the doctor's professional identity throughout medical training can inadvertently reinforce this approach [74]. Many doctors do not take leave, even when they are quite unwell. They often 'soldier on' when others would take a day off to rest. Although the COVID-19 pandemic has increased the likelihood of doctors taking time off for flu-like symptoms, this has not necessarily translated into taking time off for other health issues.

Doctors need to maintain clear boundaries when tending to their self-care and healthcare needs. Recognising when to seek independent assistance for health issues, rather than continuing self-care, can prove challenging for doctors [22]. The boundary may be easy to identify when prescription medicine is required, but it can be more difficult to define when observing the slow evolution of symptoms of burnout or a new physical or mental health issue.

All doctors will at some point have health issues that require formal health care. Doctors may present late when seeking care for a health issue [22]. This delay has potentially serious consequences, including compromising the health of the doctor, the impact it has on their healthcare team and a potential reduction in the quality of care being delivered [21].

Knowing who to turn to is a key enabler when maintaining appropriate self-care boundaries. As a first step, all doctors benefit from having their own GP. This is recognised in the Medical Board of Australia's code of conduct and by the professional colleges [75]. Many doctors report having a GP, but many do not actively maintain this relationship [76]. Doctors' health services across Australia can provide doctors with assistance to access care (see section 12.13).

12.9.2 Barriers to access

Doctors may experience many barriers along their pathway to receiving formal health care [21]. Understanding these barriers enables all doctors to support their colleagues to seek formal care in a timely manner when needed and to provide a supportive environment that reduces stigma (Box 12.1).

Doctors should reflect on their own personal barriers to accessing formal health care and develop strategies to address these, ideally before significant health issues arise.

Stigma

Stigma (and self-stigma) is a significant barrier that doctors face when seeking medical treatment [50,51]. There is often a negative perception (real or not) of doctors who seek treatment, as they are expected to be the experts on health and not need medical attention themselves. This perception can create a culture of shame and guilt, making doctors hesitant to seek care for their own health issues. Some doctors can take the phrase 'Physician, heal thyself' (Luke 4:23) too much to heart.

Doctors may feel ashamed or embarrassed about their health conditions or worry about being judged by their peers [22,74]. Some doctors worry about being perceived as weak or not capable of handling their own health issues, or as lacking in knowledge or expertise, which can make them reluctant to seek medical care. This can lead to avoidance of seeking care and a delay in diagnosis and treatment that could result in increased health complications or longer recovery times.

Confidentiality and reporting concerns

Some doctors also report that they have concerns about confidentiality of the healthcare provider when being treated by colleagues or members of close social networks [21]. This anxiety and fear can be compounded if the doctor being treated fears their medical or mental health concern may result in a finding of impairment, which may be reported to regulators or involve medicolegal issues (see sections 12.11 and 12.12).

Underlying health knowledge

Despite their medical training, doctors may not have a comprehensive understanding of their own health conditions or the treatments available to them in a particular specialist area. This potential lack of knowledge can make it challenging for doctors to make informed decisions about their care or to feel comfortable asking their treating doctor about their options. On the other hand, having a detailed knowledge of medicine may keep some doctors from consulting other medical professionals, as they may think they know the best course of action or treatment to take.

Time and cost

Time and cost may also play a role in doctors not seeking formal medical treatment [21]. The demands of their work schedules can make it difficult for doctors to find the time to schedule and attend medical appointments. They may feel guilty for taking time away from their patients or worry about being perceived as unreliable. The high cost of medical treatment can be a deterrent for doctors, as they may not have adequate insurance coverage or the financial resources to pay for their medical care.

Box 12.1 The 'corridor consultation'

It is not uncommon for doctors to consult with their colleagues informally, often in hallways or other non-private settings. The 'corridor consultation' can sometimes replace a formal medical review [21].

Much has been written about the corridor consultation, which can sometimes result in the doctor with the health issue inappropriately persisting with self-treatment. However, seeking wisdom from a knowledgeable acquaintance or from family and friends (who may be health professionals) is a well-described part of the normal pathway to care across all cultures [22].

It is important not to demonise the corridor consultation; instead, all doctors should be well versed in identifying when this occurs and recognising the potential risks. Supplying scripts or advising on investigations when a formal history and examination have not been performed, for example, will always be fraught with risk.

All doctors should be aware of the role of the corridor consultation in facilitating appropriate care. A doctor approached in an informal manner can use this interaction as an opportunity to facilitate the help-seeker's pathway to formal care with an independent health professional [22].

Developing a compassionate language of appropriate response during the corridor consultation is an important professional skill. Simply encouraging all doctors to have their own GP is an appropriate start but inadequate as the only response. The doctor seeking advice may require additional support to identify and overcome barriers to accessing formal care, and this necessitates a sensitive approach. It can be helpful to encourage colleagues who are struggling to access care to seek support from their local doctors' health service (see section 12.13).

12.9.3 Becoming a doctor-patient

Even after overcoming the barriers to accessing health care, doctors may find the experience of 'becoming a patient' challenging [76,77]. It can take time to build rapport with the treating doctor.

The process of becoming a doctor-patient requires several decisions: who to see, when to go to the doctor, what health issues to take to the doctor and how to develop a therapeutic relationship with the doctor (Table 12.1) [22].

Table 12.1 Considerations for the doctor when becoming a patient

Question	Points to consider
Who?	• A general practitioner (GP) can coordinate care and be the doctor-patient's advocate. • The GP should be independent and accessible. • There are benefits to having a GP who cares for the doctor-patient's whole family.
When?	• Determining when to go to the GP involves active reflection and prioritisation of personal health needs. Support for the decision to seek care from compassionate peers and family can help. • There are advantages if the relationship with the GP is established before a serious health issue emerges. • Scheduling regular visits to discuss preventive health care can ensure timely care.

Continued over page

Question	Points to consider
What?	• Determining what health issues to take to the GP can be difficult for a doctor. Doctors do not want to 'waste' another doctor's time with a minor health issue. Routine investigations, repeat prescriptions of regular medications and routine referrals provide ideal opportunities to navigate the expectations and boundaries of the therapeutic relationship as it is strengthened. • Over time, as rapport develops, it is easier for the doctor-patient to be comfortable about what health issues to seek care for. • Attendance for a 'check-up', without specific clinical concerns, is an accepted and common reason for individuals to visit a GP, and this also applies to doctor-patients.
How?	• Doctors need to be prepared to be uncomfortable. Having an open and frank discussion with a GP will help them navigate the boundaries related to self-care and costs. An open relationship is valued. • Most doctor-patients find it helpful to reassure their treating doctor that they want to be treated as a 'normal patient'. Expectations of special or privileged treatment need to be addressed, as they can result in poorer care. • The doctor-patient can expect to engage in the shared decision-making process with their treating doctor, and their health literacy may increase their engagement with this process. • Follow-up is an important part of the plan to enable the future strengthening of the therapeutic relationship.

The GP is often supported by other healthcare professionals who form part of the healthcare team. Psychologists, specialists and allied health providers may be required to support doctor-patients with acute and chronic healthcare needs. Sometimes, the doctor-patient is already linked to other health professionals. It is important that the treating GP is aware of other healthcare providers involved in the doctor-patient's care, to enable coordination of care.

12.10 Being a treating doctor and caring for the doctor-patient

All doctors need to ensure they have the necessary knowledge and skills to manage a consultation in which the patient is another doctor.

It is a professional responsibility for all doctors to acquire the necessary skills to deliver quality care to their doctor-patients. All doctors, including GPs and other specialists, need to have the skills to treat a doctor-patient. Senior doctors need to support junior doctors who are caring for doctor-patients.

Specific education is available to enable doctors to upskill to enhance their delivery of care to doctors and medical students. It is helpful if both the treating doctor and the doctor-patient are aware of the guidelines of the Medical Board of Australia's code of conduct [75]. Insight into the barriers that the doctor-patient has experienced before seeking formal care can help the treating doctor to identify and address specific fears that the doctor-patient may have.

12.10.1 Challenges experienced by treating doctors when the patient is a doctor

Treating doctors can find caring for a doctor-patient challenging for several reasons:

- Doctor-patients may have navigated an unusual pathway to formal care (because of the many barriers to seeking care), and it may take time to collate the results of investigations and list of previous medications.

- Some doctor-patients seek specialist care without an independent referral from their GP (even if they have a GP).
- Doctors are health-literate patients and may have many questions about their health issues, which could challenge the treating doctor's knowledge and require extra time to discuss.
- Doctors may have specific, yet often unstated, expectations of the consultation that are different to the expectations of other patients, so the treating doctor can find it difficult to address these expectations effectively.
- Consultations for some health conditions might raise the question of whether mandatory notification needs to be considered (see section 12.11).
- Treating doctors may feel uncomfortable or insecure or fear criticism of their performance during the consultation.

Doctors need to spend time considering how they will approach a consultation with a doctor-patient and, through reflection and education, develop an understanding of how to establish and then strengthen their therapeutic relationship with a doctor-patient [76].

12.10.2 Establishing and strengthening an effective therapeutic relationship

The key role of the treating doctor is to support the establishment of the therapeutic relationship and enable this relationship to be strengthened over time [76].

Although the doctor-patient may present for a specific purpose, it is important to provide them with holistic care, recognising the need to gather a full medical history, as for all other patients. It is important to assure the doctor-patient of the confidentiality of the consultation, while also keeping full records.

Treating doctors and doctor-patients may take time to settle into their respective roles and establish rapport. Building a therapeutic relationship and naming any awkwardness that may arise is essential for providing compassionate care, while maintaining appropriate therapeutic boundaries that enable the delivery of usual care. Setting these boundaries early on results in less confusion and improves care. This may include discussions about expectations related to self-treatment, self-prescribing and self-referral.

As a treating doctor, it can be tempting to cut corners when it comes to the presentation of illness in doctor-patients. Maintaining usual practice and going through the necessary steps of history taking, examination, investigation and management can ensure delivery of quality care to the doctor-patient.

It is wise to understand the doctor-patient's clinical role and to identify any potential occupational hazards they may face. This could include inquiry about engaging in exposure-prone procedures (requiring appropriate testing) and risks of exposure to other occupational hazards, including infectious diseases or radiation. Doctor-patients also have other roles in their lives, involving family and social activities. These should be taken into account when providing treatment. The treating doctor should support the doctor-patient in their preventive health care, as well as addressing all their health issues, including those relating to mental health. Preventive health includes providing vaccinations, supporting appropriate health screening relevant to age and family history, and entering appropriate recalls. This approach will help to maximise the doctor-patient's overall health and wellbeing.

Finally, it is crucial that the treating doctor and doctor-patient engage in honest shared decision making, while avoiding assumptions about the doctor-patient's knowledge and health literacy. By working together, both healthcare professionals can achieve the best possible outcomes for the doctor-patient's health.

12.10.3 Other issues the treating doctor should look out for

Doctor-patients may be reluctant to mention mental health issues [51]. Proactive and sensitive inquiry can assist discussion in this area. Errors and medicolegal issues can arise at any time during a medical career, increasing anxiety. Issues of post-traumatic stress disorder, vicarious trauma and moral injury may need exploration (see section 12.3).

Doctors may need permission to take time off work, and offering a certificate can support this discussion.

Doctor-patients may have a role in providing health care to their family. They can be encouraged to assist their family members to engage with independent health care when it is appropriate (see Chapter 8, Sexual and other professional boundaries: being a doctor in modern society, and Chapter 30, Prescribing and administering medicines).

There may be times when a treating doctor identifies a physical or mental health issue that has led to impairment and therefore potentially requires mandatory notification, if the public is at risk (see section 12.11). All health professionals need to understand their role and responsibility under the Health Practitioner Regulation National Law (National Law) legislation in their state or territory in regard to mandatory notifications [78].

12.11 Impairment, and why this matters to all doctors

Ensuring safe practice is essential. When a doctor with a health condition is practising in a manner that puts patients at risk of harm, action must be taken to protect the public.

All doctors should expect to experience personal illness at times during their career. In most cases, and if managed appropriately, these health conditions do not result in any significant risk to the public. Occasionally, however, a health condition can affect a doctor's judgement or clinical performance, which can pose a risk to patients if the doctor continues to practise without appropriate safeguards. This would then be defined as an 'impairment'.

The Medical Board of Australia's code of conduct outlines the professional expectations of doctors in regard to management of conditions affecting their own health:

> Good medical practice involves:
>
> 11.2.8 If you know or suspect that you have a health condition or impairment that could adversely affect your judgement, performance or your patient's health:
>
> - not relying on your own assessment of the risk you pose to patients
> - consulting your doctor about whether, and in what ways, you may need to modify your practice, and following the doctor's advice [75].

12.11.1 Regulation of the medical profession

For nearly two centuries, Australia has had a formal regulatory process for monitoring the professional performance and behaviour of doctors, to protect the public from harm.

Since 2010, Australia's National Registration and Accreditation Scheme has been administered by the Medical Board of Australia and the Australian Health Practitioners Regulation Agency (Ahpra). The scope of their roles is defined by the National Law as it applies in each of the states and territories of Australia [78]. There is variation in the application of the National Law across jurisdictions, and doctors need to be aware of the relevant legislation for the jurisdictions in which they work. Chapter 21,

Regulation of the medical profession, and Chapter 22, Healthcare complaints and complaint systems, provide more detail about medical regulation in Australia.

12.11.2 Impairment

A health condition that 'detrimentally affects or is likely to detrimentally affect the person's capacity to practise the profession' is considered to be an 'impairment' under the National Law [78].

Even when doctors have a health condition that would meet this definition of impairment, they may be able to safely continue in some form of practice without the need for involvement of Ahpra or the Medical Board. If doctors follow the advice of their treating practitioners and take leave or modify their practice to ensure there is no potential for harm to patients as a result of their illness, there is usually no requirement for regulatory intervention.

Regulatory processes are usually initiated in circumstances in which a doctor with an impairment continues to practise in a manner that puts the public at risk. This may be the result of impaired judgement, with a loss of capacity to recognise the potential impact of their health condition on their practice. Regulatory intervention may also occur when a doctor demonstrates poor professional conduct, which sometimes arises in association with a health issue.

12.11.3 Mandatory notification

It is vital that all doctors recognise they have a duty—to their colleagues and to the community—to ensure they take appropriate action if they form a reasonable belief that another doctor is practising with an impairment and putting patients at risk. The prime concerns are the safety of patients, the safety of the possibly impaired doctor and the safety of the concerned individual.

In these circumstances, doctors (and other health practitioners registered with Ahpra) may have a professional obligation to submit a formal notification of their concerns to Ahpra (see also Chapter 21, Regulation of the medical profession). The relevant action required will depend on several factors, including the type of relationship between the possibly impaired doctor and the doctor identifying the concern. The requirements for a mandatory notification vary depending on where the practitioner is working and whether they are a colleague, a treating practitioner or an employer. The legislation also includes mandatory notification for health practitioner students in specific situations.

All doctors in Australia are obliged to maintain insurance cover with a medical indemnity insurer. Before making a notification, any doctor concerned about a colleague or doctor-patient is strongly encouraged to seek individual legal advice from their medical indemnity insurer based on the circumstances of the matter.

For a treating practitioner (who is looking after a doctor with an impairment as a patient), there is a very high threshold for reporting risk of harm to the public, requiring a reasonable belief that the doctor-patient is placing the public at substantial risk of harm [78]. In Western Australia, there is no obligation for treating practitioners to submit a notification of this kind, although they may submit a notification voluntarily if they hold concerns about the safety of individuals.

The Medical Board of Australia and Ahpra publish detailed guidelines explaining the responsibilities related to notifications about impairment [78].

12.11.4 Self-notification

Doctors are required to renew their professional registration with Ahpra every year. At that time, they are required to provide information about any health impairment that may affect their ability to practise safely and what they are doing to manage it.

Doctors can also make a self-notification about an impairment at any time. This may be preferable to having another individual submitting a notification about them, and it gives them a chance to provide any relevant material for consideration. Before making a notification, doctors are strongly encouraged to seek individual advice from their medical indemnity insurer.

12.11.5 What happens after notification?

Having an impairment, and being under the management of a regulatory process, does not necessarily prevent a doctor from practising. The primary role of the regulator is to protect the public from harm, and this can be achieved by various means, including some that do not prevent ongoing practice (see Chapter 21, Regulation of the medical profession).

The regulatory process can serve to ensure that doctors with impairment do not damage their own reputations or careers by practising unsafely while impaired. This process may also help doctors engage in treatment, identify necessary modifications to their practice to maintain patient safety, and facilitate their return to practice after recovery.

Being the subject of a concern raised with a regulatory organisation about the possibility of impairment is usually a stressful time for any doctor. Sometimes, the nature of the health condition can also contribute to this distress. The regulatory process may be lengthy, and many doctors understandably worry about the worst-case scenario for their career.

It is important to recognise that many confidential supports are available to individuals in these circumstances (see section 12.13). It is recommended that doctors in this situation seek support and assistance early in the process, to help them navigate this difficult time in their life. Appropriate medical treatment of any underlying health conditions and an understanding of the nature of the process and various potential outcomes can often help temper the associated distress.

The Medical Board and Ahpra publish information to assist with understanding their processes [79]. Medical indemnity insurers can provide their members with individualised advice, support and legal representation. It is important to consult them as early as possible.

12.12 Health conditions that may impair safe practice

Doctors are at risk of significant health conditions that can impair safe practice if they are not identified and managed appropriately.

Health conditions only become impairments if they are likely to detrimentally affect an individual's capacity to safely practise the profession. Some health conditions are more likely than others to result in impairment, particularly if the individual lacks insight into their condition or does not engage in treatment, or if the health condition itself has a direct impact on their judgement.

Many physical and mental health issues can temporarily affect a doctor's health so severely that the doctor is not able to practise during that time. At other times, doctors can modify their work practice to manage the impact of the health issue and ensure they are practising safely. It is wise to discuss these modifications with the health professional providing care for the doctor's condition. Whether the doctor has insight and capacity to ensure safe practice is the key question that determines the need for regulatory involvement.

Certain health conditions have greater potential to become impairments. These conditions may not become impairments if they are managed appropriately and there is no likely impact on patient safety. Examples of appropriate management include the doctor taking periods of leave from practice when unwell, attending frequent and regular reviews with treating practitioners, and changing the nature or scope of their clinical practice, if relevant.

Health conditions with greater potential to result in impairment include mental health conditions, some physical health conditions, substance use disorders and cognitive impairment. Some mental health conditions, such as severe depression, bipolar disorder, psychosis and eating disorders, may result in significant impairment, especially when the doctor's insight into the impact of their health issue is affected. Similarly, substance use may result in significant impairment because the affected individual's insight is often altered by the effects of the substance. Insight is a key factor in determining when a health condition is causing impairment. Doctors need to have a clear understanding of the distinction between having a health condition and being impaired. Substance use disorders may also trigger drug-seeking behaviour, which can result in unprofessional conduct that raises separate regulatory issues.

Cognitive impairment can be related to substance use, cerebrovascular accidents, microvascular changes, Alzheimer's-type dementia or traumatic brain injury. Again, these health conditions can affect the doctor's insight into their health issue. When cognitive impairment is suspected, it is in the practitioner's and public's best interest for a formal, comprehensive assessment to be undertaken. Age alone is not an indicator of cognitive impairment [80].

Physical conditions that affect clinical practice may require an individual to commit to a scope of practice within their physical ability and, on occasion, will require notification to the regulatory authorities.

12.13 Resources and support

A regular treating practitioner is often the best professional resource, being able to provide individualised advice and support for a doctor-patient's healthcare needs.

12.13.1 Doctors' health services

There is an independent doctors' health service in every state and territory of Australia (Box 12.2). These services specialise in doctors' and medical students' health and are available free of charge to all doctors and medical students wanting to talk confidentially with another doctor.

They operate 24/7 and provide individualised support to callers, who can remain anonymous. Advice is provided by experienced and understanding doctors, who are familiar with the local professional environment and aware of other resources and services available locally.

12.13.2 Other support organisations

Most employers and training providers, such as specialist colleges and universities, provide free counselling services (on a limited basis) to their members or employees through Employee Assistance Programs. Many medical indemnity insurers also provide this support for their members.

There are many other national or local confidential services available to members of the community that can also be accessed safely by doctors and medical students, depending on their individual needs.

GPs or doctors' health services can often advise of the availability of specific services relevant to the circumstances. Examples of services that may be relevant, with websites and contact phone numbers, are given in Box 12.2.

Box 12.2 Support services for doctors

Doctors' health services

Doctors' Health Alliance—https://doctorshealthalliance.org.au

Doctors' Health Line—1800 006 888 (this number will direct you immediately to the doctors' health service in the region from which you are calling)

Websites and 24/7 support phone numbers for the state- and territory-based doctors' health services:

Doctors' Health in Queensland	https://dhq.org.au	07 3833 4352
Doctors' Health NSW	https://doctorshealth.org.au	02 9437 6552
Drs4Drs ACT	https://www.ama.com.au/drs4drs/act	1300 374 377
Victorian Doctors Health Program	https://vdhp.org.au	1300 330 343
Drs4Drs Tasmania	https://www.ama.com.au/drs4drs/tas	1300 374 377
Doctors' Health SA	https://www.doctorshealthsa.com.au	08 8366 0250
Doctors' Health NT	https://www.doctorshealthnt.com.au	08 8366 0250
Doctors' Health Advisory Service WA	https://www.dhaswa.com.au	08 9321 3098

Other supports

CRANA Bush Support Line (for the remote and isolated health workforce)—1800 805 391

Drs4Drs national telecounselling service—1300 374 377

The Essential Network for Health Professionals, Black Dog Institute (online or personalised support)—https://www.blackdoginstitute.org.au/the-essential-network

Hand-n-Hand Peer Support—https://www.handnhand.org.au

Community support organisations

Lifeline	https://www.lifeline.org.au	13 11 14
Suicide Call Back Service	https://www.suicidecallbackservice.org.au	1300 659 467
Relationships Australia	https://www.relationships.org.au	1300 364 277
MensLine Australia	https://mensline.org.au	1300 78 99 78
1800 Respect	https://www.1800respect.org.au	1800 737 732
Butterfly Foundation	https://butterfly.org.au	1800 33 4673
PANDA	https://panda.org.au	1300 726 306
StandBy—Support After Suicide	https://standbysupport.com.au	1300 727 247

Summary

A career in medicine can be rewarding and provides many opportunities for a doctor to find a place in the profession that suits their values, personality and individual circumstances. Working as a doctor, however, should not be to the detriment of personal wellbeing. Recognising when things are not going well, asking for support, proactively managing wellbeing and prioritising self-care are important steps.

The health of all doctors is important, not only to themselves but also to the communities they serve. Doctors' health should be a high priority for the profession as a whole. Every doctor has an important role in supporting colleagues to maximise their health.

Public and private health services, including health administrators, should be aware of how their health systems affect the health and wellbeing of doctors and proactively address any issues to improve the safety of their service and the wellbeing of their medical (and other) staff.

Doctors' health should be seen as being integral to the health care they deliver, rather than as an add-on. Working together towards positive cultural change to reduce stigma, acknowledge vulnerability and facilitate access to care will provide a strong foundation for a healthy medical profession.

References

1. Huth EJ, Murray TJ, editors. Medicine in quotations: views of health and disease through the ages. 2nd ed. Philadelphia: American College of Physicians, 2006.
2. World Medical Association. Declaration of Geneva. Adopted by the 3rd General Assembly of the World Medical Association, 1949; amended by the 22nd World Medical Assembly, 1968; and the 35th World Medical Assembly, October 1983; and the 46th WMA General Assembly, Stockholm, Sweden, September 1994; and editorially revised by the 170th WMA Council Session, Divonne-les-Bains, France, May 2005; and the 173rd WMA Council Session, Divonne-les-Bains, France, May 2006; and amended by the 68th WMA General Assembly, Chicago, United States, October 2017. https://www.wma.net/policies-post/wma-declaration-of-geneva/ (accessed Jun 2025).
3. World Medical Association. International code of medical ethics. Adopted by the 3rd General Assembly of the World Medical Association, London, England, October 1949; and amended by the 22nd World Medical Assembly, Sydney, Australia, August 1968; the 35th World Medical Assembly, Venice, Italy, October 1983; the 57th WMA General Assembly, Pilanesberg, South Africa, October 2006; and the 73rd WMA General Assembly, Berlin, Germany, October 2022. https://www.wma.net/policies-post/wma-international-code-of-medical-ethics/ (accessed Jul 2025).
4. World Health Organization. Constitution. Adopted by the International Health Conference, New York, signed 22 July 1946, with amendments incorporated later. https://www.who.int/about/governance/constitution (accessed Jun 2025).
5. Department of the Prime Minister and Cabinet. National strategic framework for Aboriginal and Torres Strait Islander peoples' mental health and social and emotional wellbeing 2017-2023. Canberra: Commonwealth of Australia, 2017. https://www.niaa.gov.au/resource-centre/indigenous-affairs/national-strategic-framework-mental-health-social-emotional-wellbeing-2017-23 (accessed Jun 2025).
6. Kay M, Mitchell G, Del Mar C. Doctors do not adequately look after their own physical health. *Med J Aust* 2004; 181: 368–370.
7. Medical Board of Australia. Guidelines: Registered health practitioners and students in relation to blood-borne viruses. Melbourne: Medical Board of Australia, 2020. https://www.medicalboard.gov.au/Codes-Guidelines-Policies.aspx (accessed Jun 2025).
8. Beyond Blue. National mental health survey of doctors and medical students. Melbourne: Beyond Blue, 2013. https://medicine.uq.edu.au/files/42088/Beyondblue%20Doctors%20Mental%20health.pdf (accessed Jun 2025).
9. Center C, Davis M, Detre T, et al. Confronting depression and suicide in physicians: a consensus statement. *JAMA* 2003; 289: 3161–3166.

10. Bridson TL, Jenkins K, Allen KG, McDermott BM. PPE for your mind: a peer support initiative for health care workers. *Med J Aust* 2021; 214: 8–11.e1.
11. Morishita M, Iida J, Nishigori H. Doctors' experience of becoming patients and its influence on their medical practice: a literature review. Explore (NY) 2020; 16: 145–151.
12. Wallace JE, Lemaire JB, Ghali WA. Physician wellness: a missing quality indicator. Lancet 2009; 374: 1714–1721.
13. Bodenheimer T, Sinsky C. From triple to quadruple aim: care of the patient requires care of the provider. *Ann Fam Med* 2014; 12: 573–576.
14. Shanafelt TD, Noseworthy JH. Executive leadership and physician well-being: nine organizational strategies to promote engagement and reduce burnout. *Mayo Clin Proc* 2017; 92: 129–146.
15. Shanafelt T, Goh J, Sinsky C. The business case for investing in physician well-being. *JAMA Intern Med* 2017; 177: 1826–1832.
16. Shanafelt TD. Physician well-being 2.0: where are we and where are we going? *Mayo Clin Proc* 2021; 96: 2682–2693.
17. Kemp S, Hu W, Bishop J, et al. Medical student wellbeing - a consensus statement from Australia and New Zealand. *BMC Med Educ* 2019; 19: 69.
18. Maslach C, Leiter MP. New insights into burnout and health care: strategies for improving civility and alleviating burnout. *Med Teach* 2017; 39: 160–163.
19. Shanafelt T, Trockel M, Rodriguez A, Logan D. Wellness-centered leadership: equipping health care leaders to cultivate physician well-being and professional fulfillment. *Acad Med* 2021; 96: 641–651.
20. Riley R, Kokab F, Buszewicz M, et al. Protective factors and sources of support in the workplace as experienced by UK foundation and junior doctors: a qualitative study. *BMJ Open* 2021; 11: e045588.
21. Kay M, Mitchell G, Clavarino A, Doust J. Doctors as patients: a systematic review of doctors' health access and the barriers they experience. *Br J Gen Pract* 2008; 58: 501–508.
22. Kay M, Dawes V. Working together to ensure health care access for doctors. *Med J Aust* 2019; 211: 497–498.e1.
23. Jaradat R, Lahlouh A, Mustafa M. Sleep quality and health related problems of shift work among resident physicians: a cross-sectional study. *Sleep Med* 2020; 66: 201–206.
24. Epstein S, Sparer EH, Tran BN, et al. Prevalence of work-related musculoskeletal disorders among surgeons and interventionalists: a systematic review and meta-analysis. *JAMA Surg* 2018; 153: e174947.
25. Dorevitch S, Forst L. The occupational hazards of emergency physicians. *Am J Emerg Med* 2000; 18: 300–311.
26. Ryu RC, Behrens PH, Malik AT, et al. Are we putting ourselves in danger? Occupational hazards and job safety for orthopaedic surgeons. *J Orthop* 2021; 24: 96–101.
27. Ravi A, Gorelick J, Pal H. Identifying and addressing vicarious trauma. *Am Fam Physician* 2021; 103: 570–572.
28. Kherbache A, Mertens E, Denier Y. Moral distress in medicine: an ethical analysis. *J Health Psychol* 2022; 27: 1971–1990.
29. Mantri S, Jooste K, Lawson J, et al. Reframing the conversation around physician burnout and moral injury: "we're not suffering from a yoga deficiency". *Perm J* 2021; 25: 21.005.
30. Gottlieb M, Chung A, Battaglioli N, et al. Impostor syndrome among physicians and physicians in training: a scoping review. *Med Educ* 2020; 54: 116–124.
31. Gupta M, Chedrawy E. An ontological, anthropological, and psychoanalytic perspective on physician burnout. *Cureus* 2023; 15: e34282.
32. Shanafelt TD, West CP, Sinsky C, et al. Changes in burnout and satisfaction with work-life integration in physicians and the general US working population between 2011 and 2017. *Mayo Clin Proc* 2019; 94: 1681–1694.
33. West CP, Dyrbye LN, Shanafelt TD. Physician burnout: contributors, consequences and solutions. *J Intern Med* 2018; 283: 516–529.
34. Smallwood N, Karimi L, Bismark M, et al. High levels of psychosocial distress among Australian frontline healthcare workers during the COVID-19 pandemic: a cross-sectional survey. *Gen Psychiatr* 2021; 34: e100577.
35. Scott KM, Caldwell PH, Barnes EH, Barrett J. "Teaching by humiliation" and mistreatment of medical students in clinical rotations: a pilot study. *Med J Aust* 2015; 203: 185e.1-6.

36. Hu YY, Ellis RJ, Hewitt DB, et al. Discrimination, abuse, harassment, and burnout in surgical residency training. *N Engl J Med* 2019; 381: 1741–1752.
37. Royal Australasian College of Surgeons. Building respect. https://www.surgeons.org/en/about-racs/about-respect (accessed Jun 2025).
38. Holm K, Jönsson S, Muhonen T. How are witnessed workplace bullying and bystander roles related to perceived care quality, work engagement, and turnover intentions in the healthcare sector? A longitudinal study. *Int J Nurs Stud* 2023; 138: 104429.
39. Llewellyn A, Karageorge A, Nash L, et al. Bullying and sexual harassment of junior doctors in New South Wales, Australia: rate and reporting outcomes. *Aust Health Rev* 2019; 43: 328–334.
40. Babenko O, Mosewich AD, Lee A, Koppula S. Association of physicians' self-compassion with work engagement, exhaustion, and professional life satisfaction. *Med Sci (Basel)* 2019; 7(2): 29.
41. Forbes M, Byrom L, van der Steenstraten I, et al. Resilience on the Run: an evaluation of a well-being programme for medical interns. *Intern Med J* 2020; 50: 92–99.
42. Robertson JJ, Long B. Suffering in silence: medical error and its impact on health care providers. *J Emerg Med* 2018; 54: 402–409.
43. Rowe L, Kidd M. Every doctor: healthier doctors = healthier patients. Boca Raton: CRC Press, 2019.
44. Albuquerque J, Tulk S. Physician suicide. *CMAJ* 2019; 191: E505.
45. Menon NK, Shanafelt TD, Sinsky CA, et al. Association of physician burnout with suicidal ideation and medical errors. *JAMA Netw Open* 2020; 3: e2028780.
46. Woods R. Physician heal thyself: the health and mortality of Victorian doctors. *Soc Hist Med* 1996; 9: 1–30.
47. Dutheil F, Aubert C, Pereira B, et al. Suicide among physicians and health-care workers: a systematic review and meta-analysis. *PLoS One* 2019; 14: e0226361.
48. Bourne T, Wynants L, Peters M, et al. The impact of complaints procedures on the welfare, health and clinical practise of 7926 doctors in the UK: a cross-sectional survey. *BMJ Open* 2015; 5: e006687.
49. Horsfall S. Doctors who commit suicide while under GMC fitness to practise investigation. London: General Medical Council, 2014. https://www.gmc-uk.org/-/media/documents/internal-review-into-suicide-in-ftp-processes_pdf-59088696.pdf (accessed Jun 2025).
50. Henderson M, Brooks SK, Del Busso L, et al. Shame! Self-stigmatisation as an obstacle to sick doctors returning to work: a qualitative study. *BMJ Open* 2012; 2: e001776.
51. Wijeratne C, Johnco C, Draper B, Earl J. Doctors' reporting of mental health stigma and barriers to help-seeking. *Occup Med (Lond)* 2021; 71: 366–374.
52. Jones-Schenk J. R U OK? *J Contin Educ Nurs* 2021; 52: 500–501.
53. Shanafelt TD, Dyrbye LN, West CP, et al. Suicidal ideation and attitudes regarding help seeking in US physicians relative to the US working population. *Mayo Clin Proc* 2021; 96: 2067–2080.
54. McDowell AK, Lineberry TW, Bostwick JM. Practical suicide-risk management for the busy primary care physician. *Mayo Clin Proc* 2011; 86: 792–800.
55. Oates A, Gibbons R. After a patient dies by suicide: an illustrative case for trainee psychiatrists and trainers. *BJPsych Bull* 2022; 46: 293–297.
56. Miller D. When a patient dies by suicide - the physician's silent sorrow. *N Engl J Med* 2019; 380: 311–313.
57. Hawton K, Brand F, Croft A, et al. If a patient dies by suicide: a resource for psychiatrists. Oxford: University of Oxford Centre for Suicide Research, 2020. https://www.rcpsych.ac.uk/docs/default-source/members/supporting-you/if-a-patient-dies-by-suicide/when-a-patient-dies-by-suicide-a-resource-for-psychiatrists-2020.pdf?sfvrsn=10e72fdc_2 (accessed Jun 2025).
58. Australian Institute for Suicide Research and Prevention & Postvention Australia. Postvention Australia guidelines: a resource for organisations and individuals providing services to people bereaved by suicide. Brisbane: Australian Institute for Suicide Research and Prevention, 2017. https://www.griffith.edu.au/__data/assets/pdf_file/0038/359696/Postvention_WEB.pdf (accessed Jun 2025).
59. StandBy – Support After Suicide. Find support. https://standbysupport.com.au/find-support/ (accessed Jun 2025).
60. Mount GR, Kahlke R, Melton J, Varpio L. A critical review of professional identity formation interventions in medical education. *Acad Med* 2022; 97 (11 Suppl): S96–S106.

61. Thomas M, Bigatti S. Perfectionism, impostor phenomenon, and mental health in medicine: a literature review. *Int J Med Educ* 2020; 11: 201–213.
62. Lovell B. What do we know about coaching in medical education? A literature review. *Med Educ* 2018; 52: 376–390.
63. Mulder H, Ter Braak E, Chen HC, Ten Cate O. Addressing the hidden curriculum in the clinical workplace: a practical tool for trainees and faculty. *Med Teach* 2019; 41: 36–43.
64. Roberts L, Warner T, Trumpower D. Medical students' evolving perspectives on their personal health care: clinical and educational implications of a longitudinal study. *Compr Psychiatry* 2000; 41: 303–314.
65. Lane A, McGrath J, Cleary E, et al. Worried, weary and worn out: mixed-method study of stress and well-being in final-year medical students. *BMJ Open* 2020; 10: e040245.
66. Henry-Noel N, Bishop M, Gwede CK, et al. Mentorship in medicine and other health professions. *J Cancer Educ* 2019; 34: 629–637.
67. Kjeldmand D, Holmström I. Balint groups as a means to increase job satisfaction and prevent burnout among general practitioners. *Ann Fam Med* 2008; 6: 138–145.
68. Lefebvre C, Hartman N, Tooze J, Manthey D. Determinants of medical specialty competitiveness. *Postgrad Med J* 2020; 96: 511–514.
69. Institute of Medicine Committee on Quality of Health Care in America. Kohn LT, Corrigan JM, Donaldson MS, editors. To err is human: building a safer health system. Washington, DC: National Academies Press, 2000.
70. Szafran O, Woloschuk W, Torti JMI, Myhre D. Well-being of family medicine graduates. *Can Fam Physician* 2017; 63: e432–e439.
71. Australian Health Practitioner Regulation Agency. Social media: how to meet your obligations under the National Law. Melbourne: Ahpra, 2019. https://www.ahpra.gov.au/Resources/Social-media-guidance.aspx (accessed Jun 2025).
72. Benson NM, Chaukos D, Vestal H, et al. A qualitative analysis of stress and relaxation themes contributing to burnout in first-year psychiatry and medicine residents. *Acad Psychiatry* 2018; 42: 630–635.
73. Kay M. I know to look after myself – I'm a doctor! *O&G Magazine* 2020; 22 (2). https://www.ogmagazine.org.au/22/2-22/i-know-to-look-after-myself-im-a-doctor/ (accessed Jun 2025).
74. Gerada C. Doctors' identity and barriers to seeking care when unwell. *Br J Psychiatry* 2022; 220: 7–9.
75. Medical Board of Australia. Good medical practice: a code of conduct for doctors in Australia. https://www.medicalboard.gov.au/Codes-Guidelines-Policies/Code-of-conduct.aspx (accessed Jun 2025).
76. Kay M, Mitchell G, Clavarino A. What doctors want? A consultation method when the patient is a doctor. *Aust J Prim Health* 2010; 16: 52–59.
77. Kay M, Mitchell G, Clavarino A, Frank E. Developing a framework for understanding doctors' health access: a qualitative study of Australian GPs. *Aust J Prim Health* 2012; 18: 158–165.
78. Australian Health Practitioner Regulation Agency. Making a mandatory notification. Melbourne: Ahpra, 2020. https://www.Ahpra.gov.au/Notifications/mandatorynotifications/Mandatory-notifications.aspx (accessed Jun 2025).
79. Australian Health Practitioner Regulation Agency. How we manage concerns. Melbourne: Ahpra, 2022. https://www.Ahpra.gov.au/Notifications/How-we-manage-concerns.aspx (accessed Jun 2025).
80. Wijeratne C, Peisah C, Earl J, Luscombe G. Occupational determinants of successful aging in older physicians. *Am J Geriatr Psychiatry* 2018; 26: 200–208.

PART TWO

Supporting individuals, groups and communities

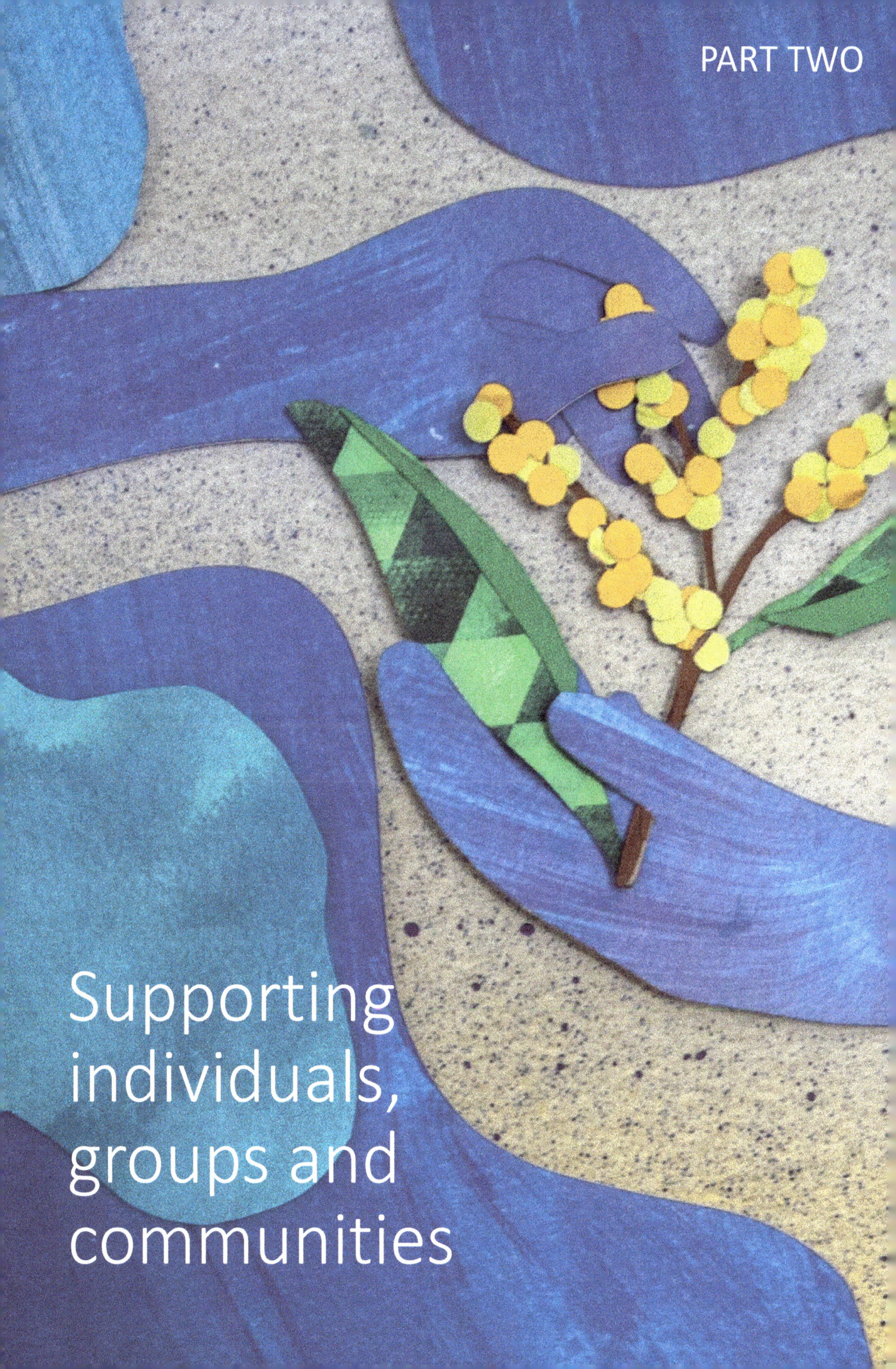

13 Infertility and assisted reproductive treatment

Louise Johnson, Karin Hammarberg

Introduction

The use of assisted reproductive treatment (ART) to conceive is increasing in Australia and other high-income countries. In 2020, almost 5% of babies born in Australia were ART conceived. Doctors need sufficient knowledge about ART and the regulation of its use to ensure they can fulfil any statutory duties related to their medical practice, make referrals when appropriate, and be aware of some of the ethical and social issues that may affect their patients. In hearing about a patient's fertility difficulties, doctors are in an excellent position to discuss the benefits of optimal parental preconception health as this is known to improve fertility and the chance of ART success. This chapter describes what ART is, outlines the legal and regulatory aspects related to the use of ART, and discusses some of the challenges faced by patients experiencing infertility and undergoing ART.

13.1 What is assisted reproductive treatment?

'Assisted reproductive treatment' is an umbrella term for infertility treatments where eggs, sperm and/or embryos are handled in a laboratory for the purpose of assisting conception.

Artificial insemination, where a partner's or a donor's sperm is placed in a woman's uterus just before ovulation, is a simple form of ART. More advanced ART includes in vitro fertilisation (IVF) and embryo transfer. In IVF, the woman has hormone injections to stimulate her ovaries to produce multiple eggs. When the eggs are mature, they are retrieved in an ultrasound-guided procedure under light anaesthetic. The eggs and the partner's or donor's sperm are placed in a culture dish in the laboratory. Three to five days later, if embryos have formed, one is transferred to the woman's uterus. If there is more than one embryo, the others can be frozen and used later.

In some circumstances, all embryos that result from a stimulated cycle are frozen. For women who have had a large number of eggs retrieved and for those with polycystic ovarian syndrome, avoiding embryo transfer in the stimulated cycle reduces their risk of ovarian hyperstimulation syndrome (OHSS). OHSS is a potentially severe complication of ovarian stimulation where the ovaries swell and fluid leaks into the abdominal cavity.

Where infertility is caused by a sperm problem, intracytoplasmic sperm injection (ICSI) can be used. ICSI follows the same process as IVF, except that a single sperm is injected directly into each egg to achieve fertilisation.

As a result of advances in cryopreservation technology, women are increasingly freezing their eggs to preserve their fertility. This can be for medical or non-medical reasons. Medical reasons for freezing eggs or ovarian tissue include undergoing gonadotoxic cancer treatments such as chemotherapy or radiation. The main reason for non-medical egg freezing is to avoid age-related infertility. Women who decide to use their eggs to attempt conception in the future will require IVF treatment. Egg freezing is costly, and several stimulated cycles may be needed to collect enough eggs to give the woman a reasonable chance of having a baby. Freezing sperm is a well-established step before artificial insemination or IVF treatment, and is also done to preserve fertility in men undergoing gonadotoxic treatments.

Sometimes donated eggs, sperm or embryos are used in IVF or ICSI. Sperm, egg and embryo donors undergo rigorous screening before donating. Evaluation of potential donors involves testing for sexually transmitted infections and genetic diseases, and assessment of family history, general health and psychological health.

Surrogacy also involves ART. Individuals and couples may seek surrogacy arrangements overseas as well as in Australia. Surrogacy is usually used by women who are unable to carry a pregnancy, same-sex male couples and single men. In traditional surrogacy, the surrogate is genetically related to the child and conceives through artificial insemination with sperm from the intended father or a donor. In gestational surrogacy, an embryo created from the intended parents' and/or donors' gametes is transferred to the surrogate, who carries the pregnancy but is not genetically related to the child.

While it is up to individual clinicians working in ART clinics to decide whether to treat a patient, some clinics have policies around the upper age limit of the patients they will treat (e.g. 50 years for women, unless there are exceptional circumstances).

The Australian Government provides Medicare rebates for ART services for people with an infertility diagnosis. This means that people in same-sex relationships and women who freeze their eggs may not have access to the same rebates as those in heterosexual relationships.

13.2 Regulation of assisted reproductive treatment in Australia

All ART clinics operating in Australia are required to be accredited by the Reproductive Technology Accreditation Committee (RTAC) through a self-regulatory system operated by the Fertility Society of Australia and New Zealand. For accreditation, ART clinics need to comply with the RTAC Code of Practice [1]. This Code of Practice requires compliance with the National Health and Medical Research Council's (NHMRC's) ethical guidelines [2]. The purpose of these guidelines is to 'provide an overarching framework for the conduct of ART in both clinical practice and research and, when read in conjunction with federal and state or territory legislation, create a robust framework for the conduct of ART in Australia'.

Commonwealth laws also regulate ART practice. The *Research Involving Human Embryos Act 2002* (Cth) stipulates the regulation of activities that involve the use of human embryos created as part of ART treatment. Organisations wishing to conduct research on excess embryos that have been donated by patients who have undertaken ART need to apply for a licence from the NHMRC's Embryo Research Licensing Committee.

The *Prohibition of Human Cloning for Reproduction Act 2002* (Cth) addresses concerns, including ethical concerns, about scientific developments in relation to human reproduction and the use of human embryos, by prohibiting certain practices such as the creation and use of a human clone.

In March 2022, the Commonwealth Mitochondrial Donation Law Reform (Maeve's Law) Bill 2021 was passed by the federal parliament [3]. It amends the Prohibition of Human Cloning for Reproduction Act and the Research Involving Human Embryos Act to make mitochondrial donation legal in Australia.

ART clinics in jurisdictions with ART legislation (Australian Capital Territory, New South Wales, Queensland, South Australia, Victoria and Western Australia) have additional requirements. Jurisdictional laws are shown in Table 13.1. South Australian legislation guides ART practice in the Northern Territory.

Table 13.1 Jurisdiction-based legislation relating to the use of assisted reproductive treatment

State or territory	ART legislation	Registration or licensing of ART clinics
Australian Capital Territory	*Assisted Reproductive Technology Act 2024* (ACT)	Registration by ACT Health
New South Wales	*Assisted Reproductive Technology Act 2007 No. 69* (NSW)	Registration by NSW Health
Queensland	*Assisted Reproductive Technology Act 2024* (Qld), passed September 2024, to be enacted	Registration by Queensland Health, when enacted
South Australia	*Assisted Reproductive Treatment Act 1988* (SA)	Registration by SA Health
Victoria	*Assisted Reproductive Treatment Act 2008* (Vic) Health Legislation Amendment (Regulatory Reform) Bill 2024 (Vic)	Registration by Victorian Department of Health
Western Australia	*Human Reproductive Technology Act 1991* (WA)	Licensing by the Reproductive Technology Council of Western Australia

13.2.1 Surrogacy

For surrogacy arrangements undertaken in Australia, jurisdiction-based surrogacy legislation exists in all jurisdictions except the Northern Territory (see Table 13.2). Surrogacy laws vary slightly between states but include the same basic principles that:

- surrogacy must be altruistic (unpaid)—commercial (paid) surrogacy is illegal
- the intended parents must have a medical or social need for surrogacy (i.e. they are unable to either conceive or carry a baby themselves)
- intended parents must cover the surrogate's costs relating to the pregnancy
- the surrogate has the final say about what happens to her body
- all parties must get legal advice before attempting pregnancy.

If a baby is born after surrogacy, the surrogate and her partner (if she has one) are registered as the parents on the birth certificate. The intended parents then apply to the court for a parentage order to transfer parentage to them. The birth certificate is then reissued with the intended parents listed.

The surrogate is usually recruited by the intended parents. When an egg or sperm donor is needed for a surrogacy arrangement, this donor may be known to the intending parents or recruited by the treating clinic.

People who undertake surrogacy in international destinations may face challenges when bringing the baby back to Australia. For a child born overseas to live in Australia, parents need to apply for Australian citizenship by descent or a permanent visa on behalf of the child. An application for Australian citizenship by descent requires parents to provide details of the surrogacy contract, including consent from the surrogate and her identity documents. Depending on the surrogacy contract, DNA testing to establish genetic relatedness to one parent may be required. If there is no surrogacy legislation in the overseas country, the surrogate remains the responsible parent and will need to sign the application. Furthermore, in some states (ACT, NSW, Queensland) it is an offence for an Australian resident to make a commercial surrogacy arrangement outside Australia. With this degree of complexity, legal advice is crucial for any patients considering overseas surrogacy arrangements.

Table 13.2 Jurisdiction-based surrogacy legislation

State or territory	Surrogacy legislation
Australian Capital Territory	*Parentage Act 2004* (ACT)
New South Wales	*Surrogacy Act 2010 No. 102* (NSW)
Queensland	*Surrogacy Act 2010* (Qld)
South Australia	*Assisted Reproductive Treatment Act 1988* (SA) *Family Relationships Act 1975* (SA)
Tasmania	*Surrogacy Act 2012* (Tas)
Victoria	Part 4 of the *Assisted Reproductive Treatment Act 2008* (Vic) makes provisions in relation to surrogacy arrangements in Victoria. The *Status of Children Act 1974* (Vic) outlines presumption of parentage in relation to children born as a result of a surrogacy arrangement. This Act also outlines the requirements for making a substitute parentage order by the parents of a child born from a surrogacy arrangement. The *Births, Deaths and Marriages Registration Act 1996* (Vic) outlines the requirements for birth registration of a child conceived via a surrogacy arrangement.
Western Australia	*Surrogacy Act 2008* (WA)

13.2.2 Donor conception

Throughout Australia, anonymous gamete (sperm or egg) and embryo donation is prohibited. This means that donors must consent to their identifying information being made available to their donor-conceived offspring when they reach adulthood. Some states with legislation also hold donor conception registers to enable more comprehensive service provision and information exchange between the parties involved in donor procedures.

The first legislation in the world to establish a central donor conception register was implemented in Victoria in 1988—the *Infertility (Medical Procedures) Act 1984* (Vic). The intention behind this legislation was that the details of children born after donor procedures, their parents and the donor are recorded so that these children can apply for information about their donor when they become an adult. Since that time, donor conception registers have been established in NSW, SA and WA (see Table 13.3). The rights of donor-conceived adults, their parents and donors to make applications for identifying or non-identifying information from a central register vary from state to state.

Voluntary registers also exist in some states (see Table 13.3). They enable donor-conceived people, their parents, donors and relatives to register information about themselves. If there is a match (via the same donor code) between people who are related, then information can be exchanged, and people can meet if they wish. For example, in Victoria, matches between parents of young children who have used the same donor have enabled them to link up and meet. Adults conceived from the same donor have also been able to meet via matches on a voluntary register.

In states without donor conception registers, donor-conceived adults can apply directly to ART clinics for information about their donor. However, success relies on records being available, the donor consenting to provide information, and appropriate support from the ART clinic where the donor procedure occurred. ART clinic capacity to undertake complex searches for contemporary contact details of a donor can also be constrained, and success in linking parties is very mixed.

In jurisdictions with legislation, there may be a prescribed limit on the number of families that can be created using the same donor.

Table 13.3 Australian donor conception registers

State or territory	ART legislation stipulating donor conception registers	Donor conception registers
Australian Capital Territory	*Assisted Reproductive Technology Act 2024* (ACT)	Not enacted at time of writing; it is intended that ACT Health will establish and run a central and voluntary register
New South Wales	Part 3, *Assisted Reproductive Technology Act 2007 No. 69* (NSW)	Central register (from 2010) and voluntary registers managed by NSW Health
Queensland	*Assisted Reproductive Technology Act 2024* (Qld), to be enacted	At the time of writing, under new legislation, the Registrar-General of the Registry of Births, Deaths and Marriages must establish and maintain a new register
South Australia	Part 3, *Assisted Reproductive Treatment Act 1988* (SA) *Assisted Reproductive Treatment (Donor Conception Register) Amendment Act 2021* (SA) *Assisted Reproductive Treatment (Posthumous Use of Material and Donor Conception Register) Amendment Act 2024* (SA)	Donor conception register established in 2021 managed by SA Health. At the time of writing, amendments to regulations were under consideration to support administration of the Act and the operation of the donor conception register.

Continued over page

State or territory	ART legislation stipulating donor conception registers	Donor conception registers
Victoria	Part 6, *Assisted Reproductive Treatment Act 2008* (Vic)	Central register (from 1988) and voluntary registers managed by the Victorian Department of Health
Western Australia	Division 5 Information, Section 45, *Human Reproductive Technology Act 1991* (WA) At the time of writing, legislative change was under consideration	Central register (established 1993) and voluntary registers managed by the Reproductive Technology Council of Western Australia
Other jurisdictions	No legislation in operation to establish donor conception registers	Australian NHMRC guidelines [2] have recognised since 2005 that donor-conceived children are entitled to information about their donor. Under the RTAC Code of Practice, ART units are required to retain records related to donor treatment and to assist donor-conceived adults to gain access to non-identifying information about their donor on application. Release of identifying information requires the donor's consent.

13.3 Clinical practice points when caring for patients with infertility

13.3.1 Suspecting infertility

Around 85% of couples who try for pregnancy conceive within 12 months. If a couple has been unable to achieve pregnancy after 12 months of trying (6 months if the woman is older than 35 years), an infertility investigation is warranted. About one-third of cases of infertility are due to a male factor and one-third are due to a female factor; in one-third of cases both partners have a fertility problem, or the cause of infertility is unknown (unexplained infertility).

Irrespective of the cause, the experience of infertility is distressing. Unlike other adverse life events, infertility is uniquely distressing because it can last for many years and the outcome is uncertain. Therefore, in addition to good and timely medical care, people need psychological support throughout the investigation and treatment of infertility.

Treatment options depend on the results of the infertility investigations. Where there is a clear cause of infertility, people should be referred to a fertility specialist without delay. This is because a woman's age is the most important determinant of the chance of success with ART. However, not everyone will need to resort to ART. A holistic approach in which general health, timing of intercourse and potential exposure to factors that may affect fertility are assessed may reveal simple solutions to a fertility problem.

In all discussions about fertility, it is important to inform patients about the benefits of optimal parental preconception health for fertility, pregnancy health and the health of the baby. Women and men who plan pregnancy, with or without ART, should be offered pre-conception care to ensure they are in the best possible health before conception.

13.3.2 Choosing a clinic and fertility specialist

Accredited ART clinics are required to have access to a clinician with a Certificate in Reproductive Endocrinology and Infertility (CREI). Some clinics have several CREI-qualified clinicians. Although ART is subsidised by Medicare and the Pharmaceutical Benefits Scheme, the out-of-pocket costs for patients are still significant. Patients need comprehensive and transparent information about all costs that they will incur for a treatment cycle and should be aware that a significant amount must be paid upfront before the Medicare benefit has been received.

Cost is a barrier to accessing ART, particularly for people from low socioeconomic backgrounds, culturally and linguistically diverse people, Aboriginal and/or Torres Strait Islander people, and people living with disabilities.

Some clinics offer low-cost services where the ART procedures are bulk-billed and out-of-pocket costs are mostly for services that are not covered by Medicare. Low-cost services may not offer donor sperm or donor egg options or be suitable for patients with complex infertility. In NSW, Victoria and WA, government-funded low-cost services are available for people from disadvantaged backgrounds.

When choosing a clinic, patients may wish to compare clinic success rates. A government-funded website launched in 2020, YourIVFSuccess (https://yourivfsuccess.com.au), allows them to do this. This website has information about all clinics in Australia, the services they provide, and how their success rates compare with the national average. There is also an interactive feature where patients can enter their personal information (such as age, cause of infertility and whether they have had a previous pregnancy) and get an estimate of their chance of having a baby after one or more treatment cycles. The estimates are based on the data clinics are required to submit annually to the Australian and New Zealand Assisted Reproduction Database.

People considering ART may want to explore a clinic's approach to person-centred care as clinics vary in their commitment to ensuring care is respectful of and responsive to the preferences, needs and values of patients and those supporting them. In choosing a fertility specialist or ART clinic, single women and same-sex couples may also wish to consider whether the clinic environment is sympathetic to and meets their specific needs and the needs of their donors or surrogates.

13.3.3 Psychosocial aspects of assisted reproductive technology

ART is physically, emotionally and financially demanding. Treatment involves several steps and things can go wrong in each of these steps. The woman might not respond to the fertility drugs, eggs may not be recovered, and embryos may not develop or implant. And even if the embryo does implant and a clinical pregnancy is established, there is still a risk of miscarriage. While most people manage the emotional ups and downs of ART, for some individuals, treatment adversely affects their mental health and they may benefit from speaking to an infertility counsellor.

13.3.4 Managing expectations

Patients need transparent and individualised information so that they have realistic expectations of their chance of having a baby with IVF. Since the woman's age is the most important determinant of ART success, information about the chance of a live birth needs to be age specific.

An example of information that can help people understand what is possible with IVF is the cumulative live-birth rate (CLBR), which measures the birth rate for all complete ART cycles a woman might undergo. The information is based on research tracking 56,652 women who started IVF between 2009 and 2012, and shows how many had a baby after between one and eight stimulated cycles [4]. A stimulated IVF cycle means a cycle where eggs are collected and all the embryos created from that cycle, including fresh and frozen embryos, are transferred one by one.

The research, conducted by the National Perinatal Epidemiology and Statistics Unit at UNSW Sydney, followed these women for a minimum of three years and a maximum of four years. The results showed an overall CLBR of 33% for the first complete cycle, increasing to 54% for the eighth cycle [4].

One of the major influences on CLBR is the age of the woman, with CLBR declining with increasing age. For example, the CLBR after the first complete cycle was 44% for women who commenced ART before the age of 30, declining to 31% for women aged 35–39 and 11% for women aged 40–44 years [4]. The corresponding CLBR results after the third cycle were 66%, 48% and 18% respectively [4].

This demonstrates that, when considering ART, patients need to be aware that several treatment cycles may be required to have a reasonable chance of having a baby. The financial implications of multiple cycles should be discussed with patients before they start treatment.

13.3.5 Add-ons

A number of so called 'add-ons', or 'adjuvant therapies', are offered by ART clinics. They are procedures or medications that are added to ART treatment to try to improve the chance of success. Examples include endometrial scratching; time-lapse imaging of embryos; preimplantation genetic testing for aneuploidy; and the prescription of steroids, testosterone and growth hormones.

Patients need to know that most of these often costly add-ons have not been properly tested in clinical trials and therefore it is not known whether they improve the chance of having a baby, or whether they are safe. Choosing Wisely Australia (https://www.choosingwisely.org.au) suggests patients should ask their doctor the following five questions before agreeing to any test, treatment or procedure:

- Do I really need this test, treatment or procedure?
- What are the risks?
- Are there simpler, safer options?
- What happens if I don't do anything?
- What are the costs?

In the context of ART, we suggest that patients also ask whether the add-on will improve their chance of having a baby.

13.3.6 Deciding what to do with excess stored embryos

People who have stored embryos or gametes that they do not intend to use are required to decide what to do with them. With appropriate counselling and consent, patients with excess embryos can donate them to research, donate them to another patient, or dispose of them (clinics thaw the embryos and allow them to succumb in the laboratory). Many patients find this decision challenging and can take some time to come to a resolution. Not all clinics offer the option of donating excess embryos to research, as research using excess embryos is only conducted in ART clinics that are licensed to do so.

13.3.7 Donor treatment and surrogacy

In an ART clinic, gamete donors are carefully screened and receive counselling about the long-term implications of donation. The intending parent(s) are also counselled and have legal certainty about parentage following donor treatment in a clinic. ART clinics sometimes advise single women who intend to have regular contact or co-parenting arrangements with a sperm donor to seek legal advice, as legal parentage and access arrangements can be affected.

Due to a shortage of sperm and egg donors in Australia, some people resort to searching for a donor on online forums. These forums are not currently regulated and there are some risks associated with using them. Risks include more than the recommended number of children being born from one sperm donor; a lack of protection, with some women pressured for sex; a lack of information about donors for the children born; risk of sexually transmitted infections; and lack of legal certainty about parentage.

The shortage of donor gametes also drives some people to seek donor treatment in overseas destinations. Some of the risks associated with international arrangements include wide variation in professional standards, particularly in unregulated jurisdictions; children not having access to information about their donor; and barriers for importing embryos created using donor gametes into Australia. During the COVID-19 pandemic travel restrictions, many people were unable to access embryos or gametes stored overseas and unable to import the embryos or gametes into Australia for local treatment.

While around 75 babies are born annually from domestic surrogacy arrangements, most people who need surrogacy travel to international destinations due to the challenges of finding a surrogate and an egg donor (where this is needed) in Australia. Common overseas destinations for surrogacy arrangements use anonymous surrogates and donors, providing no opportunity for children born as a result to access information about the woman who gave birth to them or the woman who provided the egg. In unregulated destinations, quality of treatment can vary. To increase success rates, more than one embryo is sometimes transferred to the surrogate. This increases the risk of multiple birth and the associated risks of adverse outcomes for the surrogate and the babies. In addition, there have been instances of sperm mix-ups associated with surrogacy treatment in parts of Asia, with parents discovering they are not related to their baby on receiving DNA test results for travel back to Australia.

Summary

The use of ART to have children is increasing in Australia. While there are slight differences between states and territories, the laws and regulations that govern ART practice in Australia offer protection for those involved in treatment and the children who are born as a result. The overarching principles that govern the practice of third-party reproduction are altruism on the part of the third party; the right of donor-conceived people to be informed of their biological origins; and the provision of comprehensive counselling about the social, psychological, physical, ethical, financial and legal implications of third-party reproduction to those considering donating or receiving gametes or embryos and entering surrogacy arrangements.

Infertility is a distressing experience. Medical practitioners have an important role to play in helping patients access ART when they need it and in supporting them before, during or after a treatment journey. ART treatment is physically, emotionally and financially demanding, and around half of those who use ART end treatment without a baby. Directing people to independent, evidence-based and transparent information about what treatment involves and the chance of success with ART helps people make well-informed decisions and to have realistic expectations if they decide to pursue treatment.

Note: Views in this chapter are those of the authors and do not necessarily reflect the views of organisations they have worked for.

References

1. Reproductive Technology Accreditation Committee. Code of practice. 2018. https://www.fertilitysociety.com.au/art-regulation/rtac (accessed Jun 2025).
2. National Health and Medical Research Council. Ethical guidelines on the use of assisted reproductive technology in clinical practice and research. 2023. https://www.nhmrc.gov.au/about-us/publications/art (accessed Jun 2025).
3. Storen R, Smith E. Mitochondrial Donation Law Reform (Maeve's Law) Bill 2021 (Bills Digest No. 65, 2020–21). Canberra: Parliament of Australia, 2021. https://www.aph.gov.au/Parliamentary_Business/Bills_Legislation/bd/bd2021a/21bd065 (accessed Jun 2025).
4. Chambers GM, Paul RC, Harris K, et al. Assisted reproductive technology in Australia and New Zealand: cumulative live birth rates as measures of success. *Med J Aust* 2017; 207: 114–118.

Further reading

ART legislation in NSW, independent information about aspects of ART: NSW Health https://www.health.nsw.gov.au

ART legislation in SA, independent information about aspects of ART: SA Health https://www.sahealth.sa.gov.au

ART legislation in Victoria, independent information about aspects of ART: Victorian Assisted Reproductive Treatment Authority https://www.varta.org.au; Health.vic https://www.health.vic.gov.au

ART legislation in WA, independent information about aspects of ART: Reproductive Technology Council https://www.rtc.org.au

Choosing Wisely for health professionals, consumers and carers: https://www.choosingwisely.org.au

Choosing Wisely, 5 questions to ask your doctor: https://www.choosingwisely.org.au/resources/consumers-and-carers/5questions

For information about the accreditation scheme and technical bulletins for ART clinics, including topics of patient-centred care and adjuvants: Fertility Society of Australia and New Zealand https://www.fertilitysociety.com.au

National Health and Medical Research Council ethical guidelines on the use of ART: https://www.nhmrc.gov.au/research-policy/ethics/ethical-guidelines-use-assisted-reproductive-technology

Person-centred care in ART: Victorian Assisted Reproductive Treatment Authority https://www.varta.org.au/sites/default/files/2021-02/varta-guidance-on-person-centred-care-012021.pdf

Person-centred care, general guidance: Australian Commission on Safety and Quality in Health Care https://www.safetyandquality.gov.au

Resources about men's reproductive health: Healthy Male (formerly Andrology Australia) https://www.healthymale.org.au

Resources and information about optimising chance of conception and having a healthy baby: Your Fertility https://www.yourfertility.org.au; Royal Australian College of General Practitioners https://www1.racgp.org.au/ajgp/2018/july/preconception-care

Resources for trans and diverse families: Rainbow Families https://www.rainbowfamilies.com.au

14 Termination of pregnancy and related issues

Julie Hamblin, David Ellwood AO

Introduction

This chapter aims to provide guidance about a range of aspects of clinical practice. It should be read in conjunction with any state or territory local guidelines as there are some legal and policy differences that impact clinical practice across Australia.

Termination of pregnancy is one of the most common medical procedures performed in Australia yet has always been treated differently from other procedures from a regulatory perspective. For many decades, Australia bore the legacy of British criminal law, adopted in Australia in the 19th century, which made abortion a crime both for the person performing it and the woman undergoing it. Long after the UK had updated its abortion law, termination of pregnancy remained a crime in most Australian states and territories. Indeed, it was only in 2019 that the last Australian state to review its original criminal law on termination of pregnancy (New South Wales) passed abortion law reform legislation, and Western Australia further updated its legislation as recently as 2023.

14.1 The current legal framework for termination of pregnancy

Because termination of pregnancy is regulated by state rather than Commonwealth legislation, each of the eight states and territories has its own separate abortion law. While the approach is broadly similar across jurisdictions, the detail of the legislation varies significantly. Health practitioners need to be aware of the relevant legal requirements in their jurisdiction, as well as applicable clinical practice guidelines on termination of pregnancy.

Table 14.1 provides an overview of the current law governing termination of pregnancy in each Australian state and territory. The key features can be summarised as follows:

(a) Termination of pregnancy is lawful on request, subject to gestational limits.

In all states and territories, except the Northern Territory, termination of pregnancy can be lawfully performed on request with the informed consent of the patient up to a specified gestational limit. The applicable limit varies from 16 weeks (Tasmania) to 22 weeks (NSW and Queensland), 23 weeks (South Australia and Western Australia) and an upper limit of 24 weeks in Victoria. Only in the Australian Capital Territory is there no limit on when termination of pregnancy can be performed at the request, and with the informed consent, of the pregnant woman.

The NT has retained a requirement for a medical practitioner to certify that the termination of pregnancy is appropriate, even for earlier-gestation terminations. After 24 weeks' gestation, two medical practitioners must provide this certification.

(b) Additional legal requirements apply for later-term terminations of pregnancy.

The states/territories that have a gestational limit for termination of pregnancy on request allow for later terminations to be performed if certain conditions are met. Most commonly, as set out in Table 14.1, this is a certification by either one or two medical practitioners that the termination is considered appropriate or is necessary to prevent a risk to the patient's physical or mental health. There are additional requirements in Tasmania, where one of the two medical practitioners providing the certification must be a specialist in obstetrics and gynaecology.

(c) There are restrictions on where later-term terminations of pregnancy can be performed in some jurisdictions.

In NSW, terminations of pregnancy after 22 weeks must be performed by a specialist medical practitioner at an approved health facility. In SA, terminations after 23 weeks must be performed at a prescribed hospital. There are no similar requirements in other jurisdictions.

(d) Counselling should be considered.

As part of the health practitioner's general duty of care to the patient, consideration should always be given to whether additional support should be offered by way of counselling or psychological referral. Many patients have already made up their minds before requesting a termination. However, in some cases, offering counselling or psychological referral may be part of the process necessary to ensure that the patient is able to provide full and informed consent to the termination of pregnancy.

This duty has been legislated in NSW, where the law requires a medical practitioner to consider whether counselling would be beneficial to the patient and, if so, offer it. In SA, information about available counselling must be provided to all patients seeking a termination of pregnancy.

(e) Health practitioners have the right of conscientious objection to performing terminations.

All states and territories have given statutory recognition to the right of health practitioners to refuse to perform terminations of pregnancy if they have a sincere moral or religious objection to doing so. In all jurisdictions except the ACT, a health practitioner exercising this right of conscientious objection is required to refer the patient to another practitioner who is able to provide the treatment or provide information about where a termination can be obtained.

It is always important for a health practitioner exercising a right of conscientious objection to ensure that patients are nonetheless able to access the health care they need by way of appropriate referral. This is explicitly stated in the Medical Board of Australia's *Good medical practice: a code of conduct for doctors in Australia*:

> 3.4.6 Being aware of your right to not provide or directly participate in treatments to which you conscientiously object, informing your patients and, if relevant, colleagues of your objection, and not using your objection to impede access to treatments that are legal. In some jurisdictions, legislation mandates doctors who do not wish to participate in certain treatments, to refer on the patient.
>
> 3.4.7 Not allowing your moral or religious views to deny patients access to medical care, recognising that you are free to decline to personally provide or directly participate in that care [1].

In some cases, particularly in smaller, remote communities, and at later gestations, the referral options may be more limited for medical practitioners wishing to exercise a right of conscientious objection. The importance of ensuring patients are able to access the health care they need must always be the paramount consideration, and care must be taken to support the patient to find an alternative practitioner.

It should also be noted that the right of conscientious objection does not apply in cases of emergency, where medical treatment is necessary to save the patient's life or avert a serious risk to their health.

(f) Legislation in each jurisdiction defines safe access zones.

All Australian states and territories have enacted laws establishing 'safe access zones' around premises where terminations of pregnancy are performed. These laws are directed at anti-abortion protesters who have gathered outside abortion clinics in the past, often causing distress to women seeking terminations of pregnancy. The detail of these laws varies between jurisdictions, but they generally establish a minimum distance—most commonly 150 metres—around premises where terminations are performed, within which conduct that could harass or intimidate women seeking terminations of pregnancy is prohibited.

Table 14.1 Overview of abortion laws across Australia

	Australian Capital Territory	New South Wales	Northern Territory	Queensland	South Australia	Tasmania	Victoria	Western Australia
Relevant legislation	*Health Act 1993* (ACT)	*Abortion Law Reform Act 2019* (NSW)	*Termination of Pregnancy Law Reform Act 2017* (NT)	*Termination of Pregnancy Act 2018* (Qld)	*Termination of Pregnancy Act 2021* (SA)	*Reproductive Health (Access to Terminations) Act 2013* (Tas)	*Abortion Law Reform Act 2008* (Vic)	*Abortion Legislation Reform Act 2023* (WA)
Termination lawful on request and gestational limit (if relevant)	Yes No gestational limit	Yes Up to 22 weeks	No Only if a doctor certifies the termination as appropriate	Yes Up to 22 weeks	Yes Up to 23 weeks	Yes Up to 16 weeks	Yes Up to 24 weeks	Yes Up to 23 weeks
Termination lawful in other circumstances	N/A	After 22 weeks if two doctors certify there are sufficient grounds to perform the termination	Up to 24 weeks if a doctor considers the termination is appropriate in all the circumstances. After 24 weeks if two doctors consider it is appropriate.	After 22 weeks if two doctors agree the termination should be performed	After 23 weeks if two doctors agree it is necessary to save life, prevent risk to physical or mental health, or there is a risk of serious foetal anomaly	After 16 weeks if two doctors (including one obstetrics and gynaecology specialist) reasonably believe the continuation of the pregnancy involves a greater risk to the physical or mental health of the woman than a termination	After 24 weeks if two doctors reasonably believe the termination is appropriate in all the circumstances	After 23 weeks by an authorised doctor if that doctor and another doctor consulted about the termination both consider the termination is appropriate in the circumstances

Continued over page

	Australian Capital Territory	New South Wales	Northern Territory	Queensland	South Australia	Tasmania	Victoria	Western Australia
Right of conscientious objection recognised	Yes No obligation to refer on	Yes, with obligation to refer the patient on or provide information about services that provide terminations	Yes, with obligation to refer the patient on	Yes, with obligation to refer the patient on	Yes, with obligation to refer the patient on	Yes, with obligation to refer the patient on	Yes, with obligation to refer the patient on	Yes, with obligation to refer the patient on or provide information approved by the Chief Health Officer about how to locate a health practitioner who can provide the termination
Counselling requirement	No	Doctor must consider whether counselling would be beneficial and, if so, offer it	No	No	Information about counselling must be provided	No	No	No
Where terminations can be performed		After 22 weeks, terminations can only be performed by a specialist at an approved facility			After 23 weeks, terminations must be performed at a prescribed hospital			
Safe access zones	Yes	Yes	Yes	Yes	Yes	Yes	Yes	Yes

14.2 Terminations of pregnancy for children and young people

Each state and territory has its own legal requirements for consent to medical treatment for children and young people (see Chapter 7, Consent and informed decision making). As a general rule, the question of whether a young person can provide valid consent for a termination of pregnancy will follow the same principles applying to all medical treatment.

14.3 Methods for terminating pregnancy

Methods for termination of pregnancy have changed over time. In early pregnancy (up to 9 weeks or 63 days), medical abortion using a combination of mifepristone and misoprostol administered at home by the patient is increasingly common [2]. Early medical abortion is a safe and effective alternative to surgical abortion and can be provided in the primary care setting. Although patients have a choice of method for termination, in some regions of Australia availability may limit this. Early medical abortion can help to improve access to termination of pregnancy in remote and regional areas, particularly since the service can be provided safely via telehealth as long as appropriate backup medical support is available in the event of complications. In the late first and early second trimester, surgical methods provided in a day surgery setting are most commonly used [2], including vacuum aspiration up to 14 weeks, and dilatation and evacuation at later gestations; however, the upper limit of gestational age is dependent on the skill and experience of the surgeon. For terminations later in the second trimester, medical methods are more common, and these can involve hospital admission and induction of labour. For terminations after 22 weeks, most jurisdictions recommend a feticide procedure using intracardiac potassium chloride prior to induction of labour or an operative procedure.

As with the regulation of surgical termination of pregnancy, however, the use of mifepristone for medical abortions is subject to regulatory requirements different from other medications. Although the Therapeutic Goods Administration approved mifepristone in 2012 for use in Australia for first trimester abortion up to 9 weeks' gestation, the approval is subject to special conditions. Medical practitioners who wish to use mifepristone must first register with MS Health (the company that sponsors the drug in Australia) and complete an online training program. Fellows and diplomates of the Royal Australian and New Zealand College of Obstetricians and Gynaecologists are exempt from the requirement to undergo training, but they must still be registered providers. This requirement exists in both private practice and in public hospitals, and regardless of the gestational age at which the drug is prescribed.

14.4 Ethical considerations in relation to late-term terminations

The changes in the laws in all states and territories have brought with them some certainty for clinicians and patients as to what is possible to be done within the law. This has certainly made a difference in difficult cases of severe foetal anomalies, which can sometimes only be diagnosed with certainty in the late second or even early third trimester. However, these cases can lead to some ethical dilemmas for both clinicians and patients. The degree of individual comfort and preparedness of some practitioners to perform terminations may vary with gestational age, and also the indication for the procedure. This can be very challenging as it is different from the more usual conscientious objection in which there is opposition to all forms of termination of pregnancy, which is generally recognised in law. A refusal by a skilled, competent practitioner to perform a requested termination of pregnancy at later gestations because of the practitioner's own view of the appropriateness of the procedure is both legally and ethically problematic. In more complex cases, it may be appropriate for concerned practitioners to seek help and support through referrals for second opinions, consulting with local clinical ethics committees and, in some cases, seeking legal advice.

Summary

As community attitudes and legal restrictions on termination of pregnancy have become more liberal, there are more choices available to women faced with this difficult decision. Doctors must be aware of the legal framework that applies in their own health jurisdiction and have sufficient knowledge and understanding to be able to refer patients to the appropriate services with confidence. The emotional impacts of termination of pregnancy decisions on some women are significant, and knowledge and understanding of the availability of support services, such as My Options (https://www.1800myoptions.org.au), are also required to support decision making and wellbeing.

References

1. Medical Board of Australia. Good medical practice: a code of conduct for doctors in Australia. 2020. https://www.medicalboard.gov.au/Codes-Guidelines-Policies/Code-of-conduct.aspx (accessed Jun 2025).
2. Royal Australian and New Zealand College of Obstetricians and Gynaecologists. Clinical guideline for abortion care: an evidence-based guideline on abortion care in Australia and Aotearoa New Zealand. 2023. https://ranzcog.edu.au/resources/abortion-guideline (accessed Jun 2025).

15 Family violence, child maltreatment and elder abuse

Sue Dawson, Vanessa Ballard, Nicole Lawless, Prue McEvoy

Introduction

Doctors play an important frontline role in the identification and prevention of family and domestic violence, child maltreatment and elder abuse, and intervention for patients who experience or are at risk of experiencing any of these. This chapter will discuss the nature and prevalence of family and domestic violence and outline the various roles of the medical practitioner. It will also discuss approaches to clinical assessment, as well as the roles and obligations of doctors in documenting and reporting abuse, and in ongoing care.

15.1 What are family and domestic violence, child maltreatment and elder abuse?

15.1.1 Definitions and statistics

Family violence refers to violent, threatening or other behaviour by a person who coerces or controls a member of their family or causes a family member to be fearful [1].

Domestic violence is considered to be a subset of family violence and includes behaviour within a domestic relationship that causes physical, emotional, sexual, economic and/or social harm. A person is considered to be in a domestic relationship with another person if they are or were:

- married, or in a de facto or intimate relationship, whether or not it is of a sexual nature
- living together in the same house or residential facility
- relatives by birth, marriage or adoption
- in the case of an Aboriginal and/or Torres Strait Islander person, part of the same extended family or kinship group
- in a relationship involving dependence on the ongoing paid or unpaid care from the other person
- married to, or in a de facto or intimate relationship with the same person; for example, a woman's ex-partner and current partner are in a domestic relationship with each other even if they have never met [2].

Family and domestic violence affects people of all races, ages, religious groups, sexualities, socioeconomic status and cultures. It is complex, traumatic and an insidious problem because the violence often occurs in the privacy of homes where perpetrators are in a position of trust and there is a power imbalance within relationships. The overwhelming majority of people who experience such violence are women and children [3].

Elder abuse often occurs in the context of family and domestic violence, and refers to an act occurring within a relationship where there is an implication of trust, which results in harm to an older person [4]. In Australia, an older person is generally considered to be 65 years of age or over [4] (60 years or over internationally [5]), or over 50 years of age for Aboriginal and/or Torres Strait Islander people due to their substantially lower life expectancy [6]. Elder abuse may occur at home, in the community or in institutions such as nursing homes and long-term care facilities.

Child maltreatment includes physical abuse, sexual abuse, emotional abuse, neglect and exposure to domestic violence of children under the age of 18 years (16 years in New South Wales and 17 years in Victoria) [7]. It is most commonly perpetrated by someone within the child's family or known to the child [8].

Family and domestic violence, child maltreatment and elder abuse are significant and increasing public health and welfare issues as they are deeply traumatic and often have lifelong impacts resulting in serious illness, injury, disability or death [9]. Child maltreatment is associated with negative impacts on the child's development, physical and mental health, wellbeing, and ongoing relationships that continue into adult life [10].

See Box 15.1 for statistics related to family and domestic violence, child maltreatment and elder abuse.

Box 15.1 What the statistics say

Family and domestic violence

- One in six women and one in 18 men have experienced physical or sexual violence by a current or previous partner [11].
- One in four women and one in seven men have experienced emotional abuse by a current or previous partner [11].
- One in five women and one in 16 men have experienced sexual violence [11].
- 54% of women and 65% of men who experience violence by a current partner experience more than one incident of violence [11].
- Over 29,000 people in Australia (excluding Western Australia and the Northern Territory) were hospitalised for family and domestic violence between 2010 and 2018. Of these, two in three were female and more than one in four were Aboriginal and/or Torres Strait Islander people [12].

Child maltreatment

- The Australian Child Maltreatment Study using nationally representative data found that among 16–24-year-olds, 28.2% have experienced physical abuse, 25.7% have experienced sexual abuse, 34.6% have experienced emotional abuse and 43.8% have been exposed to domestic violence during their childhood. 40.2% of young people have experienced more than one form of abuse, and 25.4% have experienced 3–5 types of abuse. Those who experience maltreatment are 2.8 times more likely to have a mental disorder during adulthood [13].
- The majority of children who experience abuse know the perpetrator and experience multiple incidents of abuse [14].

Continued over page

- Data linkage studies such as the South Australian BEBOLD (Better Evidence, Better Outcomes, Linked Data) platform highlight that one in three children will be notified to child protection services by the age of 10 years [15].
- Infants and small children who have child protection notifications will exhibit vulnerabilities across all developmental domains by 5 years of age [15].
- The most common notifications involve neglect, and half the notifications occur by 3 years of age. Aboriginal and/or Torres Strait Islander children are vastly over-represented: 25% of notifications versus 4% of the population [15].

Elder abuse

- One in six older Australians (14.8%) are reported to be victims of elder abuse annually [16].
- The most common form of abuse is psychological abuse (11.7%), followed by neglect (2.9%) and financial abuse (2.1%) [16].
- The perpetrators of elder abuse are often family members, mostly adult children, but they can also be friends, neighbours and acquaintances [16].
- Elderly men are more likely to experience physical abuse, and elderly women are more likely to experience sexual abuse and neglect [16].

15.1.2 Who is most at risk?

Groups and communities in Australia that are known to be at higher risk of experiencing family violence include Aboriginal and/or Torres Strait Islander women; women with disabilities and mental health issues; women from culturally and linguistically diverse communities; gay, lesbian, bisexual, transgender, intersex and queer people; and women in rural and remote communities [3]. There may also be barriers to disclosure for victims in small, rural or remote communities, such as fear of reprisal by the perpetrator and the stigma of shame and judgement [11].

People with a disability have been found to be 1.8 times more likely to experience sexual or physical violence than those without a disability, and Aboriginal and/or Torres Strait Islander people are 32 times more likely to be hospitalised due to family violence, more likely to be murdered by a family member and more likely to have their children removed [11].

An increase in both the prevalence and severity of family or domestic violence was reported during the COVID-19 pandemic, due to a combination of victims and perpetrators spending an increased amount of time together, increased social isolation, decreased social movement, and a higher incidence of financial stress and job insecurity [17].

The risk of child maltreatment is increased by psychosocial adversities including young parental age, parental mental illness, parental substance use, and poverty. Aboriginal and/or Torres Strait Islander children are overrepresented in notifications to statutory child protection services and in out-of-home care [14].

15.1.3 What role do medical practitioners play?

There is a strong imperative for medical practitioners to recognise and offer intervention for all types of violence and abuse in the community. There are many touchpoints in the healthcare system where it is possible to do this, including hospital presentations, aged care assessments, admissions to residential care facilities, community nursing and allied care home visits, and encounters in mental health services and outreach services.

The Australian Medical Association position statement on family and domestic violence makes broad reference to the expectations of medical practitioners:

> Medical practitioners should have systems in place to help them deal with family and domestic violence in their practice, and understand the different referral pathways to help patients find safety and begin healing. This is why it is so important that medical practitioner training includes personal attitudes and assumptions about abuse and violence, as they can affect the way medical practitioners respond to patients experiencing abuse and violence [18].

General practitioners (GPs) particularly are in a strong position to identify violence and abuse because they work with entire family units and develop strong connections and rapport with patients, building trust over a long period.

Not only do doctors have a duty of care to their patients to identify situations of abuse so they can intervene early, they also have a legal obligation in all states and territories to report concerns that a child has been a victim, or is at risk of being a victim, of abuse or neglect. In the NT, this obligation extends to reporting concerns that a person has been a victim, or is at risk of being a victim, of family and domestic violence. Accordingly, doctors should be familiar with the mandatory reporting obligations in the state or territory in which they practice (see section 15.4).

15.2 Identifying family violence, child maltreatment and elder abuse

When working with children and families, the key steps for doctors in identifying violence or abuse are recognising risk factors and vulnerability, noting early signs and symptoms, and assessing harm. Doctors can intervene at three levels:

- Recognise risk factors and intervene early to ameliorate adversity and prevent harm.
- Recognise harm and respond appropriately to mitigate future harm.
- Support the ongoing wellbeing of the patient or child to manage the long-term negative impacts of harm [7].

Doctors who fail to consider the possibility of child maltreatment in children who present with repeated or unexplained injuries or illnesses, or with emotional disturbances, have been subject to criticism by coroners and disciplinary action by medical boards and other regulators.

GPs are in a unique position as they are often aware of changing dynamics, circumstances and stresses within a family unit. They may be involved in antenatal shared care, which is an opportunity for strengthening their understanding of the mother's circumstances. It is estimated that a full-time GP sees around five women per week who have experienced family violence or abuse [19], and the children of these women will also be impacted by this violence, either directly or indirectly. GPs also have increased opportunities to be alert to the possibility of elder abuse as more than a third of GP encounters are with patients over the age of 65 years.

15.2.1 Recognising the behaviours and signs of violence or abuse

The clinical indicators of family and domestic violence, child maltreatment and elder abuse are broad and varied. Doctors must be astute observers as family violence and abuse are often hidden, and patients may have no physical injuries. Chronic mental and physical conditions can be caused by violence. Common behaviours and signs of violence or abuse to look out for are outlined in Tables 15.1–15.5.

Table 15.1 Behaviours and signs of physical abuse

Behaviours	Signs
• Pushing, shoving or rough handling • Kicking, beating, hitting, punching, slapping, biting or burning • Restraining, physically or mentally • Locking the person in a room or home • Intentional injury with a weapon or object • Overuse or misuse of medications • Smashing property, and killing and/or hurting family pets	• Internal or external injuries (sprains, dislocations and fractures, pressure sores, unexplained bruises or marks on the body) • Broken or healing bones • Lacerations to mouth, lips, gums, eyes or ears • Missing teeth • Signs of physical restraint • Evidence of hitting, punching, shaking or pulling, e.g. bruises, lacerations, choke marks, hair loss • Burns • In infants and children: failure to progress (developmental delay) or regression of developmental milestones, school failure or refusal, or any significant behavioural disturbance

Table 15.2 Behaviours and signs of sexual abuse

Behaviours	Signs
• Forced intercourse or penetration • Sexual coercion • Reproductive coercion • Sexual contact without consent • Non-contact sexual interaction • Any completed or attempted sexual act without consent • Filming or prostitution	• Bruising around the breasts, genital area or peri-anal region • Unexplained genital or urinary tract infections • Damaged or bloody underclothing • Unexplained vaginal or anal bleeding • Bruising on the inner thighs • Difficulty in walking or sitting • Chronic pelvic pain • In infants and children: failure to progress (developmental delay) or regression of developmental milestones, school failure or refusal, or any significant behavioural disturbance

Table 15.3 Behaviours and signs of emotional or psychological abuse

Behaviours	Signs
• Subtle or overt verbal abuse • Pressuring, bullying, intimidating and harassing • Humiliating, blaming, belittling, conveying to the person they are worthless • Frightening and/or threatening to harm someone or break belongings • Threatening to harm a pet • Threatening to place a person in an aged care facility • Making threats of suicide, extreme jealousy, stalking or harassment • Treating an older person as if they are a child • Engaging in emotional blackmail • Preventing contact with family or friends • Denying access to services, or religious or cultural events • Misusing the function of enduring guardianship • Screening telephone calls, listening in or disconnecting the telephone without consent, or withholding mail • Taking control of the person's home • Moving a person far away from family or friends • Withholding affection	• Feelings of helplessness, shame and powerlessness • Changes in levels of self-esteem and loss of confidence • Sadness or grief at loss of important relationships • Depression, withdrawal or listlessness • Worry or anxiety after a visit by a specific person • Reluctance to talk, fear, anxiety, nervousness, apathy, resignation, withdrawal, avoidance of eye contact • Rocking or huddling up • Loss of interest in self or environment • Insomnia/sleep deprivation • Unusual behaviour or confusion not associated with illness • Difficulty concentrating and making decisions • Suicidal ideation • Somatoform disorder • Post-traumatic stress disorder • Drug and alcohol use • In infants and children: failure to progress (developmental delay) or regression of developmental milestones, school failure or refusal, or any significant behavioural disturbance

Table 15.4 Behaviours and signs of neglect

Behaviours	Signs
• Failing to provide adequate food, shelter, clean clothing, heating, cooling, medicines, or medical or dental care • Under- or over-medicating • Refusing to permit others to provide assessments or appropriate care to the person • Preventing the person from accessing services and/or equipment and support • Exposing the person to danger or lack of supervision • Overly attentive care in the company of others; the 'hovering' carer • Misusing the role of the guardian • Allowing children to miss long periods of school • Failing to protect children from violence in the home or neighbourhood	• Poor hygiene, bad odour, urine rash • Malnourishment, weight loss, dehydration (dark urine, dry tongue, lax skin) • Bed sores (sacrum, hips, heels, elbows) • Being over-sedated or under-sedated • Inappropriate or soiled clothing, overgrown nails, decaying teeth • Broken or missing aids such as spectacles, dentures, hearing aids or walking frame • For infants: failure to thrive • For infants and children: developmental delays across all domains

Table 15.5 Behaviours and signs of financial abuse

Behaviours	Signs
• Threatening, coercing or influencing a person to change their will or sign documents relating to their assets • Taking control of a person's finances against their wishes and denying them access to their own money • Abusing powers of attorney by taking money or property • Stealing goods, e.g. jewellery, credit cards, cash, food or other possessions • Stealing money, such as pension-skimming, and selling belongings without the person's permission • Recently adding a signature on a bank account • Restricting access to money and essential needs	• Unexplained disappearance of belongings • Unauthorised use of banking and financial documents • Inability to pay bills • Significant bank withdrawals • Changes to wills • Inability of a person to access bank accounts or statements • Stockpiling of unpaid bills • Insufficient food in the fridge • Disparity between living conditions and financial resources • Insufficient money to pay for essentials for the home including food, clothing or utilities • Cancelling or refusing community services

15.2.2 Risk assessment

Doctors should be aware of evidence-based strategies and available screening tools to assist in assessing a patient's risk for future harm from family or domestic violence or abuse. The Victorian Government's Family Violence Multi-Agency Risk Assessment and Management Framework [20] provides several guides and tools for risk identification, screening and assessment of family violence and child abuse, as does the NSW Government's Domestic Violence Safety Assessment Tool [21].

Generally speaking, some of the broader risk factors for future family or domestic violence or abuse include:

- pregnancy or following a recent birth [22]
- previous violence by the perpetrator
- the victim leaving or planning to leave the relationship
- the perpetrator having a history of alcohol or drug abuse, mental health problems, or violent behaviour outside the household including violence towards animals
- the perpetrator being unemployed or having financial difficulties
- previous intimate partner sexual violence
- obsessive, jealous or controlling behaviour by the perpetrator, including stalking
- self-harm, suicide attempts or threats of suicide by the perpetrator
- access to weapons or previous use of weapons by the perpetrator [20].

Children in households where there is family violence, or where one or both caregivers are abusing alcohol, are at high risk of neglect and other forms of child maltreatment [7]. Other common risk factors for child maltreatment include:

- the child having medical needs or a disability
- an unstable housing or financial situation in the family or household
- a risky social or family context (including poverty or poor housing, or social contexts involving intergenerational trauma)
- lack of social support
- the child's caregivers having a mental illness, intellectual disability or substance abuse issues that impact the tasks of parenting [23].

A useful risk assessment tool for suspected elder abuse is the Elder Abuse Suspicion Index (EASI) questionnaire [24]. This tool is for use in cognitively intact patients; screening for cognitive impairment should be performed before screening for abuse in older persons [25].

Risk factors for elder abuse include factors related to the circumstances of the older person, including:

- social isolation from family and friends
- cognitive impairment and other forms of disability causing capacity issues
- confusion about property, belongings or surroundings
- physical or verbal violence or aggression because of cognitive impairment or another condition
- a history of family dysfunction, domestic or family violence

- insecure accommodation
- low income or financial difficulties [5].

Other risk factors for elder abuse relate to the circumstances of potential perpetrators, such as carer stress, mental health problems, alcohol abuse and financial dependency on the older person [7].

Within institutions, elder abuse is more likely to occur where the standards of care facilities are low, staff are overworked and poorly trained, and the physical environment is poorly maintained [7].

15.2.3 Asking patients about abuse

Research suggests that the majority of family violence victims do not object to a health professional asking them about violence, but only a minority are actually asked. As a doctor, raising the issue can be challenging, but patients are significantly more likely to disclose violence and abuse if they are asked directly [26]. When a patient presents with any of the common behaviours and signs of violence or abuse, or if any risk factors are identified, doctors should inquire further. If language is a barrier, communication should occur through a suitable and qualified interpreter, and not through the patient's family.

There should be a low threshold for asking about abuse. When making inquiries, doctors should ensure that the patient is alone and separated from family members or potential perpetrators. If the perpetrator is present, the patient may become uneasy, which may act as a barrier to disclosure, and any suspicion or questioning on the part of the doctor may put the patient in danger. It is appropriate to ask the patient's partner or family member to wait in the waiting room and explain that it is usual practice for doctors to consult or examine their patients alone [7]. If necessary, make a follow-up appointment with the patient on their own.

Doctors should ask questions of the patient sensitively, in a non-judgemental and empathetic way, and should begin with open-ended questions [7]. Questions and statements that may be helpful in inquiring about suspected family violence include:

- How are things at home?
- Do you feel safe at home?
- Often people who have these types of health problems are experiencing difficulties at home. Is this happening to you?
- Sometimes these symptoms can be associated with having been hurt in the past. Did that ever happen to you?
- Has your partner physically threatened or hurt you?
- Is there a lot of tension in your relationship?
- How do you resolve arguments?
- Sometime partners react strongly in arguments and use physical force. Is this happening to you?
- Are you afraid of your partner? Have you ever been afraid of any partner?
- Have you ever felt unsafe in the past at home?
- Has your partner ever controlled your daily activities?
- Has your partner ever threatened to physically hurt you? [7]

Telehealth has been effective in improving the accessibility of doctors for victims of family violence, especially during the COVID-19 pandemic; however, it is not always possible to ascertain who is present with the patient during a telehealth consultation. If inquiring about violence or abuse during a telehealth consultation, it is advisable to start with yes or no questions to ensure the safety of the patient and determine whether they are alone. It may be necessary to call back or find a safe time to call when family members or potential perpetrators will not be present [7].

15.2.4 Asking children about abuse

In cases of child maltreatment, some children may present with bruising or injuries that raise suspicion, but the majority do not. Physical injuries cause less morbidity in children than the effect of violence on neurological and emotional development. As such, it is often difficult for doctors to know whether the child's symptoms have resulted from abuse or neglect. Additionally, the family may also be actively trying to hide the abuse or neglect [7].

It is imperative that the child is not in the presence of a potential perpetrator when asked about abuse, which is often challenging. The child may be reluctant to disclose even if the perpetrator is waiting outside the consulting room, and it may be necessary to see the child at another time with a different caregiver. Depending on the developmental stage of the child, it may be appropriate for a doctor to consult a child alone (child experts consider this to be approximately 8 years of age). In order to consult the child alone, a doctor must feel comfortable explaining to the parents or guardian that it is standard practice to see the child alone. It may be helpful to say, 'It is part of my practice to see children alone for part of the consultation to get their views and so I can do the best job for you and your child' [7].

Questions and statements that may be helpful in inquiring about potential abuse of a child include:

- How do the people in your family get along?
- Has anyone made you feel afraid? Can you tell me about that?
- What happens when you get into trouble or don't listen to your [caregiver]?
- I notice you have a bruise on your [body part]. How did it happen?
- Do people in your family ever make you feel bad about yourself? Tell me what that looks like; does anything else happen? What's the worst thing that happens?
- Who takes care of you?
- Has anyone made you feel afraid? Can you tell me about that?
- What happens when your parents are angry with you?
- Has any child or adult touched or hurt your private parts? Has anyone made you touch or look at their private parts?
- Does anything happen that makes it hurt for you to wee? [7]

Children may feel shame or guilt about abuse or may not recognise that their experience is abuse. They may also be attached to the person who is abusive and fear the consequences of disclosing any abuse or neglect [7].

Doctors should inquire about child abuse only to the extent needed to determine that there is a reason to suspect a risk of harm. It is not necessary to confirm or investigate whether child abuse has occurred. Once a doctor suspects that a child is at risk of abuse, a mandatory report to the relevant child protection service must be made in accordance with the laws in the state or territory of practice. The doctor's task then becomes supporting the child and their family and addressing, where appropriate, some of the identified adversities. Only 20% of notifications proceed to statutory intervention so a broader community response must be considered.

15.2.5 Asking elderly patients about elder abuse

In the case of suspected elder abuse, the doctor should first establish the patient's cognitive capacity. If the patient has lost capacity, it may be necessary to discuss concerns with the carer unless this person is the potential perpetrator. As with all potential victims of violence or abuse, it is preferable to interview the patient alone.

If the patient's carer is a potential perpetrator, the doctor should contact a family member or an advocacy group in the relevant state or territory for advice (see section 15.4.3). A potential red flag is a carer who often interrupts to answer on behalf of a patient, although this behaviour does not always indicate mistreatment or abuse. Doctors must also consider potential medical conditions and medication effects that can mimic abuse in older patients [25].

When consulting a patient who is at risk of elder abuse, doctors should start by asking open-ended, non-judgemental questions, and encourage patients and carers to provide detailed information. Some helpful questions include:

- Has anyone limited your daily activities?
- How did you get this bruise?
- Has someone talked to you in a threatening way?
- Has someone forced you to give them money or sign papers?
- Has anyone touched you in a way that you didn't like or that made you feel uncomfortable? [7]

15.3 Responding to a disclosure of suspected violence or abuse

The World Health Organization recommends that GPs should provide first-line support to patients who make a disclosure of domestic or family violence. In addition to their mandatory reporting obligations, doctors need to manage the consequences of abuse to minimise morbidity and mortality for the patient. This includes supporting the patient and their family by listening, providing ongoing supportive and trauma-informed care, and connecting them to referral services and community resources as required.

15.3.1 Validation and safety plans

It is important for doctors to respond to all disclosures or identification of violence and abuse of adults, children or older persons in a way that validates the victim's experience and assures the patient that violence is unacceptable [26]. Any response to a disclosure should be non-judgemental, supportive and believing. A doctor should offer support that involves collaboration, choice and empowerment of the patient. This includes identifying the patient's strengths, and helping to minimise self-blame and doubt [7].

Validation statements may include:

- What is happening to you is not okay, and it is not your fault.
- Everyone deserves to be safe at home.
- I am concerned about your safety and wellbeing.

- It took you a lot of courage to disclose and discuss this with me.
- You are not alone. I will be with you through this, whatever you decide.
- You are not to blame; abuse is common and happens in all types of relationships.

Doctors should ascertain whether the patient is in any immediate danger or there is an imminent risk of violence or abuse. If so, the police should be contacted on 000. Ideally, a patient should consent to report the matter to police; however, if they are not capable of giving consent for any reason, including intimidation, then confidentiality may be breached to ensure the patient's and their children's immediate safety [7]. Infants are particularly vulnerable to harm when there is suspected family violence.

If immediate safety is not an issue, doctors should facilitate referrals to appropriate organisations to ensure the patient has financial stability, appropriate housing and relationship support. A safety plan should be created to avoid any future potential situations where violence or abuse may occur and to ensure the safety of children. Fundamentals of a safety plan include:

- identification of a safe house such as a shelter, or the home of a family member or friend
- ensuring adequate money and essential items are available if the patient is required to leave at short notice
- strategies for reducing harm if the patient is going to continue to have contact with the abuser
- a checklist of essential items and emergency contact numbers
- facilitation of transportation needs or a referral to the police, a legal service or victim support services [7].

15.3.2 Victim support services and ongoing care

There are many national and local support organisations that may be of benefit to patients who are experiencing or at risk of experiencing domestic and family violence, child abuse or elder abuse. Patients may be entitled to free counselling and financial support.

Doctors need to be aware of the relevant services and resources in their state or territory. Some Australia-wide telephone support services include:

- National Domestic Family and Sexual Violence Counselling Service—1800 737 732 (1800RESPECT)
- Kids Helpline—1800 55 1800
- Lifeline—13 11 14
- MensLine Australia—1300 78 99 78
- Family Relationship Advice Line—1800 050 321

In addition to safety planning and facilitating referrals to appropriate support services, many patients may benefit from counselling strategies such as trauma-informed cognitive behavioural therapy, motivational interviewing and mindfulness. It is also essential for doctors to be familiar with appropriate referral services in their state or territory, such as social workers, counsellors, psychologists or psychiatrists, and women's and children's services.

15.3.3 Documentation

Appropriate record keeping relating to concerns, suspicions or disclosures of family and domestic violence, child maltreatment or elder abuse is vital as it may be considered evidence in future criminal proceedings or other legal matters.

Doctors should document a patient's history and examination findings, including every injury and symptom. Documentation of each injury should include its appearance, location, size and age (if applicable). Statements from the patient about violence or abuse should be documented word for word using quotation marks. It is important to record only the facts and not personal or general opinions. Any behaviour of the patient that the doctor witnesses should also be recorded (e.g. shaking or crying). The safety and management plan and any referrals that have been made should also be documented [7].

15.3.4 Dealing with perpetrators of violence or abuse

Like victims, perpetrators of family or domestic violence or other abuse come from all socioeconomic, cultural and religious backgrounds. Although violence is perpetrated by both men and women, perpetrators are more commonly men [11]. Physical, sexual, emotional, social and financial violence or abuse is most often used to maintain dominance, power and control within a relationship [7].

Doctors, particularly GPs, have an important role in identifying patients who are at risk of perpetrating violence and abuse against family members or children. Some of the risk assessment strategies outlined above can be used to identify potential perpetrators. Addressing the issue directly with the patient may help reduce the risk for their family members, but it may also increase the risk. Therefore, care is needed when approaching this subject. Doctors should inquire without using accusatory questions. Some useful questions include:

- How are things at home?
- When you feel angry, what do you do?
- Do you think [victim] is ever scared or frightened of you?
- How do your children react when you get angry?
- Do you do things that you later regret?
- Do you ever get worried about your thoughts and feelings and how they make you behave? [7]

The immediate safety of the patient's family members, partner or children is of utmost importance, as is compliance with any mandatory reporting obligations. It is recommended that doctors do not provide care for both the victim and the perpetrator of violence or abuse, and a referral of one of the parties to another doctor can manage this scenario [27].

A referral to a behaviour change program, such as a Men's Behaviour Change Program or similar services for women or transgender people, is the preferred referral option for potential perpetrators of violence or abuse, and has been shown to have positive effects. Referrals to other health professionals or services, such as psychologists or psychiatrists, counselling, cognitive behavioural therapy, and alcohol and drug treatment programs, may also be considered, along with telephone-based information and support lines. A referral for couple or family counselling is not appropriate until the perpetrator has ceased using violent and abusive behaviours [7].

15.4 Legal obligations

As a matter of public policy, mandatory reporting aims to protect people from family and domestic violence and children from abuse and neglect by making it a criminal offence to fail to report certain behaviours to the relevant authority. Comparative studies between countries with and without mandatory reporting systems have found that substantially more cases of child abuse are identified in countries with a mandatory reporting system [28].

The mandatory reporting laws differ between Australian states and territories. The relevant legislation defines the circumstances and the threshold at which the statutory child protection service is legally able to intervene to protect a child.

15.4.1 Mandatory reporting of family and domestic violence

At the time of writing, the only state or territory to require mandatory reporting of domestic violence is the NT. The NT requires any adult to make a report to police if they believe on reasonable grounds that:

- another person has caused, or is likely to cause, harm to someone else with whom the person is in a domestic relationship; or
- the life or safety of another person is under serious or imminent threat because domestic violence has been, is being or is about to be committed.

The relevant provision is provided in the *Domestic and Family Violence Act 2007* (NT).

15.4.2 Mandatory reporting of child abuse

All states and territories have enacted laws to protect children from abuse by mandating doctors and others to report suspected child abuse. These laws vary between jurisdictions (see Table 15.6). It is important that doctors are familiar with the circumstances in which reporting is required by law in the state or territory in which they practise. These laws protect doctors (and other reporters) from civil litigation when such reports are made in good faith. It is also important that forms of abuse not covered by mandatory reporting laws in some jurisdictions are still reported when suspected.

Table 15.6 Mandatory reporting requirements by state and territory

State/territory	Authority to be notified	Abuse and neglect types that must be reported
Australian Capital Territory	Community Services Directorate Phone: Children, Youth and Families on 1300 556 729 (mandatory reporters) or ACT Policing on 131 444 (general public) Website: https://www.act.gov.au/community/child-protection-and-youth-justice/report-risk-of-significant-harm-to-a-child	*Children and Young People Act 2008* A belief, on reasonable grounds, that a child (under the age of 12 years) or young person (under the age of 18 years) has experienced non-accidental physical injury or sexual abuse.
New South Wales	Department of Communities and Justice Phone: Child Protection Helpline on 13 21 11 Website: https://dcj.nsw.gov.au/	*Children and Young Persons (Care and Protection) Act 1998* Suspicion on reasonable grounds that a child (under the age of 16 years) is at risk of significant harm. At risk of significant harm means: • basic physical or psychological needs are not being met or are at risk of not being met • the parents or caregivers have not arranged, or are unable or unwilling to arrange, necessary medical care • the parents or caregivers have not arranged, or are unable or unwilling to arrange, an education • the child has been, or is at risk of being, physically or sexually abused or ill-treated • the child is living in a household where there have been incidents of domestic violence and is at risk of serious physical or psychological harm • the child has suffered, or is at risk of, serious psychological harm • the child was the subject of a prenatal report and the caregiver did not engage with support services.
Northern Territory	Department of Children and Families Phone: Child Abuse Hotline on 1800 700 250 Website: https://nt.gov.au/law/crime/report-child-abuse	*Care and Protection of Children Act 2007* A belief, on reasonable grounds, that a child (a person under the age of 18 years) has been the victim of a sexual offence, or is likely to suffer harm or exploitation.

Continued over page

State/territory	Authority to be notified	Abuse and neglect types that must be reported
Queensland	Department of Families, Seniors, Disability Services and Child Safety Child protection telephone numbers depend on the location within the state. For further information refer to https://www.families.qld.gov.au/	*Child Protection Act 1999* A reasonable suspicion that a child (a person under the age of 18 years) has suffered, is suffering or is at an unacceptable risk of suffering significant harm caused by physical or sexual abuse and may not have a parent able and willing to protect the child from the harm.
South Australia	Department for Child Protection Phone: Child Abuse Report Line on 13 14 78 Website: https://www.childprotection.sa.gov.au/reporting-child-abuse	*Children and Young People (Safety) Act 2017* Reasonable grounds to suspect a child or young person (a person under the age of 18 years) is, or may be, at risk of harm; and the suspicion was formed in the course of the person's employment. Harm is taken to be physical harm or psychological harm caused by sexual, physical, mental or emotional abuse or neglect.
Tasmania	Department for Education, Children and Young People Tasmania Phone: Advice and Referral Line on 1800 000 123 Website: https://strongfamiliessafekids.tas.gov.au	*Children, Young Persons and Their Families Act 1997* A belief or suspicion on reasonable grounds that: • a child (a person under the age of 18 years) has been, or is being, abused or neglected within the meaning of the *Family Violence Act 2004* (a child whose safety, psychological wellbeing or interests are affected or likely to be affected by family violence) • there is a reasonable likelihood of a child being killed, abused or neglected by a person with whom the child resides • while a woman is pregnant, there is a reasonable likelihood that after the birth the child will suffer abuse or neglect, may be killed, or will require medical treatment or other intervention as a result of the behaviour of the woman or another person with whom the woman resides, or is likely to reside, before the birth of the child.

Continued over page

State/territory	Authority to be notified	Abuse and neglect types that must be reported
Victoria	Department of Families, Fairness and Housing Child protection telephone numbers depend on the location within the state. For further information refer to https://services.dffh.vic.gov.au	*Children, Youth and Families Act 2005* A belief, on reasonable grounds, that a child (a person under the age of 17 years) is in need of protection, if any of the following grounds exist: • the child has been abandoned • the child's parents are dead or incapacitated and there is no other suitable person to care for the child • the child has suffered or is likely to suffer significant harm as a result of physical injury, sexual abuse, or emotional or psychological harm • the child's physical development or health has been significantly harmed due to not receiving basic care, or effective medical, surgical or other remedial care.
Western Australia	Department of Communities Phone: Central Intake Team on 1800 273 889 or, after hours, the Crisis Care Unit on 1800 199 008 Website: https://www.wa.gov.au/organisation/department-of-communities	*Children and Community Services Act 2004* A belief, on reasonable grounds, that a child (a person under the age of 18 years) has been the subject of sexual abuse or is the subject of ongoing sexual abuse.

15.4.3 Abuse of older persons or persons who have lost decision-making capacity

While there are no mandatory obligations for reporting suspected elder abuse, there are designated pathways to report elder abuse in some jurisdictions.

In NSW, the Ageing and Disability Commission has the role of receiving and responding to reports or allegations of abuse, neglect and exploitation of older persons with a disability, to investigate these as required and to provide support and information to those in need. There is a NSW Ageing and Disability Abuse Helpline at 1800 628 221, and reports can be lodged to nswadc@nsw.gov.au or online at www.ageingdisabilitycommission.nsw.gov.au.

In Victoria, information and resources about elder abuse are available from Seniors Rights Victoria (SRV) via the SRV Helpline on 1300 368 821 (https://seniorsrights.org.au). If abuse is occurring in an aged care facility, the Aged Care Quality and Safety Commission is the primary body to contact.

If a doctor suspects a case of elder abuse or neglect where the patient has lost capacity to make decisions in their own best interest, they should first determine whether there is a substitute decision maker. If not, or if that person is the suspected abuser, the doctor can contact the public guardian, public advocate or appropriate body in the relevant state or territory to make decisions on behalf of the person [7] (see Table 15.7).

Table 15.7 Bodies able to make decisions on behalf of older people with impaired decision-making capacity

State or territory	Body
Australian Capital Territory	ACT Human Rights Commission Phone: 02 6205 2222 Website: https://www.hrc.act.gov.au/advocacy
New South Wales	The Public Guardian Phone: 1300 109 290 Website: https://www.tag.nsw.gov.au/public-guardian
Northern Territory	The Public Guardian and Trustee Phone: 1800 810 979 Website: https://pgt.nt.gov.au
Queensland	The Public Advocate Phone: 07 3738 9513 Website: https://www.justice.qld.gov.au/public-advocate
South Australia	The Public Advocate Phone: 1800 066 969 Website: https://www.opa.sa.gov.au
Tasmania	The Public Guardian Phone: 1800 955 772 Website: https://www.publicguardian.tas.gov.au
Victoria	The Public Advocate Phone: 1300 309 337 Website: https://www.publicadvocate.vic.gov.au
Western Australia	The Public Advocate Phone: 1300 858 455 Website: https://www.publicadvocate.wa.gov.au

15.5 Regulatory attitudes towards doctors as perpetrators of family and domestic violence or abuse of children or older persons

Trust is fundamental to the doctor–patient relationship, particularly given the high level of dependence and often vulnerability of patients, and this has been recognised in the law in Australia for many decades. In 1993, the Court of Appeal observed in *Richter v Walton* [29],

> even in regard to the most commonplace medical matters the trust a patient places in a doctor is considerable. In some cases, of which the present seems to me to be an example, the patient's trust cannot help but be almost absolute.

Trust is intimately tied to public confidence and the reputation of a profession, and the question of how to manage a clinician who is a perpetrator of family violence is a live issue for regulators nationwide. Therefore, the question is: Can we ask the public to have confidence in doctors if those treating the most vulnerable are, at times, themselves perpetrators?

While there are Medical Board of Australia guidelines on sensitive behavioural issues, such as *Guidelines: Sexual boundaries in the doctor–patient relationship* [30], there are currently no guidelines relating to domestic or family violence scenarios.

In a regulatory context, a complaint can be made about a doctor who is alleged to have been a perpetrator of family or domestic violence, and evolving regulatory responses over the past decade need to be understood by doctors. In response to allegations of family or domestic violence, two streams of regulatory activity may arise: immediate action under the Health Practitioner Regulation National Law (the National Law), and disciplinary action before a tribunal under the National Law or relevant state law. (See Chapter 21, Regulation of the medical profession.)

In relation to immediate action, the Medical Board of Australia or the relevant state-based regulator (in NSW the Medical Council of NSW, and in Queensland the Office of the Health Ombudsman) has powers to take immediate action to suspend a doctor's registration, or impose conditions on a doctor's registration if this is considered necessary for the protection of public health and safety, or it is considered to be in the public interest.

There are many cases where doctors have been found guilty of domestic violence and the relevant regulator has determined that immediate action is required in the public interest; however, the law in this area is not yet settled. Somewhat more settled is whether disciplinary action can be taken before a relevant tribunal and the possible outcomes of this. There is now strong legal authority that a doctor found guilty of domestic violence can be found guilty of unsatisfactory professional conduct or professional misconduct, even though the behaviour has not occurred within the practice of medicine. See Box 15.2 and Box 15.3 for examples of legal proceedings related to domestic violence perpetrated by doctors.

Where a tribunal makes a finding of unsatisfactory professional conduct or professional misconduct, the outcome and orders imposed (reprimand, conditions on registration, or suspension or cancellation of registration) will generally be influenced by a number of factors, including:

- the seriousness of the incident(s)
- whether there is a pattern of violent behaviour or propensity to violence
- whether the practitioner is remorseful
- whether the practitioner has been open and truthful and shown insight
- whether significant steps have been taken in a genuine attempt to change the conduct
- the general character and standing of the practitioner.

In cases where there are aggravating factors, the tribunal will consider general deterrence in the form of a suspension or cancellation of the doctor's registration.

Box 15.2 *Health Care Complaints Commission v Haasbroek* [2018] NSWCATOD 177

This case [31] explores the issue of domestic violence by a doctor. It represents a distinct recognition by the NSW Civil and Administrative Tribunal of the heightened gravity of domestic violence–related offences, and is authority for the proposition that 'practitioners must act, both personally and professionally, with integrity and with respect for the law, in all aspects of their behaviour'.

The case related to three situations:

- In 2011, the doctor punched a relative in the face during a family dispute and swore at him. He was subsequently found guilty of common assault occasioning actual bodily harm, although no conviction was recorded.
- In February 2015, an Apprehended Domestic Violence Order (ADVO) was made against the doctor in respect of Person A and their three children. On 16 June 2015, the doctor was involved in a verbal and physical altercation with Person A at the family home in front of the children. He also damaged Person A's clothes and mobile phone and was subsequently found guilty of common assault.
- In May 2016, Person A requested that the police apply for an ADVO, which provided that the doctor was not to contact Person A unless for the purposes of arranging a supervised visit with their children. On 30 May 2016 and 31 May 2016, the doctor breached the ADVO.

In considering whether the doctor was or was not a suitable person to hold registration under the National Law, the tribunal noted the foundational tenets to be considered were protecting public health and safety, upholding community standards, reinforcing public confidence, and deterring doctors and other health practitioners from engaging in similar conduct, noting:

> The practitioner's conduct is of the kind which could be found to render him unsuitable to practice. Violence, particularly against women, in a domestic situation is well recognised in the Australian community as abhorrent, but tragically it continues to occur.

Although the tribunal noted that the conduct of the practitioner in committing domestic violence offences was conduct of the kind 'which could be found to render him unsuitable to practice', the tribunal was of the view that the doctor was genuinely remorseful for his conduct, had insight and understood his failings. The tribunal determined the appropriate protective order was that the practitioner be reprimanded.

Similar decisions have been repeated across multiple jurisdictions in Australia.

Box 15.3 *Medical Board of Australia v PYP (Review and Regulation)* [2021] VCAT 876

These proceedings [32] related to a doctor who was charged with intentionally causing injury, recklessly causing injury and unlawful assault due to an incident at the doctor's home in which he punched his wife in the face, breaking her nose, in proximity to their 1-year-old child.

The Victorian Civil and Administrative Tribunal characterised the practitioner's conduct as professional misconduct, stating:

> In essence we considered that a violent, unprovoked assault on a defenceless woman, in front of their young child, is conduct inconsistent with possessing the required moral integrity and rectitude of character to hold registration as a medical practitioner. Such violence on the part of a doctor has particular resonance because of the role medical practitioners, and especially general practitioners, have as first responders for women who are the victims of family violence.

The tribunal delegates held that such conduct was inconsistent with the qualities associated with fitness to hold registration, observing in particular that:

> Our community rightly expects that medical practitioners will not commit a crime of this nature. Conduct of this kind impacts on the standing of and the trust that the community holds in the medical profession.
>
> Medical practitioners are and need to be seen by the community as people who are law abiding, trustworthy, safe to be in proximity to, and respectful, including of women.
>
> An offence of this kind has particular resonance for medical practitioners who may be the first point of contact for a person who is themselves a victim of an act of family violence. This is because the public expects that they will be able to provide good medical care for those who are experiencing abuse and violence, as well as to identify and respond appropriately to the perpetrators of same.

The tribunal stated that the practitioner had expressed remorse for his conduct and held that the likelihood of his re-offending was low, although they did note that such offences most often happen in private and in the absence of witnesses. However, the tribunal stated that:

> We consider that a factor here, adding to the gravity of the conduct, is the presence of the small child. We agree with the submission of the Board that the seriousness of family violence and the manifest need for general deterrence has continued to grow.

The tribunal suspended the practitioner's registration 'primarily in the interests of general deterrence'.

Summary

Doctors have a very important role in the prevention of serious physical and psychological injury to their patients who may be at risk of domestic or family violence or elder abuse. All doctors need to be aware of the warning signs of violence or abuse, be familiar with the appropriate ways to explore the issue with a potential victim, and know the referral pathways and reporting pathways in their own jurisdiction. It is crucial that victims feel believed and supported by the person to whom they disclose their situation, and doctors are very well placed to provide this support.

Child maltreatment is now considered to be a public health crisis with immediate, medium-term and longer-term consequences extending into adulthood. A doctor's role in recognising maltreatment is critical in infancy, childhood and into adolescence. Early identification can ensure that appropriate supports for the family and the child are put in place to ameliorate ongoing harm. Mandatory reporting is a legal responsibility but ensuring that ongoing trauma-informed care is provided to the child and their family or caregivers is paramount.

Regulatory approaches to doctors who are perpetrators of domestic and family violence have evolved over recent years, and such reports are now taken very seriously and may result in significant consequences for the doctor's registration.

References

1. *Family Law Act 1975* (Cth), s 4AB.
2. *Crimes (Domestic and Personal Violence) Act 2007* (NSW), s 5.
3. Australian Institute of Health and Welfare. Family, domestic and sexual violence in Australia: continuing the national story. 2019. https://www.aihw.gov.au/reports/family-domestic-and-sexual-violence/family-domestic-sexual-violence-australia-2019/contents/summary (accessed Jun 2025).
4. Australian Institute of Family Studies. Elder abuse: understanding issues, frameworks and responses. 2016. https://aifs.gov.au/research/research-reports/elder-abuse-understanding-issues-frameworks-and-responses (accessed Jun 2025).
5. World Health Organization. Abuse of older people. 2024. https://www.who.int/news-room/fact-sheets/detail/abuse-of-older-people (accessed Jun 2025).
6. Australian Institute of Health and Welfare. Older Australians. 2024. https://www.aihw.gov.au/reports/older-people/older-australians/contents/health/health-status-and-functioning (accessed Jun 2025).
7. Royal Australian College of General Practitioners. Abuse and violence: working with our patients in general practice (the White Book) (5th ed). 2022. https://www.racgp.org.au/clinical-resources/clinical-guidelines/key-racgp-guidelines/view-all-racgp-guidelines/abuse-and-violence/about-this-guideline (accessed Jun 2025).
8. Hanson RF, Kievit LW, Saunders BE, et al. Correlates of adolescent reports of sexual assault: findings from the National Survey of Adolescents. *Child Maltreat* 2003; 8: 261–272.
9. NSW Government Department of Communities and Justice. The effects of domestic and family violence. 2022. https://dcj.nsw.gov.au/children-and-families/family-domestic-and-sexual-violence/about-domestic-and-family-violence/the-effects-of-domestic-and-family-violence.html (accessed Jun 2025).
10. World Health Organization; International Society for Prevention of Child Abuse and Neglect. Preventing child maltreatment: a guide to taking action and generating evidence. 2006. https://www.who.int/publications/i/item/preventing-child-maltreatment-a-guide-to-taking-action-and-generating-evidence (accessed Jun 2025).
11. Australian Bureau of Statistics. Personal safety, Australia. 2022. https://www.abs.gov.au/statistics/people/crime-and-justice/personal-safety-australia/latest-release (accessed Jun 2025).
12. Australian Institute of Health and Welfare. Examination of hospital stays due to family and domestic violence 2010–11 to 2018–19. 2021. https://www.aihw.gov.au/reports/family-domestic-and-sexual-violence/examination-of-hospital-stays-due-to-family-and-do/summary (accessed Jun 2025).

13. Mathews B (Coordinating author). The Australian Child Maltreatment Study: national prevalence and associated health outcomes of child abuse and neglect. *Med J Aust* 2023; 218(6 Suppl): S1–S51.
14. Australian Bureau of Statistics. Characteristics and outcomes of childhood abuse. 2019. http://www.abs.gov.au/articles/characteristics-and-outcomes-childhood-abuse (accessed Jun 2025).
15. Segal L, Nguyen H, Mansor M, et al. Lifetime risk of child protection system involvement in South Australia for Aboriginal and non-Aboriginal children, 1986–2017 using linked administrative data. *Child Abuse Negl* 2019; 97: 104145.
16. Qu L, Kaspiew R, Carson R, et al. National Elder Abuse Prevalence Study: final report. Australian Institute of Family Studies. 2021. https://aifs.gov.au/research/research-reports/national-elder-abuse-prevalence-study-final-report (accessed Jun 2025).
17. Boxall H, Morgan A, Brown R. Statistical Bulletin, No. 28: The prevalence of domestic violence among women during the COVID-19 pandemic. Australian Institute of Criminology. 2020. https://www.aic.gov.au/publications/sb/sb28 (accessed Jun 2025).
18. Australian Medical Association. Position statement: family and domestic violence. 2016. https://www.ama.com.au/position-statement/family-and-domestic-violence-2016 (accessed Jun 2025).
19. Hegarty K. What is intimate partner abuse and how common is it? In: Roberts G, Hegarty K, Feder G, editors. Intimate partner abuse and health professionals: new approaches to domestic violence. London: Elsevier, 2006: 19–40.
20. State Government of Victoria. Family Violence Multi-Agency Risk Assessment and Management Framework. 2023. https://www.vic.gov.au/family-violence-multi-agency-risk-assessment-and-management (accessed Jun 2025).
21. NSW Government Department of Communities and Justice. Domestic Violence Safety Assessment Tool. 2022. https://dcj.nsw.gov.au/service-providers/supporting-family-domestic-sexual-violence-services/dfsv-tools-and-resources/domestic-violence-safety-assessment-tool.html (accessed Jun 2025).
22. Campo M. Domestic and family violence in pregnancy and early parenthood: overview and emerging interventions. Australian Institute of Family Studies. 2015. https://aifs.gov.au/resources/policy-and-practice-papers/domestic-and-family-violence-pregnancy-and-early-parenthood (accessed Jun 2025).
23. World Health Organization. Child maltreatment. 2024. http://www.who.int/news-room/fact-sheets/detail/child-maltreatment (accessed Jun 2025).
24. NSW Government Ageing and Disability Commission. Elder Abuse Suspicion Index (EASI). https://ageingdisabilitycommission.nsw.gov.au/documents/tools-and-resources/for-professionals/Elder-Abuse-Suspicion-Index-EASI.pdf (accessed Jun 2025).
25. Hoover RM, Polson M. Detecting elder abuse and neglect: assessment and intervention. *Am Fam Physician* 2014; 89: 453–460.
26. Hegarty K. The hidden epidemic of domestic violence: when to ask and how to respond. *Medicine Today* 2012; 13: 54–57.
27. Hegarty K, Forsdike-Young K, Tarzia L, et al. Identifying and responding to men who use violence in their intimate relationships. *Aust Fam Physician* 2016; 45: 176–181.
28. Mathews B. Mandatory reporting laws for child sexual abuse in Australia: a legislative history. Report for the Royal Commission into Institutional Responses to Child Sexual Abuse. 2014. https://www.childabuseroyalcommission.gov.au/research (accessed Jun 2025).
29. *Richter v Walton* [1993] NSWCA 233.
30. Medical Board of Australia. Guidelines: sexual boundaries in the doctor–patient relationship. https://www.medicalboard.gov.au/codes-guidelines-policies/sexual-boundaries-guidelines.aspx (accessed Jun 2025).
31. *Health Care Complaints Commission v Haasbroek* [2018] NSWCATOD 177.
32. *Medical Board of Australia v PYP (Review and Regulation)* [2021] VCAT 876.

16 Achieving full health potential: health equity

Jen Desrosiers, Tim Usherwood, Dinesh Palipana OAM

Introduction

Events both overseas and in Australia illustrate how inequities disproportionately affect women, Indigenous people, members of cultural minority groups, people with disabilities, people with low socioeconomic status, members of LGBTIQ+ communities, and others who experience marginalisation or oppression [1,2]. For example, the climate crisis has catalysed a health crisis, which has widened inequities and disproportionately affected the health and wellbeing of Aboriginal and/or Torres Strait Islander people [1]. Similarly, marginalised populations have been disproportionately affected by the COVID-19 pandemic due to inequitable access to prophylaxis, care and supplies, alongside higher population density and prevalence of chronic health conditions [3].

Health equity is a 'state in which everyone has the opportunity to attain full health potential and no one is disadvantaged from achieving this potential because of social position or any other socially defined circumstance' [4]. Conversely, health inequity is defined as avoidable and unfair differences in health that result from differential distribution of resources and opportunities within society [2]. Social factors, such as racism, sexism, ableism and poverty are the drivers of health inequity by influencing who becomes ill, who has access to care, and who has access to safety nets [2,5]. Despite the well-established relationship between social factors and health equity, few practical frameworks exist that link social analysis with medical training, clinical practice or health system reform [5,6]. This chapter will provide the rationale for health equity, identify the populations at risk of experiencing inequity, describe the mechanisms that produce and maintain inequity, and offer some practical actions that health practitioners can take to contribute to health equity.

16.1 The rationale for equity

Health practitioners are uniquely positioned to make meaningful contributions to health equity within and outside the health system. An equitable society is of benefit to everyone [7,8]. For example, closing the equity gap improves social cohesion, community safety, mental health and quality of life for the whole population [9]. Also, financial rationale for equity includes reduced short- and long-term direct medical costs such as emergency department visits, avoidable hospitalisation and tertiary care; and reduced indirect costs to society such as incarceration, reductions in human capital, lost productivity and opportunity costs [10]. Conversely, inequity is associated with social issues such as violence, crime, incarceration, drug dependence, teenage pregnancy and mental illness alongside reduced life expectancy, literacy, social mobility and trust [11,12].

16.2 Inequity in Australia

Populations that experience health inequity in Australia include Aboriginal and/or Torres Strait Islander peoples, refugees, cultural minority groups, people who are sexually or gender diverse, people living with mental illness, unhoused people, people with disability, incarcerated people, or members of other socially marginalised groups [13–15]. Stark health inequities between populations exist across a range of health outcomes including burden of disease, life expectancy, avoidable hospitalisation and preventable death. Inequities also exist across engagement measures such as healthcare access, uptake, acceptability and quality of care [15–19].

16.3 Mechanisms of health inequity

Avoidable differences in health are often positioned as unavoidable consequences of poor lifestyle choices, genetic differences, or internal risk factors, instead of as a result of social and structural forces such as colonisation [20–23]. These narratives position groups that experience inequity as having or being the problem that needs to be fixed with a focus on deficit, pathology or victimhood. This is sometimes encapsulated within a discourse of 'they're sicker because they don't look after themselves or don't seek care'. This narrative blames the groups that experience inequity and thereby distracts from its social and structural origins. This narrative also undermines the agency and self-determination of individuals and populations.

When health inequity is positioned as an unavoidable consequence, systems of oppression such as colonisation, racialisation, patriarchy, paternalism, ableism and social exclusion go unnoticed. This allows oppression to go unexamined, and to continue without intervention [5,23–27]. Conversely, reframing social and structural forces as risk factors for avoidable health differences allows them to be deconstructed and modified within society and within health care [22,23,28–30].

16.4 The social determinants of health

Health equity is influenced by the social, cultural, political and economic conditions in which people are born, grow, work, age and seek health care [8]. Collectively, these conditions are called the social determinants of health [7]. Conditions that promote health include employment, fair wages, safe housing, quality education, access to health care, nutritious food, green space, transportation and social support. Conditions that damage health include oppression, marginalisation, discrimination, institutional racism, violence, lack of safety, isolation and financial insecurity [2,7].

The social determinants of health include:

- socioeconomic status
- education
- gender
- employment and working conditions
- physical environment such as food availability, water, safety, housing, green space, transport, urban planning and sanitation
- social exposures including discrimination and racism
- social inclusion and social support
- culture
- access, acceptability and quality of health care [7,8].

The social determinants of health can influence, intersect and compound one another [8,31]. Membership in more than one marginalised group tends to exacerbate inequities, a process described as 'intersectionality' [31]. Also, disadvantage is likely to lead to further disadvantage, a concept called 'corrosive disadvantage'. For example, low socioeconomic status is a disadvantage, but can be corrosive when it leads to further disadvantage such as food and housing insecurity, transport restrictions, barriers to accessing health care, and social stigma [31]. Intersectionality and corrosive disadvantage can also be illustrated by women who experience intimate partner violence in remote areas of Australia. In this example, the corrosive and intersectional combination of geographical isolation, possible socioeconomic disadvantage, and distance to social support and effective services can compound the health inequity of women who experience intimate partner violence and live in remote areas [32].

Box 16.1 Case study 1: Health inequity and gender-diverse youth

Alex is an 11-year-old whose sex assigned at birth was male, but who identifies as non-binary and uses 'they' as a preferred pronoun. Alex discussed their gender identity with their family, and although supportive, the family is unsure how to navigate the health system, and is still in the early stages of learning about gender diversity. Alex has an appointment with their GP to discuss accessing puberty-blocking medication. They have never discussed their gender with a doctor before and are feeling anxious about it. Alex has been subject to threats, bullying and violence at school, and as a consequence, has difficulty concentrating, has been skipping classes, has been feeling anxious and has considered suicide.

Background: Gender-diverse young people are more likely to experience health inequity alongside compromised safety and social support compared to their cisgender counterparts [33,34]. For example, gender-diverse young people are more likely to experience health-damaging exposures such as harassment, violence, discrimination, marginalisation, parental rejection, and compromised safety and support at school. Consequently, gender-diverse youth are also more likely to experience food insecurity, diminished academic achievement and homelessness. These exposures may precipitate increased contact and greater need from health and social services. However, gender-diverse people commonly report delaying seeking care due to fears of discrimination and concerns that health practitioners lack the knowledge, training and cultural competence to provide them with equitable care [35]. Likewise, those working in health and social services report being ill-prepared to effectively care for people who are gender diverse.

Practice points:

- Health practitioners are very likely to care for gender diverse patients in their daily practice. Practice, clinic and hospital registration forms should include fields for: preferred name; preferred pronouns; and gender identity, including non-binary options.
- Training for administrative and clinical staff about topics relevant to gender diversity including chosen name and pronouns can contribute to a welcoming and affirming environment, which may contribute to improved interactions.
- Eligibility for preventive services such as cervical and prostate screening, mammography and contraception will be unique to each patient's anatomy, medication use and behaviours, and should be discussed sensitively and where relevant.

Continued over page

- Access to gender-affirming care, including appropriate medication, can improve mental health outcomes for people who are gender diverse, and can increase their likelihood of ongoing engagement with health services for preventive and routine care [36].
- Depression and anxiety are common for those who are gender diverse, and are not contraindications to the commencement of gender-affirming hormones [37,38].
- Young people also experience barriers and enablers when accessing health care.

16.5 The elements of health equity

Health practitioners play a critical role in shaping access, uptake and quality and safety of health services. Equitable, accessible, high-quality and safe care are markers of a strong health system, and timely access to care is essential. Strong health systems place priority on these elements rather than patients' ability to pay for services [27,39]. Likewise, quality and safety literature highlights the importance of accessing the right care, in the right place, at the right time and cost within all areas of the health system [40]. However, groups that experience health inequity often experience reduced access and quality of care, resulting in greater unmet health needs, and consequentially, differential outcomes [41–44].

16.5.1 Access

Timely access to health care underpins health equity. Conversely, delayed access to health care and delayed or restricted use of prescription medication can have serious health and mental health implications [45,46]. For example, delayed access increases risk of complications, requirements for specialist care, avoidable emergency department visits, hospital admissions, longer hospital stays and tertiary care needs [44,46–48].

Access to health care may be inequitably distributed due to financial, geographical, language or attitudinal barriers [48]. Financial barriers are typically out-of-pocket costs to the consumer, such as costs for transport, care, childcare and time off from work, which can be prohibitive to accessing care. Those with financial barriers to accessing care also may experience opportunity costs—when money allocated to other areas such as housing, food or electricity needs to be put toward healthcare costs—which also have consequent effects on health.

Access to health care may also be limited by geographical barriers. Geographical barriers exist when health resources and facilities are distributed unevenly; for example, shortages of GPs in rural and remote areas of Australia [49]. Consequently, rural and remote populations face disproportionate challenges accessing appropriate services due to lack of facilities, geographical restrictions, limited access to culturally safe care, transport issues, cost of accessing care and shortages of healthcare staff [49,50]. Situations where the availability of quality medical care is inversely associated with health need are referred to as the inverse care law [51]. The inverse care law involves higher concentration of health resources in urban and higher income areas, which makes health resources less likely to be available in the areas of the greatest need. This disproportionate allocation of health resources creates and maintains health inequity. For more on resource allocation and rationing in health care, see Chapter 24.

Box 16.2 Case study 2: Intersectionality—equitable care for refugees living with a disability

Susu is a refugee from a country where English is not widely spoken. She trained as a lawyer in her country of origin, but now accessing employment is difficult. Susu has a spinal cord injury affecting her hands and all the function below her chest. Language barriers have made obtaining optimal disability funding in Australia difficult for Susu. Consequently, the wheelchair Susu uses is not ideal, and she is not able to afford to pay for the support she needs due to budgetary constraints.

Susu has been experiencing some complications from her spinal cord injury. These include pressure ulcer and bladder problems for which she uses a suprapubic catheter. She lives in a regional town where many refugees have settled, but access to health care and specialist care is challenging. She has been given an appointment to the closest tertiary public hospital to review the complications. It is two hours away, scheduled for 9 am. Due to distance, cost and planning requirements, this is the first doctor she has seen in a year.

Susu generally requires two hours to get ready in the morning. Therefore, she has to access home support at 4:30 am in order to leave the house at 6:30 am and get to the appointment at 8:30 am. Susu requires an extra 30 minutes to transfer in and out of the vehicle and get into the building. Susu is unable to afford a car, and therefore has to secure transport to get to her appointment.

Once at the appointment, an interpreter is not available. The consult is managed as well as possible. The care provider helps Susu to transfer into the bed in order for the doctor to examine her, which takes five to ten minutes. The specialist notes that Susu will require regular wound reviews and dressing changes by a community nurse. Susu is unsure how to access a service like this in her regional town. However, the team reinforces that this will be important because the location and nature of the wound is now putting her at a high risk of osteomyelitis. The team also lets her know that a new wheelchair is required to resolve some pressure issues. The appointment runs out of time so Susu is unable to ask a number of other questions that she has wanted to ask over the previous year between appointments.

Background: Disability can intersect with other elements including culture, gender, sexuality, physical environment, socioeconomic status and access to high-quality health care [31,52,53]. For example, people from a refugee background are more likely to experience poor health if they also have a disability [54]. In this case study, disability intersects with culture, gender, physical environment, socioeconomic status and access to quality health care. Also, living in a regional location further compounds Susu's circumstances, and limits her access to quality health care. See Figures 16.1 and 16.2 for a visual representation and breakdown of the intersections of identity and determinants of health that Susu might experience.

Continued over page

Figure 16.1 Intersections of determinants of health and identity

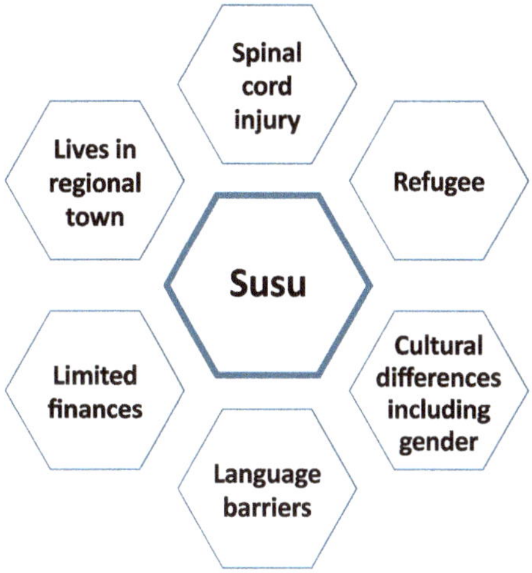

Source: Amanda Frier, chapter contributor.

Figure 16.2 Breakdown of intersectional elements

Spinal cord injury	Refugee	Budgetary contraints	Regional living
• Function affected (hands and everything below chest • Pressure ulcers • Bladder issues • Extended preparation time for appointments • Extra time required to physically access appointments • Requires additional time at appointments • Support required to attend appointments • Unsuitable wheelchair • Reduced independence • Requires home support	• Cultural differences • Gender role within culture • Cultural perspectives on disability • Language barrier • Requires interpreter • Reduced health literacy • Reduced access to family support • Difficulty accessing culturally safe support	• Difficulty obtaining disability funding in Australia • Difficulty accessing employment • Limited capacity for healthcare expenditure • Difficulty affording sufficient support • Limited capacity to afford suitable transport • Limited capacity to purchase suitable AT	• Limited access to specialist care • Extended travel time to appointments • Lack of required services • Lack of local knowledge about suitable follow-up support

Source: Amanda Frier, chapter contributor.

Approximately one in six Australians experience disability [55]. People living with disability are more likely to experience health disparities including lower life expectancy and increased incidence of comorbidities, overweight or obesity, and hypertension [15,55,56]. Despite increased health need, people living with disability are more likely to have unmet health needs and have difficulty accessing health care. People with disability also report delaying or avoiding visiting a GP because of cost or other barriers to access such as difficulty accessing transport or healthcare support.

People from a refugee background also commonly have significant unmet physical and psychosocial health needs. For example, people from a refugee background often have higher prevalence of communicable and noncommunicable diseases, oral health needs, injuries, mental health issues, prior experience of sexual and gender-based violence, reproductive health complications and nutritional deficiencies [57–60]. Despite higher health needs, people from refugee backgrounds also face a range of barriers to accessing timely and appropriate health care [61,62]. Barriers to access include language and communication differences, financial restrictions, unfamiliarity with the health system, lack of transport, varying cultural health beliefs and decision-making responsibilities [61,63,64]. Clinical and system barriers include insufficient use of interpreters, time constraints, limited knowledge and competency addressing refugee health needs [65].

Women from a refugee background are more likely to experience challenges to healthcare access due to the sociocultural norms around gender that manifest as language barriers, limited literacy, transport barriers and isolation [64]. Women from a refugee background are also more likely to be primary caregivers for children and dependents, which increases the need for access to health care. These intersections can lead to inequities in healthcare access and health outcomes, and compounding disadvantage.

Practice points:

- Addressing barriers to care may include ensuring accessibility needs are met for people living with disability. This can involve making changes to physical barriers such as the built environment, geographical accessibility and transport. For example, providing support with transport and ensuring the practice is accessible for people who use a wheelchair can address access barriers to care. Time barriers can include scheduling and time spent with patients. Ways to address time barriers could include flexibility in appointment length or appointment time and adjusting appointment formats to include video or phone consultations. Financial barriers can include direct, indirect and opportunity costs. Ways to address financial barriers can include linking patients to community services or bulk-billing options. Language and communication barriers can be addressed by accessing professional interpreters, and adapting communication to fit the patient's preferred communication. Use of friends, neighbours, relatives or medical students rather than professional interpreters can be dangerous and is not advised.
- People from a refugee background may have additional care needs and could require longer appointment times or more frequent visits, mental health support, trauma-informed care, catch-up screening, catch-up immunisations, referrals to other services, access to health information in their first language, and social support. Connections with community groups could also help with settlement tasks like banking, education, transport, employment and social services [54].
- Addressing barriers to care for people from a refugee background may include training on the use of interpreters, cultural sensitivity or cultural competence training in order to maximise opportunities for effective communication, and the development of rapport.

16.5.2 Engagement

Patients who have access to health services may decide not to engage with some services due to their or their family's previous experience of negative interaction, language barriers or perceived lack of cultural safety [28,66]. For example, perceived lack of cultural safety or equitable care may be a barrier to engagement with breast and cervical screening for some communities [67–70]. Likewise, people with a disability, people who are sexually or gender diverse, and people who have experienced sexual violence or genital mutilation are less likely to engage with sensitive examinations including breast and cervical screening and colorectal examination [71–73].

Social barriers, including stigma and fear of discrimination, may also limit healthcare engagement and open disclosure during healthcare interactions [74]. For example, patients may not disclose their ethnicity, sexuality, gender identity, HIV status, experience of sexual or domestic violence, drug use, or use of traditional or complementary medicine to their healthcare providers if they do not feel safe to do so [75–79]. Reasons for nondisclosure may include previous negative healthcare experiences; fear of discrimination or differential treatment; or legal, child protection, immigration, employment, cultural or housing ramifications [75,79,80]. Nondisclosure may compromise quality of care, accuracy of diagnoses, and treatment or management which can lead to preventable morbidity and mortality [81,82]. Thus, creating a safe environment for patients is important for optimal communication and engagement.

16.5.3 Quality and safety

Although most doctors want to provide good care to all patients, some patients receive better quality care than others due to structural biases in the healthcare system and implicit bias among healthcare professionals [83]. Implicit bias involves a 'dissociation between what a person explicitly believes and wants to do (e.g. provide good care to everyone) and the hidden influence of negative implicit associations on their thoughts and action (e.g. perceiving certain patients as less competent and thus deciding not to prescribe the patient a medication)' [84]. Implicit bias is therefore a mechanism of unconscious discrimination without conscious intent and can be present even when health practitioners are not aware of it, explicitly support equity, or intend to separate their personal values from the care they provide [85–87].

Members of marginalised groups are more likely to experience negative implicit bias during healthcare interactions and are consequently less likely to receive good-quality care, which consequently impacts health outcomes [14,29,67,85,88–91]. Areas where implicit bias is prevalent include ethnicity, culture, gender, socioeconomic status, age, mental health, HIV status, intravenous drug use, disability and social circumstances [84]. For example, it is well documented that Aboriginal and Torres Strait Islander populations experience implicit bias and resultant differential health outcomes in health care in a variety of settings including primary care, the emergency department, cancer care and surgical care [92–94]. Implicit bias is most likely to influence behaviour when an individual is fatigued, ill, anxious, distracted, or under stress or time pressure [30].

Biases affect the quality of care provided to patients from marginalised groups via suboptimal patient–provider interactions, clinical assessments and judgements, and treatment decisions [88]. Implicit bias also influences systematic differences in healthcare decision making including shortened consultations, number of questions asked of the patient, number and timing of tests ordered, reduced likelihood of referral, different prescribing practices and differential diagnoses [30,84]. Implicit bias also manifests through changes to verbal communication and nonverbal behaviour such as eye contact, and indicators of friendliness [66]. For example, research suggests that decision making around offering or withholding pain medication may be more likely to be influenced by the appearance of a patient than on clinical judgement [95].

Experiencing implicit bias during a healthcare interaction also affects patient satisfaction, trust, and future health-seeking behaviour, and reduces adherence, continuity of care and future disclosure [66,88,89,96]. For example, experiencing low-quality care acts as a barrier to future health-seeking behaviour because patients begin to expect substandard care or lose trust in the system, resulting in delayed presentation or reduced health-seeking behaviour.

Delayed presentation or reduced engagement may in turn result in judgement from health practitioners, based on narratives that associate healthcare engagement with taking responsibility for one's health. This in turn can further increase patients' reluctance to access services, which consequently results in poorer health outcomes. Overall, experience of implicit bias in health care can create cyclical implications of health disparity for individuals and their families.

16.6 Contributing to health equity: what doctors can do

Health practitioners can have a significant impact on health equity through advocating for changes in the health system, actions with individual patients, and more broadly as citizens. Actions that contribute to health equity include recognising inequities and committing to reducing them through enhanced access, uptake, and quality and safety of care.

16.6.1 Recognise inequities and commit to reducing them

Lee Jong-wook, the former Director-General of the World Health Organization, said, 'To make people count, we first need to be able to count people' [97]. The health needs, experiences and outcomes of populations that experience inequity are often not well documented. Thus, the inequities that populations experience can go unnoticed and therefore can persist. Recognising that health inequity is present in one's own practice is often a catalyst and motivator to addressing it. Practice-based data or clinical audit data can be useful for understanding practice- and community-level needs and inequities [98]. For example, equity audits have been used to evaluate access to diabetic retinopathy screening programs, management of chronic disease, cancer care and stop-smoking services, among others [98,99]. Work by Chin et al. also positions equity as a fundamental element of quality, safety and health system performance, and thus encourages integrating equity measures into quality and safety frameworks and quality improvement processes [10].

Recognition of patient-level inequities can be facilitated through discussing social history with a patient. A social history can explore questions about individual characteristics, life circumstances, emotional health, perceptions about health care, health-related behaviours, and previous experiences with access and engagement with health care. For example, sensitively asking about language, culture, ethnicity, safety at home, disability, gender identity, sexuality, income, and access to social services and housing can be helpful if relevant and appropriate at the time [100–102]. Likewise, asking patients about Aboriginal and/or Torres Strait Islander status, and responding appropriately, is important to the provision of culturally safe care, and necessary for determining eligibility for Pharmaceuticals Benefits Scheme and Medicare Benefits Schedule items. A detailed understanding of the patient's sociocultural background and personal story can support shared decision making about care and treatment, and inform referrals to other services where required.

16.6.2 Enable equitable access

Population-level data and patient experiences can provide insight into the access barriers and enablers that marginalised groups experience. Offering options to enable equitable access might include bulk-billing options, appointments during times that are accessible outside regular business hours, assistance with access to subsidised care or prescriptions, providing prescription refills without an appointment where appropriate, and prescribing generic products [103,104]. Health practitioners can also consider whether there are equitable ways to enable patients to attend their appointments rather than using missed appointment fees.

Flexible consultation formats including video, email, text and telephone appointments may be more convenient for people with a disability, with restricted access to transport, or who live in remote or rural locations. Enhancing accessibility also includes ensuring the building is accessible to those who use public transportation, and for people who use a wheelchair or have mobility limitations. Also, accessibility considerations could include making the space safe and supportive for sexually and gender-diverse people, and creating a physical environment that is comfortable for neurodiverse people. Enabling equitable access can also include ensuring that administrative forms include more than binary options for gender and a place for preferred pronouns. Also, flexible length of appointments, confidential spaces and alternative waiting rooms can enhance health equity for those for whom cultural or language considerations, mobility limitations or disability might require more time [105].

Enhancing accessibility may also include taking public health messages, screening buses or testing opportunities to places where people gather, such as festivals, or creating a festival atmosphere around a health initiative to encourage participation. Enhancing accessibility could also include using technology to bring services to rural and remote areas. For example, people in rural and remote areas often struggle to access the dentist, but now can have access to free dental check-ups through the Pearlii app, which uses artificial intelligence to detect issues including tooth decay, gum redness, staining, calculus and white spots.

16.6.3 Enable uptake

Health practitioners can explore the reasons that people who have access to services may not engage, which could include discussing barriers to uptake with patients and investigating how healthcare delivery can be made more acceptable. For example, patients may be more likely to engage with sexually transmitted infection and cervical screening if they are given the option to take a self-collected sample rather than have the sample collected by a health provider. These options increase screening among groups who experience the most barriers, while having sensitivity comparable to clinician-collected samples [68,71,106].

16.6.4 Provide culturally safe care

Culturally safe care contributes to health equity for Aboriginal and Torres Strait Islander patients [28,107] (see Chapter 17, Culturally safe health care for Aboriginal and/or Torres Strait Islander peoples). Cultural safety training for health practitioners and administrative staff can lead to improvements to access, engagement, and quality and safety. The entities operating in the National Registration and Accreditation Scheme, including the Medical Board of Australia and the Australian Medical Council, define culturally safe practice as 'the ongoing critical reflection of health practitioner knowledge, skills, attitudes, practising behaviours and power differentials in delivering safe, accessible and responsive healthcare free of racism' [108]. Similarly, Curtis et al. define cultural safety as a requirement for 'healthcare professionals and their associated healthcare organisations to examine themselves and the potential impact of their own culture on clinical interactions and healthcare service delivery. This requires individual healthcare professionals and healthcare organisations to acknowledge and address their own biases, attitudes, assumptions, stereotypes, prejudices, structures and characteristics that may affect the quality of care provided. Healthcare professionals and healthcare organisations hold themselves accountable for providing culturally safe care, as defined by the patient and their communities, and as measured through progress towards achieving health equity' [28].

Culturally safe care is therefore determined by Aboriginal and/or Torres Strait Islander individuals, families and communities. Provision of culturally safe care involves ongoing engagement, self-reflection and self-awareness, while examining and addressing bias, upskilling where necessary, and being accountable for providing care as defined by patients and communities. Project Implicit designed the Implicit Association Test, accessible at https://implicit.harvard.edu/implicit/takeatest.html, to assess implicit bias in a range of constructs including gender, sexuality, ethnicity and disability. Participation in these tests can be a valuable self-reflection tool, and can be a first step in recognising and addressing implicit bias.

'Ethical space' is also a philosophical and physical framework, designed by Cree scholar Willie Ermine, in which groups with differing world views come together to share knowledge and engage in cross-cultural conversations and collaboration in pursuit of ethically problem solving together [109]. Creating ethical space with patients and colleagues can help to bridge the gap between world views and contribute to ethical and collaborative decision making in medicine.

16.6.5 Provide structurally competent care

Structural competency is defined as 'the capacity for health professionals to recognize and respond to health and illness as the downstream effects of broad social, political, and economic structures' [110]. Structural competency places emphasis on interventions at the institutional level, such as partnering with community organisations, civil society, institutions outside the health sector, and policymakers to influence population health outcomes and advance health equity. A structural competency approach links the role of the determinants of health to broader social context alongside policy, economic, legislative and cultural factors [111].

For example, structurally competent care might look like working with a tenants protection agency and a social worker to ensure that a patient's housing conditions do not exacerbate their asthma. Structurally competent care also might look like performing a disability audit of a health service, making the appropriate adjustments, and partnering with community and allied health services to ensure that patients with disability have the appropriate level of care and support at home.

16.6.6 Encourage and support diversity in health care and healthcare leadership

Diversity within the medical and medical leadership workforce is important to the provision of equitable care, improved health outcomes and reduced health disparities [112–114]. For example, diversity in the medical workforce is associated with improved clinical care, accuracy of clinical decision making and patient satisfaction [115–117]. Diversity within teaching faculty and medical student cohorts may also contribute to health equity by providing new perspectives during training, increasing focus on equity, and better preparing students to provide marginalised groups with culturally safe and patient-centred care [118].

Despite the advantages of diversity in medicine and medical leadership, it has been slow to materialise in Australia. For example, although more than half of medical graduates are women, women remain significantly under-represented in medical leadership positions [119]. Indigenous and cultural minority groups are also under-represented in medicine and medical leadership [117,120,121]. These inequities are even more pronounced for Aboriginal and/or Torres Strait Islander women and women with disability [122].

Bullying, harassment and discrimination are systemic problems during medical training, and are associated with stress, mental health issues, impaired performance and compromised provision of care. Female, Indigenous, sexually and gender-diverse, and cultural-minority trainees are more likely to experience discrimination, bullying or harassment. Those perpetrating sexual harassment, discrimination and bullying during medical training include supervisors, other members of staff, colleagues and patients. Although medical training is rife with discrimination, bullying and harassment, it is seldom reported.

Doctors can contribute to health equity by ensuring their conduct and the conduct of their colleagues is free from discrimination, bullying and harassment. The Medical Board of Australia's code of conduct expects doctors not to discriminate against, bully or harass others and to contribute to the management of discrimination, bullying or sexual harassment by others [123]. Actions in this area might include familiarising oneself or educating others about their health service's policy and current legislation in relation to discrimination, bullying and harassment. For example, familiarity with legislation around prohibited interview questions can ensure that candidates do not experience discrimination by being asked about their culture, religion, sexuality, or plans to have a family. Other actions can include ensuring that accessible, confidential and appropriate reporting pathways are available for people who experience or witness discrimination, bullying or harassment. Simulation, including role play, and targeted medical and professional education have been successful in providing people with the confidence and opportunity to practise speaking up when they witness harassment, bullying or discrimination [124,125].

Supporting and encouraging diversity can also include advocating for diversity in recruitment, selection, remuneration and promotion decisions. For example, actions can include recommending diverse representation on selection panels, and ensuring equitable access to mentors, role models and experiences that contribute to promotion decisions. Supporting and encouraging diversity also includes contributing to a culturally safe environment and being an ally. Being an ally means recognising and challenging injustice and promoting equity through supportive personal relationships and public acts of solidarity, sponsorship and advocacy [126,127]. For example, this can include educating others, challenging exclusionary practice and ensuring that everyone is invited to speak at meetings.

Summary

Health inequity is unfair and avoidable. Health inequity results from social and structural factors, and disproportionately affects marginalised populations. There is strong evidence to support the health, social and financial benefits of equitable health care. Health practitioners can make a significant contribution to health equity through enabling access and engagement with health care, and providing high-quality, safe care that is culturally safe and structurally competent.

References

1. Islam N, Winkel J. Climate change and social inequality. New York (US): UN Department of Economic and Social Affairs (DESA) Working Papers, No. 152; 2017.
2. Braveman P, Arkin E, Orleans T, et al. What is health equity? *Behav Sci Policy* 2018; 4: 1–14.
3. Shadmi E, Chen Y, Dourado I, et al. Health equity and COVID-19: global perspectives. *Int J Equity Health* 2023; 19: 1–16.
4. Baciu A, Negussie Y, Geller A, et al., editors. The need to promote health equity. In: Communities in action: Pathways to health equity. Washington (DC): National Academies Press (US), 2017.
5. Farmer PE, Nizeye B, Stulac S, Keshavjee S. Structural violence and clinical medicine. *PLoS Med* 2006; 3: e449.
6. Westerhaus M, Finnegan A, Haidar M, et al. The necessity of social medicine in medical education. *Acad Med* 2015; 90: 565–568.
7. Marmot M, Friel S, Bell R, et al. Closing the gap in a generation: health equity through action on the social determinants of health. *Lancet* 2008; 372: 1661–1669.
8. Marmot M, Allen JJ. Social determinants of health equity. *Am J Public Health* 2014; 104: S517–519.
9. King TL, Kavanagh A, Scovelle AJ, Milner A. Associations between gender equality and health: a systematic review. *Health Promot Int* 2020; 35: 27–41.
10. Chin MH, Clarke AR, Nocon RS, et al. A roadmap and best practices for organizations to reduce racial and ethnic disparities in health care. *J Gen Intern Med* 2012; 27: 992–1000.
11. Wilkinson R, Pickett K. The spirit level. London: Penguin, 2010.
12. Wilkinson RG. The impact of inequality: How to make sick societies healthier. Oxfordshire: Routledge, 2020.
13. Aldridge RW, Story A, Hwang SW, et al. Morbidity and mortality in homeless individuals, prisoners, sex workers, and individuals with substance use disorders in high-income countries: a systematic review and meta-analysis. *Lancet* 2018; 391: 241–250.
14. Galli G, Lenggenhager B, Scivoletto G, et al. Don't look at my wheelchair! The plasticity of longlasting prejudice. *Med Educ* 2015; 49: 1239–1247.
15. Australian Institute of Health and Welfare. Australia's welfare 2021. Canberra: AIHW, 2021. (AIHW Cat. No. AUS 237.) https://www.aihw.gov.au/reports/australias-welfare/australias-welfare-2021-in-brief/contents/summary (accessed Oct 2024).
16. Mackenbach JP. Socioeconomic inequalities in health in high-income countries: the facts and the options. In: Detels R, et al., editors. Oxford textbook of global public health. Oxford, 2015; 1: 106–126.
17. Pulok MH, van Gool K, Hall J. Inequity in physician visits: the case of the unregulated fee market in Australia. *Soc Sci Med* 2020; 255: 113004.
18. Sajjad MA, Holloway-Kew KL, Mohebbi M, et al. Association between area-level socioeconomic status, accessibility and diabetes-related hospitalisations: a cross-sectional analysis of data from Western Victoria, Australia. *BMJ Open* 2019; 9: e026880.
19. Whitehead M. The concepts and principles of equity and health. *Health Promot Int* 1991; 6: 217–228.
20. Smith LT. Decolonizing methodologies: Research and indigenous peoples. London: Zed Books Ltd, 2013.
21. Tuck E, Yang KW. R-words: refusing research. In: Paris D, Winn MT, editors. Humanizing research: Decolonizing qualitative inquiry with youth and communities. SAGE Publications, 2014; 223–248.
22. Galtung J, Höivik T. Structural and direct violence: a note on operationalization. *J Peace Res* 1971; 8: 73–76.
23. Rylko-Bauer B, Farmer P. Structural violence, poverty, and social suffering. In: Brady D, Burton LM, editors. The Oxford handbook of the social science of poverty. Oxford Academic, 2016: 47–74.
24. Barr DA. The childhood roots of cardiovascular disease disparities. *Mayo Clin Proc* 2017; 92: 1415–1421.
25. Desrosiers J, Wilkinson T, Abel G, Pitama S. Curricular initiatives that enhance student knowledge and perceptions of sexual and gender minority groups: a critical interpretive synthesis. *Can Med Educ J* 2016; 7: e121.
26. Foucault M. Power/knowledge. New York: Pantheon, 1980: 90.
27. Ghidina M. Deconstructing victim-blaming, dehumanization, and othering: using empathy to develop a sociological imagination. *Teaching Sociology*. 2019; 47: 231–242.
28. Curtis E, Jones R, Tipene-Leach D, et al. Why cultural safety rather than cultural competency is required to achieve health equity: a literature review and recommended definition. *Int J Equity Health* 2019; 18: 1–17.

29. Peterkin A, Risdon C. Caring for lesbian and gay people: a clinical guide. Toronto: University of Toronto Press, 2003.
30. Van Ryn M, Saha S. Exploring unconscious bias in disparities research and medical education. *JAMA* 2011; 306: 995–996.
31. Crenshaw KW. On intersectionality: essential writings. New York: The New Press, 2017.
32. Sandberg L. Backward, dumb, and violent hillbillies? Rural geographies and intersectional studies on intimate partner violence. *Affilia* 2013; 28: 350–365.
33. Bretherton I, Thrower E, Zwickl S, et al. The health and well-being of transgender Australians: a national community survey. *LGBT Health*. 2021; 8: 42–49.
34. Rew L, Young CC, Monge M, Bogucka R. Puberty blockers for transgender and gender diverse youth—a critical review of the literature.*Child Adolesc Ment Health* 2021; 26: 3–14.
35. Lykens JE, LeBlanc AJ, Bockting WO. Healthcare experiences among young adults who identify as genderqueer or nonbinary. *LGBT Healt*h 2018; 5: 191–196.
36. Turban JL, King D, Kobe J, et al. Access to gender-affirming hormones during adolescence and mental health outcomes among transgender adults. *PLoS One* 2022; 17: e0261039.
37. Cundill P, Wiggins J. Protocols for the initiation of hormone therapy for trans and gender diverse patients. Fitzroy, Vic: Equinox: Gender Diverse Health Centre, 2017.
38. Cundill P. Hormone therapy for trans and gender diverse patients in the general practice setting. *Aus J Gen Pract* 2020; 49: 385–390.
39. Jatrana S, Crampton P. Do financial barriers to access to primary health care increase the risk of poor health? Longitudinal evidence from New Zealand. *Soc Sci Med* 2021; 288: 113255.
40. Australian Institute of Health and Welfare. Health care safety and quality. Canberra: AIHW, 2024. https://www.aihw.gov.au/reports/health-care-quality-performance/health-care-safety-and-quality (accessed Oct 2024).
41. Bernardes CM, Diaz A, Valery PC, et al. Unmet supportive care needs among Indigenous cancer patients across Australia. *Rural Remote Health* 2019; 19: 4660.
42. Bartram M, Stewart JM. Income-based inequities in access to psychotherapy and other mental health services in Canada and Australia. *Health Policy* 2019; 123: 45–50.
43. Cronin TJ, Pepping CA, Halford WK, Lyons A. Mental health help-seeking and barriers to service access among lesbian, gay, and bisexual Australians. *Australian Psychologist* 2021; 56: 46–60.
44. Detollenaere J, Van Pottelberge A, Hanssens L, et al. Patients' financially driven delay of GP visits: is it less likely to occur in stronger primary care systems? *Med Care Res Rev* 2018; 75: 292–311.
45. Schäfer WL, Boerma WG, van den Berg MJ, et al. Are people's health care needs better met when primary care is strong? A synthesis of the results of the QUALICOPC study in 34 countries. *Prim Health Care Res Dev* 2019; 20: e104.
46. Harriss LR, Thompson F, Lawson K, et al. Preventable hospitalisations in regional Queensland: potential for primary health? *Aust Health Rev* 2019; 43: 371–381.
47. Lexchin J, Grootendorst P. Effects of prescription drug user fees on drug and health services use and on health status in vulnerable populations: a systematic review of the evidence. *Int J Health Serv* 2004; 34: 101–122.
48. Carrillo JE, Carrillo VA, Perez HR, et al. Defining and targeting health care access barriers. *J Health Care Poor Undeserved* 2011; 22: 562–575.
49. Bourke L, Humphreys JS, Wakerman J, Taylor J. Understanding rural and remote health: a framework for analysis in Australia. *Health Place* 2012; 18: 496–503.
50. Fennell KM, Hull M, Jones M, Dollman J. A comparison of barriers to accessing services for mental and physical health conditions in a sample of rural Australian adults. *Rural Remote Health* 2018; 18: 4155.
51. Woolfenden S, Galea C, Badland H, et al. Use of health services by preschool-aged children who are developmentally vulnerable and socioeconomically disadvantaged: testing the inverse care law. *J Epidemiol Community Health* 2020; 74: 495–501.
52. Samra R, Hankivsky O. Adopting an intersectionality framework to address power and equity in medicine. *Lancet* 2021; 397: 857–859.

53. Kline N. Syndemic statuses: Intersectionality and mobilizing for LGBTQ+ Latinx health equity after the Pulse shooting. *Soc Sci Med* 2020; 295: 113260.
54. Dowling A, Enticott J, Kunin M, Russell G. The association of migration experiences on the self-rated health status among adult humanitarian refugees to Australia: an analysis of a longitudinal cohort study. *Int J Equity Health* 2019; 18: 1–10.
55. Australian Institute of Health and Welfare. People with disability in Australia. Canberra: AIHW, 2024. (AIHW Cat. No. DIS 72.) https://www.aihw.gov.au/reports/disability/people-with-disability-in-australia/contents/about (accessed Oct 2024).
56. Krnjacki L, Priest N, Aitken Z, et al. Disability-based discrimination and health: findings from an Australian-based population study. *Aust N Z J Public Health* 2018; 42: 172–174.
57. Tiong AC, Patel MS, Gardiner J, et al. Health issues in newly arrived African refugees attending general practice clinics in Melbourne. *Med J Aust* 2006; 185: 602–606.
58. Murray RJ, Davis JS, Burgner DP, et al. The Australasian Society for Infectious Diseases guidelines for the diagnosis, management and prevention of infections in recently arrived refugees: an abridged outline. *Med J Aust* 2009; 190: 421–425.
59. Murray L, Windsor C, Parker E, Tewfik O. The experiences of African women giving birth in Brisbane, Australia. *Health Care Women Int* 2010; 31: 458–472.
60. James K. Domestic violence within refugee families: intersecting patriarchal culture and the refugee experience. *Australian and New Zealand Journal of Family Therapy* 2010; 31: 275–284.
61. Sheikh-Mohammed M, MacIntyre CR, Wood NJ, et al. Barriers to access to health care for newly resettled sub-Saharan refugees in Australia. *Med J Aust* 2006; 185: 594–597.
62. Au M, Anandakumar AD, Preston R, et al. A model explaining refugee experiences of the Australian healthcare system: a systematic review of refugee perceptions. *BMC Int Health Hum Rights* 2019; 19: 1–23.
63. Taylor J, Haintz GL. Influence of the social determinants of health on access to healthcare services among refugees in Australia. *Aust J Prim Health* 2018; 24: 14–28.
64. Mengesha ZB, Perz J, Dune T, Ussher J. Refugee and migrant women's engagement with sexual and reproductive health care in Australia: a socio-ecological analysis of health care professional perspectives. *PLoS One* 2017; 12: e0181421.
65. Timlin M, Russo A, McBride J. Building capacity in primary health care to respond to the needs of asylum seekers and refugees in Melbourne, Australia: the 'GP Engagement' initiative. *Aust J Prim Health* 2020; 26: 10–16.
66. Cooper LA, Roter DL, Carson KA, et al. The associations of clinicians' implicit attitudes about race with medical visit communication and patient ratings of interpersonal care. *Am J Public Health* 2012; 102: 979–987.
67. Miller BC, Bowers JM, Payne JB, Moyer A. Barriers to mammography screening among racial and ethnic minority women. *Soc Sci Med* 2019; 239: 112494.
68. Brewer N, Bartholomew K, Grant J, et al. Acceptability of human papillomavirus (HPV) self-sampling among never- and under-screened Indigenous and other minority women: a randomised three-arm community trial in Aotearoa New Zealand. *Lancet Reg Health West Pac* 2021; 16: 100265.
69. Guimond ME, Salman K. Modesty matters: cultural sensitivity and cervical cancer prevention in Muslim women in the United States. *Nurs Womens Health* 2013; 17: 210–217.
70. Padela AI, Vu M, Muhammad H, et al. Religious beliefs and mammography intention: findings from a qualitative study of a diverse group of American Muslim women. *Psychooncology* 2016; 25: 1175–1182.
71. Wise J. DIY smear tests: are they the answer to falling cervical screening rates? *BMJ* 2019; 364: l361.
72. Razi T, Walfisch A, Sheiner E, et al. #metoo? The association between sexual violence history and parturients' gynecological health and mental well-being. *Arch Gynecol Obstet* 2021; 304: 385–393.
73. Conder J, Mirfin-Veitch B, Payne D, et al. Increasing the participation of women with intellectual disabilities in women's health screening: a role for disability support services. *Research and Practice in Intellectual and Developmental Disabilities* 2019; 6: 86–96.
74. Brinsdon A, Abel G, Desrosiers J. 'I'm taking control': how people living with HIV/AIDS manage stigma in health interactions. *AIDS Care* 2017; 29: 185–188.

75. Ludlam A, Saxton P, Dickson N, Hughes A. General practitioner awareness of sexual orientation among a community and internet sample of gay and bisexual men in New Zealand. *J Prim Health Care* 2015; 7: 204–212.
76. Gall A, Anderson K, Adams J, et al. An exploration of healthcare providers' experiences and perspectives of Traditional and complementary medicine usage and disclosure by Indigenous cancer patients. *BMC Complement Altern Med* 2019; 19: 1–9.
77. Sequeira GM, Ray KN, Miller E, Coulter RW. Transgender youth's disclosure of gender identity to providers outside of specialized gender centers. *J Adolesc Health* 2020; 66: 691–698.
78. Meckler GD, Elliott MN, Kanouse DE, et al. Nondisclosure of sexual orientation to a physician among a sample of gay, lesbian, and bisexual youth. *Arch Pediatr Adolesc Med* 2006; 160: 1248–1254.
79. Neale J, Tompkins C, Sheard L. Barriers to accessing generic health and social care services: a qualitative study of injecting drug users. *Health Soc Care Community* 2008; 16: 147–154.
80. Klitzman RL, Greenberg JD. Patterns of communication between gay and lesbian patients and their health care providers. *J Homosex* 2002; 42: 65–75.
81. Stoové MA, Dietze PM, Aitken CK, Jolley D. Mortality among injecting drug users in Melbourne: a 16-year follow-up of the Victorian Injecting Cohort Study (VICS). *Drug Alcohol Depend* 2008; 96: 281–285.
82. Davies A, Wood LJ. Homeless health care: meeting the challenges of providing primary care. *Med J Aust* 2018; 209: 230–234.
83. Baum FE, Bégin M, Houweling TA, Taylor S. Changes not for the fainthearted: reorienting health care systems toward health equity through action on the social determinants of health. *Am J Public Health* 2009; 99: 1967–1974.
84. FitzGerald C, Hurst S. Implicit bias in healthcare professionals: a systematic review. *BMC Med Ethics* 2017; 18: 1–18.
85. Gonzalez CM, Kim MY, Marantz PR. Implicit bias and its relation to health disparities: a teaching program and survey of medical students. *Teach Learn Med* 2014; 26: 64–71.
86. Dovidio JF, Kawakami K, Gaertner SL. Implicit and explicit prejudice and interracial interaction. *J Pers Soc Psychol* 2002; 82: 62.
87. Sabin JA, Greenwald AG. The influence of implicit bias on treatment recommendations for 4 common pediatric conditions: pain, urinary tract infection, attention deficit hyperactivity disorder, and asthma. *Am J Public Health* 2012; 102: 988–995.
88. Hall WJ, Chapman MV, Lee KM, et al. Implicit racial/ethnic bias among health care professionals and its influence on health care outcomes: a systematic review. *Am J Public Health* 2015; 105: e60–e76.
89. Chapman EN, Kaatz A, Carnes M. Physicians and implicit bias: how doctors may unwittingly perpetuate health care disparities. *J Gen Intern Med* 2013; 28: 1504–1510.
90. Van Ryn M, Burgess DJ, Dovidio JF, et al. The impact of racism on clinician cognition, behavior, and clinical decision making. *Du Bois Rev* 2011; 8: 199–218.
91. Gatwiri K, Rotumah D, Rix E. BlackLivesMatter in healthcare: racism and implications for health inequity among Aboriginal and Torres Strait Islander peoples in Australia. *Int J Environ Res Public Health* 2021; 18: 4399.
92. Quigley A, Hutton J, Phillips G, et al. Implicit bias towards Aboriginal and Torres Strait Islander patients within Australian emergency departments. *Emerg Med Australas* 2021; 33: 9–18.
93. D'Costa I, Hunt I, Russell L, Adams K. A racial bias test with tertiary cancer centre employees: why anti-racist measures are required for First Nations Australians cancer care equity. *Aust Health Rev* 2022; 47: 5–12.
94. O'Brien P, Bunzli S, Lin I, et al. Addressing surgical inequity for Aboriginal and Torres Strait Islander people in Australia's universal health care system: a call to action. *ANZ J Surg* 2021; 91: 238–244.
95. Browne AJ, Smye VL, Rodney P, et al. Access to primary care from the perspective of Aboriginal patients at an urban emergency department. *Qual Health Res* 2011; 21: 333–348.
96. Cooper LA, Beach MC, Johnson RL, Inui TS. Delving below the surface. Understanding how race and ethnicity influence relationships in health care. *J Gen Intern Med* 2006; 21: 21–27.
97. Jong-wook L. Address to WHO staff. Geneva: World Health Organization; 2003.
98. van Daalen KR, Davey F, Norman C, Ford JA. Health equity audits: a systematic review of the effectiveness. *BMJ Open* 2021; 11: e053392.

99. Badrick E, Hull S, Mathur R, et al. Health equity audits in general practice: a strategy to reduce health inequalities. *Prim Health Care Res Dev* 2014; 15: 80–95.
100. Pinto AD, Glattstein-Young G, Mohamed A, et al. Building a foundation to reduce health inequities: routine collection of sociodemographic data in primary care. *J Am Board Fam Med* 2016; 29: 348–355.
101. de Leeuw S. Physician activism and prescribing against poverty. *Can Fam Physician* 2016; 62: 332–335.
102. Paterno MT, Draughon JE. Screening for intimate partner violence. *J Midwifery Womens Health* 2016; 61: 370–375.
103. Di Law H, Marasinghe D, Butler D, et al. Progressivity of out-of-pocket costs under Australia's universal health care system: a national linked data study. *medRxiv* 2022.
104. Pulok MH, van Gool K, Hall J. Horizontal inequity in the utilisation of healthcare services in Australia. *Health Policy* 2020; 124: 1263–1271.
105. Hampson M. Redefining consultations: changing relationships at the heart of health. London: Nesta, 2013.
106. Yared N, Horvath K, Fashanu O, et al. Optimizing screening for sexually transmitted infections in men using self-collected swabs: a systematic review. *Sex Transm Dis* 2018; 45: 294.
107. Laverty M, McDermott DR, Calma T. Embedding cultural safety in Australia's main health care standards. *Med J Aust* 2017; 207: 15–16.
108. Australian Health Practitioner Regulation Agency. Aboriginal and Torres Strait Islander Health Strategy. Ahpra, 2023. https://www.ahpra.gov.au/About-Ahpra/Aboriginal-and-Torres-Strait-Islander-Health-Strategy.aspx (accessed Oct 2024).
109. Ermine W. The ethical space of engagement. *Indigenous LJ* 2007; 6: 193.
110. Metzl JM, Hansen H. Structural competency: theorizing a new medical engagement with stigma and inequality. *Soc Sci Med* 2014; 103: 126–133.
111. D'Eon M. Systems thinking and structural competence in and for medical education. *Can Med Educ J* 2017; 8: e1.
112. Crampton P, Weaver N, Howard A. Holding a mirror to society? Progression towards achieving better sociodemographic representation among the University of Otago's health professional students. *N Z Med J* 2018; 131: 59–69.
113. Ruzycki SM, Freeman G, Bharwani A, Brown A. Association of physician characteristics with perceptions and experiences of gender equity in an academic internal medicine department. *JAMA Netw Open* 2019; 2: e1915165.
114. Ruzycki SM, Franceschet S, Brown A. Making medical leadership more diverse. *BMJ* 2021; 373.
115. Marcelin JR, Siraj DS, Victor R, et al. The impact of unconscious bias in healthcare: how to recognize and mitigate it. *J Infect Dis* 2019; 220: S62–S73.
116. Bristow LR, Butler AS, Smedley BD, editors. In the nation's compelling interest: ensuring diversity in the health-care workforce. Washington (DC): National Academies Press (US), 2004.
117. Whiteford G, Shah M, Nair CS. Equity and excellence are not mutually exclusive: a discussion of academic standards in an era of widening participation. *Quality Assurance in Education* 2013; 21: 299–310.
118. Whitla DK, Orfield G, Silen W, et al. Educational benefits of diversity in medical school: a survey of students. *Acad Med* 2003; 78: 460–466.
119. Teede HJ. Advancing women in medical leadership. *Med J Aust* 2019; 211: 392-4. e1.
120. Curtis E, Wikaire E, Stokes K, Reid P. Addressing indigenous health workforce inequities: a literature review exploring 'best' practice for recruitment into tertiary health programmes. *Int J Equity Health* 2012; 11: 1–15.
121. Garvey G, Rolfe IE, Pearson SA, Treloar C. Indigenous Australian medical students' perceptions of their medical school training. *Med Educ* 2009; 43: 1047–1055.
122. Hempenstall A, Tomlinson J, Bismark MM. Gender inequity in medicine and medical leadership. *Med J Aust* 2019; 211: 475.
123. Medical Board of Australia. Good medical practice: a code of conduct for doctors in Australia. 2020. https://www.medicalboard.gov.au/codes-guidelines-policies/code-of-conduct.aspx (accessed Oct 2024).
124. Pattni N, Arzola C, Malavade A, et al. Challenging authority and speaking up in the operating room environment: a narrative synthesis. *Br J Anaesth* 2019; 122: 233–244.

125. Raemer DB, Kolbe M, Minehart RD, et al. Improving anesthesiologists' ability to speak up in the operating room: a randomized controlled experiment of a simulation-based intervention and a qualitative analysis of hurdles and enablers. *Acad Med* 2016; 91: 530–539.
126. Arndt K, English-Sand P. Being an ally. In: Ben-Moshe L, Cory RC, Feldbaum M, Sagendorf K, editors. Building pedagogical curb cuts: incorporating disability in the university classroom and curriculum. Syracuse: The Graduate School—Syracuse University, 2005: 131.
127. Gaffney C. Anatomy of an ally. *Learning for Justice* 2016; 53.

Further reading

The social determinants of health

Best practices in relation to patient-centred care for gender-diverse patients are evolving rapidly. Several resources exist to assist health practitioners to provide this care, which include:

Cheung AS, Wynne K, Erasmus J, et al. Position statement on the hormonal management of adult transgender and gender diverse individuals. *Med J Aust* 2019; 211: 127–133.

Cundill P, Wiggins J. Protocols for the initiation of hormone therapy for trans and gender diverse patients. Fitzroy, Vic: Equinox: Gender Diverse Health Centre, 2017.

Resources around providing person-centred care for youth include:

Booth ML, Bernard D, Quine S, et al. Access to health care among Australian adolescents: young people's perspectives and their sociodemographic distribution. *J Adolesc Health* 2004; 34: 97–103.

Hetrick SE, Bailey AP, Smith KE, et al. Integrated (one-stop shop) youth health care: best available evidence and future directions. *Med J Aust* 2017; 207: S5–18.

The elements of health equity

Australian Institute of Health and Welfare. Access to health services by Australians with disability. Canberra: AIHW, 2017. https://www.aihw.gov.au/reports/disability/access-health-services-disability/contents/content

Australian Refugee Health Practice Guide. Approach to consultation and management. Victorian Foundation for Survivors of Torture Inc (Foundation House), 2024. https://refugeehealthguide.org.au/consultation-and-management/

CheckUP. Access for All: Disability Awareness for Health Providers. 2024. https://www.checkup.org.au/page/Training/NDIS_-_Access_for_All/

Miller KK, Brown CR, Shramko M, Svetaz MV. Applying trauma-informed practices to the care of refugee and immigrant youth: 10 clinical pearls. *Children (Basel)* 2019; 6: 94.

Sackville R, Bennett B, Galbally R. Royal Commission into Violence, Abuse, Neglect and Exploitation of People with Disability. Report - Public hearing 10 – Education and training of health professionals in relation to people with cognitive disability. Commonwealth of Australia 2022. http://disability.royalcommission.gov.au/publications/report-public-hearing-10-education-and-training-health-professionals-relation-people-cognitive-disability

World Health Organization. Disability. Geneva: WHO, 2023. https://www.who.int/news-room/fact-sheets/detail/disability-and-health

17 Culturally safe health care for Aboriginal and/or Torres Strait Islander peoples

Helen Milroy AM, Jemma Collova, Mark Wenitong, Tamara Mackean, Talila Milroy

Introduction

Doctors have a duty to make the care of patients their first concern [1]. This duty includes care to people of all cultural backgrounds and thus requires cultural safety. The concept of cultural safety can be applied broadly and is relevant to people from any culture. In this chapter, we focus specifically on its application for First Nations people of Australia; that is, Aboriginal and/or Torres Strait Islander people.

The aim of this chapter is to introduce doctors to the concept of cultural safety and to highlight the importance of cultural safety across the healthcare sector as a mechanism to eliminate health inequities and to improve outcomes. Health inequities are systematic differences in health status or the distribution of health resources between different populations, as a result of social conditions (e.g. where people are born). In this context, health inequities are avoidable and could be reduced through the right mix of changes at the systems, organisational, service and individual levels [2]. Cultural safety is a vehicle for this necessary change. See also Chapter 16, Achieving full health potential: health equity.

In this chapter, we first provide a brief history and overview of the concept of cultural safety. Second, we outline the historical, political, social and cultural contexts that impact the health of Aboriginal and/or Torres Strait Islander people. This understanding is an essential step towards achieving cultural safety at the individual level. Third, we discuss how cultural safety must be nested within the healthcare sector, including at the individual (i.e. doctor or healthcare professional), service, organisational and systems levels. Lastly, we expand on the practical application of cultural safety, drawing on case study examples across these different levels and providing some useful resources. Although this chapter is aimed at doctors, clinical education pertaining to Aboriginal and/or Torres Strait Islander people needs to start long before graduation and continue as part of a lifelong journey.

17.1 Cultural safety: an introduction

'You people talk about legal safety, ethical safety, safety in clinical practice and a safe knowledge base, but what about cultural safety?' [3]

The term cultural safety originated in Aotearoa New Zealand in the 1980s [4]. The term was first proposed by a Māori nurse and scholar, Irihapeti Ramsden, following observed inequity in mainstream healthcare services for Māori people. Ramsden challenged the idea that all people should be cared for in the same way 'regardless of who they were' [3]. Instead, Ramsden proposed a shift towards care that accounted for people's unique needs.

The term cultural safety has only recently been adopted in the context of health care for Aboriginal and/or Torres Strait Islander people in Australia. Following public consultations, the Australian Health Practitioner Regulation Agency (Ahpra) agreed on the first nationally consistent baseline definition of cultural safety within Australia:

> Cultural safety is determined by Aboriginal and Torres Strait Islander individuals, families and communities. Culturally safe practice is the ongoing critical reflection of health practitioner knowledge, skills, attitudes, practising behaviours and power differentials in delivering safe, accessible and responsive healthcare free of racism [5].

The definition of cultural safety has also been debated in academic literature. A prominent review on the current evidence associated with cultural safety recommends that the following definition is adopted by healthcare organisations:

> Cultural safety requires healthcare professionals and their associated healthcare organisations to examine themselves and the potential impact of their own culture on clinical interactions and healthcare service delivery. This requires individual healthcare professionals and healthcare organisations to acknowledge and address their own biases, attitudes, assumptions, stereotypes, prejudices, structures and characteristics that may affect the quality of care provided. In doing so, cultural safety encompasses a critical consciousness where healthcare professionals and healthcare organisations engage in ongoing self-reflection and self-awareness and hold themselves accountable for providing culturally safe care, as defined by the patient and their communities, and as measured through progress towards achieving health equity. Cultural safety requires healthcare professionals and their associated healthcare organisations to influence healthcare to reduce bias and achieve equity within the workforce and working environment [6].

Aboriginal and/or Torres Strait Islander clients of health services have described culturally safe care as:

- kind services
- health staff who care about people
- health staff who treat people respectfully
- health staff who understand people's culture [7].

Although the above definitions vary, they highlight shared important characteristics of culturally safe care:

1. Cultural safety requires reflexivity of caregivers, including reflection of any cultural differences, implicit biases, power imbalances and privileges.
2. Cultural safety requires an appreciation of the context of colonisation, and existing racism at the individual and institution level.
3. Only the consumers of care (and not the caregiver) can determine whether a service is culturally safe.
4. Culturally safe practice is an ongoing process, as opposed to a tick-box exercise that can be achieved after training.
5. Cultural safety is the responsibility of all health practitioners, across the whole healthcare system. That is, cultural safety is not an issue only for Aboriginal Community Controlled Health Services (ACCHS); it is also important for mainstream and specialist services.

Cultural safety refers to the cultural appropriateness of healthcare providers, and also of healthcare services, organisations and systems. In this context, a culturally safe practitioner/service/organisation/system is one that enhances the collective empowerment of Aboriginal and/or Torres Strait Islander people and communities [8].

Simply put, however, cultural safety in health care is about ensuring that a person has a safe and healing journey through services, regardless of their cultural background.

Terms such as cultural safety, cultural awareness, cultural competency and cultural responsiveness are often used interchangeably, probably because the evolution of these terms has occurred quite rapidly. These terms do have important differences (see the *Cultural respect framework 2016–2026 for Aboriginal and Torres Strait Islander health* [9] for a list of definitions). Generally speaking, cultural safety is seen as a step beyond cultural awareness and competency (see Box 17.1: Related definitions). However, some academics reject the view of cultural safety existing on a continuum, and argue that cultural safety requires a paradigm shift and deeper understanding of power imbalances [10].

Box 17.1 Related definitions

Cultural awareness refers to a basic understanding that someone you are working with has a different culture to you. Cultural competency refers to congruent behaviours, attitudes and policies that come together and enable someone (or an organisation) to work effectively in cross-cultural situations. Cultural responsiveness is the process by which cultural safety is achieved [11]. That is, cultural responsiveness is the active approach that can be adopted by individuals, organisations and systems in order to achieve and maintain cultural safety.

Cultural safety is important to achieve across the whole healthcare system [12]. This includes in the context of mental health care services, where a lack of cultural safety can be especially damaging. For instance, understanding that it can be culturally appropriate for Aboriginal people to hear the voices of their ancestors could prevent misdiagnosis of psychosis, and this understanding is critical to providing appropriate and safe care [13]. Although the general guiding principles of cultural safety apply to mental health care, cultural safety in the mental health care system is associated with additional complexities that are not specifically covered in this chapter.

17.2 The Australian policy context

Internationally, cultural safety has informed policy, accreditation standards and professional competencies for several years, particularly within Aotearoa New Zealand (e.g. the Medical Council of New Zealand's *Statement on cultural safety* [14] and the Nursing Council of New Zealand's *Guidelines for cultural safety, the Treaty of Waitangi and Māori health in nursing education and practice* [15]). In these instances, cultural safety is a standard for doctors to adhere to, enforced through legislation and registration requirements. Similar movements are starting to occur in Australia. Indeed, there has been a recent increase in the recognition of cultural safety for improving access to, and the quality of, health care for Aboriginal and/or Torres Strait Islander people. The importance of cultural safety is outlined in frameworks for healthcare accreditation purposes [16–18], and also in leading Australian policy and government documents, including the National Agreement on Closing the Gap [19], the *Cultural respect framework 2016–2026 for Aboriginal and Torres Strait Islander health* [9], and the *National Aboriginal and Torres Strait Islander health plan 2021–2031* [12]. The latter proposes several objectives focused specifically on cultural safety, including:

- improving cultural safety in workplaces across health, mental health, disability and aged care systems
- enhancing data collection to improve measurement of racism and cultural safety across the health system
- delivering flexible, culturally safe, place-based and person-centred health care across allied health, community health and primary care settings
- ensuring access to person-centred, culturally safe and responsive acute care.

17.3 Tools for measuring cultural safety

As discussed above, government and other health organisations have identified the need for cultural safety across the whole healthcare system. However, we currently lack appropriate audit tools designed to reliably measure cultural safety in Australia [20]. Furthermore, many policy documents fail to define cultural safety, or do so in a culturally unsafe way [21]. Indeed, there remains a substantial amount of work to be done in this space.

Since 2019, the Australian Institute of Health and Welfare has been developing the *Cultural safety in health care for Indigenous Australians: monitoring framework* [22], which aims to measure progress in achieving cultural safety. The data reported on is pooled from a range of available national- and state-level sources to provide a broad picture of cultural safety, through identifying 1) how healthcare services are provided, 2) Indigenous patients' experience of health care, and 3) access to health care. However, there are significant data gaps and limitations to these measures, including pooling data together from different resources, and a lack of data from mainstream health services [22]. Further, these statistics provide limited insight into the experiences of Aboriginal and/or Torres Strait Islander consumers of health services. Since cultural safety is determined by the consumer/client, this perspective is crucial in providing an accurate measure of cultural safety. Existing power imbalances between consumers and systems/services/doctors may also limit consumers' ability to recognise or identify culturally safe (or unsafe) practices.

At the time of writing this chapter, only one study has aimed to create a survey to measure cultural safety within hospitals from the perspective of Aboriginal patients [23]. This survey by Elvidge et al. includes questions such as: 'During your stay in hospital, how often did the hospital staff listen carefully to you?', 'How often did hospital staff explain your treatment in a way that was difficult to understand?', 'Do you trust the hospital staff with your medical care?', and 'Do you feel that the hospital staff genuinely respect your cultural values and practices?' [23]. Building on this work, the New South Wales Bureau of Health Information released survey questions for assessing Aboriginal and/or Torres Strait Islander inpatients' experiences [24]. These surveys provide an important first step towards developing indicators for cultural safety, which will be critical in objectively assessing whether or not services are deemed to be culturally safe by the recipients of care.

17.4 Understanding cultural safety for Aboriginal and/or Torres Strait Islander people

Cultural safety requires an understanding of different cultural views of health and wellbeing, as well as an understanding of how historical, political and social contexts influence health outcomes and experiences. In this section, we provide a brief overview of these topics.

17.4.1 Aboriginal and Torres Strait Islander models of health and wellbeing

Aboriginal and Torres Strait Islander peoples have always had an understanding and appreciation of health as holistic social and emotional wellbeing (SEWB). For Aboriginal and Torres Strait Islander people, health does not just refer to the physical wellbeing of one individual but reflects the social and emotional wellbeing of a whole community. This multidimensional view of health has been visually conceptualised as the SEWB framework (Figure 17.1) [25,26]. This conceptualisation highlights the interconnected relationships between an individual and their family and kin, community, culture, country and land, spirit and ancestors, and mind and emotions. These seven social and emotional wellbeing domains are influenced by social, historical and political determinants of health and wellbeing.

Figure 17.1 A social and emotional wellbeing (SEWB) model of health

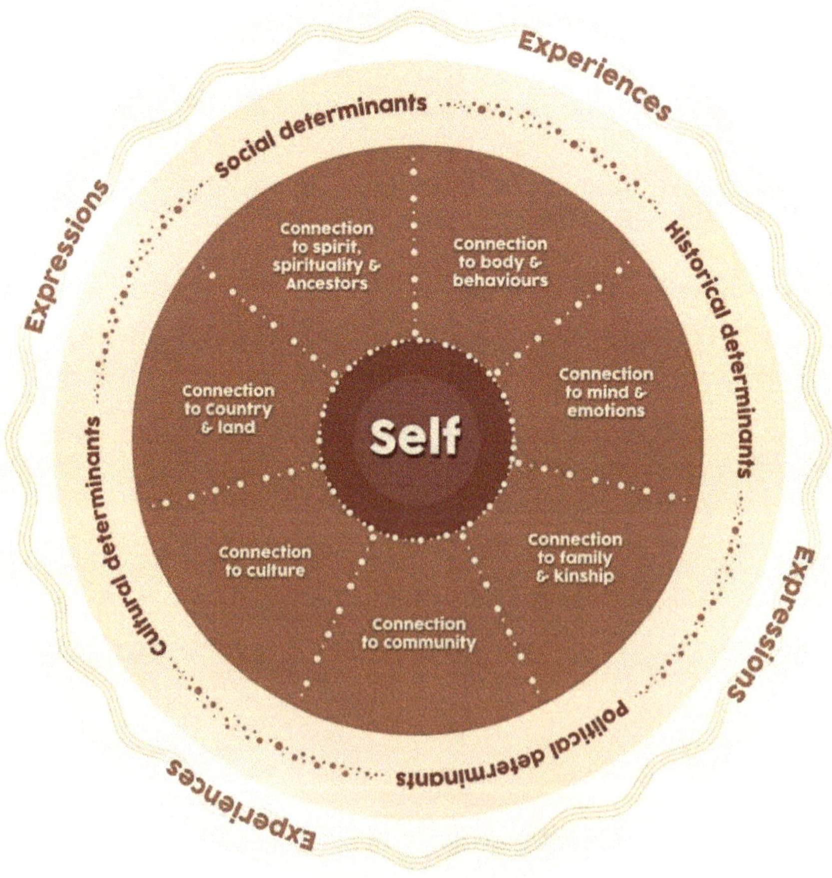

Source: Transforming Indigenous Mental Health and Wellbeing Project. Social and Emotional Gathering Report: 30–31st March 2021. The University of Western Australia, 2021. Figure 1, SEWB; p. 9.

A SEWB approach considers the broader context of family, community, culture, spirituality and country connections that contribute to health. For example, if an individual was to present to their general practitioner with ongoing epigastric discomfort, a SEWB model would consider how cultural practices, such as Sorry Business, might be linked to the client's symptoms. In Aboriginal cultures, Sorry Business can involve an array of cultural protocols, behaviours and emotions related to the death of a loved one or community member. Sorry cuts, which are deliberate but non-harmful cuts on the body to show the extent of someone's distress, should not be mistaken for self-harm behaviours. Grief can present in a variety of culturally mediated ways, including physical ailments. A holistic approach to health would provide a better understanding of the source of the epigastric discomfort once physical causes had been excluded. As another example, it can be normal in some Aboriginal cultures to hear the voices of deceased relatives, although this could be a diagnostic feature of psychosis in a Western context. An SEWB approach provides an understanding of how culture can influence the development of symptoms from a physical, psychological, spiritual or cultural perspective. Understanding how culture ascribes meaning, impacts on communication and acceptability of treatment will assist in the consultation. Being prepared to work with Elders and Cultural Healers as well as promoting a strong cultural identity will assist in all aspects of care.

Aboriginal and Torres Strait Islander peoples have effectively nurtured their own SEWB for thousands of generations. However, the SEWB of Aboriginal and Torres Strait Islander people has been impacted by colonisation and its ongoing consequences. In particular, colonisation has had broad impacts on the historical (e.g. oppression, genocide, past government policies), political (e.g. land rights, government control, right to self-determination) and social (e.g. education, employment, housing, trauma) determinants of SEWB [25,27]. In order to achieve cultural safety, we must understand how historical, political and social determinants impact Aboriginal and/or Torres Strait Islander people and their SEWB [28].

17.4.2 Historical and political context

To provide culturally safe practice, it is important to understand how historical and political contexts continue to influence health outcomes and experiences today. Australia was traditionally inhabited by two First Nations populations: Aboriginal peoples from mainland Australia, and Torres Strait Islander peoples from the islands in the Torres Strait. These two populations were (and are) ethnically and culturally very different [28]. For example, Torres Strait Islander people are of Melanesian origin from the Indonesian archipelago, with their own rich and diverse cultural histories, languages and traditions. Despite these differences, Aboriginal and Torres Strait Islander peoples successfully adapted and thrived in their physical and social environments for thousands of years. Today, Aboriginal and/or Torres Strait Islander peoples share a history of strength and resistance against the impacts of colonisation.

Aboriginal and/or Torres Strait Islander peoples are not simply predisposed to poor health and wellbeing. Before the arrival of Europeans, Aboriginal and/or Torres Strait Islander peoples lived healthy lives with little evidence of widespread illness or disease. Contemporary health inequities experienced by Aboriginal and/or Torres Strait Islander peoples have been directly shaped by the historical and continued impact of colonisation [25,29]. Colonisation, and the subsequent genocide that occurred in Australia, has left a legacy of trauma, loss and psychological distress for Aboriginal and/or Torres Strait Islander peoples [30]. This trauma transcends multiple generations and is still felt today [29,31].

The forced removal of Aboriginal and/or Torres Strait Islander children from their families and communities, known as the Stolen Generations, is just one example of the systemic oppression experienced by Aboriginal and/or Torres Strait Islander peoples over generations. The aim of this removal was the assimilation or absorption of First Nations children into the non-Indigenous community so that their identity would disappear [32]. These traumatic events affected whole families and communities. In this context, the trauma experienced by Aboriginal and/or Torres Strait Islander peoples was both collective and cumulative [29,33]. The *Bringing them home report* [32] was produced following the National Inquiry into the Separation of Aboriginal and Torres Strait Islander Children from their Families. The report was the first of its kind to clearly link the many issues facing Aboriginal and/or Torres Strait Islander peoples (including health disadvantages, mental illness and substance abuse) to the forced removal of children and its associated trauma.

Trauma also occurred in the context of powerlessness and a loss of control [29]. Control was placed over almost all aspects of Aboriginal and/or Torres Strait Islander people's lives. Colonial control occurred via massacres, slave labour, incarceration, and legislations that excluded the rights of Aboriginal and/or Torres Strait Islander peoples. Government policies also oppressed and controlled Aboriginal and/or Torres Strait Islander peoples through imposing restrictions on social interactions and physical movement. Aboriginal and/or Torres Strait Islander people were also forbidden from practising culture. Connection to culture is a key component of SEWB, and is a protective factor against suicide [34]. These historical experiences of trauma, powerlessness and helplessness continue to impact contemporary health and wellbeing outcomes for Aboriginal and/or Torres Strait Islander people.

Given this context, it is easy to understand why some Aboriginal and/or Torres Strait Islander communities may not readily trust information and interventions imposed by authorities and government. As a result, Aboriginal and/or Torres Strait Islander people may not seek appropriate medical care, especially if it is not culturally safe. In addition, contemporary events and changes can also occur at the sociopolitical level that impact on cultural safety within systems of care. Royal commissions, other inquiries or referendums can have either a positive or negative impact depending on their findings or outcomes, and this can contribute to feelings of acknowledgement, acceptance and inclusion in society. These events can also influence experiences of racism and discrimination more broadly.

17.4.3 Social determinants of health

The role of social determinants in influencing health outcomes is now well documented [27,35,36]. In Australia, social determinants explain more than one-third of the health gap between Aboriginal and/or Torres Strait Islander people and their non-Indigenous counterparts [37]. There are several social factors which may contribute to this gap. These include demographic factors, income, family life, employment, poverty, housing, education, social exclusion and racism. For example, Aboriginal and/or Torres Strait Islander people are more likely than non-Indigenous Australians to live in regional and remote areas, often with limited or inadequate access to health infrastructure [38].

Demographic factors, such as population age distributions, can also impact health and wellbeing outcomes. The population age distribution for Aboriginal and/or Torres Strait Islander people has a relatively young age structure, with a median age of 24 years [39]. In contrast, non-Indigenous Australians have a more evenly distributed age population, with a median age of 38.5 years [40]. Furthermore, it is estimated that just 5% of Aboriginal and/or Torres Strait Islander Australians are aged 65 years and over, in comparison to 17% of non-Indigenous Australians (see Figure 17.2) [41,42]. The shape of this population pyramid resembles the age distribution of a developing nation where a significant proportion of the population live in poverty. This distorted population pyramid reflects the historical and ongoing impacts of colonisation on health, such as the burden of chronic disease and lowered life expectancy. However, this age distribution also reveals social challenges for Aboriginal and/or Torres Strait Islander peoples. That is, a relatively large number of young people may lack the appropriate number of healthy adults and older people to support and guide them [43]. Furthermore, the usual buffering and support for families provided through extended family networks may also be lacking, leaving the burden of care to fall on children and young people. Children and young people are required to take on more parental responsibilities and roles, placing them at increased risk of experiencing mental wellbeing stressors.

Figure 17.2 Age structure of First Nations and non-Indigenous populations, 2021

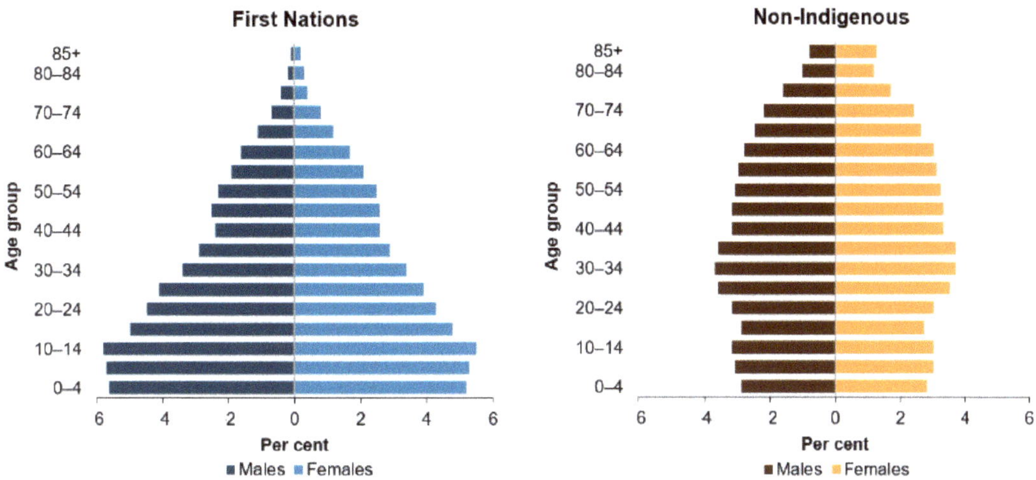

Source: Australian Institute of Health and Welfare. Aboriginal and Torres Strait Islander Health Performance Framework—Summary report 2025. https://www.indigenoushpf.gov.au/report-overview/overview/summary-report/2-demographic-and-social-context

17.4.4 Contemporary health issues

The historical, political and social determinants discussed above continue to contribute to the contemporary health issues faced by Aboriginal and/or Torres Strait Islander peoples. Despite many attempts to improve Aboriginal and Torres Strait Islander health, there remains a significant health gap between Aboriginal and/or Torres Strait Islander peoples and their non-Indigenous counterparts. For example:

- The life expectancy at birth for Aboriginal and/or Torres Strait Islander people is about eight years less than non-Indigenous Australians [44].
- Out of all deaths among Aboriginal and/or Torres Strait Islander adolescents, 80% were considered potentially avoidable in the current health system [45]. Aboriginal and/or Torres Strait Islander people are less likely to report excellent or very good health, as compared to non-Indigenous Australians [44].
- Aboriginal and/or Torres Strait Islander people experience a burden of disease more than twice the rate of non-Indigenous Australians. This burden is mostly accounted for by chronic diseases, including cardiovascular disease, mental and substance use disorders, cancer, diabetes and respiratory diseases [44].
- Aboriginal and/or Torres Strait Islander people die from avoidable causes at three times the rate of non-Indigenous Australians [46].
- In the 2018–19 period, 30% of Aboriginal and/or Torres Strait Islander people who needed to go to a health provider did not go [47].
- In 2020, over 20% of Aboriginal and/or Torres Strait Islander people, or their families, were racially discriminated against by doctors, nurses and/or medical staff [22].

Improving the health and social outcomes for Aboriginal and/or Torres Strait Islander peoples is a national priority in Australia (e.g. National Agreement on Closing the Gap [19]). If we are to close this health gap, we must address the barriers that Aboriginal and/or Torres Strait Islander people face in accessing and receiving appropriate health care. One such barrier is the limited availability of culturally safe healthcare services that meet the needs of Aboriginal and/or Torres Strait Islander people.

It is important to note here that despite the above challenges, Aboriginal and/or Torres Strait Islander people have fought hard to reject deficit narratives of their people and communities as a 'health problem' to be solved. Indeed, deficit discourse may have an impact on health and be a barrier for appropriate care [48]. Instead, Aboriginal and/or Torres Strait Islander people advocate for strengths-based approaches, which are led by Aboriginal and/or Torres Strait Islander people [48,49]. In this chapter, we adopt this strengths-based approach to explore ways of effectively improving cultural safety and therefore health outcomes for Aboriginal and/or Torres Strait Islander people.

17.5 Nested cultural safety: a systems approach

17.5.1 Nexus of care

Cultural safety occurs via a 'nexus of care'. That is, culturally safe care requires a dynamic and interactional approach, whereby individual-, organisation- and systems-level care needs to adapt in order to be responsive to the needs of the consumer. Figure 17.3 shows how cultural safety occurs within a 'nexus of care' and is influenced by complex relationships between the health professional and team, patient and family, and healthcare systems and services. In this section we unpack the various components at play in healthcare interactions in order to demonstrate how different actions and different ways of thinking can be changed at the individual and collective level, with the purpose of promoting cultural safety.

Figure 17.3 Factors contributing to the 'nexus of care' influencing cultural safety

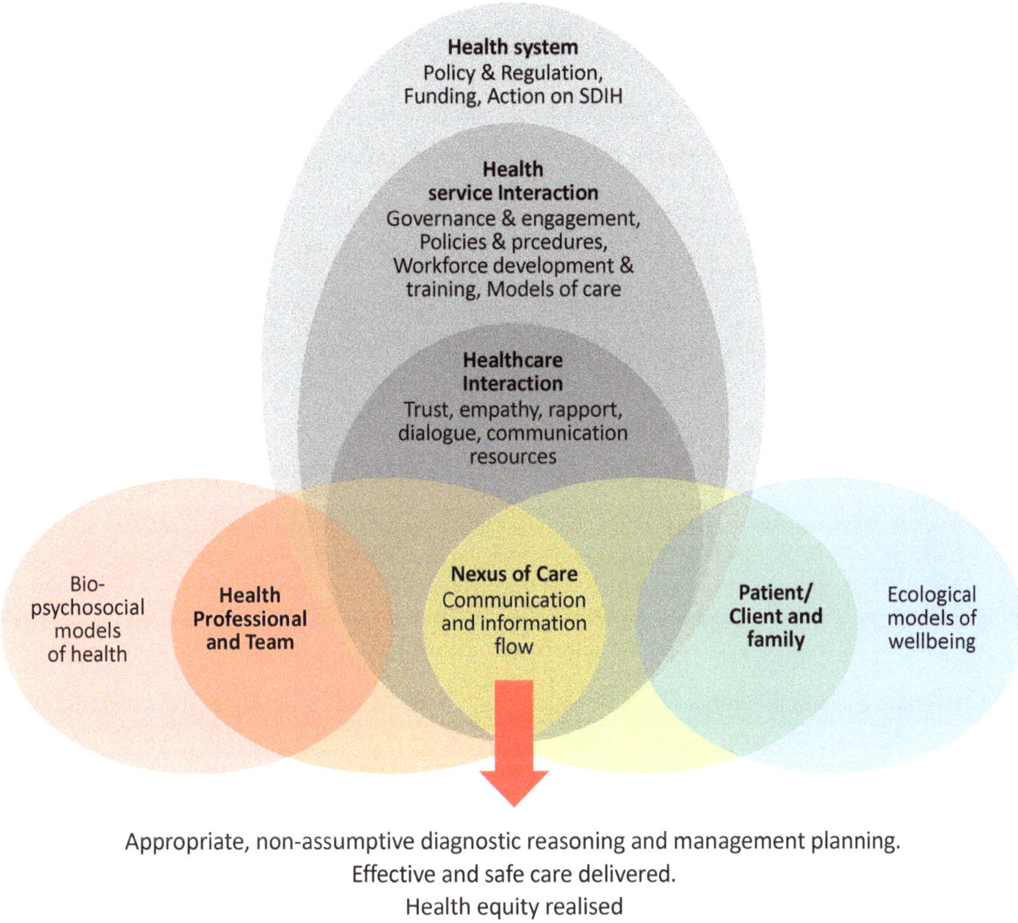

Source: Authors.

17.5.2 Health professional and team

Health professionals in Australia predominantly use a biopsychosocial model of health, and team dynamics can influence what models dominate care processes. Hierarchies of professions and 'master/apprentice' ways of learning and working together may mean that a single senior doctor's perspective can drive the way care is delivered, at the expense of a more culturally safe approach. For example, a senior doctor who favours a dominant biological model over a more holistic ecological model would focus on biological factors during the delivery of care. Determinants of health captured by an ecological model (which recognises the role of the environmental, policy and social contexts) may then be ignored in the care delivery, to the detriment of the consumer.

Similarly, implicit bias and racism born of colonisation may not be evident to a doctor with low levels of cultural awareness, and if pointed out, may be resisted. Unfortunately, racism is common in health settings, with a national survey revealing over 30% of Aboriginal and/or Torres Strait Islander people experiencing racial discrimination in medical settings, most or all of the time [50]. Aboriginal and/or Torres Strait Islander doctors are also more than five times more likely to report bullying as a major source of stress, and are 10 times more likely to experience racism than non-Indigenous doctors [51].

'Hidden curriculum' experiences such as bedside teaching and role modelling also influence teaching and learning, and this is another example of how unhelpful colonial notions of Aboriginal and/or Torres Strait Islander people can be reproduced and reinforced in health care. Doctors need to be courageous and tackle their own and others' ignorance and racism to maintain high professional standards of care and respect.

In addition, many international medical graduates are recruited to Australia from overseas to provide medical services in areas of need where large Aboriginal and/or Torres Strait Islander populations may reside. It is essential that cultural safety training and orientation to Aboriginal and Torres Strait Islander health is included in their introduction to working in Australian communities.

17.5.3 Patient/client and family

As described earlier, many Aboriginal and/or Torres Strait Islander people use a SEWB model of health based on the interconnectedness of all living things [25]. However, many health professionals within mainstream services do not have a basic understanding of this model of health. Unless the possibility of different explanatory models of health and wellbeing are explicitly considered, unsafe healthcare interactions can occur without mutual understanding. For example, conversations between doctors and patients often focus heavily on medical discourse and assume dominance of biomedical knowledges over other knowledges (including Aboriginal and/or Torres Strait Islander knowledges about SEWB). However, working with cultural belief systems and ways of understanding and communicating are more likely to improve engagement, understanding and outcomes. These conversations also exclude non-medical aspects (e.g. social or economic factors) which may impact the likelihood of a patient seeking treatment or the treatment being effective [52].

Ideally, doctors would consider the broader context of wellbeing (including connections to kinship and culture) as well as any primary issues of concern that are not health related but may require cross-agency input. Doctors should also recognise the agency and strength within Aboriginal and/or Torres Strait Islander families, which is often underappreciated. For example, Aboriginal family groups are typically governed by complex kinship systems that securely place each person in relation to every other person in the group. These kinship structures ensure that each person is supported, which enhances mental and physical wellbeing [53]. Doctors should recognise the role of kin as a protective factor in health care.

17.5.4 Healthcare interaction

Given experiences of colonisation, trauma and racial discrimination, it is important to recognise that some Aboriginal and/or Torres Strait Islander people are reluctant to seek medical help in the first instance and are unlikely to return if they experience a negative healthcare interaction. Healthcare interactions are influenced by education and social contexts, as well as assumptions, stereotypes and significant power imbalances. These factors can interfere with building rapport and effective communication between a doctor and patient.

Culturally safe care requires effective communication between doctors and patients. However, shared understandings of key medical concepts between doctors and some Aboriginal and/or Torres Strait Islander patients can be difficult to achieve, and this miscommunication often goes unrecognised. This is clearly demonstrated in a case study example described by Cass et al., in which a doctor was explaining the treatment required to an Aboriginal patient. The doctor explained the need for the Aboriginal patient to relocate to Darwin to address their chronic renal disease. However, the patient misunderstood this conversation and believed that they had been told they were cured [52]. Furthermore, the doctor had felt they had done a good job at explaining the situation and was unaware of this miscommunication.

Miscommunication in healthcare interactions can occur for several reasons, including simple differences in discourse. For example, question-and-answer routines are not common in some Aboriginal and/or Torres Strait Islander discourses. Factors such as the cultural appropriateness of who should ask certain questions, and how to respond, can further complicate question-and-answer conversations. An Aboriginal patient may not respond honestly to the question 'do you understand the need for dialysis?', as it can be seen as impolite to contradict or respond negatively to a question [52]. An alternate way of checking understanding is through a yarning or conversational style, such as asking, 'can you tell about your kidneys/illness/treatment?', aiming to seek their opinion or explanation rather than a direct yes/no response.

Aboriginal and/or Torres Strait Islander health workers and liaison officers can play an important role in improving communication between patients, doctors and team members. These workers can have positive effects on communication, rates of discharge against medical advice, and continuity of care [54]. For these reasons, Aboriginal and/or Torres Strait Islander health workers and liaison officers are a critical part of the workforce and can help to build trust and empathy.

Aboriginal and Torres Strait Islander communities are diverse and have a range of community-specific protocols regarding engagement and communication. It is always important to understand and learn what the local protocols are when working in health care.

In summary, some common considerations include:

- using clear language, considering English may be a second or third language, and literacy skills may also reflect this
- only using traditional language words with permission in the community of origin as words can have a different meaning in other language groups
- using an interpreter or cultural worker to assist
- giving an Acknowledgement of Country or a welcome ceremony in greeting protocols, depending on the circumstances
- making introductions in a yarning style to work out family relationships, obligations and protocols for behaviour
- avoiding too many direct questions, which may result in disengagement; instead, try to allow the person to tell you their story
- understanding that not all family members may speak, depending on who is in the room; these are features of 'avoidance relationships'
- other kin sometimes being responsible for decisions and needing to be consulted
- understanding that eye contact will vary across communities, with many communities avoiding direct eye contact at all times; establishing rapport will need to be gauged in a culturally appropriate manner
- being aware of your body language as this will form part of the communication
- understanding that long silences or pauses are common and may mean a sign of respect
- saying yes often may be a way of avoiding conflict and should alert you to checking if this is the correct response
- considering the appropriateness of age and gender out of respect for Eldership and men's and women's business.

17.5.5 Health service interaction

The Australian health system is made up of services across the care spectrum and across geographical settings, and thus may vary widely. Notwithstanding this variability, colonisation has greatly shaped the Australian healthcare system and facilitated a view of Aboriginal and/or Torres Strait Islander people as inherently deficient and problematic. More recently, critiques of the healthcare system have surfaced systemic problems such as racism and dominance of biomedical views. The limitations of mainstream health care for Aboriginal and/or Torres Strait Islander people led to the development of ACCHS, which in turn have influenced the evolution of comprehensive primary health care worldwide and health care in Australia. Today, ACCHS play a significant role in training the medical workforce, and can demonstrate superior performance over mainstream general practices for Aboriginal and/or Torres Strait Islander patients [55]. Current Primary Health Networks and Local Health Districts/Networks are also required by legislation and quality healthcare standards to provide culturally responsive health care. Health service policies and procedures also have an important role to play in facilitating partnerships between ACCHS and Primary Health Networks, and in promoting workforce development and the implementation of appropriate models of care.

17.5.6 Health system

The health system provides the legislative and policy frameworks which set standards of care and allocation of resources. Culturally safe policy development is critical for culturally safe practice. At the policy level, cultural safety applies to how policies are created and actioned. Cultural safety means ensuring Aboriginal and/or Torres Strait Islander leadership and empowerment, proper resource allocation, accountability for implementation and appropriate monitoring, and privileging the perspectives of Aboriginal and/or Torres Strait Islander patients [56]. Culturally unsafe policy can occur due to a lack of political will, entrenched deficit framing and ongoing marginalisation and exclusion of Aboriginal and/or Torres Strait Islander knowledge and peoples.

Quality of care standards, service and professional accreditation, and jurisdictional public health acts represent levers for change for cultural safety. However, these levers need to be uncoupled from colonial constructs of who and what Aboriginal and/or Torres Strait Islander peoples are, and the value they (and their knowledge systems) can bring to health and social care. Health professional bodies (such as Australian Indigenous Doctors' Association and Indigenous Allied Health Australia) are vehicles for advocacy in this endeavour.

17.6 Cultural safety in practice

As discussed above, the concept of cultural safety encompasses positive and multi-level approaches to the integration of Aboriginal and/or Torres Strait Islander–led models of care and understandings of health and wellbeing to improve patient care and outcomes. Cultural safety is relevant at the individual level, but also at systems and policy levels. If a culturally safe experience for Aboriginal and/or Torres Strait Islander people is the aim, then cultural safety must be adopted throughout all these levels.

Doctors should view cultural safety as a continuous and lifelong process that is strengthened with self-education, clinical experience and formal training, as well as self-reflection and personal commitment [57]. The practical application of cultural safety can be fully realised in all clinical settings and by all health professionals. In what follows, we outline how doctors can practically engage with and apply cultural safety principles throughout their professional lives and across their developing roles as clinicians, supervisors, advocates and leaders. We also discuss specific roles and challenges for Aboriginal and/or Torres Strait Islander practitioners. Finally, we provide case study examples of culturally safe practice.

17.6.1 Role as a junior doctor

Australian medical school accreditation standards mandate the integration of Indigenous health curricula. It is expected that junior doctors begin their professional roles with a set of core competencies and knowledge surrounding Aboriginal and Torres Strait Islander health, with the expectation that this knowledge advances with time.

Junior doctors experience important steps in learning through immersion in clinical practice. They often spend more time with health consumers and their families in hospitals and clinics and can play a very important role in advocacy. Close doctor–patient contact means that cultural safety at the interpersonal level is needed. In addition, and across the entirety of a doctor's professional life, self-reflection is essential in advancing knowledge and skills. Reflective tools encourage the doctor to consider how they apply cultural safety through the domains of creating culturally safe workplaces, understanding and supporting Aboriginal and Torres Strait Islander self-determination, and through leadership and accountability (e.g. see the Victorian Government Department of Health's *Aboriginal and Torres Strait Islander cultural safety framework: Part 1* [57]).

17.6.2 Role as a consultant/senior doctor

Professional progression and advancement come with increased responsibility and additional roles in mentorship, supervision, leadership and management. Senior doctors act as important role models to junior doctors and clinical teams with regards to demonstrating culturally safe practice. Senior doctors are encouraged to leverage their professional privilege and power to influence change and advocate for cultural safety in their workplaces, and also within other professional bodies where they may be employed. In building on the experience as junior doctors, reflective tools encourage senior doctors to also consider how they create culturally safe practices and systems through their role in leading clinical teams and modelling safe practice, higher level decision making, resource allocation, system reform and through education and training of staff. The overall approach is one of lifelong learning and reflective practice to enable innovation and change over time.

17.6.3 Recommendations for culturally safe practice

Provide care that is free of judgement, bias and racism, and that addresses inequity of health outcomes for Aboriginal and/or Torres Strait Islander people.

Racism has far-reaching impacts on the physical and mental health of Aboriginal and/or Torres Strait Islander people and is a social determinant of health that contributes significantly to health inequity [9,58]. Doctors should be taught about the impacts of racism and how their own biases and preconceptions may impact patient care. Doctors should strive to take an anti-racist approach whereby they actively reflect on their own attitudes and provide individualised care without basis in stereotypical or biased views. They can also actively advocate and engage in activities that combat racism, such as ameliorating the ways racist systems impact Aboriginal and/or Torres Strait Islander patients [59], and respecting specific cultural needs of Aboriginal and/or Torres Strait Islander patients when relevant; for example, being aware of gender protocols, allowing patients to have ward leave and spend time outside, and permitting additional visitors who fall outside of the immediate family structure.

Senior doctors can model appropriate behaviour and should be accountable for their actions towards Aboriginal and/or Torres Strait Islander patients, as well as the actions of those under their supervision. Senior doctors should use their influence to embed systems changes through their own good practice and advocacy. Everyone is responsible for calling out racism and discrimination. Senior doctors should also be supported to continuously develop culturally safe practice, acknowledging that they may not have received this training during their earlier education.

Use appropriate language and terminology when discussing Aboriginal and/or Torres Strait Islander patients, families and communities.

All doctors should be aware of the correct terminology and respectful language of the peoples of the lands on which they live and work. Familiarity with protocols, language and Aboriginal/Torres Strait Islander English will reduce misunderstandings and interpersonal barriers with patients and families. For example, understanding that some Aboriginal and/or Torres Strait Islander people tend to agree with questions even if they don't understand them should alert the clinician to seek greater assurances that the information has been understood or agreement has been reached.

Table 17.1 How to demonstrate inclusive and respectful language

Don't	Do
Do not shorten 'Aboriginal and/or Torres Strait Islander people(s)' to 'ATSI' or 'Indigenous peoples', as this is perceived as lacking respect. Terms such as 'Aboriginals' and 'Aborigine' can be highly offensive and should not be used.	Use 'Aboriginal and/or Torres Strait Islander people(s)', unless specifically referring to an individual who is known to be either Aboriginal or Torres Strait Islander. When in doubt, ask Aboriginal and/or Torres Strait Islander people how they would like you to refer to them. Preference may be for their clan group names.
Do not use universalising or homogenising labels. For example, Noongar culture is different to Larrakia or Koori culture.	Acknowledge the diversity of Aboriginal and/or Torres Strait Islander communities by using pluralisation for words such as 'peoples' and 'cultures'.
Do not perpetuate deficit or paternalistic language, such as 'in need of being rescued', or a 'vulnerable minority with health issues'.	Acknowledge strengths and resilience.

Information adapted from *Demonstrating inclusive and respectful language* by Reconciliation Australia [60].

Build rapport during interactions.

Relationships are very important for Aboriginal and/or Torres Strait Islander peoples. Doctors should introduce themselves in a friendly way and ask where the patient's people are from. They should allow time to explain, and not rush the patient. If time is taken to establish rapport properly in the first instance, the consultation will be far more efficient and effective. Senior doctors should be proactive in demonstrating positive engagement with Aboriginal and/or Torres Strait Islander people; for example, with bedside teaching.

Engage in self-education regarding cultural protocols, languages and communities in the region where you live and work.

There is great diversity across Aboriginal and Torres Strait Islander communities, and cultural protocols vary between communities. Self-education is essential, as it is not acceptable to always rely on Aboriginal and/or Torres Strait Islander staff to educate others on these matters. Aboriginal and/or Torres Strait Islander staff may be living outside of their own community and may not be aware of or in a position to speak about the specific cultural protocols for that community. Furthermore, relying on Aboriginal and/or Torres Strait Islander staff for education can be burdensome for those individuals and not necessarily part of their role. Local resources from libraries, museums, websites and cultural tours can improve understanding of the languages and cultural protocols of surrounding Traditional Custodian groups (see this chapter's further reading list). Visiting local services and getting to know the community can establish your interest and commitment to cultural safety. Share learning through team meetings and in supervision to build service capability.

Support self-determined and patient-centred management that does not challenge or deny Aboriginal and/or Torres Strait Islander concepts of health and wellbeing.

Aboriginal and/or Torres Strait Islander conceptualisations of health within a SEWB model should be at the forefront of developing patient focused management plans [9]. Doctors should be aware of the SEWB model, and the importance of connection to community, culture and country in the provision of care. Senior doctors may have influence to change various systems in their workplaces, such as admission protocols, performance data collection and accountability of hospital performance regarding Aboriginal and/or Torres Strait Islander people's health. Senior doctors should be receptive to recommendations by other staff that support Aboriginal and/or Torres Strait Islander people.

Be allies and advocates for Aboriginal and/or Torres Strait Islander people through personal commitment and dedication.

Being an advocate is not just about doing one specific thing to meet the needs of Aboriginal and/or Torres Strait Islander clients. Striving towards cultural safety requires lifelong learning, and behaviours that become part of one's personal and professional 'core business'. To start this process, doctors could consider joining or attending conferences and educational opportunities led by Aboriginal and/or Torres Strait Islander health bodies such as the Australian Indigenous Doctors' Association, the Leaders in Indigenous Medical Education (LIME) Network or the RACGP Aboriginal and Torres Strait Islander Health faculty. Doctors should also continue this learning and advocacy outside of work, in their everyday lives.

Promote the voice of Aboriginal and/or Torres Strait Islander people and perspectives in professional bodies, colleges, boards or committees.

Doctors should use their position of power to influence policies and protocols. A starting point could be to review college policies for cultural training and professional development of cultural safety (e.g. see the LIME accreditation tools for specialist medical colleges [61]). If no such policy exists, it is essential to question this absence, and advocate for well-resourced and minimum engagement for all trainees and college members.

Set standards within workplaces for engagement with Aboriginal and Torres Strait Islander health issues and cultural safety training.

Embedded, consistent and accountable policies surrounding cultural safety education and training are essential. If these are lacking, or present but not being actioned, advocate for change within the workplace.

17.6.4 Specific roles and challenges for Aboriginal and/or Torres Strait Islander doctors

Aboriginal and/or Torres Strait Islander doctors play an integral and unique role in cultural safety. Indeed, the growth of the Aboriginal and Torres Strait Islander health workforce is essential for cultural safety and improvement in Indigenous health outcomes [62]. However, the challenges of cultural loading must be recognised in the context of a minority workforce who are asked to bear the responsibility and obligation to their families, communities and other Aboriginal and/or Torres Strait Islander people, while also maintaining their own clinical learning and practice.

There has been a significant focus on recruitment of Aboriginal and/or Torres Strait Islander people into medical careers, as well as factors that promote retention, career progression and the ways in which the Aboriginal and/or Torres Strait Islander health workforce can aid a deeper understanding of how race operates in health systems to perpetuate inequities [63,64]. Bullying, embedded institutionalised racism, and a lack of cultural safety have been highlighted as pervasive barriers to growth and retention of the Aboriginal health workforce [64,65]. The Australian Indigenous Doctors' Association found that only half of the Indigenous doctor survey respondents felt that their workplace was culturally safe. In response, the association has proposed mandatory and regular cultural training, along with clearer procedures for racial discrimination complaints and follow-ups [65].

Aboriginal and/or Torres Strait Islander junior doctors benefit from leadership that fosters professional development in culturally safe spaces, provision of Aboriginal and/or Torres Strait Islander mentors, and the inclusion of Aboriginal and/or Torres Strait Islander health curricula and education [66]. Retention of Aboriginal and/or Torres Strait Islander staff would also be improved through strong managerial leadership, support from peers, and opportunities for debriefing, reflection and recognition of workload [64]. The practical steps outlined in this chapter can also directly and indirectly improve the professional wellbeing and workplace experiences of Aboriginal and/or Torres Strait Islander doctors.

17.6.5 Organisational approaches

As explained above, doctors can influence the cultural safety of their organisations. However, the ability for doctors to provide culturally safe care can also be influenced by the organisation in which they work. At a minimum, all organisations should have a constitution that recognises Aboriginal and/or Torres Strait Islander peoples and commits to equitable service provision. Organisations should have auditable and measurable goals in relation to cultural engagement and services for Aboriginal and/or Torres Strait Islander people. For example, the Kimberley Aboriginal Health Planning Forum developed a cultural security framework for Kimberley mental health/social and emotional wellbeing [67]. The framework includes targets and key performance indicators for culturally safe care, focused on four key result areas: professional development of the workforce, the workplace environment, work practices, and systems and processes. Through this framework, the organisation and its staff are held accountable for the provision of culturally safe care through a continuous quality improvement approach. Another example of organisational change is the Congress of Aboriginal and Torres Strait Islander Nurses and Midwives, which promotes lifelong learning towards cultural safety through providing targeted professional development. Through the Murra Mullangari program, participants gain an understanding of the concept of cultural safety and insights into the culture of power, and how to address inequities in nursing and midwifery [68].

Cultural safety can be embedded at the organisational level through:

- having an Acknowledgement of Country on public display (e.g. in waiting rooms)
- displaying Aboriginal and/or Torres Strait Islander artwork
- providing culturally appropriate resources and messaging (e.g. patient handouts)
- providing a means for patients to identify as Aboriginal and/or Torres Strait Islander through standard and safe processes applied to all patients
- actively promoting and championing the importance of Aboriginal and/or Torres Strait Islander people's knowledge and skills in the core work of the organisation (e.g. see the Victorian Government Department of Health's *Aboriginal and Torres Strait Islander cultural safety framework: Part 1* [57])

- offering and embedding a range of resources, education and training to allow staff engagement with Aboriginal and/or Torres Strait Islander cultures and knowledges
- remaining accountable to goals set surrounding cultural safety and engagement with Aboriginal and/or Torres Strait Islander people
- ensuring policies and protocols reflect best practice in relation to cultural safety
- ensuring continual review of policies and protocol in relation to the above
- employing Aboriginal and/or Torres Strait Islander people, and providing them opportunities for development and leadership
- ensuring an organisational commitment to employment and professional development of Aboriginal and/or Torres Strait Islander staff that does not challenge or deny their identity and upholds their own cultural safety as an employee
- including a statement about the organisation's commitment to culturally safe care and zero tolerance for racism within practice position descriptions and job advertisements
- acknowledging and promoting significant Aboriginal and/or Torres Strait Islander events (e.g. NAIDOC Week, Reconciliation Week, Sorry Day).

17.6.6 Systems approaches

Systemic and structural change cannot occur without attention to the systems, organisational and service levels in addition to the individual level. Doctors must leverage their position of privilege to influence change in the multitude of systems in which they are involved. This includes—but is not limited to—the public health system, medical education systems, local health districts, private health systems, professional bodies, guidelines, and peak bodies that inform clinical practice, political systems and policy.

Cultural safety requires deliberate embedding of Aboriginal and/or Torres Strait Islander perspectives and knowledges into accreditation, education and policies to achieve integrated and accountable responses [69]. Clinical guidelines, health service policies and specialty college standards should commit to accountable processes that promote cultural safety through all systems in which they operate. Political and educational systems must be influenced to address racism and systemic-born challenges that are faced by Aboriginal and Torres Strait Islander patients and doctors.

Systems-level change can occur through:

- higher representations of Aboriginal and/or Torres Strait Islander people in decision-making and policy positions
- changes to accreditation that focus on cultural safety
- changes to legislation that mandate culturally safe practices; for example, ensuring hospital access to Traditional Healers [70].

17.6.7 Case study examples

Box 17.2 Case Study 1—Role as a junior doctor

Emma is a junior doctor on the respiratory medicine team at a tertiary hospital. She is preparing to discharge Travis, a 35-year-old Noongar man from Perth after he was transferred from the rural hospital for management of a severe exacerbation of asthma. Travis has received asthma education, including the correct use of his devices, and has been provided a culturally specific asthma action plan via Asthma Australia. This culturally specific asthma action plan includes instructions that are easy to understand, and which are accompanied with visual illustrations of an Aboriginal person taking the medicine. Throughout his stay, Emma made sure Travis was seen by the Aboriginal Liaison Officer, who assisted with further communication, education and allied health support. In addition, Emma has spoken to the local Aboriginal Community Controlled Health Organisation senior medical officer to provide a handover and arranged a follow-up appointment for Travis. Emma has also spoken to the pharmacist to ensure the new medicines will be in stock. With permission from Travis, Emma has spoken to his wife and extended family about the discharge plan and the action plan should he become unwell. Emma has also made sure his family will be available to pick him up on return home.

Box 17.3 Case Study 2—Role as a consultant/senior doctor/leader

Dr J is a consultant physician at a major teaching hospital. She facilitates fortnightly bedside teaching for a small group of medical students and junior doctors. She has planned to see an Aboriginal patient today. Before seeing the patient, she tells the students and junior doctors which language group the patient is from, as well as the way the patient prefers to be addressed. She discusses the concepts of SEWB with the students and asks them to focus their social history taking around this. When students become unclear on how to proceed, Dr J models a yarning style of history taking, which includes indirect questioning, allowance for silences, use of narrative and metaphor, and explorations of family and social circumstances. This style helps the interview to continue. Following the interview, students are given the opportunity to ask questions. Realising the students and junior doctors had limited knowledge about SEWB principles, Dr J adds this to the agenda of the next Hospital Education Committee meeting. Her advocacy at this meeting leads to allocation of funding for mandatory cultural safety education with a local training group for all new medical staff.

Box 17.4 Case Study 3—Organisational role

Brad is the new registrar at an urban general practice. When he commenced his new position, he saw several patients who identified as Aboriginal and/or Torres Strait Islander but found that the practice was not meeting the needs of this patient cohort. Brad organised a meeting with his supervisor and practice manager who agreed with his assessment. Brad performed a clinical audit of the number of preventative health assessments that had been conducted for Aboriginal and/or Torres Strait Islander patients in the previous 12 months. He also researched what Medicare Benefits Schedule (MBS) item numbers were available for Aboriginal and/or Torres Strait Islander people. In an all-staff meeting, goals were established to improve the rates of preventative health assessments for Aboriginal and/or Torres Strait Islander patients, with a plan to review this in 12 months. The practice manager arranged mandatory cultural training at the nearest Aboriginal Community Controlled Health Organisation. Culturally appropriate patient handouts and resources were added to the practice desktops for easy access. In addition, an Acknowledgement of Country was displayed at the front desk. The practice will now have biannual meetings to review policies and protocols in relation to their Aboriginal and/or Torres Strait Islander clients to ensure best practice in service provision. Cultural safety training will also continue for all staff on a regular basis.

Box 17.5 Case Study 4—Systems approaches

Institutional racism is a significant barrier in the delivery of health care to Aboriginal and/or Torres Strait Islander people [12]. As part of the northern Queensland response to complaints of racism in the hospital system, a consultancy group (including both Aboriginal and/or Torres Strait Islander and non-Indigenous people) was contracted by the local health and hospital services (HHS) to do a desktop review of their services. The review highlighted a failure of basic cultural safety, and systemic racism. In response to these findings, an advisory group was developed, which consisted of CEOs from local ACCHS. The review broadened to a statewide review of Queensland's 16 HHS and developed the *Matrix for identifying, measuring and monitoring institutional racism within public hospitals and health services* (the Matrix) [71]. Results from the Matrix revealed that 10 of the 16 HHS scored very high levels of institutional racism, and the remaining six HHS scored high.

The Matrix surfaced many important issues at a systems level. While the state was actively working to address these issues, the advisory group highlighted macro, policy and structural issues that were crucial for systemwide reform. The group suggested that leadership in cultural safety, equity and racism started at the top. Although some HHS had Aboriginal and/or Torres Strait Islander board members, many did not. There were also no set processes in place for ensuring Aboriginal or Torres Strait Islander representation on the board.

In response to the above, there was a push for change to ensure that Aboriginal and/or Torres Strait Islander people were legislated to sit on each HHS board. Indeed, this was followed by legislation ensuring each HHS has a health equity plan for Aboriginal and/or Torres Strait Islander health in the service area. While not the end game, it is important to ensure that any positive changes to improving cultural safety for Aboriginal and/or Torres Strait Islander people are not ad hoc and are sustained in health systems.

Summary

This chapter explores cultural safety as a mechanism for eliminating health inequities. In Australia, culturally safe health care is necessary to improve the health outcomes for Aboriginal and/or Torres Strait Islander peoples. However, many mainstream health services are not culturally safe. It is important to frame understandings of cultural safety within individual, organisational and systemic levels. Cultural safety requires a reflective assessment of power, privilege and bias across these different levels. It also requires an understanding and incorporation of Aboriginal and Torres Strait Islander views of health (including SEWB).

References

1. Medical Board of Australia. Good medical practice: a code of conduct for doctors in Australia. 2020. https://www.medicalboard.gov.au/Codes-Guidelines-Policies/Code-of-conduct.aspx (accessed Apr 2025).
2. World Health Organization. Health inequities and their causes. Geneva: WHO, 2018. https://www.who.int/news-room/facts-in-pictures/detail/health-inequities-and-their-causes (accessed Feb 2022).
3. Ramsden IM. Cultural safety and nursing education in Aotearoa and Te Waipounamu [PhD thesis]. Wellington (NZ): Victoria University of Wellington, 2002. https://www.croakey.org/wp-content/uploads/2017/08/RAMSDEN-I-Cultural-Safety_Full.pdf (accessed Apr 2025).
4. Papps E, Ramsden I. Cultural safety in nursing: The New Zealand experience. *Int J Qual Health Care* 1996; 8: 491–497.
5. Australian Health Practitioner Regulation Agency. Consultation report – Report on findings from the public consultation on the definition of 'cultural safety' for use within the National Scheme. Ahpra, 2019. https://www.ahpra.gov.au/News/Consultations/Past-Consultations.aspx (accessed Apr 2025).
6. Curtis E, Jones R, Tipene-Leach D, et al. Why cultural safety rather than cultural competency is required to achieve health equity: a literature review and recommended definition. *Int J Equity Health* 2019; 18: 1–17.
7. Apunipima Cape York Health Council. Community primary health care consultations, Community Engagement, Apunipima Family Centered Model of Care. 2014. https://www.apunipima.org.au/model-of-care/ (accessed Jul 2025).
8. Walker R, Schultz CR, Sonn C. Cultural competence – transforming policy, services, programs and practice. In: Dudgeon P, Milroy H, Walker R, editors. Working together: Aboriginal and Torres Strait Islander mental health and wellbeing principles and practice. Commonwealth of Australia, 2014: 195–220.
9. Australian Health Ministers' Advisory Council. Cultural respect framework 2016–2026 for Aboriginal and Torres Strait Islander health. 2016. https://apo.org.au/node/256721 (accessed Apr 2025).
10. Brascoupé S, Waters C. Cultural safety – exploring the applicability of the concept of cultural safety to Aboriginal health and community wellness. *J Aborig Health* 2009; 5: 6–41.
11. Indigenous Allied Health Australia. Cultural responsiveness in action framework. https://iaha.com.au/workforce-support/training-and-development/cultural-responsiveness-in-action-training/ (accessed Jul 2025).
12. Commonwealth of Australia. National Aboriginal and Torres Strait Islander health plan 2021–2031. 2021. https://www.health.gov.au/resources/publications/national-aboriginal-and-torres-strait-islander-health-plan-2021-2031 (accessed Apr 2025).
13. Parker R, Milroy H. Schizophrenia and related psychosis in Aboriginal and Torres Strait Islander people. *Aboriginal and Islander Health Worker Journal* 2003; 27: 17–19.
14. Medical Council of New Zealand. Statement on cultural safety. MCNZ, 2019. https://www.mcnz.org.nz/our-standards/current-standards/cultural-safety/ (accessed Apr 2025).
15. Nursing Council of New Zealand. Guidelines for cultural safety, the Treaty of Waitangi and Māori health in nursing education and practice. Wellington (NZ): 2011. https://www.nursingcouncil.org.nz/Public/NCNZ/About-section/Cultural_Safety_Guidelines.aspx (accessed Apr 2025).
16. Royal Australasian College of Physicians. Indigenous strategic framework 2018-2028. Australia: RACP, 2018. https://www.racp.edu.au/about/board-and-governance/governance-documents/indigenous-strategic-framework-2018-2028 (accessed Apr 2025).

17. Royal Australasian College of Surgeons. Surgical competence and performance. East Melbourne (VIC): RACS, 2020. https://www.surgeons.org/-/media/Project/RACS/surgeons-org/files/Louise-Pfrunder/Surgical-Competence-and-Performance-Framework_V16.pdf (accessed Apr 2025).
18. Royal Australian College of General Practitioners. Standards for general practices 5th edition. East Melbourne (VIC): RACGP, 2020. https://www.racgp.org.au/running-a-practice/practice-standards/standards-5th-edition/standards-for-general-practices-5th-ed/table-of-contents (accessed Apr 2025).
19. Commonwealth of Australia, Department of the Prime Minister and Cabinet. National Agreement on Closing the Gap. Canberra, 2020. https://www.closingthegap.gov.au/national-agreement/national-agreement-closing-the-gap (accessed Apr 2025).
20. Green M, Cunningham J, Anderson K, et al. Measuring health care experiences that matter to Indigenous people in Australia with cancer: identifying critical gaps in existing tools. *Int J Equity Health* 2021; 20: 1–10.
21. Lock M, Williams M, Lloyd-Haynes A, et al. Are cultural safety definitions culturally safe? A review of 42 cultural safety definitions in an Australian cultural concept soup. Research Square, 2021.
22. Australian Institute of Health and Welfare. Cultural safety in health care for Indigenous Australians: monitoring framework. Canberra: AIHW, 2023. https://www.aihw.gov.au/reports/indigenous-australians/cultural-safety-health-care-framework (accessed Apr 2025).
23. Elvidge E, Paradies Y, Aldrich R, Holder C. Cultural safety in hospitals: validating an empirical measurement tool to capture the Aboriginal patient experience. *Aust Health Rev* 2020; 44: 205–211.
24. Bureau of Health Information. Development report – Aboriginal patient experience question set. NSW: BHI, 2020. https://www.bhi.nsw.gov.au/topics/aboriginal-patient-experience (accessed Apr 2025).
25. Gee G, Dudgeon P, Schultz C, et al. Aboriginal and Torres Strait Islander social and emotional wellbeing. In: Dudgeon P, Milroy H, Walker R, editors. Working together: Aboriginal and Torres Strait Islander mental health and wellbeing principles and practice. Canberra: Commonwealth of Australia, 2014: 55–68.
26. Transforming Indigenous Mental Health and Wellbeing Project. Social and Emotional Gathering Report: 30-31st March 2021. The University of Western Australia, 2021. https://timhwb.org.au/blog/2021/05/01/social-and-emotional-wellbeing-gathering-march-2021/ (accessed Aug 2025).
27. Zubrick SR, Shepherd CCJ, Dudgeon P, et al. Social determinants of social and emotional wellbeing. In: Dudgeon P, Milroy H, Walker R, editors. Working together: Aboriginal and Torres Strait Islander mental health and wellbeing principles and practice. Canberra: Commonwealth of Australia, 2014: 93–112.
28. Dudgeon W, Wright M, Paradies Y, et al. Aboriginal social, cultural and historical contexts. In: Dudgeon P, Milroy H, Walker R, editors. Working together: Aboriginal and Torres Strait Islander mental health and wellbeing principles and practice. Canberra: Commonwealth of Australia, 2014: 3–24.
29. Milroy H, Dudgeon P, Walker R. Community life and development programs–Pathways to healing. In: Dudgeon P, Milroy H, Walker R, editors. Working together: Aboriginal and Torres Strait Islander mental health and wellbeing principles and practice. Canberra: Commonwealth of Australia, 2014: 419–436.
30. Raphael B, Swan P, Martinek N. Intergenerational aspects of trauma for Australian Aboriginal people. In Danieli Y, editor. International handbook of multigenerational legacies of trauma. New York (USA): Springer, 1998: 327–339.
31. Atkinson J, Nelson J, Atkinson C. Trauma, transgenerational transfer and effects on community wellbeing. In: Dudgeon P, Milroy H, Walker R, editors. Working together: Aboriginal and Torres Strait Islander mental health and wellbeing principles and practice. Canberra: Commonwealth of Australia, 2014: 135–144.
32. National Inquiry into the Separation of Aboriginal and Torres Strait Islander Children from their Families (Australia), Wilson RD. Bringing them home: Report of the national inquiry into the separation of Aboriginal and Torres Strait Islander children from their families. Sydney, Australia: Human Rights and Equal Opportunity Commission, 1997.
33. Menzies K. Understanding the Australian Aboriginal experience of collective, historical and intergenerational trauma. *International Social Work* 2019; 62: 1522–1534.
34. Chandler MJ, Lalonde CE. Cultural continuity as a protective factor against suicide in First Nations youth. *Horizons* 2008; 10: 68–72.
35. Marmot M. Social determinants of health inequalities. *The Lancet* 2005; 365: 1099–1104.
36. Marmot M. Social determinants and the health of Indigenous Australians. *Med J Aust* 2011; 194: 512–513.

37. Australian Institute of Health and Welfare. Australia's health 2024: in brief. Canberra: AIHW, 2024. https://www.aihw.gov.au/reports/australias-health/australias-health-2024-in-brief/summary (accessed Apr 2025).
38. Australian Institute of Health and Welfare. Rural and remote health. Canberra: AIHW, 2024. https://www.aihw.gov.au/reports/rural-remote-australians/rural-and-remote-health (accessed Apr 2025).
39. Australian Bureau of Statistics. Estimates of Aboriginal and Torres Strait Islander Australians. Canberra: ABS, 2021. https://www.abs.gov.au/statistics/people/aboriginal-and-torres-strait-islander-peoples/estimates-aboriginal-and-torres-strait-islander-australians/latest-release (accessed Apr 2025).
40. Australian Bureau of Statistics. Population projections, Australia, 2022 (base)—2071. Canberra: ABS, 2023. https://www.abs.gov.au/statistics/people/population/population-projections-australia/latest-release (accessed Apr 2025).
41. Australian Institute of Health and Welfare. Profile of First Nations people. Canberra: AIHW, 2024. https://www.aihw.gov.au/reports/australias-welfare/profile-of-indigenous-australians (accessed Apr 2025).
42. Australian Institute of Health and Welfare. Aboriginal and Torres Strait Islander Health Performance Framework – Summary report 2025. https://www.indigenoushpf.gov.au/report-overview/overview/summary-report/2-demographic-and-social-context (accessed Jul 2025).
43. Milroy HW, Watson M, Kashyap S, Dudgeon P. First Nations People and the law. *Australian Bar Review* 2021; 50: 510-522.
44. Australian Institute of Health and Welfare. Health and wellbeing of First Nations people. Canberra: AIHW, 2024. https://www.aihw.gov.au/reports/australias-health/indigenous-health-and-wellbeing (accessed Apr 2025).
45. Azzopardi PS, Sawyer SM, Carlin JB, et al. Health and wellbeing of Indigenous adolescents in Australia: a systematic synthesis of population data. *The Lancet* 2018; 391: 766–782.
46. Australian Institute of Health and Welfare. Aboriginal and Torres Strait Islander health performance framework 2020 summary report. Cat. no. IHPF 2. Canberra: AIHW, 2020.
47. Australian Bureau of Statistics. National Aboriginal and Torres Strait Islander health survey (2018–19). Canberra: ABS, 2019. https://www.abs.gov.au/statistics/people/aboriginal-and-torres-strait-islander-peoples/national-aboriginal-and-torres-strait-islander-health-survey/2018-19 (accessed Apr 2025).
48. Fogarty W, Lovell M, Langenberg J, Heron M-J. Deficit discourse and strengths-based approaches: Changing the narrative of Aboriginal and Torres Strait Islander health and wellbeing. Melbourne (VIC): The Lowitja Institute, 2018.
49. Dudgeon P, Bray A, Walker R. Self-determination and strengths-based Aboriginal and Torres Strait Islander suicide prevention: an emerging evidence-based approach. In Page AC, Stritzke WGK, editors. Alternatives to suicide. Academic Press, 2020: 237–256.
50. Cunningham J, Paradies YC. Patterns and correlates of self-reported racial discrimination among Australian Aboriginal and Torres Strait Islander adults, 2008–09: analysis of national survey data. *Int J Equity Health* 2013: 12: 1–15.
51. Australians for Native Title and Reconciliation. Health equality. Sydney (NSW): ANTaR, 2024. https://antar.org.au/issues/closing-the-gap/health-equality (accessed Apr 2025).
52. Cass A, Lowell A, Christie M, et al. Sharing the true stories: improving communication between Aboriginal patients and healthcare workers. *Med J Aust* 2002; 176: 466–470.
53. Dietsch E, Martin T, Shackleton P, et al. Australian Aboriginal kinship: a means to enhance maternal well-being. *Women Birth* 2011; 24: 58–64.
54. Mackean T, Withall E, Dwyer J, Wilson A. Role of Aboriginal Health Workers and Liaison Officers in quality care in the Australian acute care setting: a systematic review. *Aust Health Rev* 2020; 44: 427–433.
55. Panaretto KS, Wenitong M, Button S, Ring IT. Aboriginal community controlled health services: leading the way in primary care. *Med J Aust* 2014; 200: 649–652.
56. Mackean T, Fisher M, Friel S, Baum F. A framework to assess cultural safety in Australian public policy. *Health Promot Int* 2020; 35: 340–351.
57. Department of Health. Aboriginal and Torres Strait Islander cultural safety framework: Part 1. Victoria: Victorian Government Department of Health, 2021. https://www.health.vic.gov.au/publications/aboriginal-and-torres-strait-islander-cultural-safety-framework-part-1 (accessed Apr 2025).

58. Paradies Y, Ben J, Denson N, et al. Racism as a determinant of health: a systematic review and meta-analysis. *PloS One* 2015; 10: e0138511.
59. Kairuz CA, Casanelia LM, Bennett-Brook K, et al. Impact of racism and discrimination on physical and mental health among Aboriginal and Torres Strait islander peoples living in Australia: a systematic scoping review. *BMC Public Health* 2021; 21: 1302.
60. Reconciliation Action Plan (RAP). Demonstrating inclusive and respectful language. Reconciliation Australia, 2018. https://www.reconciliation.org.au/wp-content/uploads/2018/05/language-guide.pdf (accessed Apr 2025).
61. The LIME Network. LIME accreditation tools for specialist medical colleges. Melbourne (VIC): LIME Network, 2018. https://limenetwork.net.au/colleges-hub/accreditation-tool (accessed Apr 2025).
62. Department of the Prime Minister and Cabinet. National strategic framework for Aboriginal and Torres Strait Islander peoples' mental health and social and emotional wellbeing 2017–2023. Canberra: National Indigenous Australians Agency, 2017. https://www.niaa.gov.au/resource-centre/national-strategic-framework-aboriginal-and-torres-strait-islander-peoples-mental (accessed Apr 2025).
63. Bond C, Brough M, Willis J, et al. Beyond the pipeline: a critique of the discourse surrounding the development of an Indigenous primary healthcare workforce in Australia. *Aust J Prim Health* 2019; 25: 389–394.
64. Deroy S, Schütze H. Factors supporting retention of aboriginal health and wellbeing staff in Aboriginal health services: A comprehensive review of the literature. *Int J Equity Health* 2019; 18: 70.
65. Australian Indigenous Doctors' Association. Report on the findings of the 2016 AIDA member survey on bullying, racism and lateral violence in the workplace. AIDA, 2017. https://aida.org.au/app/uploads/2021/01/Report-on-AIDA-Member-Survey_Final.pdf (accessed Apr 2025).
66. Taylor EV, Lalovic A, Thompson SC. Beyond enrolments: a systematic review exploring the factors affecting the retention of Aboriginal and Torres Strait Islander health students in the tertiary education system. *Int J Equity Health* 2019; 18: 1–19.
67. Kimberley Aboriginal Health Planning Forum. A cultural security framework for Kimberley mental health/social and emotional well-being and alcohol and other drug services. https://kahpf.org.au/cultural-security-framework (accessed Apr 2025).
68. Congress of Aboriginal and Torres Strait Islander Nurses and Midwives. Murra Mullangari: Introduction to cultural safety and cultural humility. CATSINaM, 2022. https://catsinam.org.au/murramullangari (accessed Apr 2025).
69. Laverty M, McDermott DR, Calma T. Embedding cultural safety in Australia's main health care standards. *Med J Aust* 2017; 207: 15–16.
70. Government of Western Australia. New Mental Health Act benefits regional WA. 2015. https://www.wa.gov.au/government/media-statements/Barnett%20Liberal%20National%20Government/New-Mental-Health-Act-benefits-regional-WA-20151130 (accessed Apr 2025).
71. Marrie H. A matrix for identifying, measuring and monitoring institutional racism within public hospitals and health services. CQUniversity; 2014. https://hdl.handle.net/10018/1254540 (accessed Apr 2025).

Further reading

Department of Health. Aboriginal and Torres Strait Islander cultural safety framework: Cultural safety continuum reflective tool. Victoria: Victorian Government Department of Health, 2021. https://www.health.vic.gov.au/publications/aboriginal-and-torres-strait-islander-cultural-safety-framework-part-1

Medical Deans Australia and New Zealand. Indigenous health strategy 2021-2025. Sydney (NSW): MDANZ, 2021. https://medicaldeans.org.au/indigenous-health/

NSW Department of Education. Racism. No way! NSW, 2000. https://racismnoway.com.au

Royal Australian College of General Practitioners, National Aboriginal Community Controlled Health Organisation. Supporting effective, culturally safe primary healthcare: NACCHO-RACGP Resource Hub. https://www.racgp.org.au/the-racgp/faculties/aboriginal-and-torres-strait-islander-health/guides/cultural-safety

Royal Australian College of General Practitioners, National Aboriginal Community Controlled Health Organisation. NACCHO RACGP Good practice tables. RACGP/NACCHO, 2022. https://www.racgp.org.au/the-racgp/faculties/aboriginal-and-torres-strait-islander-health/guides/naccho-racgp-good-practice-tables

Royal Australian College of General Practitioners. An introduction to Aboriginal and Torres Strait Islander health cultural protocols and perspectives. South Melbourne (VIC): RACGP, 2012. https://www.racgp.org.au/the-racgp/faculties/aboriginal-and-torres-strait-islander-health/guides

Transforming Indigenous Mental Health and Wellbeing Project. The Dance of Life. University of Western Australia, 2022. https://doi.org./10.5281/zenodo.10042685

18 People with mental illness and the law

Roy Donnelly

Introduction

Although psychiatrists and other mental health professionals have specialised knowledge and skill in the care of patients with mental illness, all practising doctors should be capable of recognising a serious mental illness or disorder. Legislation in all states and territories provides that any medical practitioner may authorise the temporary detention of a person who meets relevant mental health criteria, pending a more comprehensive assessment by a specialist psychiatrist. It is therefore important that doctors be broadly familiar with the principles of mental health law, particularly the criteria upon which they may authorise the detention of patients.

Doctors hold substantial powers under mental health laws to require detention and assessment of persons with mental health conditions. These powers are a significant impingement upon a person's normal rights of freedom and consent. It is therefore important that doctors are familiar and compliant with the legal processes that exist to make sure those powers are exercised fairly, properly and within the scope of the law.

All Australian states and territories have specific legislation governing the care of patients with mental illness. The relevant Acts are listed in Table 18.1. The basic aims and principles of the various Acts are similar, but there are considerable differences of detail, particularly in the procedural aspects and terminologies adopted.

Mental health legislation is frequently updated. In particular, reviews are underway to reform mental health laws to provide greater protection of individual rights and ensure patients have input into their care and treatment wherever possible.

This chapter provides an overview of the general principles of mental health laws across Australia. This chapter should not be relied on as an authoritative guide to the details of the legislation in each state or territory.

Table 18.1 State-based mental health legislation and mental health review tribunals

State or territory	Legislation	Tribunal
New South Wales	*Mental Health Act 2007*	Mental Health Review Tribunal (http://www.mhrt.nsw.gov.au)
Victoria	*Mental Health and Wellbeing Act 2022*	Mental Health Tribunal (https://www.mht.vic.gov.au)
Queensland	*Mental Health Act 2016*	Mental Health Review Tribunal (http://www.mhrt.qld.gov.au)
South Australia	*Mental Health Act 2009*	South Australian Civil and Administrative Tribunal (https://www.sacat.sa.gov.au/case-type/mental-health)
Western Australia	*Mental Health Act 2014*	Mental Health Tribunal (https://www.mht.wa.gov.au)
Tasmania	*Mental Health Act 2013*	Tasmanian Civil and Administrative Tribunal (https://www.tascat.tas.gov.au/mental-health)
Northern Territory	*Mental Health and Related Services Act 1998*	Mental Health Review Tribunal (https://nt.gov.au/law/courts-and-tribunals/mental-health-review-tribunal)
Australian Capital Territory	*Mental Health Act 2015*	ACT Civil and Administrative Tribunal (https://www.acat.act.gov.au/case-types/mental-health-cases)

18.1 Definition of mental illness

Mental health laws in each state and territory include a definition of the term 'mental illness'. However, the definition is not uniform across jurisdictions. For example, in New South Wales, the *Mental Health Act 2007* (NSW) defines mental illness as follows:

> Mental illness means a condition that seriously impairs, either temporarily or permanently, the mental functioning of a person and is characterised by the presence in the person of any one or more of the following symptoms—
>
> (a) delusions,
>
> (b) hallucinations,
>
> (c) serious disorder of thought form,
>
> (d) a severe disturbance of mood,
>
> (e) sustained or repeated irrational behaviour indicating the presence of any one or more of the symptoms referred to in paragraphs (a)–(d) [1].

The Australian Capital Territory and the Northern Territory have almost identical definitions. The other states have definitions that are similar in concept, being focused on conditions that cause disturbances of thought, mood, perception or other cognitive processes, such as memory or orientation. In South Australia, the Mental Health Act 2009 (SA) has a broad definition that simply states: '"mental illness" means any illness or disorder of the mind' [2].

The legislation of some states and territories includes an additional definition for persons who do not have a mental illness but who exhibit certain disturbances of their mind, or whose behaviour is sufficiently irrational to justify detaining them against their will. These additional definitions include 'mentally disordered' (NSW) [3], 'mental disorder' (the ACT) [4] and 'mental disturbance or complex cognitive impairment' (the NT) [5].

All jurisdictions declare certain criteria or circumstances that cannot of themselves be used as the basis for making a definition of mental illness. These include:

- expressions of particular political, religious or cultural beliefs
- sexual preferences or orientation
- participation in immoral or illegal conduct
- a developmental, intellectual or physical disability
- use of alcohol or any other drugs
- having a personality disorder
- engaging in antisocial behaviour [6].

18.2 Voluntary admission

Most patients admitted for mental health care are admitted on a voluntary basis—that is, at the patient's request or with their consent. Voluntary patients are afforded the same rights as a person admitted to a general hospital for medical or surgical treatment.

The legal principles for voluntary admission will not be considered further here, other than to make two comments. First, where safe and clinically appropriate, voluntary admission is preferred, to avoid both impinging upon a person's rights and the potential legal implications of having a past involuntary admission on a person's clinical record. Second, if a person is admitted as a voluntary patient but their mental health deteriorates, the admission may be converted to an involuntary one, provided the appropriate requirements for involuntary admission are met.

18.3 Involuntary admission

Mental health legislation in all states and territories provides broadly similar criteria for involuntary admission and detention of patients, but with significant differences in terminology and procedures.

18.3.1 Criteria governing involuntary admission

The general criteria that need to be met in all states and territories to authorise detention, assessment, involuntary admission, and mental health treatment may be broadly summarised as follows:

- The person is considered likely to be at risk of harming themselves or others if not detained for assessment or treatment.
- The risk of harm arises because of the presence of a mental illness or other mental condition as defined in the legislation of the relevant state or territory (i.e. a person cannot be detained under mental health legislation for dangerous or objectionable behaviour that falls outside of behaviour consistent with mental illness or other defined mental disturbances).

- In many jurisdictions, the person must be assessed as lacking the capacity to consent to appropriate mental health treatment.
- No treatment of a less restrictive basis is available, and any restrictions placed on the person must be the minimum necessary for the safe and effective care of the person (e.g. a mandatory community treatment order, rather than inpatient admission, should be considered where appropriate).

18.3.2 Presentation of a person with mental illness for review

Requests to review a person for possible mental illness may come from the person themselves or from the person's carer, relative or friend, or someone with an interest in or concern about the person [7].

The various state and territory Acts authorise certain people to arrange for the transportation of a person who may require acute mental health review to a relevant health facility. Police officers and ambulance officers are generally granted authority to transport people who appear to be mentally ill and in need of review to a hospital or other authorised location for assessment under the relevant mental health Act [8–11].

Judicial officers, such as magistrates, may also refer an accused person for mental health review if they determine the person may have a mental illness [12,13].

18.3.3 Procedures for assessment and involuntary admission of patients with mental illness by medical practitioners

Each state and territory has developed its own complex laws to define the procedures for detaining, assessing and treating persons as involuntary mental health patients. It is beyond the scope of this chapter to describe each of these laws in detail.

There may be additional considerations for Aboriginal and/or Torres Strait Islander people (see the *Mental Health Act 2014* [WA] and Chapter 17, Culturally safe health care for Aboriginal and/or Torres Strait Islander peoples, for further details). However, with respect to the role of medical practitioners, each law has a similar framework, as follows.

Initial review and referral for assessment

The mental health Acts provide for a medical practitioner to compulsorily examine and detain a person and have the person transported to an authorised mental health facility for examination by a psychiatrist. The medical practitioner must find that the person meets the relevant criteria (as described in section 18.3.1) for involuntary admission; in particular, that the person is likely at risk of harming themselves or others because of the presence of a mental illness (or, in some jurisdictions, another defined mental disturbance).

The medical practitioner must make the assessment based on their own observations but may rely on reports of others about the person's behaviour, where appropriate. They must document the assessment under the required rules in each jurisdiction; this generally requires completion of a formal certificate or other prescribed document.

Time limits apply to the validity of assessment orders or recommendations for review, after which they cease to have effect. The time limits can vary from 24 hours to 14 days, depending on the jurisdiction and the basis of the order.

The specific procedures are defined differently in each jurisdiction's mental health Act, as are the definitions and terminology used. The following is provided as a broad overview:

- **In NSW**, the process allows a person to 'be taken to and detained in a declared mental health facility on the basis of a certificate about the person's condition issued by a medical practitioner or accredited person' [14].
- **In Victoria** and **Tasmania**, the process requires the making of an assessment order, which authorises examination of the person and, if required, referral to an authorised mental health facility for assessment by a psychiatrist [15,16].
- **In Queensland**, the *Public Health Act 2005* (Qld) authorises the assessment of a person whom the police or ambulance officers have made subject to an emergency examination authority. A medical practitioner may examine such a person to assess whether a recommendation for assessment by a psychiatrist under the *Mental Health Act 2016* (Qld) is required [17].
- **In SA**, the process is known as making a level 1 inpatient treatment order, which authorises a person to receive involuntary inpatient mental health treatment, pending review by a psychiatrist or authorised medical practitioner.
- **In Western Australia**, a medical practitioner may refer a person for examination by a psychiatrist if they reasonably suspect the person meets the criteria for an involuntary treatment order [18].
- **In the NT**, a medical practitioner makes a recommendation for psychiatric examination based upon the person meeting the required criteria [19].
- **In the ACT**, a medical practitioner is authorised to 'apprehend a person' and take the person 'to an approved mental health facility' if they believe on reasonable grounds that the person meets the relevant criteria [8].

Despite similarities in the criteria and broad principles applied, there is little uniformity in the procedures and terminology used between states and territories. Medical practitioners therefore need to be aware of the particular rules and procedures that apply in their jurisdiction.

Psychiatrist review

Following authorisation for initial detention and assessment, the person will need to be assessed by a psychiatrist or other approved practitioner in an authorised mental health facility. The aim of this assessment is to determine whether the patient requires involuntary admission and/or mental health treatment. Where this is the case, in general the psychiatrist can authorise involuntary admission and, where clinically required, treatment, pending formal review by the relevant mental health tribunal (see next subsection).

As with the initial review and referral phase, there is great variability in the procedures and terminology used between jurisdictions. In general, the decision to admit a person for involuntary care and treatment is based on the assessment of at least two independent medical practitioners, one of whom must be a psychiatrist or equivalently recognised mental health specialist medical practitioner. However, the legal requirements and procedures for authorising involuntary admission differ significantly between states and territories. Medical practitioners need to be aware of the particular procedures and referral pathways that apply to their jurisdiction. A brief summary of the procedures in each state and territory is as follows:

- **In NSW**, an assessment as to whether the person meets the relevant criteria for involuntary admission must be undertaken at the declared mental health facility by two authorised medical officers, one of whom must be a psychiatrist [20].
- **In Victoria**, an authorised psychiatrist must assess a person subject to an assessment order (an 'assessment patient') to determine whether they meet the criteria for a temporary treatment order [21].

- **In Tasmania**, an approved medical practitioner (psychiatrist or other approved mental health doctor) must confirm that the person referred under an assessment order meets the treatment criteria, then apply to the tribunal for a treatment order. However, where no prior assessment order was made, two approved medical practitioners must confirm the person meets the required criteria [22].
- **In the ACT**, two psychiatrists or another relevant doctor working in consultation with a psychiatrist (as defined in the Act) must both assess the person and determine that the relevant criteria for involuntary admission and treatment are met [23].
- **In Queensland**, an authorised doctor must assess a patient referred for assessment to determine if they meet the treatment criteria for involuntary admission and, if so, make a treatment authority for the person [24].
- **In SA**, a psychiatrist or authorised medical practitioner may make a level 2 inpatient treatment order for a patient already under a level 1 order made by another practitioner [25].
- **In WA**, a psychiatrist must assess the person at the mental health facility to ascertain if they meet the criteria for involuntary admission—alternatively, the psychiatrist may request a further examination of the patient to confirm the need for involuntary admission [26].
- **In the NT**, a person detained at a mental health facility under the authority of a doctor (or other authorised health practitioner) must be assessed by an authorised psychiatric practitioner to determine if they meet the criteria for involuntary admission [27].

Each jurisdiction places time limits on how soon the person must be assessed by a psychiatrist or other relevant doctor after being taken to a mental health facility. These are generally very short, ranging from 4 hours to 24 hours; however, extensions may be authorised where provided for in the relevant legislation. There are requirements for ongoing and regular psychiatry reviews while the person remains an involuntary patient.

Mental health tribunal review and supervision

Every state and territory has a form of mental health tribunal that is responsible for the authorisation and supervision of persons requiring involuntary admission and treatment for mental health conditions (see Table 18.1). The tribunals generally comprise legal practitioners, psychiatrists and consumer representatives.

The authority provided to medical practitioners (including psychiatrists) to detain and treat persons on an involuntary basis is temporary. The ultimate authority to continue detention and involuntary mental health treatment rests with the relevant mental health tribunal.

All persons admitted for involuntary mental health treatment under the authority of a psychiatrist or other doctor must be notified to the relevant mental health tribunal. The mental health tribunal has an obligation to hold a hearing to authorise the continued involuntary admission and treatment of such persons. Hearings are required to occur within defined time frames that vary widely between jurisdictions. For example, in NSW, 'the person must be brought before the Tribunal as soon as practicable' after their admission to a mental health facility [28]. By contrast, in Victoria, the tribunal hearing must occur before the expiry of the initial psychiatry order authorising involuntary admission and treatment (the temporary treatment order), which occurs 28 days after it was made [29].

Where a tribunal has authorised ongoing involuntary admission and treatment, the mental health Acts require the tribunal to regularly review and renew the orders, usually at six-monthly intervals. The supervising psychiatrists are also required to undertake regular reviews of the person's progress and their need for continued involuntary admission. If a person no longer meets the criteria for involuntary admission, the orders for involuntary admission are revoked. However, if clinically indicated, the patient may consent to remain under a voluntary admission.

Patients, their family or representatives may appeal to the relevant tribunal with respect to the making of an involuntary treatment order or other aspects of the patient's care and treatment. An appeal or review procedure to protect patients' rights is legislated in all states and territories and can be accessed by patients, their representatives or official community visitors.

18.3.4 Authorised treatment locations

The mental health Acts generally provide that the involuntary admission and treatment of persons who have a mental illness can only occur within 'authorised' or 'designated' mental health facilities. These facilities are required to meet certain standards and be subject to various assessments and inspections, such as inspections by regulatory authorities and mental health advocates.

Purpose-built mental health units treating involuntary patients in the public or private sector are required to be authorised. Public hospital emergency departments are usually defined as an authorised facility for the purpose of initial assessment and detention, as are some other public hospital locations. In some cases, where a person under an involuntary admission requires transfer to a general hospital for treatment, diagnostic tests or surgery not available in the psychiatric hospital, involuntary detention orders may be extended to general hospital care.

As described above, there are time limits by which the person must be transferred to an authorised location for psychiatric assessment and, if appropriate, involuntary admission. Doctors need to be aware of the particular requirements in their state or territory, especially if considering the need for detention of persons with mental illness outside public hospitals or defined mental health facilities.

18.4 Community treatment orders

A person may be placed under a community treatment order when they are able to live in the community, but they must comply with certain obligations, such as attending regular mental health reviews and adhering to prescribed treatment. A community treatment order is still a form of involuntary treatment, but one which does not require detention in a mental health facility. Consistent with the obligation to provide care on the least restrictive basis, psychiatrists must consider whether a community treatment order is a suitable option before recommending a person be admitted as an involuntary inpatient.

The making of a community treatment order generally requires:

- a diagnosis of a mental illness requiring the use of compulsory treatment
- an assessment that neither the patient nor the community is at serious physical risk if the patient is not detained in a mental health facility
- a structure or organisation that enables monitoring of the patient's treatment.

If the person does not comply with the community treatment order, it may be revoked, and the person admitted to hospital as an involuntary inpatient.

18.5 Patients in the forensic mental health system

Forensic mental health is concerned with the management of persons with mental illness who come into contact with the criminal justice system. This includes persons who have been charged with criminal offences and those already convicted and serving a custodial sentence. It is also concerned with the care and treatment of persons detained in forensic mental health facilities for commission of a crime for which they are not legally responsible, by reason of mental illness.

A high proportion of persons who come into contact with the criminal justice system have some form of mental illness or cognitive impairment. States and territories have specific laws that govern patients in the forensic mental health system; these laws account for the particular circumstances and risks raised by the management of these patients. They include procedures to facilitate diversion of people from the criminal justice system for mental health assessment and treatment where this is deemed more appropriate, as well as governing the provision of mental health services to persons in custody.

It is beyond the scope of this chapter to describe these laws in detail. Medical practitioners should be aware of the need to seek specialist forensic psychiatry advice regarding treatment options for persons with mental illness who have come into contact with the criminal justice system.

18.6 Electroconvulsive therapy and other restricted or prohibited treatments

18.6.1 Electroconvulsive therapy

Most mental health laws include specific sections governing the consent for and administration of electroconvulsive therapy (ECT) to persons with mental health conditions. In those jurisdictions, approval to perform ECT on minors or persons subject to involuntary treatment orders must be obtained from the relevant mental health tribunal [30–36].

18.6.2 Psychosurgery and neurosurgery

Psychosurgical or neurosurgical treatment for mental illness is prohibited in NSW and the NT [37,38]. In Victoria, Queensland, SA, WA, Tasmania and the ACT, there are specific provisions governing the use of psychosurgical or neurosurgical techniques to treat mental illness. The requirements are complex and vary between jurisdictions [39–44].

18.6.3 Other therapies

Discredited therapies, such as insulin-induced coma and deep-sleep therapy, are specifically prohibited in some state and territory mental health laws [45–48].

18.7 Use of seclusion and restraint

Most mental health laws include provisions regulating the use of either restraint or seclusion techniques for patients with mental illness. In addition, local policies that provide mandatory guidance and rules governing the use of such techniques often exist. The laws vary between jurisdictions but generally include a requirement that the use of these techniques must be deemed necessary to manage serious risks to the patient or staff, as well as requiring strict monitoring and supervision of patients subject to such orders.

18.8 Consent to non-psychiatric treatment

Involuntarily admitted patients may experience other non-psychiatric illnesses that require treatment. In seeking consent for such treatment, the doctor is entitled to, and should first, seek consent directly from the patient, as mental illness will not necessarily invalidate such consent.

Where valid consent cannot be obtained from the patient, the state or territory guardianship provisions will normally apply. However, some mental health laws contain specific provisions regarding consent for non-psychiatric treatment, which should be followed where relevant (see also Chapter 5, Communication in clinical practice, and Chapter 7, Consent and informed decision making) [49–52].

18.9 State-based resources to assist medical practitioners

All states and territories have resources available to assist and advise medical practitioners about the relevant mental health laws, including the processes for initiating involuntary assessment and admission where appropriate. These resources include various mental health crisis services, as well as consultant liaison psychiatry services in hospitals or public mental health services (see also Chapter 26, Medicolegal examinations and reports, court procedures and expert evidence, and Chapter 32, Legal frameworks: rights, responsibilities and protections).

It is beyond the scope of this chapter to provide contact details of such services. However, most are readily available from local public hospitals, through state and territory department of health websites and information services, or from local non-government mental health and crisis support services.

Summary

All practising doctors need to be capable of recognising serious mental illness and understanding the fundamentals of the laws relating to detention and assessment of persons with mental health conditions. These laws vary in their details between jurisdictions, and this chapter has provided an overview of some of the main differences, particularly relating to the definition of mental illness and the procedures to be followed if a doctor assesses that a person is at risk of harming themselves or others if not detained for assessment or treatment of a mental illness. The chapter has also covered the basics of community treatment orders and the management of forensic patients with mental illness who have come into contact with the criminal justice system. Laws governing the administration of ECT and other therapies are summarised, and medical practitioners are made aware of the resources available in each state and territory to advise and assist them with the relevant mental health laws in that jurisdiction.

References

1. *Mental Health Act 2007 (NSW)*, s 4.
2. *Mental Health Act 2009* (SA), s 3.
3. *Mental Health Act 2007* (NSW), s 15.
4. *Mental Health Act 2015* (ACT), s 6.
5. *Mental Health and Related Services Act 1998* (NT), ss 4, 6A(1), 15.
6. *Mental Health Act 2007* (NSW), s 16.
7. *Mental Health and Related Services Act 1998* (NT), s 32.
8. *Mental Health Act 2015* (ACT), s 80.
9. *Mental Health Act 2007* (NSW), ss 20, 22.
10. *Mental Health and Related Services Act 1998* (NT), ss 31, 32A.
11. *Mental Health Act 2014* (WA), s 156.

12. *Mental Health Act 2007* (NSW), ss 23, 24.
13. *Mental Health and Cognitive Impairment Forensic Provisions Act 2020* (NSW), ss 18, 19.
14. *Mental Health Act 2007* (NSW), s 19(1).
15. *Mental Health and Wellbeing Act 2022* (Vic), s 146.
16. *Mental Health Act 2013* (Tas), ss 24–26.
17. *Public Health Act 2005* (Qld), s 157F.
18. *Mental Health Act 2014* (WA), s 26.
19. *Mental Health and Related Services Act 1998* (NT), s 34.
20. *Mental Health Act 2007* (NSW), s 27.
21. *Mental Health and Wellbeing Act 2022* (Vic), ss 159, 180.
22. *Mental Health Act 2013* (Tas), s 37.
23. *Mental Health Act 2015* (ACT), ss 84, 85.
24. *Mental Health Act 2016* (Qld), s 43.
25. *Mental Health Act 2009* (SA), s 25.
26. *Mental Health Act 2014* (WA), ss 55, 56.
27. *Mental Health and Related Services Act 1998* (NT), ss 38, 39.
28. *Mental Health Act 2007* (NSW), s 27(1)(d).
29. *Mental Health and Wellbeing Act 2022* (Vic), s 183.
30. *Mental Health Act 2007* (NSW), Pt 2, Div 3.
31. *Mental Health and Wellbeing Act 2022* (Vic), Pt 3.5.
32. *Mental Health Act 2015* (ACT), Pt 9.2.
33. *Mental Health and Related Services Act 1998* (NT), Pt 9, Div 2.
34. *Mental Health Act 2016* (Qld), Ch 12, Pt 9, Div 1.
35. *Mental Health Act 2014* (WA), Pt 21, Div 6.
36. *Mental Health Act 2009* (SA), Pt 7, Div 1.
37. *Mental Health Act 2007* (NSW), s 83(1)(c).
38. *Mental Health and Related Services Act 1998* (NT), s 58(2).
39. *Mental Health and Wellbeing Act 2022* (Vic), Pt 3.6.
40. *Mental Health Act 2016* (Qld), Ch 12, Pt 9, Div 2.
41. *Mental Health Act 2009* (SA), Pt 7, Div 2.
42. *Mental Health Act 2014* (WA), Pt 21.
43. *Mental Health Act 2013* (Tas), Ch 2, Pt 6.
44. *Mental Health Act 2015* (ACT), Pt 9.3.
45. *Mental Health Act 2007* (NSW), s 83.
46. *Mental Health Act 2016* (QLD), s 240.
47. *Mental Health Act 2014* (WA), s 210.
48. *Mental Health and Related Services Act 1998* (NT), s 59.
49. *Mental Health Act 2007* (NSW), ss 99–109.
50. *Mental Health and Wellbeing Act 2022* (Vic), Pt 3.4.
51. *Mental Health and Related Services Act 1998* (NT), s 63.
52. *Mental Health Act 2014* (WA), s 242.

Further reading

Royal Australian and New Zealand College of Psychiatrists Mental health legislation Australia and Aotearoa New Zealand—Summary tables. https://www.ranzcp.org/clinical-guidelines-publications/in-focus-topics/mental-health-legislation

19 Advance care planning and end-of-life care

Will Cairns OAM

Introduction

Every one of us dies. While modern technology has been very successful in preventing and controlling illness in childhood and middle age, we have been remarkably unsuccessful in prolonging the lives of the elderly. Recent analysis suggests that we humans have a maximum possible biological life expectancy of about 87 years, on average [1]. Our genes do not include any possibility for us to live on indefinitely.

As these realities are gradually becoming recognised after more than a century of focus on life prolongation, our communities' expectations of what health care will provide for them are shifting and the roles of doctors are changing. Doctors are now expected to integrate care at the end of life into the mix of professional roles, ethical duties and legal obligations that comprise their good medical practice. While this can seem overwhelming and at odds with previous expectations, there are a few simple steps that can help doctors to incorporate the universality of mortality into their practice in the interests of their patients and the community at large.

- The first step is to embrace the fact that all lives are finite, including their own.
- The second is to accept that efforts to prolong peoples' lives do not always deliver a quality of life that would be acceptable to the person themselves.
- The third is to consider the reality that life prolongation will eventually become impossible for every patient, may not be desired by a patient, or may actually bring more harm than good.

Few of us question the need for competency in the skills that can prolong lives and sustain their quality. It seems obvious that we should also expect to maintain competency in the complementary skills necessary to recognise when further treatment is unlikely to be beneficial, to support wise decision making, and to provide care and support to those who are dying and their families.

Perhaps the most important skill that a doctor can bring to care at the end of life is to be able to communicate with compassion and humanity about the complexity of the issues that our patients are facing, and to acknowledge the emotions that are being generated as the natural human responses to loss and the threat of loss through death.

The current version (2020) of *Good medical practice: a code of conduct for doctors in Australia* [2] addresses many of these issues relating to care at the end of life:

> Doctors have a vital role in assisting the community to deal with the reality of death and its consequences. In caring for patients towards the end of their life, good medical practice involves:
>
> 4.13.1 Taking steps to manage a patient's symptoms and concerns in a manner consistent with their values and wishes.
>
> 4.13.2 Providing or arranging appropriate palliative care, including a multi-disciplinary approach whenever possible.
>
> 4.13.3 Understanding the limits of medicine in prolonging life and recognising when efforts to prolong life may not benefit the patient.
>
> 4.13.4 Understanding that you do not have a duty to try to prolong life at all cost. However, you have a duty to know when not to initiate and when to cease attempts at prolonging life, while ensuring that your patients receive appropriate relief from distress.
>
> 4.13.5 Accepting that patients have the right to refuse medical treatment or to request the withdrawal of treatment already started.
>
> 4.13.6 Respecting different cultural practices related to death and dying.
>
> 4.13.7 Striving to communicate effectively with patients and their families so they are able to understand the outcomes that can and cannot be achieved.
>
> 4.13.8 Encouraging advance care planning and facilitating the appropriate documentation, such as an advance care directive (or similar).
>
> 4.13.9 Taking reasonable steps to ensure that support is provided to patients and their families, even when it is not possible to deliver the outcome they seek.
>
> 4.13.10 Communicating bad news to patients and their families in the most appropriate way and providing support for them while they deal with this information.
>
> 4.13.11 When your patient dies, being willing to explain, to the best of your knowledge, the circumstances of the death to appropriate members of the patient's family and carers, unless you know the patient would have objected.
>
> 4.13.12 Sensitively discussing and encouraging organ and tissue donation with the patient's family, when appropriate and consistent with legislation and accepted protocols.

Finally, the nature of the guidance provided to doctors in this book, and in this chapter in particular, has continued to evolve rapidly over recent decades as a part of the evolution of our increasingly complex and culturally diverse community.

Medical professionalism is slowly disavowing paternalism (and male dominance), and doctors no longer control information and knowledge. Other than in emergencies, disasters and a limited range of special circumstances, doctors no longer simply decide on a course of action and impose it on their patients, or the community—we are collaborators. Doctors have become sources of advice and guidance about the choices that are possible and their likely consequences.

Medical ethics also continue to evolve in response to the changing expectations and values of our community in the face of the realities that medicine cannot always deliver benefits and that every life is finite. Medical ethics are also changing because there has been a rapid shift in attitudes towards individual decision making. The imposition of institutional, particularly religious, values onto patient choices is waning as the rights of individuals to make their own choices grows. This has been particularly evident in reproductive health and for end-of-life choices including voluntary assisted dying (VAD).

In the 21st century, Australia is a heterogeneous society comprising a great diversity of cultures and belief systems. Contemporary doctors should be prepared for dealing with, and respecting, significant variety in the responses of their patients and their families to death, dying, and the challenges of providing and receiving health care at the end of life. This chapter will discuss some of the issues that arise in the provision of end-of-life care.

19.1 Dealing with death as the normal end to every life

19.1.1 Understanding the normality of death

Doctors engage with patients and their families across the whole of life: from before conception through gestation, birth, childhood, growth, maturation, reproduction, ageing and death.

For doctors, developing the skills of effective communication for decision making at the end of life starts with introspection. A doctor who has reflected on their own mortality and carefully considered that their role as a clinician includes dealing with the inevitability of death will find it much easier to engage in care at the end of life and will be less vulnerable to personal distress when managing life-limiting illnesses in their patients.

Most doctors at the beginning of their training are uncomfortable dealing with the deaths of their patients, and commonly feel uncertain about contemplating their own mortality. Many people, doctors and their patients alike, struggle with the complexity of decision making about the use of modern high-tech medicine that, in spite of its great benefits, can at times result in prolongation of life with a significantly diminished quality of life and/or a long, drawn-out death.

It is only over the past hundred years that we have been very successful in avoiding premature death; death in old age has become the norm for most people in Australia. Unsurprisingly, it is for these more common deaths that we are most prepared, and this is the focus of most of this chapter. However, some people still die as infants or children from congenital or acquired illnesses, and accidents and misadventure can kill any of us at any time.

Over recent years, much of the conversation about death and dying has been in the domain of palliative care, which focuses on the final stages of peoples' lives. This ignores the reality that many of the more confronting conversations must be had, and the difficult decisions made, before care becomes palliative.

Doctors (and many other healthcare workers) across all fields of practice can find themselves expected to take on a broad range of roles in support of people who are facing life-limiting illnesses and expected death. They also need to consider how they might deal with the chaos and disorder of deaths that are unexpected, sudden and uncontrolled, whether they involve individuals and their families, or occur during disasters that cause multiple deaths in large communities.

Doctors need to consider the balance between their duties to provide treatment and prolong life where possible, and to relieve suffering in the face of the reality and normality of eventual death. Doctors must provide support for dying people and/or their bereaved family members, even when they find the circumstances of a death personally confronting. More experienced doctors have a duty as mentors to their colleagues to demonstrate how to open and lead the discussions with patients and families who need their doctor to talk about death and dying (see also Chapter 5, Communication in clinical practice).

Doctors who accept the inevitability of death find it easier to understand that they are not responsible when the treatments that they provide are not successful in preventing death, or why a patient may refuse a treatment that they have been offered.

Countless lives are prolonged by modern technologies. However, these advances have also brought with them challenging ethical and legal dilemmas for the medical profession, the community, legislators and the courts. The most common issues relate to the care of patients who lack decision-making capacity—particularly infants, children, those with severe illnesses or injuries, and older people with dementia and life-ending illnesses—for whom decisions about end-of-life care must be made by others. These challenges are made more difficult when deterioration has been rapid and unexpected, and where there has been no prior discussion of the possibility or the patient's wishes.

Good medical practice sometimes requires doctors to withhold or withdraw treatment that is desired by a patient, or their substitute decision maker, on the grounds that it will not bring the desired benefit of cure or life prolongation and/or is more likely to cause harm than bring good.

The potential for conflict in such situations can be averted or reduced by doctors who engage in early and open discussions with their patient about what might realistically be achieved and how this aligns with their hopes, wishes, goals and preferences. Advance care planning (ACP) must include clear and accessible documentation of the discussion and the resulting plan [3,4]. Doctors are encouraged to integrate discussions about death and dying into their routine interactions with well patients, including encouraging ACP that reflects the risks of sudden and unexpected death. As people grow older, or develop serious illness at any age, doctors should start to address the often-complex medical and personal issues around treatment decisions with honesty, openness and compassion, supporting and empowering patients and families to make informed choices.

Such conversations are particularly important for patients who are newly diagnosed with, or receiving treatment for, an illness that brings the very real possibility that it might cause death. Most patients who know their illness is serious are already considering challenges that they might face, including that they might die. Many are greatly relieved when their doctors are comfortable talking about mortality and assist their patients to engage in important decision making. When they are not, doctors may impede their patient from completing a range of tasks and/or fulfilling goals that are very important for both them and their family. Of course, some patients do not wish to address such issues and rebuff efforts to encourage them to do so, as is their right. Doctors should ensure that the patient knows that the door remains open to talk about these issues at a later date if the patient changes their mind.

Patients and their families commonly need appropriate guidance and care at the end of life. If a doctor feels they are unable to provide it themselves, they should refer their patient on to someone who can. Although dealing with death and dying can be emotional and difficult at times, the management of a successful engagement with a patient, their family and our colleagues in the transition to the acceptance and subsequent experience of a comfortable and peaceful death can be one of the most rewarding experiences of medical practice.

19.1.2 Personal self-care when dealing with death and dying

As one thoughtful palliative medicine trainee said at their periodic assessment:

> What I have found working in palliative care is that I have to use all parts of myself in my work, not just the technical. The challenge is to use everything you have, but not to use yourself up (anonymous, personal communication).

Like many people, doctors too have times when they struggle to find meaning in a finite life that ends in death. Frequently this emerges in late adolescence or young adulthood when we first face up to our own mortality, and that of our family and close friends. For some doctors (and other health practitioners) their first direct experience of a death is when one of their patients dies. This can pose a significant challenge for health practitioners, who are expected to deal with death as part of their day-to-day work.

Doctors in particular may face the added challenge of feeling responsible when one of their patients dies if they believe that they failed in their perceived duty to prevent a person's death, particularly when that death is a complication of treatment or the suicide of a patient they were treating. Sharing these challenges within their medical team decreases the sense of personal responsibility that doctors commonly feel for their patient's outcomes. Throughout their careers, doctors, their healthcare colleagues, and their patients will all benefit from active nurturing of the mutual support and common humanity by which they can help one another to cope with the challenges posed by dealing with death.

Sometimes doctors have difficulty making the personal transition from an all-out effort to prevent the death of their patient to a focus on the quality of their patient's life while dying. When doctors struggle, patients and their families may not receive the support they need, or perhaps even find their own journey obstructed.

A singular focus on the *quantity* of life may result in a diminished *quality* of life, even to the point that a patient (and/or their family) may perceive their life to have a negative quality. One of the core tasks of preparing for the role of doctor, both for teachers and learners, is to foster a culture that both strives to prolong life and accepts the inevitability of death at the end of every life.

Doctors commonly address this challenge successfully from within their personal relationships and belief systems, including religious beliefs and cultural beliefs. Many doctors also find great benefit from engaging with outside professional supports through reflective practice, peer supervision and participation in communities of practice. However they address these issues, many acknowledge that having done so makes them better doctors.

19.1.3 Learning to communicate about death and dying

One of the more difficult tasks for doctors is what is commonly described as 'breaking bad news' to patients and their families. Developing the skills to engage in considered and sensitive conversations and communicate openly, candidly, honestly and compassionately about matters of life and death is a necessary first step for doctors aiming to provide the best possible care at the end of life. It is one of the core responsibilities of good medical practice.

Few doctors do not feel at least some trepidation as they approach a patient and/or their family to convey confronting information and discuss issues of care at the end of life. Anxiety is an understandable and normal response in anticipation of a conversation that may cause distress for several reasons. Doctors may be challenged by the emotional responses of their patient and/or their family, and those of other healthcare workers who may be present. They may feel that their own views of themselves as healers are being challenged. Cultural differences between the doctor and their patient may result in challenges to their ability to provide information. Doctors may also be personally distressed by the information and its consequences for the patient and their family, and such news may also trigger an emotional response to a loss in the doctor's personal life and cause them to reflect on their own mortality.

Sometimes doctors take refuge behind an emotional wall that can make them seem unfeeling. At the other end of the spectrum, when doctors become too emotionally connected, they may find themselves unable to provide the wise counsel and support that the patient and their family need. Somewhere in between is a state that acknowledges the emotion of the situation, including the doctor's own responses, and yet leaves them able to continue to provide support and carefully considered, evidence-based and wise advice.

Other than in an emergency, when urgent action is essential and there is insufficient time for discussion and contemplation, effective communication about planning for matters of life and death should not be rushed. It takes time for both doctors and patients and their families to come to understand and integrate new information, and to generate a plan based on careful consideration of the health outcomes that can and cannot reasonably be achieved. This reinforces the need for ACP to be started early and continued as an ongoing and dynamic process, commonly extended into several sessions.

In addition to learning on the job from observation of skilled practitioners, opportunities for doctors to improve their skills in communication about end-of-life issues are widely available as part of undergraduate medical training, at all stages of prevocational and specialist doctor training, as part of continuing professional development, and from many healthcare system employers. It is also accessible for self-education in the medical literature and online. For example, *Clinical practice guidelines for communicating prognosis and end-of-life issues with adults in the advanced stages of life-limiting illness, and their caregivers* [5] was published in the *Medical Journal of Australia* and has been found by many to be very helpful (see also Chapter 5, Communication in clinical practice). Doctors should also cultivate their abilities to meet with families, and to be able to deal with the responses, questions and perspectives of multiple participants in group meetings.

Even doctors who have engaged in a lifetime of such conversations in emergency departments, intensive care units, oncology clinics or palliative care units commonly still feel anxiety when communicating about difficult issues. But they temper these responses with the understanding that the information that they have to communicate does not belong to them but to their patient and/or their family; that, even when the recipients vent their emotions on the messenger, it is the information that evokes distress; and that not communicating disempowers their patient and their patient's families. Only with the knowledge, understanding and guidance that they have received from their doctors are patients and their families able to choose from the options that are open to them, and plan and move on in a world wherein death remains inevitable, however tragic the circumstances might be.

As with other difficult but inescapable duties, sometimes doctors have no choice other than to take a big breath and step forward, accepting that such conversations might evoke a range of emotions from anger to gratitude, and sometimes generate tears all round. These tasks are often the doctor's duty to take on, and represent an important part of providing support for their patients.

19.1.4 Doctors preparing their community for the normality of death

The promotion of awareness that every life is finite and death is inevitable should run through all of healthcare delivery, but not in an overbearing or morbid manner. The early integration of the normality of death can support best-practice care that understands the use of modern technology in the pursuit of attainable healthcare goals and the delivery of an enhanced quality of life.

ACP is both the preparation for and the documentation of healthcare decisions with the aim of ensuring that choices are respected.

> Advance care planning involves planning for your future health care. It enables you to make some decisions now about the health care you would or would not like to receive if you were to become seriously ill and unable to communicate your preferences or make treatment decisions.

> Advance care planning gives you the opportunity to think about, discuss and record your preferences for the type of care you would like to receive and the outcomes you would consider acceptable. Advance care planning helps to ensure your loved ones and health providers know what matters most to you and respect your treatment preferences.
>
> Ideally, advance care planning will result in your preferences being documented in a plan known as an advance care directive and the appointment of a substitute decision-maker to help ensure your preferences are respected [6].

Most commonly, patients do not initiate conversations about ACP. Few understand what ACP entails and so the process generally starts with a doctor, another health practitioner, or sometimes a solicitor (in association with the creation of a will) raising the benefits of creating a plan. This creates an environment in which a person (and family) can feel encouraged to pursue an understanding of their illness, their values and goals for their life, the treatment options that are open to them, and the outcomes that they might expect, and to integrate them into their personal decision making and documents that would become active if they lost capacity. Effective ACP serves the interests of patients, patients' families, healthcare workers and the community at large.

In addition to the benefits to clinical decision making, many people, both patients and their families, are informed and empowered by the opportunity to talk about their preferred place of death, how their death might be managed, who they would like to be there, and any personal, cultural, religious or spiritual observances and funeral arrangements that are important to them. While governments and organisations tend to focus on documentation and legal issues, for clinicians and their patients ACP can be viewed simply as an essential component of the good medical practice necessary if patients are to achieve the best possible outcomes from their health care.

ACP is most effective when done early as a deliberately thoughtful and measured process, and may become quite fraught if delayed until there is little or no time for contemplation of values and hopes. ACP discussions may need to be repeated several times and documents amended as clinical circumstances change and personal preferences evolve.

19.1.5 Respecting cultural differences regarding death and dying

The Australian community includes a great diversity of cultures that shape behaviour and the choices that people make at the end of their life. People who understand that they are dying commonly prefer to shift their focus from their illness and interacting with the healthcare system to their family, their personal interests and the cultural support from and obligations to their community.

For many, particularly Aboriginal and/or Torres Strait Islander people, and many others who live in rural and remote areas who have been displaced from their country and their homes by the demands of treatment, this can mean returning to the security and support of their community even though it may mean withdrawing from therapy that might prolong their life. Doctors should recognise and respect how important culture and community can be to those dealing with their death and dying.

Box 19.1 Clinical example

A First Nations woman with complex chronic kidney disease had been required to live in a regional city for renal dialysis. She was found to have an advanced and untreatable pancreatic cancer. Her medical conditions, prognosis and options were discussed with her. Her choices were between continuing dialysis in the city and dying of pancreatic cancer in perhaps several months or stopping dialysis and returning home to her family in her remote community and dying in just a few weeks. She opted to return home and died peacefully after two weeks.

Some cultural groups in Australia do not have a tradition of talking about death and dying. This can be a significant issue because the complexity of 21st-century health care in Australia requires open communication with, and active participation by, patients and their families to achieve the best outcomes. This can be a difficult and confronting issue that requires great patience, particularly when doctors feel that they have not been able to bridge the cultural gaps that must be closed to achieve best healthcare outcomes.

Doctors have historically been somewhat limited in what they have offered to dying people and their families from cultural and linguistic backgrounds other than their own. Of course, recognising that every culture has always had to deal with death, over recent years many clinicians have become highly skilled in working with patients from the variety of cultures in their particular community. Doctors who engage with their local community (including by identifying those key people who can help to bridge the gaps) can help patients and their families to better understand what healthcare services can and cannot offer, and gain insights into how to best support the uptake of the benefits of modern medicine by their patients.

Doctors might consider that health care itself is a culture into which they are initiated during their early careers and recognise that, like all cultures, it continues to evolve. This book, *Good medical practice*, is one of the ways that the culture of medicine is communicated. All doctors are a part of that culture, as well as the cultures of their family, their friends and their community. Together, these both shape how we think and behave and limit what we can see and understand.

19.2 Decision making for care at the end of life

Over the past couple of centuries, medicine has experienced a technological revolution. A great diversity of treatments is now available to prevent or cure many diseases and to delay death by controlling and managing the manifestations of ageing in the face of a finite lifespan.

And yet, for all their tremendous benefits, every healthcare intervention also brings with it a novel combination of compounding risks that are increasingly likely in patients with more than one illness and as they grow older.

Some treatments bring benefits that are so great that little thought is required before decisions to act are made. For others, the risks and benefits are delicately balanced and need to be considered carefully. Many risks are very small, while others are common enough that they need to be discussed with every patient. While the adverse effects of treatment are often immediate, some play out over long periods of time that may not be appreciated by patients who are dealing with the immediate effects of an illness.

As medicine started on its technological journey, the glamour and promise of science and invention focused primarily on the biological benefits of treatments and life prolongation was prioritised over social, emotional, psychological and spiritual matters that were also important to many people. The norm at the beginning of the careers of some of the more senior doctors who are still working today was that doctors would choose whatever treatment they deemed was appropriate and inform their patient of their decision.

As discussed in section 19.1.1, it has become very apparent that, at times, modern technology can prolong a life with little or no quality. The goals of many people do not include living on indefinitely into old age, but to focus on other domains that contribute to their quality of life. This evolution in understanding has been matched by a rapid increase, or perhaps co-evolution, in the belief in individual autonomy: that people have the right to make choices for health care that match their personal goals for their own finite life. This change is manifest in the terms patient- or person-centred care, and whole-person care, that are coming to dominate descriptions of how healthcare workers approach their patients. They are at the core of good medical practice.

Patients with advanced and progressive diseases commonly do not have sufficient understanding of their illness and the balance of possible benefits and burdens of treatments to be able to make wise decisions unsupported. This complexity in contemporary decision making requires that doctors work closely with their patients, and/or their substitute decision makers and families, to make the best possible choices.

Discussions about decision making commonly raise the issue of futility. At its simplest, an action is futile when it cannot achieve the desired goal or is likely to be unbeneficial. However, decisions about futility in health care are commonly more complex with varying degrees of uncertainty, multiple players, and a diversity of goals [7]. Additionally, many treatments bring a range of burdens to the patient, to the community and/or to the patient's family. Some treatments are likely to be so burdensome that they are not offered to a patient, or a decision is reached by the patient in collaboration with their family and their doctor that an option of treatment will not be taken up (see also section 19.2.4).

As a response to the demands posed by this evolution in the nature of medical practice, a formative and far more effective and structured ethical and legal framework is emerging to support doctors and their patients to work together through collaborative decision making to make the best possible decisions in the complex world in which we find ourselves.

19.2.1 Communicating with patients and their families

Effective decision making at the end of life is founded on effective communication. This usually requires leadership by doctors who generally have a broader awareness of the diversity of personal, ethical and legal issues that can arise at the end of life than do patients and their families.

For much of the 20th century, doctors did not commonly explore these issues. But the growing expectations of the success of modern medicine in cure and life prolongation has highlighted those times when treatments are unsuccessful, and death is inevitable. This has led to a growing expectation that doctors will routinely explore a patient's preferences for care at the end of life as a core component of dealing with life-threatening illnesses.

However, some obstacles to effective discussions about death, dying and care at the end of life remain. These include:

- doctors and their patients focusing solely on the biology of disease and the goals for cure or life prolongation
- doctors' and patients' reluctance to acknowledge that a person is deteriorating towards their death and make appropriate decisions to change the goals of care

- doctors and their patients not being comfortable to discuss the social, psychological and spiritual domains that may actually be most important to patients and their families
- discomfort and/or lack of skill or confidence among senior doctors to initiate and lead the necessary discussions, particularly if they believe that the patient or their family will become distressed and oppose any proposed limitation of treatment
- lack of training, experience and role models for junior doctors who need effective communication skills to address the issues that arise in care at the end of life
- lack of understanding of the legal requirements, processes and documents of ACP
- failure to have elicited and documented a patient's preferences through ACP when/if that had been possible, poor documentation and/or communication of the previously expressed wishes of the patient, and/or not-for-resuscitation decisions [8]
- failure to respect ACP documents when they do exist
- failure to engage with family members who are expected to make decisions on the patient's behalf, particularly when the patient's preferences have not previously been discussed [9].

Most effective care at the end of life is founded in 'shared decision making' with the patient, if they have capacity (or 'supported decision making' if they are cognitively impaired), the family (unless the patient refuses), and the doctors and other healthcare workers all working collaboratively to decide what will fulfil the patient's will and preferences. This requires doctors to communicate effectively (see Chapter 5, Communication in clinical practice).

Early conversations and planning with patients may be predominantly hypothetical but are still very important and require candour with a patient about their death at some time in the future. More specific discussions with a patient about their care at the end of life commonly start when it becomes necessary for their doctor to tell them that they have an illness that may or will cause their death. Initiating such difficult conversations is an art in itself, but it does not end there. After they have dealt with the shock of the news, even if it simply confirmed what they expected anyway, patients soon are understandably concerned to know what happens next. Patients commonly want to know how long they are likely to live, whether there are any treatments that might prolong their life, what would those treatments entail, how their illness will progress and how they will die.

The doctor needs to understand the medical issues of their patient as much as is possible, but must also be open with their patient about what they don't know, and the uncertainties. They need to know what the patient knows and understands and what they may have misunderstood. They then need to use language the patient can understand to offer an accurate description of their illness, their prognosis and their medical options. Finally, they must confirm that the person has understood well enough to be able to make any necessary decisions.

The doctor can then open the door to an exploration of the patient's wishes, goals, values, expectations and preferences for the remainder of their life. While the progression of life-ending illnesses is commonly inexorable (but not predictable), patients who are well supported by their doctors can exercise a significant measure of agency in how they can choose to experience their dying and their death—the location, with whom, the cultural context, and, where VAD has been legalised and they are eligible, how and when.

It is generally unwise to make specific numerical predictions of life expectancy. Life expectancy can be honestly expressed as hours to days, days to weeks, weeks to months, or months to years. Any estimation should include the proviso that some people live for a far longer, or a far shorter time than expected, perhaps adding that, given the intrinsic uncertainties, if there are things that a person feels they must do it is better to do them earlier rather than miss the opportunity.

Good communication about care at the end of life is most commonly not a single event but a process that can unfold over a long time. In fact, slowing down the process, or starting early, supports thoughtful decision making. Unless a decision is required urgently, it is generally most effective to start by clarifying the issues, and then to pause while all participants take time to absorb the diagnosis and prognosis, and weigh up the options, including the uncertainties and how they might play out over time. This approach supports considered decisions, and is always subject to the proviso that adaptation may be necessary if events do not pan out as expected.

Doctors should also be comfortable communicating with substitute decision makers and family members, either together with the patient or separately if the patient does not have capacity. Discussions being held with substitute decision makers and family about difficult decisions (e.g. withholding or withdrawing treatment—see section 19.2.4) should focus on the will and preferences of the patient. This avoids the family feeling burdened by the belief they are personally responsible for the outcome and diminishes the risk that the family will adopt the default position of 'doing everything possible'.

While communication must be open and clear, in such circumstances doctors are not legally obliged to obtain consent to withhold life-prolonging treatment that they believe is futile or unbeneficial (though this is not the case in Queensland where, other than in an emergency, consent from a substitute decision maker must be obtained to withdraw or withhold life-prolonging treatment when a patient lacks capacity) [10–12].

It should be acknowledged that some medical interventions that cause suffering (e.g. the side effects of chemotherapy or the post-operative pain of surgery) may be acceptable to the person if there is ultimately some benefit to their comfort or prognosis, or if they can help a person to achieve some activity, task or duty that is important to them. Conversely, it is also important to explore the potential loss of opportunities as a consequence of pursuing unbeneficial treatments. These include the opportunity to spend time with family or to achieve other goals ('bucket lists'). Many people who have pursued unbeneficial treatments have regretted that the last days, weeks or months of their life were spent unwell from treatment (e.g. chemotherapy) when the patient (and their family) might have gained far more from time engaged in other activities that were important to them.

Given that it would be very unusual for a family to want a patient to suffer, a practical approach to this discussion is to ask the family that is asking for 'everything' to be done exactly what they mean by this and what outcome they are hoping for. Not only does this reassure the family that the doctor is listening to their concerns and expectations, but it can lead to a fruitful discussion about what the family believes the patient would realistically hope to achieve. It also opens up the discussion about the likely outcome and encourages recognition that the emotional and anticipatory grief reactions of the family are separate from the interests of the patient. When discussions are not handled well, families may lose trust in the doctors, the healthcare team and the hospital, and make poor and ill-informed decisions that may later be regretted.

Sometimes, in spite of everyone's best efforts, such discussions can become gridlocked, and it then becomes important to remember that there are few, if any, absolutes in clinical medicine, and this extends to declarations of futility. When the opinions of the treating doctors are not accepted by patients and/or their families, there are strategies that can open a pathway to a resolution that satisfies all participants.

Depending on the circumstances, these can include:

- offering, or arranging, a second opinion from another specialist (ideally, the second doctor should have the opportunity to meet with the patient and/or the family to offer and explain their opinion)
- offering a trial of treatment, ensuring that there is mutual agreement about the required outcomes and time restrictions of the trial to gauge success and justification for ongoing treatment. This strategy gives the patient and family time to see for themselves whether or not there is any improvement, and to adjust emotionally as well as intellectually to a bleak message from the treating doctor.
- offering to transfer the patient's care to another doctor or another hospital if the family can find a doctor who is prepared to attempt a different approach and take over the care
- discussion with a clinical ethics service or clinical ethicist (if available), which may assist both the clinical team and the patient/family to navigate complex decisions around the possible benefit/burden of a possible treatment or intervention.

When the healthcare team and patient and family continue to disagree after mediation involving independent clinicians, clinical ethicists or ethics committees, one or the other party may seek a decision from a tribunal or a court. It may be appropriate to obtain legal opinion. The role of tribunals and courts is discussed in section 19.3.4 and in works such as *Health law in Australia 4th edition* [7].

Finally, it is vitally important to document all communications with patients and their families, and the strategies that have been applied. Although effective communication and good working relationships make it extremely unlikely that a case will end up in court, documentation of good process and clear communication is most reassuring to the court that due process has been followed and that the patient and family have been dealt with respectfully and with dignity (see also Chapter 5, Communication in clinical practice; Chapter 27, Medical records, reports and certificates; and Chapter 32, Legal frameworks: rights, responsibilities and protections).

This approach to communication is also consistent with the common-law duty of doctors to always act in a manner that respects their patient's will and preferences. In such situations, full and careful discussion with the patient (if competent to understand and to consent to treatment) or their substitute decision maker about the available treatment options and goals and preferences is likely to pre-empt problems and provide satisfactory outcomes. While these suggestions may seem time-consuming, engaging in early and effective communication is an investment that will be rewarded if subsequent actions and conversations require far less effort and lead to less distress.

19.2.2 Decisions and consent for treatment at the end of life

Even during palliative care at the very end of life, when the primary goal has become comfort, there are times when medical interventions may benefit the patient (e.g. thoracocentesis, fixation of a pathological fracture). When the goals, risks and potential benefits have been explained carefully and are clear, most patients or their substitute decision makers will accept measures that might provide comfort. These require documentation of informed consent as for all interventions (see Chapter 7, Consent and informed decision making).

19.2.3 Refusal of medical treatment—the patient's right to choose

One of the core principles of health care in Australia is that competent and informed patients are entitled to refuse medical treatment or request that medical treatment be withdrawn even though such refusal or withdrawal may lead to their death. Adult patients are assumed to have decision-making capacity unless there is evidence to the contrary (see Chapter 7, Consent and informed decision making, for advice on assessing capacity/competence). Generally speaking, and in the absence of advance care directives (ACDs), those who are empowered to act on behalf of patients lacking capacity can make such decisions so long as they are acting in a manner that respects the patient's will and preferences.

The use of technology to maintain or prolong life, and the increasing prevalence of dementia in an ageing population, have increased the numbers of patients who are unable to make decisions about their own health care. All Australian jurisdictions have created guardianship legislation to strengthen patient autonomy in the face of concerns that technological advances may be used to unduly prolong life of terminally ill patients and most states and both territories have created legislation for the making of ACDs (except in New South Wales—see section 19.3). Legislation also protects the interests of doctors who might be accused either of prematurely withdrawing treatment from, or overtreating, the terminally ill.

While a person with capacity might choose to refuse palliative treatment designed to relieve pain or other suffering, a doctor should probably seek to address such a decision with the person separately from decisions about whether to refuse other medical treatment. Guardianship legislation typically does not allow a substitute decision maker to request withdrawal of palliative care. Palliative care is defined in Victorian legislation as including 'the provision of reasonable medical treatment for the relief of pain, suffering and discomfort' and 'the reasonable provision of food and water' [13]. A court in Victoria also determined that feeding provided by percutaneous gastric tube was medical treatment and not palliative care, and therefore could be refused [14].

Decisions by patients to refuse or cease treatment are not considered to be suicidal. If the consequence of such refusal is death, then the cause of death is the disease, not the decision. Importantly, the right to refuse treatment is not matched by a right to insist on a treatment that a doctor does not believe is appropriate.

19.2.4 Withholding or withdrawing futile or burdensome treatment

Decisions about starting or stopping treatment may be made by patients, their substitute decision maker acting on their behalf (see section 19.3.2), their doctors, or very commonly by doctors, patients and their families working together. Doctors should have a clear understanding of their roles, rights and duties, and those of their patients and their substitute decision makers.

It is important to note that while from an ethical and legal perspective there is no difference between withholding and withdrawing an unbeneficial treatment, in the minds of patients, families and health practitioners the emotional meaning of such actions can be very different.

Doctors trying to understand for themselves whether it would be appropriate to withhold or withdraw a medical intervention might start by deciding whether a treatment falls into the relatively straightforward category of absolutely futile [15]. In such circumstances, and particularly in an emergency, doctors can simply decide not to offer or to withdraw treatment that is futile or not beneficial (i.e. treatment would not impact on the outcome, such as cardiopulmonary resuscitation [CPR] for a patient who is dying by exsanguination from the erosion of a major thoracic blood vessel by a lung cancer, or for a patient with a severe destructive head injury).

In such circumstances, the doctor's role becomes to explain to the person and their family why they have made their decision, and to shift the focus on to comfort measures including supporting the patient, their family and other healthcare workers as they face the inevitability of the person's death.

As described in section 19.2, the term 'futile' is widely used within the healthcare community and also commonly understood by many in the broader community to mean 'an action that will not achieve the desired outcome'. However, declarations of 'futility' by doctors may be understood by some as a form of medical paternalism. Therefore, as they prepare for discussions about poor outcomes, doctors might consider whether their patient and/or their family are likely to be distressed by the concept of 'futility', so that they should avoid using it because of its negative connotations, subjectivity and potential for misinterpretation. A broad discussion of these issues may be of interest [7,16,17].

As an alternative approach in their communication with patients and families, doctors might use terms such as treatment being 'unlikely to bring any benefit', or 'more likely to cause significant harm than any benefit' or 'not indicated' to provide a clear message that the decision under discussion is about the effectiveness of the treatment, not the person's worth. Such discussions should also reference the continuation of treatment that remains in the best interests of the patient and has been accepted by them (e.g. anticonvulsants or insulin), as well as good palliative care including medicines to control symptoms.

Far more commonly, doctors find themselves facing choices where there is significant uncertainty about the outcome of the medical interventions, including whether or not they may be beneficial. In day-to-day practice, doctors commonly use statistics and their clinical assessment to gauge the likelihood that a treatment will have an impact that benefits the patient. Patients and their families, on the other hand, may prefer to assess benefit based on the likelihood that they will achieve their personal interests, preferences and goals over the possibility of disease control and life prolongation.

The key factors that should be addressed in discussions with patients and/or decision makers include:

- the likelihood of producing a benefit that is desired by the patient
- the burden of suffering of the patient (and perhaps their family) with or without the treatment
- the financial cost of the treatment to the patient and/or the community
- and the opportunity costs for the patient of not having completed other activities that they might have preferred to engage in and that would be better dealt with before their inevitable death.

This approach to decision making requires that the doctor encourage the patient (or the decision maker) to consider their own preferences and goals for treatment, if that has not been done already. A patient's preferences take precedence over those of the doctor or the goals or interests of the patient's family.

As discussed in sections 19.2 and 19.2.1, many, if not most treatments come with a balance of risks and benefits, and even simple discussions about straightforward therapeutic decisions require acknowledging that balance before proceeding. Caution and hesitancy are important human traits that should be recognised as supporting thoughtful choices, but can at times paralyse decision making (e.g. vaccine hesitancy).

Doctors may or may not agree with their patient's decision because either they believe the patient's goals may not be achievable, or because they personally do not find the patient's goals appropriate. Nonetheless, a patient's choices from what they are being offered must be respected. Patients have no legal right to insist on treatment that their doctor believes is futile (assuming that such a belief is generally supported by their colleagues), and generally, doctors are not legally obliged to offer treatment that they believe is futile. Doctors do not require consent to stop futile treatment and doing so does not breach the law (except in Queensland, where consent must be obtained from the patient's substitute decision maker) [18,19]. However, other than in an emergency [7,19], the unilateral imposition of a doctor's assessment can evoke distress and anger from the patient and/or their family. Careful and considered explanation, seeking a second opinion, discussion with a clinical ethics service where available, and offering time for reflection can all help the acceptance of confronting decisions.

Australian courts have noted that, in the first instance, what constitutes 'futile' treatment is a matter for medical practitioners [20,21]. As is clear from the Medical Board of Australia's code of conduct, doctors have an ethical obligation not to provide treatment that is burdensome and of little or no value [2]. Many professional and healthcare organisations have recognised the importance of this issue and have issued similar statements on withholding and withdrawing treatment [22].

Over the past few decades, the legal framework and documents for end-of-life decision making have become far more effective. These include processes for the appointment of substitute decision makers, ACP and ACDs, and the creation of end-of-life care plans. Almost all healthcare facilities use some form of what have commonly been called not-for-resuscitation (NFR) or do-not-resuscitate (DNR) orders. More recently it has been suggested that NFR/DNR be replaced by the softer term 'allow natural death', but still with the intent that this description would mean that resuscitation should not be attempted. Queensland's Acute Resuscitation Plan (ARP) document can do both and supports the alternative choice of life prolongation if that is the patient's will and preference, and is achievable.

19.3 Documentation: advance care planning, advance care directives and the law

The common law has long recognised the right of a patient to make an ACD in regard to their medical treatment. This is now reinforced by legislation in all states and territories except NSW. Doctors should familiarise themselves with the relevant laws and regulations that apply in the state or territory in which they are practising.

ACP is central to whole-person care and wise decision making. ACP is based on the ethical principle of respect for the dignity and autonomy of all patients. ACP may include the creation of 'advance care directives' (known as 'advance health directives' in Queensland and Western Australia, 'health directions' in South Australia and the Australian Capital Territory, and 'advance personal plans' in the Northern Territory) which are also commonly known as living wills. In NSW, which has not legislated for ACDs, only common-law directives exist and because there aren't any formal requirements, they can be verbal.

The ethical and legal premise of such directives is that they give effect to the person's wishes at a time when those wishes cannot otherwise be established because a person has lost the capacity to communicate their choices themself. In ethics, this allows for respect for autonomy. In law, it respects the legal right of a competent person to refuse treatment.

ACD documents commonly include the patient's goals and preferences, and can specify which treatments the person does and does not wish to be provided to them in certain clinical situations. They are the means by which a patient's prior decisions are communicated and implemented by doctors should they become unable to speak for themselves, except in the ACT where health directions are valid at all times [7]. They also guide the patient's substitute decision makers (who must also respect ACDs) and enhance effective decision making and communication between healthcare workers and patients' families.

People may prepare advance care plans and directives without medical assistance and support (although they sometimes require a doctor's signature). However, the process and outcome are likely to be much more effective with medical participation. The preceding discussion is almost more important than the final paperwork because the preferences that are subsequently documented are more likely to accurately match the person's preferences and the realities of the clinical context of the decisions that must be made [23,24]. Doctors can also seek to address any of their patient's broader emotional, spiritual, cultural or religious needs [25] that might influence their preferences. If a doctor finds themselves outside the domains within which they are comfortable, or if the discussion reveals more complex issues, referral to a social worker, counsellor, pastoral care service or cultural support service should be considered (see also Chapter 17, Culturally safe health care for Aboriginal and/or Torres Strait Islander peoples).

In response to non-uniform legislation and terminology across Australia, in 2021 the Australian Health Ministers' Advisory Council published the *National framework for advance care planning documents* [26], which is an update of the *National framework for advance care directives 2011*. This document defines advance care plans and directives, outlines best practice and offers remedies to improve acceptance of directives across jurisdictions.

The value of ACP has been demonstrated in an Australian randomised controlled trial comparing facilitated ACP with standard care in elderly inpatients in a large public hospital [27]. Those who participated in ACP were much more likely to have their end-of-life wishes known and respected and were more satisfied with the quality of their care. Furthermore, their families were also more satisfied with the care provided and experienced fewer clinically significant symptoms of stress, anxiety and depression than the surviving relatives of deceased patients who had not received ACP.

In assisting often elderly and ill patients to complete a directive, the doctor must judge that the patient has capacity to understand the nature and purpose of the discussion and of the decisions that are being made, and their consequences (see also Chapter 7, Consent and informed decision making).

While ACP is rapidly becoming routine practice, plans and directives are not yet as common as perhaps they should be given the strong views that many people express for their care in old age. Probably more importantly, they are not always accessed or respected even when they are available. Some Australian doctors have argued that ACP is ethically complex and not always an unequivocal good [28]. While many people have strong opinions and prefer to document their choices about treatments that they may or may not want in the future, participation in ACP is and should always remain a person's individual choice, never mandatory. No-one should be forced to make choices before they are ready or for hypothetical events in their future.

Again, Australian doctors are encouraged to familiarise themselves with the legal framework for ACP that applies in the jurisdiction where they work. Many will find these online resources particularly helpful:

- The website of Advance Care Planning Australia (https://www.advancecareplanning.org.au) provides comprehensive practical information and guidance, as well as links to websites that can provide the documents and describe the process of ACP for all jurisdictions in Australia. These can be very helpful to doctors, other healthcare workers, and the community at large as they deal with the challenges of ACP wherever they work and live [6].
- The Australian Centre for Health Law Research at Queensland University of Technology (QUT) has created an online resource (https://end-of-life.qut.edu.au) addressing ACDs and further information which explores the broad range of issues of law at the end of life including the differences between jurisdictions [29]. It also offers online training.

All state and territory governments also have websites that provide links to the relevant resources.

19.3.1 Implementing advance care directives

Increasing numbers of Australians are creating an ACD (or the jurisdictional equivalent) to guide the care they would prefer should they lose capacity. A doctor treating a patient who lacks capacity at the time a decision must be made, and who is provided with a statutory or common-law ACD that is valid in that jurisdiction, is expected to comply with the directive as it applies to the clinical situation at hand. The law on ACDs is different in every state and territory and doctors should be familiar with the law in the jurisdiction in which they are working. It is not the doctor's role to determine if the patient was competent and adequately informed at the time of signing, or if the directive was made voluntarily. However, doctors should satisfy themselves that the directive conforms with the legislation in their jurisdiction [30].

In NSW, where ACDs are not provided for in a statute, common-law ACDs are binding on doctors and must be followed if they are valid and apply to the clinical situation [31]. In considering common-law documents, it is recommended that the doctor hold discussions with family members who may be able to clarify the patient's wishes about oral or written directives. If there is doubt about what the patient's wishes are in the current clinical situation, the patient's will and preferences must guide decision making.

Where a directive does not coincide with, or differs markedly from, the views of the healthcare team about what treatment is in the best interests (and reflects the will and preferences) of the patient, careful ethical reflection is required. The law across Australia differs on when an ACD does not need to be followed. As a general rule, a valid directive not to provide treatment must be followed, even if it conflicts with the treating doctor's view of treatment that could be provided. This is consistent with the well-established legal and ethical right of a patient to refuse medical treatment.

Conversely, in some parts of Australia a directive that requests that specific treatment be provided when certain circumstances occur, or if the doctor does not believe the patient intended the direction to apply in the circumstances before them, need not be followed when the provision of that treatment in those circumstances would be contrary to good medical practice [7].

Before acting against such a directive, effort should be made to determine if the patient's views have changed since the directive was made, and independent clinical, ethical or legal advice sought.

As ACDs become more common, other practical issues for doctors will emerge.

- In the legislation there is no time limit for which an ACD is valid. Therefore, as with a will, an ACD must be assumed to be valid indefinitely unless it is revoked.
- When a doctor finds themselves in a clinical situation where the existence of an ACD would help decision making, how much effort must a doctor make to determine whether such a document is known to exist? In the absence of a central register and where no advance directive is in the patient's medical record or held by the hospital, doctors should inquire of immediate family and friends as to whether one exists. This question also applies to the existence of a document that appoints a substitute decision maker.

Patients should be strongly encouraged to keep their legal documents up to date by creating a new document whenever their will and preferences change, and by sending a valid copy of their latest version to their healthcare providers. Patients can upload their ACP documents to My Health Record, and many health systems, hospitals and individual practitioners can also upload them into their patients' medical records.

19.3.2 Substitute decision makers

Issues relating to substitute decision makers can be complex, and for a broader legal perspective it may be helpful to refer to *Health law in Australia 4th ed* [7], Chapter 7, Adults who lack capacity: substitute decision-making.

Some people do not have capacity to make their own healthcare choices at the time decisions need to be made and have not created an ACD document to guide healthcare decision making on their behalf. 'Substitute decision makers' (sometimes also referred to by the American term 'surrogate decision makers') are the persons legally recognised to make decisions for people who have lost capacity to make decisions for themselves.

Substitute decision making for adults who lack decision-making capacity for healthcare decisions is facilitated primarily by guardianship and other related legislation which has been enacted in all Australian states and territories. This permits a range of decision makers to make different types of healthcare decisions and provides for the formal appointment of decision makers, referred to by various terms including 'enduring guardians' or as persons appointed to have 'enduring power of attorney for medical treatment'. The statutes authorise a hierarchy of 'persons responsible' or 'statutory health attorneys', which often include a guardian appointed by a tribunal, an enduring guardian, or the patient's relative, partner, carer or friend. The laws pertaining to the appointment and role of substitute decision makers and guardians are further discussed in Chapter 7, Consent and informed decision making.

Some ACDs appoint a substitute decision maker. Implementing ACDs that have invoked a substitute decision maker gives effect to the patient's preferences and is, in ethics, referred to as a substituted judgement. The decision maker bases their decisions on the views, wishes and preferences of the patient, informed by prior direct verbal or written communication, and/or their knowledge of the person. Substitute decision makers appointed by other means are also generally required to make decisions that align with the patient's ACD if one exists.

Legislation is moving away from the consideration of the person's 'best interests' and towards their 'will and preferences' as the basis upon which a substitute decision maker reaches their decisions [7]. However, for some adult patients who lack capacity and for younger children in particular, it may not be possible to determine their will and preferences and decisions can only be made based on what is in their best interests.

Whether described as respecting a person's 'will and preferences' or being in their 'best interests', the law often specifies the factors that must be considered. Typically, these include:

- the 'will and preferences' or 'best interests' of the patient
- the wishes of any nearest relative or any other family members
- the consequences to the patient if the treatment is not carried out
- any alternative treatment
- the nature and degree of any significant risks associated with the treatment or any alternative treatment
- whether the treatment is only to promote and maintain the health and wellbeing of the patient.

Of all these factors, the 'will and preferences' or 'best interests' of the patient are paramount.

Each state and territory has produced its own range of documents to guide substitute decision making and doctors are advised to familiarise themselves with the guidelines for their jurisdiction [29]. The doctor should also endeavour to confirm that a person who is purporting to be the substitute decision maker has been appointed to the role, or is legally empowered to assume that role and make the relevant decisions. Occasionally, people who have assumed themselves to be, or have claimed to be, the substitute decision maker have been found not to have the right to undertake the role—for example, because someone else had been appointed by the patient as their enduring power of attorney, or had a higher priority. Additionally, doctors in Australia should be aware that cultures vary in how they traditionally allocate the role of decision maker. Patients and their families may be surprised or distressed by what the law requires.

19.3.3 Making and documenting decisions about resuscitation

ACP is central to effective care at the end of life. But conversations about a person's decisions are meaningless if they have not been documented and communicated to those who will find themselves trying to respect them. ACDs, ARPs and NFR/DNR orders are the means by which choices become instructions for courses of action. Doctors caring for persons with serious and life-limiting illnesses should make themselves aware of their patients' existing ACP documents, and if they are inadequate for the circumstances, consider how they can be made fit for purpose.

Resuscitation, including CPR, can extend the lives of people who would otherwise have died prematurely. As a consequence, in most healthcare settings, the default response to a medical emergency is to resuscitate in the absence of an instruction from a doctor to the contrary.

However, when applied injudiciously to every person who is extremely unwell and dying, resuscitation can cause significant harm, rather than any benefit. At times, CPR turns what would have been a peaceful and dignified death into a traumatic spectacle for all concerned: the dying person, their family, healthcare workers and even passers-by.

In the past, doctors seldom translated discussions and any directive documents into the medical instructions that would inform other healthcare workers who found themselves caring for a deteriorating patient. Over the years this has led to countless futile and burdensome episodes of CPR being inflicted on people, particularly frail older people, whose natural and normal death was thus disrupted by a violent physical assault that had no chance of preventing death.

Box 19.2 Clinical example

Many years ago, a doctor who was caring for a patient dying at home from advanced cancer believed they had made all the necessary arrangements. Unfortunately, the patient collapsed suddenly and died in their bathroom with the door locked. The family called emergency services. When the fire brigade and ambulance arrived, they smashed down the door to extract the patient. Because there was no document instructing them not to engage in CPR, the corpse was subjected to resuscitation that was not wanted by anyone. Subsequently, in that community and for that doctor's dying patients at least, written NFR orders became standard practice.

CPR is at times used without clinical justification (i.e. where it is futile and the natural process of dying should not be interfered with). Studies have shown that the effectiveness of CPR for patients who suffer a cardiac arrest in hospital as measured by survival to discharge from hospital is about 30% [32], but this rate falls to about 4% in patients with significant morbidities [33].

Alternatively, decisions not to resuscitate have sometimes been made without input from the patient or the family and by a single member of the healthcare team. Not uncommonly, even when discussions have been held with patients and their families and thoughtful decisions about resuscitation have been made appropriately, they have not been clearly documented or communicated.

The progressive introduction of ACP as standard practice, particularly in residential aged care and as part of estate planning with lawyers, has also opened the door for doctors to fulfil their duty to initiate discussions about their patients' preferences. However, while ACP documents such as ACDs have changed the culture of care of people with life-limiting illnesses, by themselves they commonly do not protect dying people from unwanted or futile interventions like CPR. Because of this, over recent decades, documentation of the resuscitation status of seriously ill and older people has become the norm.

Such decisions are the personal choice of the patient or their substitute decision maker in consultation with their doctor and/or based on:

- the prognosis for the clinical condition that led to the recognition that the question of whether to initiate resuscitation might arise if or when a person deteriorated
- the likelihood of success or the potential for harm from CPR
- the quality of life that might be achieved if CPR was successful in restoring cardiorespiratory function.

However, an order not to commence CPR is generally required to be issued or created by a doctor in most healthcare settings.

Box 19.3 Clinical example

A 95-year-old woman resident of an aged care facility decided that she did not wish to be resuscitated in the event of a significant cardiac event. After several faints she was sent to the emergency department for assessment. While she was being examined in the emergency department, her heart stopped beating. As documentation of her preferences had been included in her medical record by her general practitioner, CPR was not commenced.

NFR documents based on an ACD can ensure that decisions about whether to attempt resuscitation and other potentially life-prolonging measures are respected. However, there is a move to relabel NFR orders as 'allow natural death' orders. This runs the risk of being a bit too vague and potentially hard to interpret in an emergency. Queensland has created a standard document, the ARP, that includes an up-front highlighted section for instructions on whether or not to commence CPR [34]. There is also a similar document for children that reflects the legal differences in paediatric decision making: the paediatric ARP (PARP).

The ARP is a doctor's instruction to other healthcare workers that includes a clinical assessment, a capacity assessment, a resuscitation management plan, the patient's choices and preferences, their consenting details including name and contact details of their substitute decision maker, and a description of any consenting discussions. The ARP is particularly useful because its use both opens the door to candid discussions with patients and their substitute decision makers, and communicates vital decisions to those who must implement them. Unlike an NFR order, the name 'acute resuscitation plan' does not presume that existence of the document means that resuscitation will not be attempted—an ARP is a plan and an instruction for how to respond to a deterioration in a patient's condition.

While many patients admitted to acute healthcare facilities do not require an NFR order or ARP, the same cannot be said for those admitted to residential aged care facilities, or transferred from such facilities to acute settings. Documents such as an ARP based on an ACD can avoid the need to make emergency decisions with insufficient information, and minimise the likelihood of unwanted, inappropriate and distressing intrusion in the peaceful natural deaths that many older people hope for when they do have capacity to make such choices.

Nonetheless, not all emergencies can be prepared for and sometimes decisions must be made with little or no time for contemplation. Occasionally the patient can make choices on their own behalf.

Box 19.4 Clinical example

A man who had far advanced lung cancer that was causing him significant pain suddenly developed severe but painless haematemesis and low blood pressure. His doctor, who had come to know him well over previous months, sat down with him and discussed his clinical diagnosis of a bleeding ulcer that was likely to cause his rapid death if not treated, and described his options of further investigation or simply being kept comfortable. The man said, 'Let it go.' An experienced nurse sat at his bedside throughout and administered mild intravenous sedation and analgesia as needed. He died peacefully several hours later. At autopsy the man was found to have a perforated duodenal ulcer.

At other times there is no evidence about what the person would have preferred and decisions must be made solely on clinical grounds. While the default position is to initiate CPR, a doctor may still use their clinical judgement to decide that CPR would be either futile (e.g. severe fatal injury) or excessively burdensome and likely to cause significant harm (e.g. extreme frailty in an older person with dementia).

It should always be made clear that an ARP or NFR order will not reduce the level of care otherwise provided to the patient or even necessarily mean the denial of some other treatments with curative intent (such as treating infections that are causing distressing symptoms). Doctors are encouraged to develop the skills to hold these discussions [35].

Good medical practice always involves open discussion with patient, family or substitute decision maker to the extent that is possible, even in an emergency. Even a nod or the shake of a head in response to a clear question from a doctor to a watching relative might suffice as a form of consent. As noted earlier, while consent to withhold treatment including CPR is not a legal requirement in other jurisdictions, in Queensland doctors are required by law to seek consent to withhold or withdraw life-prolonging treatment, except in an emergency when consent is not available [36,37].

Unsurprisingly, as always there remains some variation in law and terminology between the states and territories [18]. However, patients who cross borders will usually find that their documents are respected so long as they conform to the laws of the jurisdiction in which the documents are being used.

19.3.4 The role of the courts and tribunals in end-of-life care

Over time, a range of disputes or legal uncertainties about end-of-life care have come before Australian tribunals and courts, and a pattern has emerged in how they approach such matters [38]. The cases have predominantly involved instances of patients refusing medical treatment and nutrition and hydration; those caring for these individuals were uncertain as to whether they were obliged to accept the person's refusal and were concerned about their moral and legal obligations (e.g. concern that those caring for the person were not actively supporting suicide by self-starvation).

The right of patients to refuse treatment has been fully accepted, but only after their mental health and competence or capacity for decision making has been closely assessed. The tribunals and courts also require reassurance that the information provided to patients is sufficient to enable them to understand the consequences of their choices, including what they may experience without nutrition, hydration and/or medication. In these cases, the validity of advance care plans and anticipatory directions about terminal care have been endorsed, even where the planning was not documented but depended upon the oral evidence of the individual and/or of family members. In reaching decisions, tribunals and courts have applied the test of whether any treatment is in the patient's 'best interests' and have deemed treatments that are futile or overly burdensome as not meeting this test.

These issues can be complex. For a comprehensive discussion, doctors might consider reading section 14.40, Refusal of treatment (p. 615), in White et al. *Health law in Australia 4th ed* [7].

19.4 When cure or life prolongation is becoming impossible

Intensive modern medical technology offers a great but not infinite power to sustain a life, even when organ systems are failing irrevocably. However, for many if not most patients and their families, the goal of their engagement with medical treatment is to prolong, sustain or restore *a life with a quality that is acceptable to the patient.*

Doctors who are treating a patient have a duty to them to recognise when it is becoming or is no longer possible to cure disease or to prolong life with sufficient quality as defined by the patient, and that further treatment is not likely to bring desired benefits. This is only possible if the doctor has been able to establish a relationship with their patient that reaches beyond the bounds of the technical aspects of their disease and its treatment to explore with the patient (and/or their decision maker) their hopes, goals and preferences and to integrate these into decision making.

Such recognition should be communicated compassionately and openly to the patient in a manner that allows them to understand and to integrate the information.

Many people pursuing a cure have delayed a range of activities and actions that are also very important to them. Some people, recognising that their life is finite, would prefer to relinquish the possibility that a treatment might prolong their life for the certainty that before they die, they will be able to do something that is very important to them. This might include achieving a reconciliation, making a visit to a person or place, or being well enough to undertake a spiritual journey.

Too many patients have not been given timely information about their condition and prognosis. Lack of candour by doctors obstructs communication within families and has caused many people to miss out on much-needed support and the opportunity to do things that were very important to them. So, when a patient's goal of cure or significant life prolongation is becoming unattainable, they need and have a right to know. Only then, and sometimes requiring permission from their doctor, can they move on to pursue their other goals.

It is also vitally important that patients feel safe in the knowledge that they will continue to be supported, including with palliative care, whatever choices they make.

As they engage with their patients in this important phase of patients' healthcare journeys, doctors should be alert to the risks of persisting with treatment in order to validate their own role, even though it cannot meet their patients' wishes and hopes.

Additionally, doctors may also sometimes find themselves avoiding difficult conversations about end-of-life issues because of the emotions they may generate, both in themselves and in their patients and their families. While such responses are understandable, they disempower patients and deny them the opportunity to achieve their preferred personal goal(s).

19.5 End-of-life care: a 'good death'

Patients and their families usually describe a 'good death' as one that avoids or minimises suffering, does not prolong dying, provides a sense of control, relieves burdens on family and strengthens relationships with loved ones.

In 2016 and 2017, the Australian Medical Association (AMA) issued position statements on policy on euthanasia and VAD that focused primarily on the need to provide high-quality care at the end of life. While not supporting VAD at that time, it recognised that some doctors support the practice of VAD. The results of another survey of members by the AMA carried out in 2024 has led to a change in the AMA policy so that it now supports practitioners who choose to participate in a lawful VAD process, as well as those who choose not to participate [39]. The resulting position statement covers the following considerations for VAD:

- the patient is free from unnecessary suffering as far as is possible
- the patient is cared for in their environment of choice
- the patient's goals and values for end-of-life care are respected
- the patient's privacy and confidentiality are respected, even after death
- the physical needs of the patient and also the psychological, emotional, cultural, religious and spiritual needs of the patient and their family members and carers are addressed
- patients and, where appropriate, their family members and carers are empowered to participate in managing their treatment
- patients, their family members and carers are provided with access to counselling and support as necessary, including support for family members and carers after the patient's death [39].

As approximately half of all deaths take place in hospitals, the Australian Commission on Safety and Quality in Health Care has also developed detailed guidance on how hospitals and their staff should strive to ensure that all patients receive good quality end-of-life care [40].

19.6 Provision of palliative care

In any discussion about a patient's choice to refuse or withdraw from treatment, or when a doctor is suggesting withholding or withdrawing from treatment that is of little or no benefit, patients and their families must be informed that, whatever choices are made, palliative care will be maintained. Doctors must take steps to ensure that this undertaking is fulfilled by understanding and integrating the non-specialist components of palliative care into their own practice as appropriate (e.g. palliative management of end-stage cardiac failure by cardiologists) and referring to specialist palliative care services as necessary.

A helpful starting point is with the World Health Organization definition [41] of palliative care:

> Palliative care is an approach that improves the quality of life of patients (adults and children) and their families who are facing problems associated with life-threatening illness. It prevents and relieves suffering through the early identification, correct assessment and treatment of pain and other problems, whether physical, psychosocial or spiritual.

Palliative care:

- provides relief from pain and other distressing symptoms
- affirms life and regards dying as a normal process
- intends neither to hasten nor postpone death
- integrates the psychological and spiritual aspects of patient care
- offers a support system to help patients live as actively as possible until death

- offers a support system to help the family cope during the patient's illness and in their own bereavement
- uses a team approach to address the needs of patients and their families, including bereavement counselling, if indicated
- will enhance quality of life and may also positively influence the course of illness
- is applicable early in the course of illness, in conjunction with other therapies that are intended to prolong life, such as chemotherapy or radiation therapy, and includes those investigations needed to better understand and manage distressing clinical complications.

The obligation to provide appropriate palliative care is made clear in the Medical Board of Australia's code of conduct [2], the AMA's position statement [39] and legislation in some jurisdictions (e.g. Queensland). Several excellent Australian sources of guidance for the delivery of palliative care in various circumstances have been published [42,43].

Most doctors will find themselves providing at least some aspects of palliative care at some time in their career. All doctors should be familiar with the knowledge and associated skills that comprise the basic tenets of non-specialist palliative care. They are not complex or difficult, and form the basis of good clinical practice.

They are founded on recognition of the importance of holistic care, minimisation of suffering where possible, and communicating effectively and openly with patients and their families—skills that are crucial in all fields of medicine. They also include an understanding of the pathophysiology of dying, core skills of communication around death and dying, empathy and compassion, and basic symptom control in the context of the acceptance of impending death. Doctors should also familiarise themselves with their local or regional specialist palliative care services from which they might seek advice and to which they can refer their patients as appropriate.

19.6.1 Good palliative care is not voluntary assisted dying

It has long been accepted by the community, the courts and the medical profession that administering drugs such as morphine and sedatives to relieve pain and distress in dying patients is ethical and lawful. So long as the intention and the conduct of the doctor prescribing or administering the drugs is to relieve symptoms and not to hasten the death of the patient, it represents good medical practice. Palliative care specialists whose goal for their patients is comfort use the lowest effective doses to control symptoms [44,45].

Several decades ago, many felt it necessary to justify the palliative use of opioids and other medications that might have caused some sedation by invoking what is known as the 'doctrine of double effect'. This perspective had its origins in Catholic moral theology which taught that an act undertaken with good intent is moral despite the possibility of other unintended ill effects.

Physicians and nurses providing palliative care have observed that the use of opioids to control pain has little impact on the duration of life [46]. Both anecdotally, and more recently from objective evidence, it is apparent that, rather than accelerating death, good palliative care, including the use of appropriate doses of strong analgesics, sometimes extends life [47,48].

The carefully titrated use of opioids and sedatives to control severe physical, emotional and/or spiritual distress is best described as 'palliative sedation', remembering also that increasing drowsiness and eventually unconsciousness due to the progressive physiological and biochemical derangements intrinsic to dying is extremely common and the reality for many dying people.

At the same time, some patients who are receiving opioids who have a particular reason for living a little bit longer (e.g. waiting for a relative to arrive or to be present for some important event), seem to be able to sustain their life for a short time by force of will, although of course the inexorable progress of some illnesses may make this impossible.

Over recent decades, the community and the profession have come to understand the goals of care at the end of life and, increasingly, the routines of good medical practice at the end of life, including the appropriate use of medicines to relieve suffering, are being integrated into the mainstream of health care. Provided the primary aim of treatment is symptom relief, a doctor does not need to provide justification for the core activities of palliative care.

19.7 Care of children at the end of life

In theory, infants and children who are dying should not be treated differently from adults who are dying. Unsurprisingly, because it is in our evolved nature to be very highly protective of children, many doctors caring for children with life-limiting illnesses, and their families, do experience a degree of emotional distress over the conflict between their desire to protect children and their duty to act in a child's overall best interests.

In bygone times, our instincts were less likely to generate conflict because we had little to no experience or expectation of delaying death. This is not to suggest that grief was any less of an issue—for example, the prolonged and profound grief experienced by Charles Darwin after the death of his 10-year-old daughter Annie in 1851 has been documented in his biographies.

However, over the course of the 19th, 20th and 21st centuries we have gained knowledge, skills and technology that have progressively reduced the mortality of children. In high-income countries such as Australia and Aotearoa New Zealand, death in childhood has become uncommon by historical standards—from perhaps 30% before the age of 10 in England in about 1850 to less than 1% now in Australia. Nonetheless, globally there are still about 5 million deaths annually in children under 5 years of age [49].

Modern technologies have also meant that many children with life-limiting illnesses are living much longer. A focus on the successes of modern health care has changed our expectations. As a community, we have become less accepting of the reality that not all diseases in children can be treated and many doctors and other health professionals have limited experience in caring for these patients. Doctors can be unprepared for the challenges they face when a child's death has become inevitable despite the best available treatment. This can become an issue when the families of dying children wish to take them home from the super-specialty units in capital cities to the smaller communities where they live.

Modern technologies also bring with them the risk that persistence with treatment can extend the duration of a life with little or no hope of cure or improvement. Doctors, families and sometimes children themselves now face the same challenges experienced in adult medicine—knowing when to stop trying to prolong life because the child's death has become inevitable and further efforts at life prolongation will simply prolong suffering.

Box 19.5 Anecdote

One paediatric nurse expressed their sadness on the admission to a palliative care unit of a newborn baby who was dying, saying 'It is not normal for a child to die!'

Their colleague replied: 'It is normal, it's just that it has become very uncommon.'

Therefore, while remembering that, fortunately, most families are now unfamiliar with the challenges of dealing with the death of a child, doctors caring for children and their families have a particular duty to prepare themselves for this role. Doctors might consider how they fulfil their duty to children to adhere to the same moral and ethical principles of decision making on behalf of children as they do for adults, including respecting their right to make their own decisions to the degree that they have the capacity to do so.

As a child deteriorates towards their death, it becomes necessary for doctors to work closely with the child (in an age-appropriate manner) and their family, to navigate the difficult journey of letting go of their hopes and desires that the child will not die, and to prepare everyone for the child's death.

Doctors should also be aware that their need to validate their work can have an influence on the decisions that they make, particularly with regards to treatment that has become futile. At times, doctors may struggle to accept that the treatment that they have provided has not worked, and that their role has become to provide care for the dying child (or to refer on as appropriate), and to provide support for the child's parents and other family members as they face the reality that a child is dying. Failure to recognise and adapt to these issues can result in prolongation of significant suffering for the child.

Experience and research has shown that many children who are approaching the end of their life have a far greater awareness of their condition and their impending death than either their family or their doctors had realised. And sometimes they can become more active as a participant in the complexity of the management of the end of their life than the adults in the room have expected or realised.

One young preschool-aged child told the nurse who asked them how they were going: 'I am not ready to go to the Care Bears yet.'

And as an example of the highly confronting challenges that are posed for parents, healthcare workers and the law, dying teenagers have been known to say: 'I want to have sex before I die!'

Finally, doctors should also be alert to the reality that the siblings of seriously ill or dying children are at risk of being neglected. They often have little attention or support as they struggle to deal with both the challenges and tasks of their own childhood and the impact of the sick child's illness on their family and their life.

A recent article written by a parent and published in the *New York Times* describes how these issues unfolded over the course of their child's illness and death [50].

There are number of resources available for ACP in children and adolescents such as Voicing my Choices and My Wishes, and in Queensland a paediatric version of the Statement of Choices.

19.7.1 Treatment decisions for newborn infants

Irrespective of the benefits they deliver, technological advances in neonatology create difficult ethical dilemmas for parents and doctors caring for extremely premature or severely disabled newborn infants. In 1986 in *F v F* in the Supreme Court of Victoria, Justice Vincent observed: 'No parent, no doctor, no court, has any power to determine that the life of any child, however disabled that child may be, will be deliberately taken from it' [51]. This statement does not necessarily help to resolve the ethical dilemmas and practical clinical challenges that have grown more difficult over subsequent years.

However, the law also recognises the rights and responsibilities of parents, in conjunction with treating doctors, to decide whether medical intervention should commence or continue. The reserve power of the state supreme courts to review and possibly overrule such decisions has rarely been used in Australia, but may be requested when parents and doctors, or other members of the healthcare team, cannot reach an agreement, or seek authorisation for a proposed course of action.

While paediatricians around the world have developed codes of practice that forbid hastening death, these codes do allow selective treatment or non-treatment, the guiding principle being the 'best interests' of the infant, having regard to the future quality of life, the benefits and burdens of treatment and whether the treatment is futile.

Decisions about 'best interests' can be very difficult as the subject has no voice and the adult participants in collaborative decision making may have very different beliefs about what the infant's 'best interests' might be.

In reaching decisions regarding the treatment of extremely premature or severely disabled infants, informed parental involvement is essential. It is important that the following roles are clear: the doctor should act in the interests of the infant patient and as medical adviser to the parents, and the parents have legal responsibilities to act on behalf of their child. If it is agreed that treatment should be withheld or withdrawn, adequate palliative care must continue. Throughout decision making and the provision of palliative care, continuing support for the parents is required and members of the healthcare team should be involved in all these stages [40].

Where parents and clinicians disagree, or where clinicians disagree with each other, clinical ethics services can be very helpful in distilling the ethical issues and achieving resolution without the need for referral to the courts. There are several ethical frameworks that are very helpful in paediatrics; for example: the zone of parental discretion, the ethics of care which incorporates the values and relationship with parents; and the harm principle, which in some situations is more helpful than the legalistic 'best interest' approach.

Where differences of view between families and treating doctors have led to common-law decisions, the courts have considered the best interests of the child as well as their present and future quality of life, the futility of current treatment, and the burdens and benefits of present and future treatment [52]. Consideration of such issues in discussion with parents may assist decision making in this ethically difficult area.

Nonetheless, these are complex and emotional issues and when they reach the courts they commonly spill out into the public domain with intense debate in the media between groups with very strongly held and often irreconcilable opinions.

Clinicians wishing to explore the legal dimensions of this challenging area in greater depth are advised to read sections 14.270–14.340, Withholding or withdrawing life-sustaining treatment from children (pp. 648–663), in White et al. *Health law in Australia 4th ed* [7].

19.7.2 Engaging with children who have life-limiting illnesses

Many clinicians have experienced the reality that most children with life-threatening illnesses, even those who are quite young, have some degree of understanding of the significance of their condition including that it may or will cause their death: they have talked to other children in outpatient clinics; they open up with ward nurses in the middle of the night; they listen at doorways to their parents' conversations with doctors and with one another; they hear their parents crying, see the tears and listen to hushed arguments; they feel the sadness; and they are given a disproportionate number of presents and treats. They may know about death from common life experiences of losing their grandparents and their pets, and are exposed to the constant stream of news and other media.

Children who are being subjected to prolonged, repeated, unpleasant, uncomfortable or sometimes painful investigations and treatment know something serious is happening. They experience the signs and symptoms of their own bodies; they observe the emotional responses of their families and health practitioners; they closely observe the illnesses and deterioration of other children; they compare themselves to well children; and they watch children who are sick and dying and then suddenly are no longer there.

At the same time, their families and the clinicians who treat and care for them are dealing with the broad range of emotional and psychological responses to the tension between how they see their roles as protectors and carers and the realities of the impending death of the child.

These dynamics were first explored in a seminal longitudinal study by anthropologist Myra Bluebond-Langner (subsequently published as a book, The private worlds of dying children, in 1978) [53]. Her observational research followed children, their families, and the health practitioners who cared for them over the course of children's life-ending illnesses through to their deaths.

The study revealed the complexity of the interactions across the social milieu of the community and healthcare services. In particular, it documented how all the participants—the children, their families, their doctors and other healthcare workers—behaved in ways that fulfilled their roles as they saw them to protect themselves, one another, and the integrity of their social structures, so that they could maintain their sense of stability in their roles and relationships that helped them to feel safe.

This understanding has had a profound influence on the scope and quality of care of children at the end of life. Paediatric palliative care and paediatric palliative medicine have since grown to embrace a far wider range of patients with both congenital and acquired life-limiting illnesses.

19.7.3 End-of-life decision making for adolescents and younger children

The law concerning decision making for and by children is complex. For a more detailed discussion, see Health law in Australia 4th ed [7], Chapter 6, Children and consent to medical treatment. See also Chapter 7, Consent and informed decision making, of this book.

The primary decision makers for children are usually their parents. Doctors should consider carefully how to engage with both children and their families to facilitate communication about decision making. These are not easy topics for any of the participants but, as discussed above, children are generally far more aware of their own condition than is commonly realised. A failure to acknowledge what a child can see and feel is happening to them can be distressing and disempowering for them.

Historically (as described in section 19.7.2), most children were excluded from participation in decision making about their own care at the end of life, even when they were clearly of an age at which they would normally be expected to participate in deciding about other aspects of their lives. Their individual progressive acquisition of the right to participate in decision making is generally described under the umbrella term of Gillick competency [7]. Now, as the child matures and they develop the cognitive ability to participate in shared and informed decision making, their views are increasingly being taken into consideration.

Of course, infants and many older children with life-limiting and/or neurocognitive degenerative conditions do not have capacity to participate fully in these conversations as a consequence of their underlying condition. Nonetheless, seeking to understand a child's world, their joys and pleasures, their likes and dislikes, and their means of communicating is crucial to optimising their engagement in the medical actions and interventions that may be considered.

Additionally, for those times and in situations where parents are not involved, other caregivers (e.g. carers, NDIS workers or teachers) must be included if the child's voice and interests are to be heard so that harm is minimised, and to optimise symptom relief and pleasure.

Uncommonly, situations arise where parents refuse to consent to treatment that the doctor advises, or demand treatment that the doctor believes is not in the best interests of the child. In such situations, as with adult patients, the doctor must do one or more of the following: spend more time discussing all the relevant issues with the parents and other members of the healthcare team, offer the parents a second medical opinion, ensure that all possible sources of support for the parents are made available, discuss the matter with a clinical ethics committee and, as a last resort, refer the matter to the guardianship authority or apply to the relevant court [54,55]. As mentioned above in the context of adults, it is crucial that parents are informed that active palliative care will continue whatever choices are made.

Treatment decisions about children involving medical procedures that do not treat a malfunction or disease, such as sterilisation and bone marrow donation, are beyond the authority of parents and must be authorised by a court. However, it is clear that court authorisation is not needed for other actions involving withdrawal of futile or burdensome treatment in the child's best interests that will lead to the child's death [56].

Some parents also hope to protect their child by refusing to allow information to be given to the child. This must be addressed with great sensitivity. However, the child may choose to reveal to the parents (sometimes through healthcare workers) that they already know much of what the parents would like to protect them from.

19.8 Making decisions for patients with post-coma unresponsiveness

The diagnosis and appropriate management of patients with post-coma unresponsiveness (PCU) raises difficult clinical and ethical issues for health professionals and the families concerned. These situations will usually be managed by senior consultant staff in intensive care units or palliative care units, and are generally beyond the scope of this book, but a brief discussion follows.

Following a NSW Supreme Court decision in which the judge found deficiencies in a hospital's policies and procedures that were exacerbated by the lack of national guidelines [57], the National Health and Medical Research Council (NHMRC) issued two key documents to guide clinicians in the diagnosis and ongoing care of such patients [58,59]. Moving away from the somewhat pejorative term 'vegetative state', the NHMRC suggested the new term of PCU, by which it also wished to separate post-coma states from the unresponsiveness seen in the terminal phase of some progressive illnesses. Briefly, PCU is a state of apparent wakefulness with a complete lack of responsiveness.

The NHMRC management guidelines on the topic emphasise that the diagnosis must not be considered before a minimum of 4 weeks after the appearance of unresponsive wakefulness, and that the diagnosis and any estimate of prognosis made after that should be regarded as provisional, to be reviewed at regular intervals.

The guidelines cover the responsibilities of the patient's representative (particularly to pay attention to the person's best interests) and the weight to attach to past expressions of the patient's wishes. Treating clinicians have the ethical responsibility to ensure that care and treatment are serving identified medical goals and that the treatment is neither futile nor unduly burdensome. In determining who is to act as the patient's representative, guardianship legislation provides the appropriate mechanisms (see section 19.3.2).

19.9 Voluntary assisted dying

VAD is the term that has been adopted in Australia to describe the process whereby a person with decision-making capacity is able to choose to end their life. It is a *voluntary* act by the person who requests that they be *assisted* by a doctor who arranges the provision of a substance that brings forward their *dying*.

At the time of writing, all Australian states and the ACT have legalised VAD in similar but not identical legislation, and it is possible that the NT will follow in the near future. Doctors should familiarise themselves with the relevant legislation in their state or territory. Links to the VAD laws in all states and territories can be found through QUT's compilation of End of Life Law in Australia [29] at: https://end-of-life.qut.edu.au/assisteddying.

To be eligible for VAD, a person:

- must be an Australian citizen or permanent resident living in the jurisdiction in which VAD will be accessed
- must be experiencing physical, emotional or spiritual suffering from a life-limiting illness
- must be aged at least 18 years
- must have capacity to make the request and maintain capacity throughout the process
- cannot have been coerced into making the request
- must have a predicted life expectancy of less than the amount specified in jurisdictional legislation.

Of particular importance, jurisdictional legislation varies significantly in how it seeks to balance the legal rights of persons to access VAD with the rights of individual healthcare workers and of institutions that might conscientiously object to VAD and not wish to participate. Doctors and other healthcare workers should be clear about their rights and legal obligations in the event that they are approached by a patient requesting information about, or for access to, VAD.

Legislation in all jurisdictions except NSW creates an offence for coercing persons to pursue VAD, but not all do so for coercing persons to not pursue or to revoke their request to access VAD. Of course, coercion by a doctor in form any would be unethical, even if not illegal in VAD legislation.

There are two options for the administration of VAD substances in Australia, and again, the details of the legislation and regulations regarding these options vary between jurisdictions—doctors should familiarise themselves what is required in their state or territory. These options for administration are:

1. **VAD by patient self-administration:** The doctor prescribes the lethal dose of the VAD substance(s) to an eligible patient which is dispensed to the patient. The patient decides if, when and where to consume the VAD substance in order to end their life.
2. **VAD by practitioner administration:** The VAD substance(s) is administered by a clinician.

This allows equal access to VAD by persons who are unable to swallow or to keep the VAD substances down after swallowing, and, again, eligibility varies between jurisdictions.

19.9.1 The history and terminology of euthanasia and voluntary assisted dying

Globally, euthanasia is illegal in most countries. However, over recent decades community support for the right of people to control the timing of their own death has increased, and an increasing number of jurisdictions, particularly in the Western world, have legalised the practice under a variety of names. In addition to Australia, a growing number of nations have passed a variety of legislation that permits at least some forms of VAD, which use a range of terms to describe the process.

This evolution in community attitudes appears to be related to the recognition that:

- even the highest quality palliative care cannot always relieve suffering at the end of life
- despite the great benefits, modern healthcare technologies can sometimes sustain lives of poor quality and result in unnaturally prolonged and very unpleasant deaths

- many people feel disempowered by modern medicine in a time of increasing emphasis on individual autonomy, both in health care and many other aspects of life
- the influence of religious doctrine on people's choices is waning.

As a result, in some jurisdictions the majority of people have come to believe that the timing of death is a matter of personal choice for people with life-limiting illnesses.

The word euthanasia in its original use in the human context meant an easy and gentle death, and did not imply an active role in bringing about that death. Its common contemporary meaning when applied to humans is an action by a doctor with the intent of ending the life of a patient who is terminally ill and in distress. Professional and public debate about euthanasia is frequently accompanied by the use of a variety of other terminology (such as voluntary euthanasia and physician-assisted suicide) which can cause confusion.

'Voluntary assisted dying' is the terminology that has been agreed upon in Australia and describes the processes that, at the time of writing, have been legalised in all Australian states and the ACT. It describes the legal provision by a doctor of a substance with which a person with decision-making capacity can choose to end their life, either by consuming it themselves or sometimes with the direct assistance of a doctor or a nurse. Doctors are encouraged to use VAD as the agreed term that has been in adopted in legislation in all Australian jurisdictions.

It is very important to recognise the clear distinction between VAD (and euthanasia), and the withdrawal or withholding of life-sustaining treatment. The latter has long been an uncontroversial part of the daily routine of medical practice across Australia, particularly in intensive care (see sections 19.2.4 and 19.4).

19.9.2 Evolving positions of the medical profession on voluntary assisted dying

Since the previous edition of this publication, the formal positions of many organisations around the world on the issue of VAD have changed to varying degrees and are continuing to evolve. For example, the World Medical Association has changed its position from clear opposition to VAD in 1992 [60], to a focus on the right of physicians to conscientiously object to VAD in 2019 [61].

In 2016 and 2017, the AMA issued updated position statements on policy on euthanasia and VAD that focus primarily on the need to provide high-quality care at the end of life [62,63]. While not supporting VAD, it recognised that some doctors support the practice of VAD. A further updated position statement was launched in 2025 to reflect the current legal position where VAD is widely available [39]. It continues to advocate strongly for high-quality end-of-life care but recognises that some doctors will become involved in the process of VAD [39].

Similarly, in 2006 the British Medical Association (BMA) opposed assisted dying. After a 2020 survey of its members, BMA adopted a neutral stance and will continue to lobby on behalf of the rights of doctors to follow their conscience on the issue [64]. The Royal Australasian College of Physicians' 2018 *Statement on voluntary assisted dying* adopted a neutral stance [65], as did the Royal College of Physicians in the UK in 2019 [66].

The Australian and New Zealand Society of Palliative Medicine's (ANZSPM) position on VAD has fluctuated since its initial neutral statement created in about 2000. In 2012, the ANZSPM position changed and for several years described physician-assisted suicide as unethical. Subsequently, ANZSPM reverted to a neutral position until 2021, when it adopted a policy that predominantly seeks to ensure that the provision of VAD is not identified as a component of the discipline and practice of palliative medicine. It also clearly identifies those components of the routine practice of palliative medicine that should not be considered as VAD [67]. Palliative Care Australia is similarly neutral on VAD [68].

Irrespective of their views on VAD, all the organisations referenced above believe that it is unethical for doctors to fail to provide or arrange for adequate palliative and end-of-life care to patients who have requested or are planning to access VAD.

19.9.3 When patients ask their doctors about voluntary assisted dying

Like the rest of their community, Australian doctors hold a wide range of beliefs on VAD. Given this diversity, doctors will produce a variety of responses to patients requesting VAD that reflect their personal beliefs. Doctors are therefore advised to prepare in advance of their first request by understanding their obligations under the legislation that applies where they are working.

Current legislation that legalises VAD provides for the right of all healthcare workers and the organisations they work in to conscientiously object to providing VAD, with some significant differences in the details between jurisdictions. That doctors and other healthcare workers have rights to conscientious objection does not mean that they are free to obstruct access or coerce patients not to pursue VAD where it is a legal option. While legislation about coercion in the context of VAD varies between jurisdictions, coercion by a doctor of a person either to access or not to access VAD is unethical at all times. VAD is a patient's right and choice, subject to the criteria laid down in legislation.

The actions that individual doctors take must also fulfil their ongoing obligations to their patients and their duty to respect the laws in the jurisdiction where they are working.

At the time of writing there are important differences with respect to conscientious objection between the laws and regulations in effect across the states and territories of Australia. Legislation seeks to balance the right of doctors not to participate in VAD with the right of patients to participate in VAD where it is legal. Doctors still have an ethical duty of care, and may also be required by law, to continue to provide ongoing care unrelated to VAD and/or to redirect patients so that their right to access VAD is not obstructed. Doctors should familiarise themselves with how the tension between their own rights and those of their patients have been addressed in the relevant legislation in the jurisdiction where they are working. These can be found through individual state and territory health department websites that describe jurisdictional VAD regulations; see also the QUT website [29].

The doctor's second task is then to consider their personal views on VAD and how they will respond to patients wishing to discuss VAD when their first such patient is sitting in front of them. Irrespective of their own views on VAD, doctors can start by exploring why their patient is making the request, and whether their reasons are remediable. It has always been the case that some patients dealing with a life-limiting illness ponder whether they may wish to end their life. This can do so for a variety of reasons, including depression; distressing physical symptoms or very poor quality of life; loss of agency and control due to a diminishing ability to live independently; a belief that they are a burden on family or the community; loss of a sense of purpose in life (commonly described as existential distress); or simply that they are content with the sum of the life that they have lived and do not wish or feel the need to live for more time in a condition that they expect (often with some justification) may at best be unpleasant and undignified, and at worst characterised by severe and distressing symptoms that cannot be controlled by even the best palliative care.

Doctors have a duty to identify and respond to the needs of a terminally ill patient—for example, by supporting a patient to understand that they may die or are dying and providing them with access to effective pain control and/or access to available palliative care services.

Therefore, it must be stressed again that, irrespective of their views on VAD and whether or not their patient is considering seeking access to VAD, doctors have a duty to understand that the provision of palliative care (e.g. symptom relief, care and compassion, the withdrawal or withholding of unbeneficial treatment) is not VAD. Those doctors who conscientiously object to VAD have an ethical duty to continue to meet other non-VAD needs of their patients who are pursuing VAD, either by providing such care themselves or ensuring that continuity of care is maintained while transferring the responsibility for such care to another doctor.

While some patients do not wish to discuss the issues that are causing them to ponder VAD, many would benefit from a relationship with their doctor that supports them to be able to explore the challenges that they are facing or will face. Only then does it become possible to address such problems with better symptom management, increased home support, ACP, emotional support, discussion of existential issues and treatment of depression. While individual doctors may not be able to address all or even some of these issues, they are still able to mobilise such resources from within their community.

However, while no-one should find themselves choosing to pursue VAD because they are unable to access appropriate palliative care, even the best of support and specialist palliative care cannot resolve all of the issues that lead some people to request VAD. Doctors should not feel responsible for the impossibility of relieving all suffering or for failing to relieve patients of their desire for VAD.

It is important to note that VAD legislation in all Australian jurisdictions requires that the doctor completing the death certificate of a person who has died after consuming the VAD substance identifies the cause of death as being the illness or condition that qualified them for VAD. The doctor is not permitted to mention or attribute the cause of death to VAD, suicide, or the consumption/administration of the VAD substance.

Finally, doctors should not coerce or place undue pressure on their colleagues to either provide or to refuse to provide VAD. Both are choices of conscience that individual doctors are legally empowered to make.

19.10 Supporting the dying person and their family around the time of death

Many people have little experience of being present at a death. As patients, and as patients' families, they may not understand what they are either experiencing or seeing. Similarly, many people do not know how to respond to a person's death. Culturally driven responses vary greatly, and doctors should be prepared for the full range of behaviours from silent, calm acceptance to an outpouring of great distress, including anger. The doctor's presence and their own responses while a person is dying and afterwards can also serve to shape the responses of families.

Many doctors who have continued to care for patients who are dying expected deaths, and for their families, will recognise the peace that can come with acceptance by a patient and their family that death is inevitable and is no longer to be feared. They will have shared the tears and the reminiscences, and laughed at the jokes by the patient, their family and their friends, and perhaps have made a few jokes of their own when appropriate.

Of course, while palliative care tends to focus on the deaths from illnesses that have been controllable for a time and that have become the norm in Australia, not all deaths are peaceful. Some are unexpected, sudden and perhaps violent. They disrupt lives and relationships, they can cause social and financial chaos, and in some cases, disasters disrupt whole communities. There may be anger, resentment, fear and tension between family members who are forced together by social obligation. Doctors have no control over, or responsibility for, such matters that may have had their origins decades earlier.

Good medical practice means being with people as they die. Not 24 hours per day, but sufficiently frequently for patients and their families to feel that they are being watched out for, and that they are not alone.

One of the more important roles of doctors is to recognise when death is near and to explain and normalise the phenomena of dying as they unfold—fluctuating consciousness, changed breathing patterns, decreased appetite and thirst, peripheral shutdown, etc. Sometimes normalisation of the unfamiliar and the provision of reassurance that these signs do not necessarily require medical intervention is all that is necessary.

Doctors caring for dying people need to identify distressing symptoms and signs that should be addressed—agitation, pain, dyspnoea, a full bladder, haemorrhage, etc.—and to treat them in a manner appropriate to the circumstances of the moment. These are the core skills of palliative care and are well described in sources such as Therapeutic Guidelines: Palliative Care [69].

Dying runs to its own unpredictable timetable and good end-of-life care may mean waiting patiently for a person to die, or finding that they die more quickly than expected. It means being surprised along with the family when a seemingly unconscious person who has not spoken for days suddenly says, 'Good morning doctor!', or makes a joke. Or just sitting with a family at the bedside making quiet small talk. It may mean chuckling with a relative who has followed you out of the room to the sink where you are washing your hands to tell you that the person you had just said seemed 'unlikely to die today' had died as you shut the door.

Good medical practice can also mean allowing the grief to wash over you, or soaking up the anger because you know that it is directed at you simply because you are there, or maybe you did not say quite the right thing, or perhaps because you were not there after you had said you would be but the person died suddenly from something else weeks before you expected.

And years later it can mean people coming up to you in the supermarket saying, 'Thank you! You won't remember me but you looked after my mother when she died in the nursing home.' Or they may just smile at you in front of the cauliflowers—you remember their face but don't remember the details, but they do. Their lives were changed, as were countless others, because you helped to normalise the death of their relative, a change that is so important for a healthy society.

19.11 Communication and confidentiality after death

After a patient dies, it is not uncommon for family members to have questions and concerns about the circumstances surrounding their death. Doctors should be being willing to explain, to the best of their knowledge, the circumstances of the death of their patient to appropriate members of the patient's family and to carers. This is a very important duty because many people have only a very limited understanding of the process of dying, can misinterpret the normal physiological phenomena of dying as distress, and can misunderstand the use and impact of medicines in palliative care (see section 19.10). Not infrequently, they wrongly believe that the medicines used judiciously in everyday palliative care caused the death and, unless corrected, this myth becomes perpetuated in the community.

Such conversations should be started even while the patient is approaching death as explanations of what is being observed by the patient themselves, and their family and carers sitting at the bedside. However, if the doctor knows that the patient would have objected to such discussions or did not wish some matters disclosed (such as the underlying cause of death), then these wishes should be respected [2].

19.12 Providing support in bereavement

Grief is the normal reaction to a loss and grieving is the evolved process by which humans and other animals heal from a loss. Indeed, the strong bonds that form between individuals that are vital for social cohesion are sustained in part by grief being such a deterrent to their being broken. Given that these bonds between individuals are so commonly broken by death, grieving also exists as an evolved mechanism for individuals who do suffer a loss to move on in pursuit of the biological and social imperatives of their lives.

Most people who have experienced the death of a relative or a friend navigate their bereavement without the need for specific treatment. However, for some, bereavement brings with it a significantly increased risk of early impulsive suicide or major depressive illness.

A study of Swiss mortality statistics for the period 1987–2005 found very high rates of suicide in widowed persons [70]. The study found that the suicide rates were highest in the first week after bereavement, particularly in bereaved men, declining over the next few months but, except in older widows, not reaching the baseline levels during the first year.

Good medical practice means understanding that grief and grieving are normal phenomena in normal people dealing with a loss. Grief unfolds at its own pace and cannot been hurried. Most people who are grieving need support and do not require treatment. Nonetheless, doctors should also be alert to the signs and symptoms of depression and complicated grief in their patients who are bereaved. Additionally, doctors should also be alert for bereaved elderly spouses who may not be able to cope with tasks of independent living when these had been shared with their spouse who has now died.

Doctors who are not comfortable or do not have the skills to manage complicated grief themselves should consider referring their patient on to specialised services.

19.13 Triage and resource-allocation decision making in pandemics and other disasters

Doctors are expected to step forward in the face of disaster. The recent COVID-19 pandemic overwhelmed healthcare services in communities around the world, and pandemics are just one of the many forms of calamity.

Any doctor may suddenly find themselves in the midst of a disaster and having to make choices about which patients will and will not receive potentially life-saving treatments. Commonly this means doctors shifting the focus of their treatment goals from the interests of every individual patient to engage in resource allocation as triage by weighing the relative claims of numbers of patients and the broader overall interests of the community as a whole. A doctor may find themselves having to decide on what grounds patients will be chosen to receive or not to receive life-saving treatment.

Most doctors have not been prepared for such confronting tasks, and current laws and regulations offer little ethical guidance or legal support for those who have no choice other than to take on the burdensome duties of triage and resource allocation [71,72].

The distress that many healthcare workers experienced during the COVID-19 pandemic was made worse because they had not been prepared for the overwhelming nature of what was required of them. It is abundantly clear that doctors and other healthcare workers should be trained and supported to deal with the diversity of local, regional and global disasters that will inevitably occur. No doctor or global region can be sure that they will not be impacted.

At the time of writing, the Australian Medical Council was developing a guidance to integrate the core knowledge and skills of responding to disasters into medical training at all levels, to support doctors to prepare themselves for their possible roles in disaster responses, and to guide them when they suddenly find themselves having to take on these unfamiliar tasks.

Summary

This chapter has highlighted that care at the end of life is not restricted to the provision of good palliative care. It requires that doctors engage with their patients and their community to promote the broad understanding that death is the normal and inevitable end for every life. Helping our community to deal with mortality and prepare for death is a core role for doctors as part of their good medical practice.

The chapter has addressed a broad range of issues from how the law deals with death and dying to how children with life-limiting illnesses understand their own circumstances.

Ultimately, the most important tasks for doctors seeking to support their community in this most complex and emotionally challenging domain are to nurture their ability to establish good working relationships with patients, their families and colleagues, and to develop the skills to lead the effective communication and collaboration necessary to achieve the best possible outcomes, even when people are dying.

While not every doctor will face death on a regular basis, this knowledge is central to the art of good medical practice founded in the doctor's comfort with their own mortality and acceptance that modern medical technology cannot override the reality that every human life ends in death.

References

1. Olshansky SJ, Willcox BJ, Demetrius L, Beltrán-Sánchez H. Implausibility of radical life extension in humans in the twenty-first century. *Nat Aging* 2024; 4: 1635–1642.
2. Medical Board of Australia. Good Medical Practice: a code of conduct for doctors in Australia. 2020. https://www.medicalboard.gov.au/codes-guidelines-policies/code-of-conduct.aspx (accessed Jun 2025).
3. Australian and New Zealand Intensive Care Society. ANZICS statement on care and decision-making at the end of life for the critically ill (edition 1.0). Melbourne: ANZICS, 2014. https://intensivecareathome.com/wp-content/uploads/2015/05/ANZICS-Statement-on-Care-and-Decision-Making-at-the-End-of-Life.pdf (accessed Jun 2025).
4. Silvester W, Detering K. Advance care planning and end-of-life care. Med J Aust 2011; 195: 435–436.
5. Clayton JM, Hancock KM, Butow PN, et al. Clinical practice guidelines for communicating prognosis and end-of-life issues with adults in the advanced stages of a life-limiting illness, and their caregivers. *Med J Aust* 2007; 186: S77–S105.
6. Advance Care Planning Australia. Advance care planning explained. Queensland Health, 2025. https://www.advancecareplanning.org.au/understand-advance-care-planning/advance-care-planning-explained (accessed Apr 2025).
7. White B, McDonald F, Willmott L, Then S-N, editors. Health law in Australia 4th edition. Sydney: Thomson Reuters, 2023.
8. Brown M, Ruberu R, Thompson CH. Inadequate resuscitation documentation in older patients' clinical case notes. *Intern Med J* 2014; 44: 93–96.
9. Barclay S, Maher J. Having difficult conversations about the end of life. *BMJ* 2010; 341: 653–655.
10. *Powers of Attorney Act 1998* (Qld), Sch 2, s 5(2).
11. *Guardianship and Administration Act 2000* (Qld), Sch 2, ss 5(2), 79.
12. White B, Willmott L. Rethinking life-sustaining measures: questions for Queensland. Brisbane: QUT Printing Services, 2005: 69–72. https://eprints.qut.edu.au/7093/ (accessed Jun 2025).

13. *Medical Treatment Planning and Decisions Act 2016* (Vic), s 3(1), definition of 'palliative care'.
14. *Re BWV; Ex parte Gardner* (2003) 7 VR 487; [2003] VSC 173.
15. Wilkinson DJC. Futile treatment: the ethicist's perspective. *Med J Aust* 2013; 198: 223–224.
16. Kasman DL. When is medical treatment futile? A guide for students, residents, and physicians. *J Gen Intern Med* 2004; 19: 1053–1056.
17. Koczwara B. What is futile and who decides? The clinician's dilemma. *Med J Aust* 2013; 198: 221–222.
18. Willmott L, White B, Downie J. Withholding and withdrawal of 'futile' life-sustaining treatment: unilateral medical-decision making in Australia and New Zealand. *J Law Med* 2013; 20: 907–924.
19. End of Life Law in Australia. State and territory laws. Brisbane: University of Technology Queensland, 2024. https://end-of-life.qut.edu.au/treatment-decisions/adults/state-and-territory-laws (accessed Jun 2025).
20. *Messiha v South East Health* [2004] NSWSC 1061.
21. *Northridge v Central Sydney Area Health Service* [2000] NSWSC 1241.
22. Catholic Health Australia. Code of standards for Catholic health and aged care services in Australia. Red Hill (ACT): Catholic Health Australia Inc, 2001. https://cha.org.au/wp-content/uploads/2021/06/Code-of-ethicsfullcopy.pdf (accessed Jun 2025).
23. Balaban RB. A physician's guide to talking about end-of-life care. *J Gen Intern Med* 2000; 15: 195–200.
24. Ashby MA, Thornton RN, Thomas RL. Advance care planning: lessons from a study of Tasmanian enduring guardianship forms. *Med J Aust* 2013; 198: 188–189.
25. Grant L, Murray SA, Sheikh A. Spiritual dimensions of dying in pluralist societies. *BMJ* 2010; 341: 659–662.
26. Australian Government Department of Health. National framework for advance care planning documents. Canberra: Commonwealth of Australia, 2021. https://www.health.gov.au/resources/publications/national-framework-for-advance-care-planning-documents (accessed Jun 2025).
27. Detering KM, Hancock AD, Reade MC, Silvester W. The impact of advance care planning on end of life care in elderly patients: randomised controlled trial. *BMJ* 2010; 340: c1345.
28. Robins-Browne K, Palmer V, Komesaroff P. An unequivocal good? Acknowledging the complexities of advance care planning. *Intern Med J* 2014; 44: 957–960.
29. End of Life Law in Australia. Brisbane: Queensland University of Technology, Australian Centre for Health Law Research. https://end-of-life.qut.edu.au (accessed Jun 2025).
30. Biegler P, Stewart C, Savulescu J, Skene L. Determining the validity of advance directives. *Med J Aust* 2000; 172: 545–548.
31. NSW Health. Making an advance care directive—form and information booklet. Sydney: NSW Government, 2023. https://www.health.nsw.gov.au/patients/acp/Pages/acd-form-info-book.aspx (accessed Jun 2025).
32. Weerasinghe DP, MacIntyre CR, Rubin GL. The epidemiology of cardiac arrests in a Sydney hospital. *Resuscitation* 2002; 53: 53–62.
33. Weil MH, Fries M. In-hospital cardiac arrest. *Crit Care Med* 2005; 33: 2825–2830.
34. Queensland Health. Resuscitation resources for health professionals. Brisbane: Queensland Government, 2025. https://www.health.qld.gov.au/clinical-practice/guidelines-procedures/clinical-resources/resuscitation-resources-for-health-professionals (accessed Jun 2025).
35. Hayes B. Clinical model for ethical cardiopulmonary resuscitation decision-making. *Intern Med J* 2013; 43: 77–83.
36. Lawrence S, Willmott L, Milligan E, et al. Autonomy versus futility? Barriers to good clinical practice in end-of-life care: a Queensland case. *Med J Aust* 2012; 196: 404–405.
37. Stewart CL. A defence of the requirement to seek consent to withhold and withdraw futile treatments. *Med J Aust* 2012; 196: 406–408.
38. Willmott L, White B, Smith MK, Wilkinson DJC. Withholding and withdrawing life-sustaining treatment in a patient's best interests: Australian judicial deliberations. *Med J Aust* 2014; 201: 545–547.
39. Australian Medical Association. Position statement on voluntary assisted dying. 2025. https://www.ama.com.au/articles/ama-position-statement-voluntary-assisted-dying-2025 (accessed May 2025).
40. Australian Commission on Safety and Quality in Health Care. National consensus statement: essential elements for safe and high-quality end-of-life care in acute hospitals. Consultation draft—January 2014.

https://www.safetyandquality.gov.au/sites/default/files/migrated/Draft-National-Consensus-Statement-Essential-Elements-for-Safe-and-High-Quality-End-of-Life-Care-in-Acute-Hospitals.pdf (accessed Jun 2025).

41. World Health Organization. Definition of palliative care. Geneva: WHO, 2020. https://www.who.int/news-room/fact-sheets/detail/palliative-care (accessed Jul 2023).
42. National Health and Medical Research Council. An ethical framework for integrating palliative care into the management of advanced chronic or terminal conditions. 2011. https://pallcarevic.asn.au/wp-content/uploads/2015/11/Ethical-Framework-for-Integrating-Palliative-Care-Principles-.pdf (accessed Jun 2025).
43. Royal Australian College of General Practitioners. Medical care of older persons in residential aged care facilities—the silver book 5th ed. Vic: RACGP, 2019. https://www.racgp.org.au/clinical-resources/clinical-guidelines/key-racgp-guidelines/view-all-racgp-guidelines/silver-book/part-a/palliative-care (accessed Jun 2025).
44. Lo B. Euthanasia in the Netherlands: what lessons for elsewhere? *Lancet* 2012; 380: 869–870.
45. Douglas CD, Kerridge IH, Ankeny RA. Narratives of 'terminal sedation' and the importance of the intention-foresight distinction in palliative care practice. *Bioethics* 2013; 27: 1–11.
46. Thomson CJH. '... (D)eath, a necessary end, will come when it will come', (William Shakespeare, Julius Caesar, Act 2, Scene 2.). *Intern Med J* 2011; 41: 439–440.
47. Temel JS, Greer JA, Muzikansky MA, et al. Early palliative care for patients with metastatic non-small-cell lung cancer. *N Engl J Med* 2010; 363: 733–742.
48. Zimmermann C, Swami N, Krzyzanowska M, et al. Early palliative care for patients with advanced cancer: a cluster-randomised controlled trial. *Lancet* 2014; 383: 1721–1730.
49. World Health Organization. Child mortality and causes of death. Geneva: WHO. https://www.who.int/data/gho/data/themes/topics/topic-details/GHO/child-mortality-and-causes-of-death (accessed Jun 2025).
50. Wildman S. If my dying daughter could face her mortality, why couldn't the rest of us? *The New York Times*. 2024 Nov 25. https://www.nytimes.com/2024/11/25/opinion/children-cancer-grief.html (accessed Jun 2025).
51. *Re F; F v F. Vincent J* (1986) Unreported, Supreme Court of Victoria, 2 July 1986.
52. Tibballs J. Legal basis for ethical withholding and withdrawing life-sustaining medical treatment from infants and children. *J Paediatr Child Health* 2007; 43: 230–236.
53. Bluebond-Langner M. The private worlds of dying children. Princeton University Press, 1978.
54. Skene L. Law and medical practice. 3rd ed. Sydney: LexisNexis Butterworths, 2008: 346–362.
55. Wellesley H, Jenkins IA. Withholding and withdrawing life-sustaining treatment in children. *Paediatr Anaesth* 2009; 19: 972–978.
56. *Re Baby D (No.2)* (2011) FamCA 176 (16 March 2011).
57. *Northridge v Central Sydney Area Health Service* (2000) NSWLR 1241.
58. National Health and Medical Research Council. Post-coma unresponsiveness (vegetative state): a clinical framework for diagnosis. Commonwealth of Australia, 2004. https://webarchive.nla.gov.au/awa/20170817105215/https://www.nhmrc.gov.au/guidelines-publications/hpr23 (accessed Jun 2025).
59. National Health and Medical Research Council. Ethical guidelines for the care of people in post-coma unresponsiveness (vegetative state) or a minimally responsive state. Commonwealth of Australia, 2008. https://www.nhmrc.gov.au/about-us/publications/ethical-guidelines-care-people-post-coma-unresponsiveness (accessed Jul 2023).
60. World Medical Association. Statement on physician-assisted suicide. Adopted 1992. Revised 2005. https://www.wma.net/policies-post/wma-statement-on-physician-assisted-suicide/ (accessed Jul 2023).
61. World Medical Association. WMA declaration on euthanasia and physician-assisted suicide. 2019. https://www.wma.net/policies-post/declaration-on-euthanasia-and-physician-assisted-suicide/ (accessed Jul 2023).
62. Australian Medical Association. Position statement on euthanasia and physician assisted suicide. 2016. https://www.ama.com.au/sites/default/files/documents/AMA_Position_Statement_on_Euthanasia_and_Physician_Assisted_Suicide_2016.pdf (accessed Jun 2025).
63. Australian Medical Association. AMA media release: euthanasia and physician assisted suicide. 2017. https://ama.com.au/sites/default/files/documents/241116%20-%20AMA%20Position%20Statement%20on%20Euthanasia%20and%20Physician%20Assisted%20Suicide%202016.pdf (accessed Jun 2025).

64. British Medical Association. Physician-assisted dying. 2021. https://www.bma.org.uk/advice-and-support/ethics/end-of-life/physician-assisted-dying (accessed Apr 2025).
65. The Royal Australasian College of Physicians. Statement on voluntary assisted dying. 2018. https://www.racp.edu.au/docs/default-source/advocacy-library/racp-voluntary-assisted-dying-statement-november-2018.pdf (accessed Jun 2025).
66. Royal College of Physicians (UK). The RCP clarifies its position on assisted dying. 2020. https://www.rcp.ac.uk/news-and-media/news-and-opinion/the-rcp-clarifies-its-position-on-assisted-dying/ (accessed Jun 2025).
67. Australian and New Zealand Society of Palliative Medicine. Position statement: the practice of euthanasia and physician-assisted suicide. Last updated: November 2021. https://www.anzspm.org.au/common/Uploaded%20files/Position%20Statements/2%20ANZSPM_Position_Statement_Euthanasia_Physician_Assisted_Dying.pdf (accessed Jun 2025).
68. Palliative Care Australia. Palliative care and voluntary assisted dying position statement 2022. https://palliativecare.org.au/statement/palliative-care-and-voluntary-assisted-dying-position-statement-2022/ (accessed Jul 2023).
69. Palliative care [version 5]. In: Therapeutic Guidelines. Melbourne: Therapeutic Guidelines Limited, 2024. https://www.tg.org.au/products/therapeutic-guidelines/updates/palliative-care/ (accessed Jun 2025).
70. Ajdacic-Gross V, Ring M, Gadola E, et al. Suicide after bereavement: an overlooked problem. *Psychol Med* 2008; 38: 673–676.
71. Close E, Willmott L, Cockburn T, et al. Transparent triage policies during the COVID-19 pandemic: a critical part of medico-legal risk management for clinicians. *Med J Aust* 2021; 215: 71–74.e1.
72. Close E, White B, Willmott L, et al. If COVID hospitalisations increase, it's still not clear how patients will be prioritised for ICU beds. *The Conversation*. 2021 Oct 27. https://theconversation.com/if-covid-hospitalisations-increase-its-still-not-clear-how-patients-will-be-prioritised-for-icu-beds-169948 (accessed Jun 2025).

Further reading

Advance Care Planning Australia. Queensland Health. https://www.advancecareplanning.org.au

End of Life Law in Australia. Brisbane: Queensland University of Technology, Australian Centre for Health Law Research. https://end-of-life.qut.edu.au

Gawande A. Being mortal: illness, medicine and what matters in the end. London: Profile Books, 2014.

Hitchcock K. Dear life: on caring for the elderly. *Quarterly Essay*. 2015 Mar. https://www.quarterlyessay.com/essay/2015/03/dear-life

Kerridge I, Lowe M, Stewart C. Ethics and law for the health professions. 4th ed. Sydney: Federation Press, 2013.

Myra Bluebond-Langner. The private worlds of dying children. Princeton University Press, 1978.

Skene L. Law and medical practice. 3rd ed. Sydney: LexisNexis Butterworths, 2008.

Srivastava R. Tell me the truth: conversations with my patients about life and death. Melbourne: Viking Penguin, 2010.

White B, McDonald F, Willmott L, Shih-Ning Then, editors. Health Law in Australia. 4th ed. Sydney: Thomson Reuters, 2023.

PART THREE

Roles and responsibilities in the Australian health and legal systems

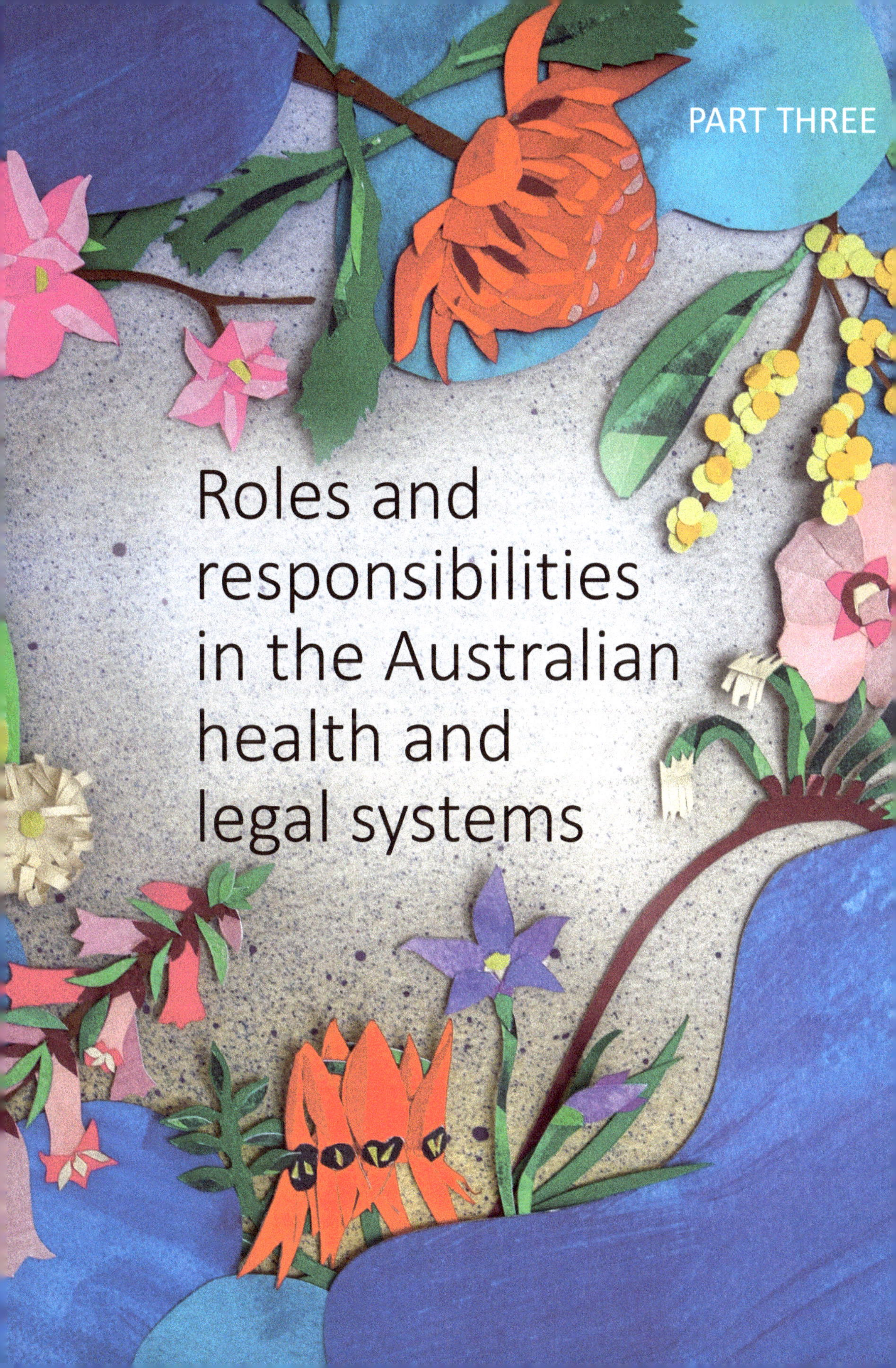

20 The Australian healthcare system

Susan Wearne

Introduction

This chapter provides an overview of the Australian healthcare system. It starts by outlining the functions of primary, secondary and tertiary care, and which governments are responsible for them. Next it discusses the funding of the health system and doctors' employment structures. Lastly, there is an introduction to the organisations and schemes that educate, support, insure and regulate medical practice and practitioners. There is a focus on topics that pose risks for doctors, especially those new to Australian medical practice. It should be noted that there are frequent reviews and changes to the healthcare system, and this chapter should be read as a general guide.

20.1 Functional levels: primary, secondary and tertiary care

The Australian health system delivers different levels of care according to peoples' health, or the frequency and severity of their illness.

20.1.1 Primary care

Primary care is the first point of contact for people accessing the health system, and provides widespread access to health promotion, preventative care and management of acute and chronic health problems. International evidence demonstrates that countries with strong primary care are associated with a more equitable distribution of health in populations [1].

Primary care is delivered by health professionals such as general practitioners (GPs), pharmacists, opticians, dentists, physiotherapists and practice nurses. Primary care practitioners combine their management of the majority of problems with monitoring for early hints of complex or serious problems that will require input from other specialists.

Primary care practitioners refer people with problems requiring specialist expertise to secondary care. Some allied health providers, such as opticians, can refer to ophthalmologists, but most often access to secondary care is through referral from GPs. See Box 20.1 for key facts about referrals.

20.1.2 Secondary care

Secondary medical care is provided by doctors who train in particular aspects of care such as psychiatry, surgery or geriatrics. Many work in public or private hospitals and/or private consulting rooms, while some are based in the community, such as community paediatricians and mental health services.

In some rural and remote areas, GPs are expected to provide secondary-level services that would usually be delivered by other specialists in urban areas. Examples include GPs with additional training in obstetrics or anaesthetics, and GPs who supervise haemodialysis in remote Aboriginal and/or Torres Strait Islander communities.

20.1.3 Tertiary care

The complexity of illnesses, and the treatments now available for them, means patients can benefit from seeing subspecialists with expertise in narrow fields of treatment or technology. Examples are vitreo-retinal surgeons, who are subspecialist ophthalmologists who treat retinal disease; and gynaecological oncology, which is a subspecialty of obstetrics and gynaecology. Subspecialists' requirements for equipment, skilled support staff and case load mean they are based in urban centres. Historically, referral to subspecialists came from specialists within the same discipline, but increasingly, GPs are referring patients directly to subspecialists, a practice contributed to by a reduction in the number of 'generalist' specialists willing to care for people with any problem within their discipline.

In rare cases, care is further specialised into quaternary care, where certain conditions are only managed by one or two national centres.

Box 20.1 Referring and requesting Medicare services [2]

Doctors can refer patients for consultations with other doctors or for pathology or diagnostic imaging. Referrals for different types of service have slightly varied legal requirements for claiming Medicare benefits. The following list is a combination of these requirements and represents good practice:

- relevant clinical information about the patient's condition for investigation, opinion, treatment and management
- the date of the referral
- the patient's name, date of birth, gender, Aboriginal and/or Torres Strait Islander status, Medicare number and contact details (address, phone number, email)
- the requesting practitioner's full name, provider number and contact details (address, phone number, fax, email)
- the physical or electronic signature of the referring practitioner
- the details of other practitioners caring for the patient who should receive a copy of any reports about the patient.

Timing of referrals

- GPs can opt to refer people to other specialists for a year or indefinitely, depending on the clinical condition.
- Non-GP specialists can refer to another specialist for a maximum of three months. After that time, patients are expected to seek review from their GP to see if ongoing non-GP specialist input is needed.
- Time counts from the date the person is first seen by the specialist doctor, not the date of the initial referral.
- Referrals cannot be backdated.

Continued over page

- Patients should choose where to present the referral. Referrals do not need to be made out to a specific specialist or consultant physician, pathology lab or imaging service.

Record keeping

- Doctors must keep adequate and contemporaneous notes of consultations and include the duration, date and time for which a rebate is claimed. The notes may be used to audit if the claim was appropriate.

20.1.4 Aboriginal and Torres Strait Islander medical services

All medical practitioners in Australia must be able to provide culturally safe care to Aboriginal and/or Torres Strait Islander people to identify and manage high-risk disease, such as rheumatic fever, in this population. However, there are also specific services for Aboriginal and/or Torres Strait Islander communities, which play an important role.

Aboriginal community controlled health services (ACCHS) provide culturally appropriate comprehensive primary health care for and run by Aboriginal and/or Torres Strait Islander people. ACCHS implement a holistic definition of health, as defined in the 2023 Constitution of the National Aboriginal Community Controlled Health Organisation (NACCHO):

> 'Aboriginal health' means not just the physical well-being of an individual but refers to the social, emotional and cultural well-being of the whole Community in which each individual is able to achieve their full potential as a human being thereby bringing about the total well-being of their Community. It is a whole of life view and includes the cyclical concept of life-death-life [3].

This whole of life view leads to ACCHS working in health promotion and programs that address the social determinants of health. ACCHS offer multidisciplinary care and train and employ Aboriginal and/or Torres Strait Islander health workers and practitioners, as well as a wide range of allied health, nursing and medical personnel. See also section 17.6.5 in Chapter 17, Culturally safe health care for Aboriginal and/or Torres Strait Islander peoples.

Aboriginal and Torres Strait Islander medical services are funded by the Australian Government. Health professionals are often employed on a salary and may also be able to claim Medicare payments.

20.2 Government responsibilities

The Australian Government is responsible for primary care, including Aboriginal and Torres Strait Islander medical services and aged care. State and territory governments are responsible for running public hospitals that provide secondary, tertiary and quaternary care. Public hospitals cannot charge fees to public patients. The funding paid by the Australian Government to states and territories for health care is negotiated periodically. Inpatient services are similar across states and territories, although there is variation in their provision of community-based primary care and outpatient non-GP specialist services.

Private hospitals and secondary care specialist consulting rooms are run as private businesses or as not-for-profit organisations, some of which have religious or charitable affiliations. Private hospitals provide a significant proportion of elective surgery.

Australia has more than 1300 public and private hospitals that, in 2022–23, collectively provided over 12 million hospital admissions and 33.2 million days of patient care. Of those, about 7.1 million (59%) were admissions to public hospitals, and about 5.0 million (41%) were to private hospitals [4].

The delineation of responsibility for primary and other care between the federal and state or territory governments was established when there was greater distinction between illnesses that could be treated in the community and those that needed hospital services. The system seems less suited to caring for an ageing population with multiple chronic comorbidities. Patients can shuttle between multiple practitioners and be at risk when the treatment recommended for one problem interacts with the treatment of another, or is recommended without knowing the patient's relevant history. All governments are considering how best to adapt the current structures to better coordinate patient care across multiple providers.

20.2.1 Legislation

National legislation

Doctors must work in accordance with national and the relevant state or territory legislation. The *Health Insurance Act 1973* (Cth) introduced Medicare as a publicly funded universal healthcare insurance scheme. The Act and its subsequent amendments legislate how Medicare currently operates. The *Private Health Insurance Act 2007* (Cth) is the main law that sets out the requirements for private health insurance and health insurers.

State/territory legislation

The relevant state or territory legislation is determined by the location of the service, not the residence of the doctor or the patient. State and territory legislation covers multiple areas of medical practice, including:

- recording of births and deaths
- termination of pregnancy
- voluntary assisted dying
- mental health standards and voluntary/involuntary admissions
- poisons and drugs, including prescription of drugs of dependence such as opiates
- driving licence standards
- management and reporting of communicable diseases.

The Health Practitioner Regulation National Law (the National Law) was enacted in each state and territory in 2009 and 2010. This created the National Registration and Accreditation Scheme for registered health practitioners (discussed in detail in Chapter 21, Regulation of the medical profession).

20.3 Australian Government funding schemes

Any single episode of care is likely to be resourced through multiple funding streams, many of which originate from taxation.

The Australian Government has responsibility for primary care but does not employ primary healthcare professionals. Instead, it funds or subsidises costs through Medicare, the Pharmaceutical Benefits Scheme (PBS) and Aboriginal and Torres Strait Islander medical services. The Australian Government also funds training programs and incentives for primary care professionals and invests in mechanisms to improve primary healthcare system management.

Australian citizens, permanent residents, refugees and humanitarian entrants can apply to Services Australia for a Medicare card. This card proves their eligibility for funding towards their healthcare costs. Visitors and temporary residents, including those working as doctors, are responsible for their own healthcare costs. Australia has reciprocal healthcare agreements with 11 countries, including Aotearoa New Zealand, the United Kingdom and Ireland. Citizens of these countries can receive some care in Australia for free and vice versa when Australians visit these countries. Other visitors are personally responsible for their costs, which they may be able to claim back from their travel insurer.

20.3.1 Medicare

Medicare is Australia's public health insurance system and is administered by Services Australia. Medicare provides refunds (called rebates) towards the cost of services to patients with a Medicare card. The Medicare Benefits Schedule (MBS) lists the rebates available for each type of consultation or activity, such as diagnostic pathology or radiology or operation. The percentage of the rebate compared with the schedule fee varies. For example, patients who see doctors working as GPs but without general practice qualifications can claim 80% rebates, whereas patients who see GPs with specialist qualifications in general practice can claim 100% rebates for some items. When a patient is admitted to hospital, the rate reduces to 75%.

Many medical, diagnostic and allied health services are provided for free, or at a subsidised cost, at the time of the service. Health professionals who 'bulk-bill' accept the Medicare rebate as full payment for their service and may be eligible for further government financial incentives for doing so. It is more common for GPs to bulk-bill than other specialists. Gap fees—the difference between the doctor's fee and the Medicare rebate—are increasing, and can be several hundred dollars for some medical specialties. The Australian Medical Association (AMA), which is the peak professional body for doctors in Australia, regardless of their specialty, publishes a list of recommended fees per specialty that is available to their members. Doctors are expected to publish their charges so that patients are aware of the likely out-of-pocket costs ahead of any consultations.

Doctors require a Medicare provider number for their patients to claim rebates from Medicare. Provider numbers are specific to a single physical location of medical practice. See also section 33.6 of Chapter 33, Entering and leaving practice and practice management.

Doctors are personally responsible for claims made using their Medicare provider number. Each claim must accurately reflect the service given to the patient. Doctors are advised to be cautious about any colleague, clinic owner, manager or supervisor who offers to make Medicare claims on their behalf. Responsibility for the accuracy of Medicare claims cannot be delegated and any error in claiming is redirected to the doctor as the holder of the provider number. Practices or hospitals may have to share responsibility for debts from inappropriate claims if it is clear that their systems coerced the doctor into making inappropriate claims.

Medicare fraud or inappropriate claiming is taken seriously and can lead to a doctor paying back inappropriate claims, being fined, losing their access to Medicare, or being deregistered by a tribunal on referral by the Medical Board of Australia. The Department of Health, Disability and Ageing monitors claims and can investigate those whose claims vary significantly from those of their peers. Overservicing, which is defined as making 80 Medicare claims per day for more than 20 days in the year, will also be identified.

Doctors whose billing raises concerns of excessive or inappropriate claims are referred to the Professional Services Review. This group of doctors, including one from the same specialty as the doctor being investigated, decides on the appropriateness of a doctor's claims and assesses whether any action is needed.

Obtaining a Medicare provider number

Access to Medicare provider numbers is legislated to promote quality practice and the geographical distribution of doctors. Section 19AA of the *Health Insurance Act 1973* (Cth) focuses on quality and section 19AB on distribution. The details of requirements can change so it is important to check the Department of Health, Disability and Ageing website prior to making career decisions [5].

Section 19AA outlines that Medicare provider numbers are available to:

1. Australian citizens and permanent resident doctors who have specialist medical qualifications, are vocationally recognised by the Australian Health Practitioner Regulation Agency (Ahpra) as a specialist, and are not Bonded Medical Scholars
2. Australian citizens and permanent resident doctors on an approved workforce program—for example, the Australian General Practice Training Program or the Approved Medical Deputising program—who are working towards Fellowship
3. international medical graduates (IMGs) who are temporary residents in Australia.

To promote distribution of the medical workforce to underserved areas, section 19AB of the Health Insurance Act provides that IMGs and foreign graduates of accredited medical schools can only obtain a provider number in areas of workforce shortage for their first 10 years after being registered to practice in Australia. This is known as the '10-year moratorium'. These doctors must have or be working towards vocational recognition.

The Department of Health, Disability and Ageing defines areas of workforce shortage and updates them regularly to reflect changes in doctor and population numbers. Information on how this is done and maps that show the classifications of areas as Distribution Priority Areas [6] (for GPs) and Districts of Workforce Shortage [7] (for other medical specialists) are on the Department of Health, Disability and Ageing website.

Annual provider numbers

Medicare provider numbers are time limited for all doctors except for Australian doctors in the first category above. Doctors are expected to apply for an update of their number before it expires and are legally obligated to tell patients ahead of any consultation if their provider number is no longer valid for Medicare rebates.

Bonded Medical Scholars

Nearly 30% of Australian Government–funded places in medical school are reserved for Bonded Medical Scholars: students who agree to work in areas of workforce shortage for defined lengths of time after graduation. Once they have completed their bonded service, they are eligible for a Medicare provider number to practise anywhere in Australia.

This introduction to Medicare is best supplemented with access to the Medicare educational resources available from Services Australia.

20.3.2 Pharmaceutical Benefits Scheme

The PBS subsidises the cost of medicine for most medical conditions. Patients pay a set fee for a supply of each medicine to last 30 or 60 days. Doctors must apply to Services Australia for a prescriber number to issue PBS medicines. Doctors keep the same unique prescriber number throughout their medical work in Australia.

The PBS indicates which medicines can be issued for what conditions, and in what quantity. Rare or expensive drugs, or drugs whose supply is restricted, may require an 'authority prescription'. Applications for authority prescriptions can be made by telephone or online to Services Australia. The latter requires doctors to apply in advance to Services Australia for a PRODA (Provider Digital Access) account. Further information about prescribing in the PBS system is provided in Chapter 30, Prescribing and administering medicines.

Therapeutic Goods Administration

The Therapeutic Goods Administration (TGA) is responsible for assessing the safety, quality and efficacy of new drugs and medical devices prior to their inclusion (or not) as registered or licensed products on the Australian Register of Therapeutic Goods. This includes some complementary medicines. The TGA also maintains databases of problems with drugs or devices, hazard alerts and recalls of therapeutic devices in Australia and overseas. Doctors are expected to report adverse events suspected to be due to medicines to the TGA. See also section 30.1 of Chapter 30, Prescribing and administering medicines.

20.3.3 Department of Veterans' Affairs

The Australian Defence Force (ADF) provides health care for currently serving personnel. The Department of Veterans' Affairs (DVA) provides a broad range of clinical, wellbeing and support services for veterans, formally defined as those who have served at least one day full-time in the ADF. Some services are funded for all veterans, such as Non-Liability Health Care for mental health diagnoses and veterans' health checks when re-entering civilian life.

Funding of other health care is determined by a person's age, type of military service, and any resulting injuries, illness or disability, and DVA allocates different cards—gold, white or orange—depending on these factors. Veterans with gold cards are eligible for clinically necessary treatment for all medical conditions, whereas a white card confers partial coverage: only accepted service-related injuries or conditions are eligible for DVA-funded treatment. Orange cards provide subsidies for medicines and wound care.

The families and partners of veterans who die in service may also be eligible for entitlements and pensions. DVA has its own contracted hospitals, programs, funding rules, and system of forms, referrals and prescriptions. The notation 'RPBS' (Repatriation Pharmaceutical Benefits Scheme) on prescribing resources indicates the clinical conditions for which a veteran can receive medication at a subsidised cost. Likewise, the RMFS (Repatriation Medical Fee Schedule) is the MBS equivalent.

20.3.4 Other insurance schemes

Private health insurance rebate

Australians who buy private health insurance can claim back the costs of certain private primary, secondary- or tertiary-level services, medicines or equipment. GP services are excluded. There are tax incentives for people to take out private health insurance in order to encourage its uptake and the use of private rather than public services. Private health insurers must classify their private hospital cover into Gold, Silver, Bronze or Basic levels to indicate what is and is not covered.

Motor vehicle accident insurance

Each state and territory government operates a compulsory third party insurance scheme for drivers of registered motor vehicles. This provides cover for the costs of injuries to pedestrians, cyclists or other road users while someone is driving. Doctors may need to complete insurance forms for patients and can claim consultation and administrative costs from the motor vehicle accident insurer. Medicare will not provide a rebate for consultations that are covered by this insurance.

Workers' compensation

Workers' compensation schemes fund medical costs separately to Medicare. Workers' compensation schemes were introduced around the turn of the 20th century so that families were no longer left destitute if working men were killed or injured in industrial accidents [8]. The main reason for a claim was that an injury occurred at work. Prior to this, injured employees had to prove in court that the employer's negligence caused their injury.

Over a century later, following the same principle, workers are compensated for injuries and the cost of treating injuries at work. The paperwork can be complicated, with forms varying between states and territories and insurance companies. Compensation schemes will pay for employees to seek medical care and receive necessary treatment. Employees may be allocated a rehabilitation provider who helps them navigate their care, accompanies them to their appointments and assists with their return to work. Patients cannot claim Medicare rebates for the same services that are paid for through workers' compensation. In recent years, compensation schemes have switched from asking doctors to certify people as not fit to work, to certifying what work they are able to do.

National Disability Insurance Scheme

The National Disability Insurance Scheme (NDIS) funds the costs associated with having a disability. It is funded by the Australian Government and was legislated in 2013. The scheme entitles people under the age of 65 with a permanent and significant disability to funding for reasonable and necessary support needs related to their disability. NDIS does not fund health care, but services such as speech pathology and physiotherapy, designed to support a disabled person, may be funded. Doctors can recommend patients apply to NDIS for assistance and may be required to verify disability to support people's claims.

20.3.5 Supplementary funding

The Australian Government runs additional schemes to support access to care for vulnerable groups of the population.

Medicare and Pharmaceutical Benefits Scheme Safety Nets

Individuals or families who have high costs for medical or pharmaceutical services in a year can apply under safety net provisions to receive prescriptions and services at lower cost for the rest of that year. The level of funding and the safety net thresholds are revised annually. Doctors do not necessarily need to know the details of the scheme but can make a difference by suggesting to patients that they may be eligible to apply. The scheme is run by Services Australia.

Health Care Cards

Students, seniors and people on low incomes may be eligible for a Health Care Card, which is issued by Services Australia. This entitles people to PBS drugs at a lower cost and changes the Medicare Safety Net threshold. Doctors may bulk-bill or offer concessional rates to Health Care Card holders.

Closing the Gap

Doctors can register Aboriginal and/or Torres Strait Islander people for the Closing the Gap PBS scheme. This gives access to any PBS medicine at the Health Care Card concessional rate. Aboriginal and/or Torres Strait Islander people who also have a Health Care Card are not required to pay for PBS medicines.

Disease-specific funding

Subsidies may be available for patients with specific illnesses. For example, the National Diabetes Services Scheme subsidises the costs of needles, syringes and testing strips for those with type 1 diabetes.

20.4 Doctors' employment

20.4.1 Primary care

The three main options for working as a GP are to own a practice, work as a contractor or be a salaried employee. Each has advantages and disadvantages, and GPs may switch from one to another at different stages of their career. The opportunities for autonomy and independence provided by owning or being a partner in a practice comes with responsibility for running a business as well as being a doctor. Contractors arrange their own hours, charge patients for services and then pay a service fee to the practice. They are considered self-employed for tax purposes and have to fund their own annual leave, sick leave, parental leave and superannuation. Salaried GPs gain these employment benefits in exchange for working hours and requirements set by their employer.

Most primary healthcare professionals—including the majority of GPs, allied health professionals and pharmacists—work in private businesses.

20.4.2 Secondary and tertiary care

Medical staff in public hospitals are usually either salaried staff specialists or appointed as visiting medical officers (VMOs) who work under contractual agreements with the hospital. Many VMOs work a certain number of sessions (half days) per week in the public hospital, and often also work in nearby private hospitals and private consulting rooms.

Staff specialists can be appointed to public positions with a right of private practice. This enables them to bill Medicare or a private health insurance provider for services delivered in public hospitals to private patients; any service claimed through Medicare cannot also be claimed through hospital funding. Staff specialists are also expected to contribute to teaching and training of medical students, early-year graduates and specialist trainees.

Doctors who work in public hospitals may also offer services as owners or contractors in private consulting rooms. Patients pay for their services and may be able to claim a Medicare rebate or costs back from their private health insurance.

Universities employ clinicians as academics in teaching and/or research positions, usually within medical schools. In addition to their salaried university work, these specialists continue their clinical work as medical practitioners in hospitals or in private rooms. Universities may offer staff specialists or VMOs honorary academic conjoint or adjunct appointments with academic institutions to recognise their contribution to research and teaching.

20.5 Organisations and programs to support medical practice

20.5.1 Medical research

Medical research is an essential component of the health system in the development, evaluation and delivery of innovations in health care. Australia's two main medical research funding organisations are the National Health and Medical Research Council (NHMRC) and the Medical Research Future Fund (MRFF). Both offer competitive research grants. The NHMRC is a government-funded independent agency, while the MRFF operates within the Department of Health, Disability and Ageing, with funding decisions being recommended by public servants and then made by the Minister for Health and Ageing. Universities, philanthropic trusts, charities and private enterprises also fund medical research. See also Chapter 31, Medical research.

20.5.2 Clinical support

Guidelines for practitioners

An ongoing challenge is linking the outcomes of research and innovation from the NHMRC, MRFF and other research with clinical practice. There are clinical support mechanisms that assist doctors to choose optimal care given the plethora of options for medical treatment. Increasingly, this support is electronic rather than in hard copy, and is beginning to be integrated into clinical practice software.

Clinical practice guidelines aim to assist by synthesising research into usable formats for clinicians. National guidelines are produced by the NHMRC, specialist medical colleges and organisations, such as the Heart Foundation, that focus on specific illnesses or systems. HealthPathways, produced by Primary Health Networks (PHNs), outline how particular conditions or patient groups can access care within local regions.

Clinical activities or medicines listed on the MBS or PBS (respectively) require some level of evidence of their efficacy and cost-effectiveness. More detailed information on prescribing is available via the *Australian medicines handbook* [9] or the Therapeutic Guidelines (https://www.tg.org.au/), and in Chapter 30, Prescribing and administering medicines.

Digital clinical support

Just as doctors access information and guidelines online, patients now expect similar access to their results and records. Seamless transfer of medical information from one clinician to another still seems to be an elusive, but important, goal. The Australian Digital Health Agency is responsible for providing digital assistance for both providers and patients, and it reported an increased use of patients' individual electronic record (My Health Record) during the COVID 19 pandemic. See also Chapter 29, Professional practice, digital technology and artificial intelligence.

Translator service

The free Translating and Interpreting Service (TIS National) helps doctors to consult with patients who speak languages other than English. Doctors need to first register with TIS National and can then book an interpreter to be available for consultations either on the phone or onsite. TIS National also offers immediate phone interpreting across the country (call 131 450).

20.5.3 Public health

The COVID-19 pandemic brought Australia's public health workforce to the fore. This group of health professionals focuses on the health of the population as a whole, not just the care of individuals. Each state and territory government has a chief health or medical officer who works with other medical officers, public health nurses, epidemiologists and environmental health experts. During disasters, outbreaks, epidemics or pandemics, chief health officers are expected to use their legislated power for the overall benefit of the community.

Less overt roles also protect the public. Doctors must report to the health department cases of communicable diseases, such as salmonella or cases of rubella, so that outbreaks can be identified and managed. Other tasks include setting and monitoring the issuing of certain drugs that can be abused or become addictive, such as sleeping tablets and opiates. The rules vary for each jurisdiction. Not knowing the rules is no defence in law if a doctor prescribes more than the allowed amount of medication, and so it is recommended that doctors check the rules on what is allowed prior to working in a new location.

20.5.4 Mental health

Each state and territory appoints a chief psychiatrist who monitors the standards of mental health care, and ensures that practitioners treat patients according to that state or territory's mental health Act. See also Chapter 18, People with mental illness and the law.

20.5.5 Safe, quality care

The whole emphasis of this book is to outline how doctors are expected to practise professionally. There are also systems to monitor that this occurs and that healthcare organisations as a whole promote safe and quality care. Further detail is provided in Chapter 23, Patient safety.

Australian Commission on Safety and Quality in Health Care

The Australian Commission on Safety and Quality in Health Care (ACSQHC) has several responsibilities:

1. Development of National Safety and Quality Health Service Standards [10] that state the level of care patients can expect from health service organisations. For example, there are standards for medication safety and infection control.
2. Development of clinical standards for particular clinical issues, such as acute stroke, and antimicrobial stewardship.
3. Coordination of the Australian Health Service Safety and Quality Accreditation Scheme [11]. This scheme monitors how health services operate to the national and clinical standards. ACSQHC also oversees an accreditation scheme that assesses general practices against standards set by the Royal Australian College of General Practitioners.
4. Publication of the Australian Atlas of Health Care Variation series [12]. This reveals how healthcare use varies according to where people live. This information is designed for use by service planners to promote more equitable access to care.

20.5.6 Professional organisations

Advocacy groups for patients

Consumer groups, such as the Consumers Health Forum of Australia, work to protect patients' rights and to improve the quality of services from their perspectives. Some groups advocate for specific demographics or people with specific illnesses, such as multiple sclerosis, kidney disease or diabetes.

Advocacy groups for health professionals

Alongside their advocacy for consumers, some groups create resources designed to assist clinicians. For example, the National Asthma Council publishes information for patients and families of someone who has asthma, as well as evidence-based guidelines for clinicians on managing asthma [13].

The AMA is the peak professional body for doctors in Australia. The AMA promotes and protects the professional interests of doctors and the healthcare needs of patients and communities. Representing its doctor members, the AMA works with governments to develop and influence health policy to provide the best outcomes for doctors, their patients and the community. The AMA publishes the *Medical Journal of Australia* (https://www.mja.com.au), the country's leading general medical journal.

Other groups advocate for doctors in particular settings, backgrounds or interests. For example, medical specialties have societies that advocate for them separately from the college's role in setting and assessing standards of practice, and the Rural Doctors Association of Australia is a membership organisation that represents the interests of rural doctors.

Primary Health Networks

PHNs are independent organisations working to streamline health services, particularly for those at risk of poor health outcomes, and to better coordinate care. The Australian Government funds PHNs to operate in 31 health regions that closely align with the state and territory local hospital networks. A board oversees their work, and clinical councils and community advisory committees provide advice. GPs are recommended to connect with their PHN when starting in a new area in order to access the resources they provide and better integrate with other health professionals and services.

Rural workforce agencies

The Australian Government also funds Rural Workforce Agencies in each state and the Northern Territory to improve the access, quality and sustainability of the regional, rural and remote health workforce. Rural workforce agencies consult with communities, practitioners and other healthcare organisations to determine the health workforce needs in their area. They then run programs and administer grants, scholarships and bursaries to meet these needs. This includes helping communities to recruit health professionals, assisting with locum placements, promoting rural careers and facilitating rural experience for students, junior doctors and registrars training in general practice or other medical specialties.

All rural workforce agencies participate in the Pre-Fellowship Program that enables doctors who are non-vocationally registered to work in rural regions and access Medicare. These doctors must work in areas of workforce shortage (as designated by the Department of Health, Disability and Ageing as a Distribution Priority Area) and receive 80% of the Medicare rebate. These doctors become eligible for 100% Medicare rebates once accepted onto a program to gain GP qualifications.

20.5.7 Medical indemnity

Medical practitioners must arrange medical indemnity insurance in order to be registered to practise by the Medical Board of Australia. Providers of this insurance offer advisory services for practitioners facing complaints or legal action and, if needed, will fund payments ordered by courts or arrived at in settlements to compensate patients for poor outcomes. The cost of insurance varies according to the practitioner's specialty, with obstetrics and other surgical specialties typically being the most expensive.

Doctors may also be required by individual hospitals or employers to have personal liability insurance in case they cause an injury outside of their medical practice. An example could be leaving a floor wet and causing someone to slip.

Income protection insurance is available to cover doctors in private practice if they are unable to work because of personal illness or injury. It may not be needed by those in salaried practice, with sick leave provisions, but those running a private practice may have ongoing costs of employing staff and paying rent or mortgages for buildings while not being able to work.

20.6 Medical education and training in Australia

20.6.1 Outline

The path from high school to practising specialist doctor usually takes 10–20 years in Australia. Students study for their primary medical degree at one of 21 medical schools. Eighteen of these are within public universities and three are in fee-paying private universities. Courses can be five or six years if taken as a first degree, and three to four years for a postgraduate degree. Approximately one-quarter of students complete clinical training at one of the University Rural Clinical Schools, designed to give students the interest and experience needed to encourage rural work once qualified.

Graduates then complete a one-year internship working under supervision to gain general registration with the Medical Board of Australia. From 2025, this is a two-year transition to practice and includes community as well as hospital placements. General registration is granted after one satisfactory year of supervised practice and a Certificate of Completion granted after the second year.

Doctors may then apply for specialist training or gain more clinical experience as a resident medical officer. Entry to specialist training can be very competitive, and an increase in the number of medical schools has intensified competition between graduates for popular specialties.

Specialist training is overseen by specialist medical colleges, and combines work-based learning with tutorials, workshops, supervisor feedback on performance, training courses and significant amounts of personal study. During this time, doctors are employed to work in general practice or hospitals (mostly public but occasionally private). All colleges assess their trainees to ensure they reach the standards expected in that specialty.

Many doctors choose not to, or are unable to, gain access to the specialist training program of their choice. These doctors may seek alternative specialties or careers, or continue to work in their chosen discipline as career medical officers without gaining specialist qualifications.

IMGs who enter the Australian system are assessed on their prior qualifications and experience to determine their equivalence with Australian graduates. Those whose qualifications are not recognised in Australia may need to sit the Australian Medical Council examinations. Doctors who successfully complete these written and clinical examinations are eligible for general registration after a period of supervised practice.

Figure 20.1 Australian medical training pathways

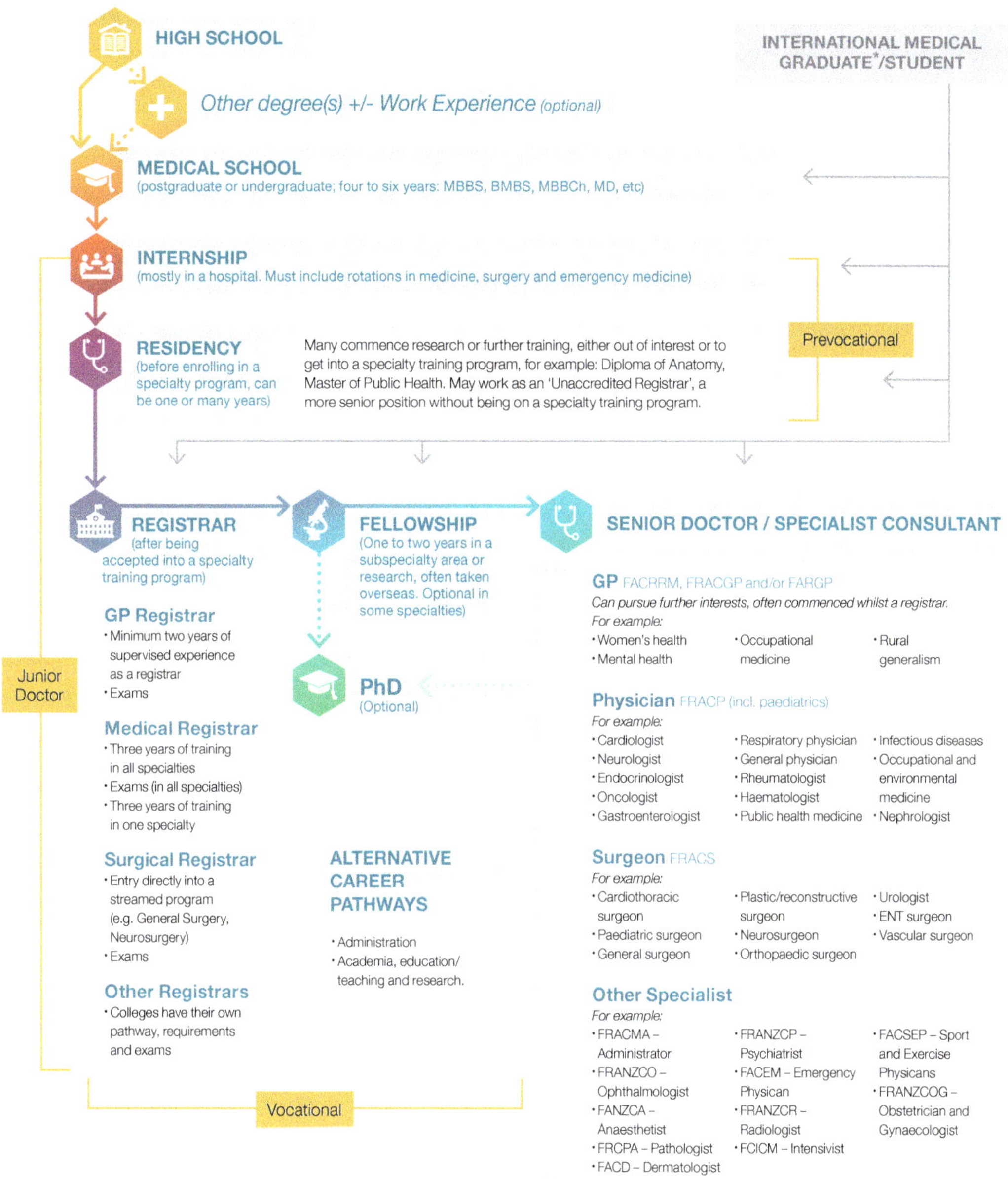

* International medical graduates' qualifications and experience determine their entry point into Australian medical training employment.

Source: Australian Government Department of Health. National Medical Workforce Strategy 2021–2031, p 46. https://www.health.gov.au/sites/default/files/documents/2022/03/national-medical-workforce-strategy-2021-2031.pdf, adapted from Australian Medical Association. How to become a doctor. Permitted for use under Creative Commons Licence - Attribution-NonCommercial-NoDerivatives CC BY-NC-ND.

20.6.2 Specialist medical colleges

Specialist medical colleges set the standards and curricula for their disciplines, and assess doctors against those standards for their Fellowship and registration as specialists. Colleges also advocate for their members and their specialty. Many conduct research, produce clinical practice guidelines to improve the quality of care provided by their members, and offer professional development programs to keep Fellows up to date with new developments. Such continuing professional development (CPD) is compulsory for all specialists. Since 1 January 2023, specialists have been required to nominate a CPD home (usually their college) and complete their CPD program guided by a professional development plan. See also Chapter 10, Continuing professional development.

Specialist medical colleges assess international specialists on their comparability to Australian-trained specialists, unless they hold a specialist qualification from a country whose health system and training are considered to be equivalent to those in Australia. In this case, an internationally qualified specialist may be eligible for registration after six months of supervised and assessed practice in Australia.

20.6.3 Australian Medical Council

The Australian Medical Council's purpose is to ensure that standards of education, training and assessment of the medical profession promote and protect the health of the Australian community. Currently, it accredits universities that offer medical degrees and specialist medical colleges against standards that they set in consultation with the Medical Board of Australia, consumers, the profession and governments. Since 1 January 2023, it has also been responsible for the accreditation and standards of CPD homes, which will oversee continuing professional development for doctors.

20.7 Regulation of medical practice

20.7.1 The Medical Board of Australia and the Australian Health Practitioner Regulation Agency

The structure and function of the regulatory system in Australia is covered in detail in Chapter 21, Regulation of the medical profession. In brief, the Medical Board of Australia works together with Ahpra to carry out the following functions:

- register medical practitioners and medical students
- develop standards, codes and guidelines for the medical profession
- investigate notifications and complaints about medical practitioners
- where necessary, conduct panel hearings and refer serious matters to Tribunal hearings
- approve accreditation standards and accredited courses of study.

The Medical Board of Australia (i.e. the national board) is supported by boards in each state and territory. They have the delegated powers to make individual registration and notification (complaints) decisions based on the national policies and standards set by the national board.

Summary

The Australian health system is complex and can seem confusing at first. There are pitfalls to avoid, and understanding how the different elements work together can help practitioners be effective in the care of their patients. Given the political structure in Australia, it is important to recognise which aspects of health care are the responsibility of the Australian Government and which are managed by state and territory governments; the latter are likely to vary significantly from one jurisdiction to another. All doctors need to be aware of the relevant laws within their own jurisdiction, as well as the rules governing their interactions with national schemes, particularly Medicare and the PBS. Checking organisations' online information as well as conferring with colleagues is time well spent to prevent falling foul of the law or professional expectations.

References

1. Starfield B, Shi L, Macinko J. Contribution of primary care to health systems and health. *Milbank Q* 2005; 83: 457–502.
2. Services Australia. Refer or request Medicare services. Australian Government, 2025. https://www.servicesaustralia.gov.au/organisations/health-professionals/subjects/referring-and-requesting-medicare-services (accessed May 2025).
3. National Aboriginal Community Controlled Health Organisation. Constitution for the National Aboriginal Community Controlled Health Organisation. Canberra (ACT): NACCHO. https://www.naccho.org.au/app/uploads/2023/09/10.-NACCHO-CONSTITUTION-Ratified-Ver-151111-for-ASIC.pdf (accessed May 2025).
4. Australian Institute of Health and Welfare. Hospitals at a glance. Canberra (ACT): AIHW, 2025. https://www.aihw.gov.au/hospitals/overview/hospitals-at-a-glance (accessed May 2025).
5. Department of Health, Disability and Ageing. Accessing Medicare for health practitioners and industry. Canberra (ACT): Commonwealth of Australia, 2024. https://www.health.gov.au/topics/medicare/access-practitioners-industry (accessed May 2025).
6. Department of Health, Disability and Ageing. Distribution Priority Area. Canberra (ACT): Commonwealth of Australia, 2024. https://www.health.gov.au/topics/rural-health-workforce/classifications/dpa (accessed May 2025).
7. Department of Health, Disability and Ageing. District of Workforce Shortage. Canberra (ACT): Commonwealth of Australia, 2024. https://www.health.gov.au/topics/rural-health-workforce/classifications/dws (accessed May 2025).
8. Purse K. The evolution of workers' compensation policy in Australia. *Health Sociology Review* 2005; 14: 8–20.
9. Australian Medicines Handbook 2025. Adelaide: AMH Pty Ltd, 2025.
10. Australian Commission on Safety and Quality in Health Care. National safety and quality health service standards. 2nd ed. – version 2. Sydney: ACSQHC, 2021. https://www.safetyandquality.gov.au/standards/nsqhs-standards (accessed May 2025).
11. Australian Commission on Safety and Quality in Health Care. Australian health service safety and quality accreditation scheme. Sydney: ACSQHC, 2018. https://www.safetyandquality.gov.au/our-work/accreditation/australian-health-service-safety-and-quality-accreditation-scheme (accessed May 2025).
12. Australian Commission on Safety and Quality in Health Care. Australian atlas of healthcare variation series. Sydney: ACSQHC. https://www.safetyandquality.gov.au/our-work/healthcare-variation/australian-atlas-healthcare-variation-series (accessed May 2025).
13. National Asthma Council. Australian Asthma Handbook version 2.2. 2022. https://www.nationalasthma.org.au/health-professionals/australian-asthma-handbook (accessed Jul 2025).

Further reading

Australian Government Department of Health, Disability and Ageing. The Australian health system. Canberra (ACT): Commonwealth of Australia, 2025. https://www.health.gov.au/about-us/the-australian-health-system

Australian Institute of Health and Welfare. Health system overview. Canberra: AIHW, 2024. https://www.aihw.gov.au/reports/australias-health/health-system-overview

Services Australia. Start with Medicare. Canberra (ACT): Commonwealth of Australia, 2024. https://www.servicesaustralia.gov.au/start-with-medicare-health-professional

21 Regulation of the medical profession

Anne Tonkin AO, Joanne Katsoris

Introduction

The medical regulatory system in Australia has the primary purpose of protecting the public when they access health care, by ensuring that only appropriately qualified people can call themselves medical practitioners, and by responding to notifications of concern about practitioners. Other goals include facilitating workforce mobility, and supporting high-quality education and training, and access to services.

This chapter describes the current structure and function of the medical regulatory system, known as the National Registration and Accreditation Scheme, and the roles of the various bodies within the scheme. It also discusses the roles of other bodies in jurisdictions where there is co-regulation (Queensland and New South Wales). The chapter concludes with an overall description of the processes involved in registration and the management of notifications of concern (complaints) about medical practitioners. It should be noted that the system is constantly evolving and changing to meet specific challenges.

21.1 National Registration and Accreditation Scheme

The current national regulatory system, known as the National Registration and Accreditation Scheme (NRAS), was formed in 2010 with the establishment by the federal and state and territory health ministers of a single Medical Board of Australia. The eight previously independent state and territory medical boards or councils became delegated decision makers of the Medical Board, with the exception of NSW (see section 21.3.1). A national agency, the Australian Health Practitioner Regulation Agency (Ahpra), was established to provide administrative, legal and policy support to the board and to 14 other national boards regulating 15 other health professions.

The legal foundation of the system is the *Health Practitioner Regulation National Law Act 2009*, as in force in each state and territory, which is usually referred to as 'the National Law'. The National Law establishes the national boards and Ahpra, and grants them the power to regulate practitioners. The National Law is not federal legislation. It is state- and territory-based legislation that depends on legislation passed by the parliaments of all states and territories. This has led to some differences between jurisdictions, which will be discussed briefly in section 21.3. The overall structure of the NRAS is shown in Figure 21.1.

Figure 21.1 Overall structure of the National Registration and Accreditation Scheme

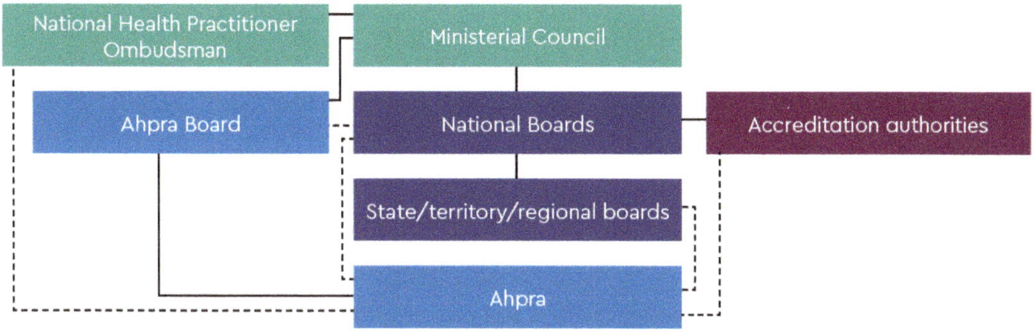

Source: Reproduced with permission from Ahpra (https://www.ahpra.gov.au/About-Ahpra/What-We-Do.aspx).

Medical regulation is funded entirely by registration fees from practitioners, and medical practitioners continue to make a significant contribution to decision making, constituting at least 50% of the members of the national and most jurisdictional boards and committees.

Registration under the NRAS is nationwide, supporting ready mobility of the medical workforce and consistency of standards across the country. For most medical practitioners, registration and annual registration renewal are the only times they interact with the regulatory system. About 5% of doctors each year have a notification of concern (which may be about their conduct, performance or health) lodged with the system. These practitioners then interact with Ahpra and the Medical Board's delegated decision makers during the processing of the notification. More detail is provided in section 21.5.

21.2 Roles of organisations within the national regulatory system

There are several organisations within this rather complex system. All of them work together to achieve the objectives of the scheme, focusing primarily on the broad goal of protecting public safety in health care.

21.2.1 Medical Board of Australia

The national board is responsible for overseeing the medical regulatory system, working in partnership with Ahpra. The Medical Board sets registration standards, which are approved by health ministers and determine which individuals are eligible for registration as a medical practitioner. It develops and maintains the profession-specific code of conduct—*Good medical practice: a code of conduct for doctors in Australia* [1]—which is available as a guide for practitioners in general and also used as a benchmark in regulatory proceedings about individuals. The board also issues guidelines for doctors about particular areas of concern, including the *Guidelines for registered medical practitioners who perform cosmetic surgery and procedures* [2], and *Sexual boundaries in the doctor–patient relationship* [3] (see section 21.5.5). The Medical Board also has the responsibility of appointing the accreditation authority for medicine, currently the Australian Medical Council (AMC), and approving qualifications as being suitable for registration, on the advice of the AMC.

The Medical Board has 12 members, all appointed by the federal and jurisdictional health ministers. Currently, eight members are registered medical practitioners and four are community members.

21.2.2 Delegated decision makers

Every year, the Medical Board receives registration applications from over 130,000 medical practitioners, some of which require individualised decision making rather than a straightforward online renewal. It also receives over 6000 notifications of concern about doctors. To manage the workload, the Medical Board has delegated its decision-making powers to a number of committees. These include state and territory boards, state-based committees and national committees.

21.2.3 Australian Health Practitioner Regulation Agency

Ahpra provides administrative, legal, policy and investigative support to the Medical Board. Staff employed by Ahpra manage the registration process and the national public register of practitioners; carry out investigations of notifications of concern; and provide advice about policy, legal and financial issues to the board. Ahpra is also the signatory on contracts on behalf of the board; for example, with the accreditation authority for medicine (the AMC) and the doctors' health services funded by the board.

Ahpra employs the staff who support the Medical Board to carry out its functions under the National Law. Ahpra's work ranges from receiving and processing registration applications and notifications, preparing reports and the agendas for meetings at which these are considered, to managing the complex IT system required to support its operations. There is a National Legal Practice within Ahpra, which provides legal advice to boards and undertakes legal processes on behalf of the boards; for example, when a matter is referred to a tribunal. Ahpra is also responsible for the day-to-day management of the board's finances, and provides advice to the board about its budget and the setting of registration fees. In short, Ahpra works in partnership with all 15 boards (including the Medical Board and the 14 other national boards) to administer the regulation of 16 health professions. The Medical Board in turn sets policy, develops codes of conduct and guidelines, and makes regulatory decisions about individual practitioners. Neither entity can do its work without the other.

Ahpra is managed by a corporate board, known as the Ahpra Board, which is appointed by, and responsible to, the federal and jurisdictional health ministers. The Ahpra Board has an executive consisting of a chief executive officer and several executive directors of key functions within Ahpra, including regulatory operations. There are Ahpra offices within each state and territory capital city, and Ahpra staff are located within each office. The national office is situated in Melbourne.

21.2.4 National Health Practitioner Ombudsman and Privacy Commissioner

The National Health Practitioner Ombudsman and Privacy Commissioner investigates complaints, facilitates resolutions and makes recommendations to improve the regulation of Australia's registered health practitioners. The Ombudsman and Commissioner accepts complaints about the way in which Ahpra and the boards have handled matters including:

- notifications about registered health practitioners
- registration matters
- personal information
- freedom of information requests.

21.2.5 Australian Medical Council

Accreditation functions within the NRAS are carried out by the AMC, which has been appointed by the Medical Board to be the accreditation authority for medicine. The AMC develops accreditation standards for primary medical education and specialist training, which are then approved by the Medical Board. The AMC assesses medical schools and specialist colleges to ensure they have good governance, adequate resources and processes, and appropriate curricula to support training. It also assesses the jurisdictional bodies that accredit intern training positions. The accreditation reports are submitted to the Medical Board, together with recommendations concerning the suitability of the relevant training program for providing a qualification for registration.

The AMC is also responsible for providing assessments for international medical graduates seeking registration via the standard pathway in Australia, awarding an 'AMC Certificate' to those who are successful. In addition, the AMC provides advice to the Medical Board on the recognition of new areas of medical specialty or endorsement for scope of practice, and the training programs that would lead to suitability for registration in that specialty or endorsement for that scope if approved. The final approval of a new specialty and protection of the title associated with it are within the power of health ministers. Finally, the AMC accredits providers of continuing professional development ('CPD homes') for medical practitioners.

21.2.6 Tribunals

Each jurisdiction has its own independent tribunal, variably named, to which serious notifications about health practitioners are required to be referred whenever a delegated decision maker of the Medical Board forms a reasonable belief that professional misconduct has occurred. The tribunals are judicial bodies that have powers to impose more severe sanctions than are available to the board, including suspension or cancellation of registration for the most serious matters. Health practitioners are also able to appeal many board decisions. These appeals are heard and decided by the tribunals.

21.3 Co-regulatory jurisdictions

21.3.1 New South Wales

When the NRAS was established in 2010, NSW decided that it would only partially enter the scheme. While registration matters continue to be managed by the Medical Board and Ahpra, notifications are handled by the Medical Council of NSW, a jurisdictional body set up specifically to manage complaints about the performance, conduct or health of doctors within NSW (see Chapter 22, Healthcare complaints and complaint systems). While some of its processes differ from those of the NRAS, the Medical Council of NSW has a close relationship with the Medical Board and uses the same code of conduct as the benchmark for performance and conduct of doctors within NSW.

21.3.2 Queensland

Queensland became a co-regulatory jurisdiction in 2013, with the establishment of the Office of the Health Ombudsman (OHO) in that state (see Chapter 22, Healthcare complaints and complaint systems). The OHO receives all complaints in Queensland, and has powers to investigate complaints about doctors relating to conduct or performance concerns. These are then either managed by the OHO itself or referred to Ahpra for management through the NRAS. Both entities have the power to take action to manage the risk to the public, including referring matters believed to include professional misconduct to the Queensland Civil and Administrative Tribunal.

21.4 Registration

Registration as a medical practitioner depends on an individual meeting the registration standards set by the Medical Board. Once registered, the person can call themselves a medical practitioner, and if they have accredited specialist training, they can call themselves a specialist in the specific field. Registration is recognised throughout Australia, regardless of where the practitioner lives or works.

It is important to note that the regulatory system operates by protecting specific titles, determined by health ministers. The scope of practice of an individual practitioner is determined by that practitioner, together with their employer where relevant through credentialing processes, taking into account the practitioner's training, expertise and experience. While the Medical Board does not regulate scope, practitioners must be able to demonstrate that they are adequately trained and experienced to undertake their selected type of practice, and must not misrepresent their capabilities to patients or the public.

Ahpra maintains a register of medical practitioners [4], which is publicly available online and can be viewed by any member of the public or employer who wishes to learn more about a potential service provider or employee. The information on the register includes the practitioner's name and principal place of practice, their qualifications and types of registration (limited, provisional, general and/or specialist), and any restrictions on their registration. Restrictions may arise from issues related to their registration, or from actions taken about notifications of concern, including conditions designed to improve the safety of their practice (more detail in section 21.5).

21.4.1 Registration of medical students

Registration of medical students has occurred since the beginning of the NRAS. Each medical school submits a list of students and Ahpra registers them on this basis. The student register is not publicly available. Registration is required for a student to undertake clinical studies that include contact with patients (see Chapter 4, Ethical and legal responsibilities of medical students).

21.4.2 Provisional registration

New graduates from Australian medical schools are required to apply for provisional registration towards the end of their final year. Applicants are required to meet qualification and registration standards, and must declare any criminal history. Each new graduate must complete 12 months of satisfactory supervised practice in accredited intern training positions before they become eligible for general registration.

21.4.3 Registration of international medical graduates

International medical graduates have various pathways to registration in Australia, depending on their country of origin [5]. Graduates from Aotearoa New Zealand medical schools, which are accredited by the AMC, who have completed an Australian or Aotearoa New Zealand internship, are eligible for general registration. Graduates from countries with regulatory systems recognised by the Medical Board as 'competent authorities' are eligible for provisional registration, and can apply for general registration after 12 months of satisfactory supervised practice. International medical graduates from all other countries who have completed the AMC assessment process and gained the AMC Certificate (called the 'standard pathway') are then eligible for provisional registration with the Medical Board, and can apply for general registration after a year of satisfactory supervised practice.

21.4.4 General registration

Medical practitioners with general registration are required to practise within the limits of their own training and competence. Many develop particular areas of interest and practise in limited scopes of practice, but need to bear in mind the ethical requirement to be adequately trained and experienced to undertake their selected type of practice, and not to misrepresent their capabilities to patients. Endorsement of registration that recognises AMC-accredited training is available for two specific scopes of practice: acupuncture and cosmetic surgery.

21.4.5 Specialist registration

Specialist registration is granted to medical practitioners who have completed training with an accredited specialist college and been awarded the relevant Fellowship qualification. This qualification allows them to use the protected title that corresponds to the specialty. International specialists are assessed by the relevant specialist college for their comparability to an Australian-trained specialist, and may be required to sit additional assessments or complete a period of supervised practice before they are eligible for registration as a specialist in Australia. Specialists from a limited number of countries may be eligible for an expedited specialist pathway requiring 6 months of satisfactory supervised practice before obtaining specialist registration. Up-to-date details are available on the Medical Board website [5].

21.4.6 Limited registration

Limited registration is available for internationally qualified doctors who are otherwise not eligible for general or specialist registration, but who may be in Australia for a specific purpose, such as postgraduate training or supervised practice, teaching or research, or to fill a position in an identified area of need.

21.4.7 Non-practising registration

The National Law allows any doctor who has held either general or specialist registration to apply for non-practising registration at a greatly reduced fee. This category of registration does not require professional indemnity insurance or continuing professional development activities. Because of these provisions, non-practising registration is suitable for doctors who wish to remain on the register, but it does not allow them to be involved in any form of medical practice, including writing referrals or prescriptions.

21.4.8 Renewal of registration

All registered practitioners are required to renew their registration on an annual basis. For most, this is an automated online process that involves making declarations that they have professional indemnity insurance, are meeting the current registration standard on continuing professional development (see also Chapter 10, Continuing professional development), are not impaired in their capacity to practise medicine, and have not been convicted of a serious crime. For a few, renewal applications require individual assessment and a decision by a registration committee of the Medical Board.

21.5 Notifications of concern (complaints)

At the time of writing, the Medical Board receives approximately 6250 notifications about medical practitioners every year. Notifications can be made about the standard of a practitioner's practice, about their conduct or about a health impairment. It is important to note that the board can only consider notifications about individual practitioners, rather than health services. Complaints about health services are handled by the health complaints entity (HCE) in each state and territory (see Chapter 22, Healthcare complaints and complaint systems). When regulatory action is taken by the Medical Board against an individual practitioner, the action is taken on the person's medical registration. For example, if a practitioner is found to be practising in a manner that causes a risk to public safety, their registration may be subjected to conditions designed to make their practice safer.

Over recent years, the Medical Board and Ahpra have been moving towards a more risk-based approach to managing notifications, so that the process is tailored to match the risk to public safety. This means that the process for a high-risk notification may be different in several respects to the process for a low-risk one. The board and Ahpra are also constantly working to improve these processes, particularly their efficiency and the time they take, recognising that practitioners experience significant stress when a complaint is made about them (discussed further in section 21.5.7).

21.5.1 Data on notifications

Approximately 5–6% of all registered medical practitioners in Australia will have a notification made about them each year. Importantly, these notifications are not distributed evenly across the population of practitioners: about 4–5% of all practitioners account for 50% of the notifications received. While it is common for an individual to receive one or two notifications during their career, the strongest predictor of a practitioner having a notification made about them is their history of notifications. Once a practitioner has been the subject of three or more notifications, the risk of a further notification is significantly increased (Ahpra, unpublished data), indicating that there may be areas within the doctor's practice that need to be improved.

The majority of voluntary notifications are made by members of the public, including patients and their relatives. About 20% are referred by an HCE, and about 10% come from other practitioners, including employers. A statutory requirement within the National Law requires registered health practitioners to make a mandatory notification about another health practitioner if they have a reasonable belief that the practitioner's practice poses a substantial risk of harm to the public. There are three major categories of concern that may lead to a requirement to make a mandatory report:

- practice that is seriously below acceptable standards
- a serious conduct issue, including sexual misconduct (see Chapter 8, Sexual and other professional boundaries: being a doctor in modern society) or practising while intoxicated with alcohol or drugs
- a health impairment that seriously affects their ability to practise (see Chapter 12, Personal health of the doctor: illness and impairment).

These mandatory notifications are uncommon (about 350 annually compared with about 6000 voluntary notifications), and they are overwhelmingly made by other practitioners or employers. The majority of them are related to conduct, particularly sexual misconduct.

Mandatory notifications about health impairments are very uncommon, and are only required if the practitioner in question has an actual impairment related to their health, and is unwilling or unable to take steps themselves to maintain public safety. There has been significant misunderstanding of this requirement over recent years, leading to concern among doctors that they face a mandatory report if they seek help for a health condition. It is very important to stress that reports are only required if the health condition has led to impairment putting the public at substantial risk of harm, *and* the practitioner is unwilling or unable to take appropriate steps to reduce the risk. This means that a practitioner seeking help for a health condition that has not yet led to impairment would not reach the threshold for being reported. Similarly, if there is potential risk but the practitioner makes the appropriate decisions—for example, to take some time off to regain their health, or to engage in treatment that mitigates the risk—there is no need for the treating practitioner to make a mandatory report. In Western Australia, treating doctors are exempt from the mandatory reporting provisions, but remain bound by ethical and moral standards to make a report if they are treating a practitioner whose ongoing practice poses substantial risks to the public and who is not willing to take steps themselves to mitigate the risk. There are guidelines for mandatory reporting on the Medical Board's website [6].

Notifications can also be made about students, but only for impairment that puts the public at risk if their studies involve contact with patients, or for criminal offences carrying a potential penalty of a year or more of imprisonment. These notifications are very uncommon.

21.5.2 Notification processes

Ahpra and the Medical Board are constantly reviewing how they manage notifications. The processes have changed significantly over the past few years with the goal of improving efficiency and reducing stress for both notifiers and practitioners (Figure 21.2). Any member of the public, including registered health practitioners, can make a voluntary notification about a practitioner, which is received by Ahpra on behalf of the Medical Board (except in Queensland, where the notification is made to the OHO in the first instance, and NSW, where the notification goes to the Health Complaints Commission). Under the National Law, once a notification is made and accepted as being based on legal grounds, it must be assessed. Ahpra is primarily responsible for the administrative processing and investigative management of notification matters, while regulatory decision making for each matter is the responsibility of the Medical Board via its delegated decision-making committees.

Delegated decision makers include the state and territory jurisdictional boards and their notifications committees, and several national committees established for specific purposes. The latter include specialised National Special Issues Committees dealing with matters that involve sexual boundary issues (see section 21.5.5) and cosmetic practice, and notifications involving Aboriginal and/or Torres Strait Islander people.

Figure 21.2 The process for handling notifications

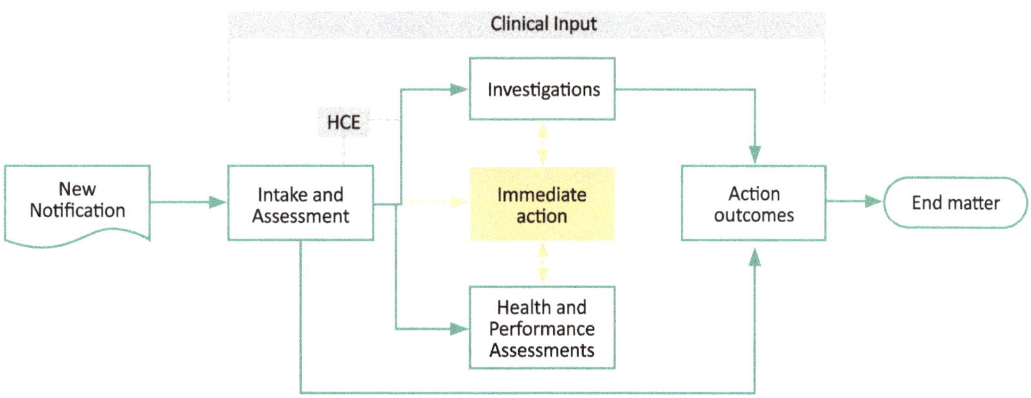

Source: Reproduced with permission from Ahpra.

Ahpra employs medical practitioners to provide clinical input into all notifications about doctors at a very early stage. The clinical input can be a very valuable part of assessing the risk of the alleged conduct or performance issue. Risk is assessed by considering the characteristics of the practitioner, including their previous regulatory history, their practice setting, the nature of their practice, the nature of the notification, and any risk controls already in place. A trained Ahpra staff member often contacts the practitioner, usually by telephone, to let them know that the notification has been received and to seek information about their practice setting, and any steps that they may have taken themselves to reduce the risk of a similar issue arising in the future. If a matter is assessed as being low risk, it will then be put to a delegated decision-making committee for early closure, usually with no further regulatory action. In some cases, where action is required to protect the public, the Medical Board can take actions such as issuing a caution or imposing conditions on registration; for example, requiring the practitioner to undertake education. In recent years, the Medical Board has established a number of processes and committees aiming to close low-risk matters early and quickly.

Higher-risk matters are progressed to the phase of investigation, which involves trained Ahpra investigators gathering information and writing an investigation report. This process may take many months, particularly if information is required from Medicare or the Pharmaceutical Benefits Scheme, or if other relevant processes are occurring, such as legal or coronial proceedings. Occasionally, if there is evidence suggesting poor professional performance or a health condition impairing practice, the Medical Board may require a performance assessment or health assessment, respectively, and these also increase the time required. The case may also need to be reviewed by an independent expert. The investigation report and associated information is then submitted to one of the Medical Board's committees which, as the delegated decision maker, decides whether any regulatory action is required, and if so, what is needed to reduce the risk to the public into the future.

Very-high-risk matters, where a decision-making committee forms a reasonable belief that the practitioner's practice represents a serious risk to the community, can result in immediate action to protect the public while further investigation occurs. For very serious matters, this may include suspension of the practitioner's registration.

21.5.3 Risk controls: individual, practice-based and regulatory

The National Law has established that the fundamental purpose of regulation of the medical profession is to protect the public, not to punish practitioners. Therefore, the key question that decision makers need to address when dealing with notifications is whether the situation as it stands at the time of the decision represents an ongoing risk to public safety. If a practitioner demonstrates that they have adequately self-regulated in response to a notification and taken appropriate steps to reduce the ongoing risk, the likelihood of imposition of regulatory action may be lowered.

For example, if there has been a misunderstanding or miscommunication, or the complaint is about a recognised complication of a procedure and the patient was adequately informed about this before giving consent, there is clearly little ongoing risk and the decision is likely to be to take no further action. In some instances, there has clearly been a problem in the management of a patient's condition, but the practitioner (often on the advice of their professional indemnity insurer) has undertaken additional education or training about the particular issue, and can make the case that there is no *ongoing* risk. In these cases, again, no regulatory action may be required. Similarly, hospitals or employers may put in place controls that reduce risk; an example would be to require a second practitioner to be present for specific procedures. Again, no regulatory action is likely to be required if the ongoing risk has been reduced adequately by these measures.

In matters where there has been poor professional performance or unprofessional conduct, and neither individual nor practice-based controls have been implemented to satisfactorily deal with the ongoing risk to patients, the Medical Board has a small number of potential regulatory controls that can be imposed. At the lower level of severity, the board may propose to caution the practitioner regarding the conduct or performance and/or impose conditions on the practitioner's registration requiring them to meet an appropriate standard of practice. Common conditions involve a requirement to undertake education about the issue of concern, or to undergo a period of supervised practice in a particular area. Less commonly, in cases of alleged sexual boundary transgression (see Chapter 8, Sexual and other professional boundaries: being a doctor in modern society), a condition may prevent a practitioner from consulting with any patients of a particular gender. In all cases, a proposal to caution or impose conditions is followed by a show cause process, in which the practitioner is invited to provide additional information and reasons why the action should not be taken. Some practitioners opt to sign a voluntary undertaking instead of conditions, and these have the same enforceability as conditions and cannot be withdrawn without the board's approval.

More serious sanctions, such as reprimands, fines and suspension or cancellation of registration, cannot be imposed by the board (except suspension as an immediate interim action), but require referral to a panel or tribunal. In any case where the board forms the reasonable belief that the conduct or performance of a practitioner constitutes professional misconduct (more serious than unprofessional conduct), the case will usually be referred to the relevant tribunal. In these cases, the board presents its arguments to the tribunal as to why the practitioner's performance or conduct represents a risk to public safety, and the practitioner presents their position. The tribunal then makes the decision and, where relevant, determines the sanctions to be imposed, which may include fines, suspension or cancellation of registration.

21.5.4 Notification outcomes

Most notifications made about doctors result in no regulatory action (over 75% in 2022–23). In many cases, this is because the Medical Board's delegated decision makers determine that the reported events do not suggest that there is an ongoing risk to public safety. In others, there may have been an indication of risk at the time of the event, but the practitioner and/or their employer have taken steps to control that risk going forward, so that there is no need for a regulatory control.

Of the remaining matters, another 10–15% are referred to an HCE within the relevant jurisdiction (see Chapter 22, Healthcare complaints and complaint systems), often because the complaint is about a health service rather than an individual practitioner. About 10% of cases result in imposition of a caution or conditions. Each year, about 1% of all matters are referred to a tribunal because the board has formed a reasonable belief that the behaviour or performance constitutes professional misconduct (the most serious category). The majority of these matters are conduct issues rather than poor clinical performance, and include sexual boundary transgressions (see Chapter 8, Sexual and other professional boundaries: being a doctor in modern society). The performance issues that result in referral to a tribunal often include an element of concern about conduct as well, such as failing to follow up patients with complications, or failing to attend when on call, resulting in poor patient outcomes.

21.5.5 Notifications about sexual misconduct

For centuries, dating back to the time of Hippocrates, the medical profession has held an agreed position that sexual contact with patients represents a very serious breach of the trust that is at the heart of the doctor–patient relationship. The reasons for this are explored further in Chapter 8, Sexual and other professional boundaries: being a doctor in modern society; however, the fundamental reason is that this behaviour by doctors is harmful to their patients. The Medical Board has issued specific guidelines for doctors about sexual boundaries [3].

The imperative to avoid crossing sexual boundaries cannot be stressed too strongly. It is very important for doctors to recognise that such crossings can include a wide range of behaviours, such as inappropriate sexualised comments (e.g. while undertaking an intimate examination), sexualised behaviour disguised as a legitimate medical examination, and establishing a consensual sexual relationship with a patient or a patient's close relative (e.g. the mother of a paediatric patient). All these behaviours have occurred over recent years and caused significant harm to the patients involved.

In 2017, in response to an independent review on the management of sexual boundary notifications (the Paterson report [7]), the Medical Board and Ahpra made significant changes to the processes for regulating these matters. The key changes included a specialised, national, delegated decision-making committee with specific training in decision making in sexual boundary allegations, and the establishment of a specialised group of Ahpra investigators with training in how to interact with potential victims/survivors of sexual abuse. In addition, recognising the rarity of false accusations of sexual misconduct against doctors, the Medical Board is now more inclined to take such accusations seriously and investigate them. Some matters of this kind in recent years have depended primarily on the testimony of one or more patients, and practitioners have been found by independent tribunals to be guilty of sexual misconduct on this basis.

21.5.6 Notifications about health impairment

Notifications of concern about a doctor's health are uncommon. These notifications are generally only made when there is an actual impact on practice (impairment) and the doctor is not taking steps to reduce the risk posed to the community. When these notifications occur, the regulatory approach is focused on encouraging the doctor to manage their condition and, where possible, return to practice safely. Physical conditions, such as visual disturbances or tremor that may affect manual dexterity, are usually managed well by individual practitioners, some of whom make self-notifications to the Medical Board. Psychiatric illness, substance use disorders and cognitive impairment are often more problematic, largely because the doctor involved may have lost a degree of insight into their condition and may not recognise that their performance is impaired. Doctors' health is discussed in more detail in Chapter 12, Personal health of the doctor: illness and impairment.

Notifications about health are generally managed by receiving reports from treating practitioners, or requiring the doctor to undergo an independent health assessment by an appropriate practitioner. If the evidence of impairment contained within the notification is seriously concerning, the matter may be submitted for immediate action to protect the public while further assessment is undertaken. Following the health assessment, a practitioner member of the board or delegated decision maker has a discussion with the doctor, usually in the presence of a representative of their professional indemnity insurer. These discussions may offer insight into the issues, and be followed by a period of restricted practice (by conditions or undertakings) while the doctor undergoes treatment as required. The removal of those restrictions requires a satisfactory progress report from the treating doctor and sometimes also a review by an independent practitioner.

Recognising the importance of doctors' health in underpinning safe health services for the community, the Medical Board strongly recommends that all doctors have their own general practitioner. It also funds doctors' health services in all jurisdictions, managed confidentially and at arm's length by an independent company owned by the Australian Medical Association. All doctors receive contact details for doctors' health services in the early correspondence they receive from Ahpra about a notification [8].

21.5.7 The stress of having a notification

For the past several years, Ahpra has been surveying both notifiers and practitioners who have been involved in the notifications process [9]. Both groups overwhelmingly find the process stressful, and many doctors report having severe anxiety, feeling that their career is in jeopardy. The Medical Board and Ahpra have been changing their processes in an attempt to reduce the level of stress. Trained Ahpra staff often make telephone contact with practitioners very early after receipt of a notification, to give them a contact person within Ahpra and to reduce the legalistic tone of some of the written communications. The wording of letters has been extensively revised to reduce their formality. Low-risk matters are being handled more efficiently and closed as quickly as possible.

Despite these changes, doctors report that receiving a notification remains extremely stressful, partly because they overestimate the risk of losing their registration (which in reality occurs in less than 1% of notifications) and partly because of the high standards that doctors set for themselves, which are challenged whenever a patient complains [9]. The fact that the majority of notifications go through assessment (as required by the National Law) is sometimes misinterpreted as an indication that the board believes that the practitioner is guilty, leading to a sense of injustice.

The data available from internal Ahpra surveys of practitioners who have been through the notifications process indicate that those who attempted to resolve the concerns raised by the notifier had a lower rate of action taken on their registration. In particular, a much smaller number had conditions imposed. This indicates that a proactive and positive approach by practitioners in dealing with direct complaints from patients and in responding to a notification to reduce the risk going forward results in a better outcome for the practitioner and for the public.

It is also important to keep in mind that, no matter how careful and diligent a practitioner may be, it is highly likely that most will experience at least one notification over their career. The great majority of these will have no negative impact on the practitioner's registration. Loss of registration is very rare and is reserved for very serious matters such as sexual boundary transgressions. For many doctors, the most punishing aspect of the notification is the stress and anxiety that accompanies it, and taking steps to reduce the impact is a very important part of the doctor's response. Professional indemnity insurers and doctors' health organisations are very well placed to provide advice and assistance, and doctors are strongly advised to make contact with one or both of these [8].

Summary

Since 2010, the medical regulatory system in Australia has been a national system (NRAS) based around a national board and its delegated decision makers (including state and territory boards and committees) working in partnership with Ahpra. Over time, the system has evolved and matured in response to various regulatory challenges. Health ministers have made it clear that the paramount goal of the NRAS is protection of the public. This is achieved by registering only appropriately trained, fit and proper individuals as medical practitioners, and managing notifications of concern about individual doctors in a way that protects the public and addresses any safety concern while having the least possible impact on the doctor's practice.

References

1. Medical Board of Australia. Good medical practice: a code of conduct for doctors in Australia. 2020. https://www.medicalboard.gov.au/Codes-Guidelines-Policies/Code-of-conduct.aspx (accessed Dec 2024).
2. Medical Board of Australia. Guidelines for registered medical practitioners who perform cosmetic surgery and procedures. 2023. https://www.medicalboard.gov.au/codes-guidelines-policies/cosmetic-medical-and-surgical-procedures-guidelines.aspx (accessed Dec 2024).
3. Medical Board of Australia. Guidelines: sexual boundaries in the doctor–patient relationship. 2018. https://www.medicalboard.gov.au/Codes-Guidelines-Policies/Sexual-boundaries-guidelines.aspx# (accessed Dec 2024).
4. Australian Health Practitioner Regulation Agency & National Boards. Register of practitioners. 2024. https://www.ahpra.gov.au/registration/registers-of-practitioners.aspx (accessed Dec 2024).
5. Medical Board of Australia. Expedited specialist pathway. https://www.medicalboard.gov.au/Registration/International-Medical-Graduates/Expedited-specialist-pathway.aspx (accessed Jul 2025).
6. Medical Board of Australia. Guidelines for mandatory notifications. 2020. https://www.medicalboard.gov.au/Codes-Guidelines-Policies/Guidelines-for-mandatory-notifications.aspx (accessed Dec 2024).
7. Paterson R. Independent review of the use of chaperones to protect patients in Australia. 2017. https://www.nhpo.gov.au/chaperone-review (accessed Jul 2025).
8. Doctors for Doctors (Drs4drs). https://www.drs4drs.com.au (accessed Dec 2024).
9. Biggar S, van der Gaag A, Maher P, et al. 'Virtually daily grief'—understanding distress in health practitioners involved in a regulatory complaints process: a qualitative study in Australia. *Int J Qual Health Care* 2023; 35: mzad076.

Further reading

General information about the Medical Board of Australia: https://www.medicalboard.gov.au

General information about the Australian Health Practitioner Regulation Agency: https://www.ahpra.gov.au

Gee C, Tonkin A, Gaby S, et al. Responding to sexual boundary notifications: the evolving regulatory approach in Australia. *J Med Regul* 2021; 107: 25–31.

22 Healthcare complaints and complaint systems

Lisa Pritchard

Introduction

The right to provide feedback, including complaints, about healthcare experiences is a fundamental part of patient-centred care. Doctors who deal well with direct complaints from patients are known to receive fewer formal complaints to health complaint agencies and the Australian Health Practitioner Regulation Agency (Ahpra). This chapter includes the background to the right to complain, the structure of the healthcare complaints system in Australia, and the processes that apply in different jurisdictions. It also identifies some specific situations that commonly result in complaints and provides information for practitioners on how to handle a complaint well.

22.1 The right to complain

Contemporary medical practice recognises person-centred care as the gold-standard approach to healthcare delivery [1]. The Australian Commission on Safety and Quality in Health Care (ACSQHC) National Safety and Quality Health Service (NSQHS) Standards [2] notes that partnering with patients in their own care is an important pillar of patient-centred care.

Partnering with patients is integral to the development, implementation and evaluation of health policies, programs and services [3–5]. On an individual level it means care that focuses on the relationship and interactions between a patient and their doctor, and acknowledges the importance of trust, mutual respect and knowledge sharing as critical to the delivery of the best health outcomes [6].

Partnering with patients also means, among many other things, being open to hearing about concerns or feedback about how their care has been delivered, or perceived to have been delivered.

The right of patients to complain about their medical care is also included in the *Australian charter of healthcare rights* [7]. The charter describes the rights that consumers, or someone they care for, can expect when receiving health care. These rights cover access, safety, respect, communication, participation, privacy and the right to complain or comment on care received. They apply to all people in all places where health care is provided in Australia. This includes public and private hospitals, day procedure services, general practice, community health services and any other place where a health service is provided; for example, in a person's home.

22.2 Benefits of complaints and feedback

22.2.1 Identifying complaints

A healthcare complaint is an expression of dissatisfaction made to or about a person or organisation, related to healthcare services, staff or the handling of a complaint, where a response or resolution is explicitly *or implicitly* expected [8].

A medical practitioner should be open to hearing feedback or complaints—they can provide useful information or insights into a patient's experience or a doctor's practice that the doctor may not otherwise have insight into. It also provides an opportunity to reflect on what can be done differently to improve patient safety, experience, quality and outcomes.

However, patients or their representatives may not always use direct, clear or specific language when making a complaint—sometimes, when a person makes a complaint, they will not explicitly use terminology such as 'complaint' or 'dissatisfaction'. Instead, they may say 'I am unhappy about ...', 'I don't like ...', 'I am concerned about ...', 'I disagree with your decision about ...', or 'Why didn't ... happen?' [9].

Patients from some cultural backgrounds may also not be accustomed to making complaints or giving direct feedback. The Centre for Cultural Diversity in Ageing [10] highlights the importance of being attuned to your patients and having cultural awareness when it comes to treating patients and hearing patient complaints and feedback. Some cultures, for example, are accustomed to giving direct feedback while other cultures may prefer more subtle indirect feedback.

Medical practitioners should also consider potential privacy concerns, particularly where there may be stigma around certain issues that could lead to reluctance for a person to share their concerns [10]. Perceptions of stigma may also lead patients to fear discrimination, making them less likely to speak up if they are not satisfied or if something is wrong; for example, where the person has a mental illness. Others may fear that making a complaint will impact on their ongoing access to health care [11].

Doctors should therefore adopt flexible approaches to inviting and receiving feedback from patients, and in particular, patients from culturally and linguistically diverse backgrounds [10]. They should consider whether the person needs an interpreter or support person present to be able to raise their concerns.

Proactively seeking feedback from patients about whether they are happy with their treatment and inviting any suggestions they may have can be empowering and strengthen respectful engagement. It will also ensure that opportunities for reflection and improvement are maximised and framed as a positive activity contributing to a relationship of trust with the patient.

22.2.2 Benefits of dealing with complaints well

Patients generally, in the first instance, direct their complaints about their health care to their health service provider. They are usually seeking an acknowledgement and understanding of their experience, an apology, and sometimes a system, policy or process change to reduce the likelihood of reoccurrence [12].

How you deal with complaints and feedback from patients will affect your ongoing treating relationship, how your patients report their experience to others and whether they escalate their complaint to, for example, a health complaints commission or other regulator. The ACSQHC reports that only a small proportion of people who are dissatisfied will lodge a complaint (less than 4%), but they will tell their family and friends about their bad experience and go elsewhere if they can [11].

Effective and responsive complaints handling can help to avoid this risk, and avoid escalation [13] and deterioration of the doctor–patient relationship.

Aside from the issue of escalated complaints, patient complaints and feedback also provide unique information about patient needs and the quality of care they receive or perceive they have received. They provide valuable insights into potential problems and opportunities for improving the way health care is delivered. Even if a complaint is not substantiated, it is important to reflect on why the patient or their representative held concerns—there may be opportunities to improve communication or to better manage patient education and expectations.

Having strong governance and a culture and mindset that encourages, listens, and responds individually and systemically to complaints and feedback is critical. Among other things, a good complaints management approach and system can help to:

- improve the safety and quality of health care by providing information about the experiences of patients and carers
- restore the trust and confidence of a patient or carer
- prevent wasteful practices and reduce costs, such as insurance
- create a more satisfactory working environment for clinicians and staff
- enhance the reputation of the medical practitioner and minimise negative comments or publicity [11].

22.2.3 Dealing with complaints and feedback

Complaints are less likely to occur if a doctor has good communication skills, employs competent staff and practises with patience, courtesy and empathy. If a complaint or the hint of a complaint arises, the medical practitioner should be willing to make time to listen to the complainant in a non-defensive manner. Often, simply acknowledging the complaint, acknowledging the patient's right to complain and (if appropriate) accepting the legitimacy of the complaint and undertaking to prevent recurrences will resolve the matter there and then, and enhance the doctor–patient relationship. In more serious matters, medical practitioners should seek advice from their medical indemnity insurer [14].

When managing a complaint, the process you follow should, among other things, be:

- accessible—make information about how to make a complaint easily accessible and encourage and support patients and their representatives to report complaints
- timely—resolve complaints in a timely way. Acknowledge the complaint within 48 hours and inform the person complaining about how, and how quickly, their complaint will be dealt with.
- responsive—seek to understand the concerns raised and the resolution that is being sought, and provide timely feedback on the analysis of complaints and actions taken. Avoid being defensive.
- free—access to your complaints process should be free of charge to patients
- confidential—make personally identifiable information concerning the patient complaint available only to people involved in managing the complaint. Take active steps to protect disclosure unless the patient consents to their information being shared. Store complaint records separately from patient records and only store and use them according to information privacy obligations (e.g. see *Privacy Act 1988* [Cth] or individual state or territory legislation for public health services).
- free of retribution—never take detrimental action against a patient because they have made a complaint

- risk aware—record the risks identified from the analysis of complaints in your risk management system [8,11]
- improvement focused—use information from the analysis of complaints to inform improvements in safety and quality.

Some health complaints commissions publish complaint-handling standards or resources to guide complaint handling. See, for example, the Victorian Health Complaints Commissioner's *Complaint handling standards* [15] or the South Australian Office of the Health and Community Services Complaints Commissioner's tips, advice and resources for providers [16].

22.2.4 Complaints and feedback about a colleague or peer

Sometimes a medical practitioner may receive feedback or a complaint about another medical or health practitioner.

If a medical practitioner receives a complaint about a colleague, member of staff or peer they should do the following:

- Obtain sufficient objective information to enable a judgement to be made about the seriousness of the complaint and the appropriate course of action or response. For example, consider whether the complaint raises concerns about professional misconduct, unprofessional conduct or unsatisfactory professional performance requiring escalation according to the medical practitioner's professional obligations (see mandatory notification requirements of the Health Practitioner Regulation National Law [the National Law] for the relevant state or territory [17]), or whether the patient should be directed to a practice manager, professional lead or patient liaison officer.
- Provide the patient with information about what you can and cannot assist with, and provide options for dealing with their concerns; for example, information about the practice or health service's complaints process, or details about the local health complaints agency.
- Ask the patient what action they would like to see as a result of their complaint or feedback. For example, they may wish to be referred to a different medical practitioner or to make a formal complaint through an established complaint process.
- Consider whether the substance of the complaint raises concerns of 'notifiable conduct' (see definition of 'notifiable conduct' in the National Law for the relevant state or territory [17]) that must be reported to the relevant regulatory agency or registration board (see Chapter 21, Regulation of the medical profession). The key question to consider here is whether or not the complaint raises concerns of risk to future patients. Let the patient know if a report will be made and explain why this must be done and why it is important.
- Avoid attempting to explain or respond on another practitioner's behalf and respect the privacy and confidentiality of both the patient and practitioner complained about (see Chapter 6, Confidentiality, privacy and disclosure).
- Avoid unsolicited criticism of a colleague; you may not have sufficient information to be able to judge their actions, and this behaviour can lead to significant distress for both the patient and your colleague if the criticism turns out to be unjustified.
- Consider whether the patient requires any additional support; for example, if the substance of the complaint, or discussing the complaint, has caused trauma or distress.

22.2.5 Anonymous and 'vexatious' complaints

A medical practitioner may be tempted not to consider anonymous or repeated complaints or to label complaints as vexatious if the complaint is perceived to have no basis, and to reject it without further consideration.

The ACSQHC notes that people may lodge anonymous complaints about their health care because they fear that making a complaint will adversely affect their future treatment or access to the service. Complaints and other feedback received anonymously should be received and properly considered—it can still be valuable in providing information about trends and specific issues, even if issues cannot be thoroughly pursued due to a lack of information [11].

When it comes to vexatious complaints, there is limited understanding among health professionals about what is *actually* a vexatious complaint. The widely accepted legal and regulatory definition refers to 'a groundless complaint *made with an adverse primary intent to cause distress, detriment or harassment* to the subject' of the complaint (emphasis added) [13]. A complaint found to have no basis, other than perhaps a misunderstanding or incorrect perception, is not of itself a vexatious complaint.

Available evidence indicates that the proportion of vexatious complaints is low [13] and it is more likely that concerns are under reported rather than there being excessive unnecessary or vexatious complaints [13].

The Medical Board of Australia's *Good medical practice: a code of conduct for doctors in Australia* [18] addresses vexatious complaints made by other medical practitioners. If doctors find themselves dealing with a truly vexatious complaint from another medical practitioner, or a patient or patient representative, they should discuss this with their medical defence organisation.

While not vexatious, some patients may have a history of repeatedly making complaints and may require a particular tailored response. Doctors should be clear but respectful, clarify and confirm the details of the complaint, and if previously dealt with, provide this information respectfully and record notes to this effect.

Doctors should also seek to understand the repeated nature of the complaints; for example, it may be attributable to a patient's diagnosis, the complexity of their treatment, unreasonable expectations or misunderstandings. Responses require identifying the most appropriate and effective means of conveying objective information to individual patients and encouraging patients to bring a support person or to make notes during consultations to avoid later misunderstandings.

22.3 Health complaints agencies in Australia

In addition to being able to raise their complaints directly with a medical practitioner or health service provider, patients and patient representatives can make their complaints to health complaints agencies or commissions. These agencies are independent, state or territory government–funded and jurisdiction-specific bodies. In general, their focus is on dealing with complaints from the 'users' or 'consumers' of health services, or their representatives.

Except for Queensland and New South Wales, health complaints agencies primarily focus on enquiring into complaints about health service organisations, unregistered practitioners and registered practitioners, but exclude issues associated with the health, conduct or performance of registered practitioners. Their primary objectives are to attempt to resolve complaints through dispute resolution processes, and to address system issues, service safety and quality improvement.

In contrast, the Medical Board of Australia, together with Ahpra (see also Chapter 21, Regulation of the medical profession), deal with complaints about individual registered medical practitioners, with a focus on their health, conduct and performance through a process of registration, complaints handling, investigations and compliance monitoring. In this context, complaints and concerns are referred to as 'notifications' and are generally received from members of the public (patients or their relatives), medical practitioners or other registered practitioners, employers, or other authorities or regulators (e.g. the coroner, the police, Medicare or health departments). Unlike state/territory-based health complaints agencies, Ahpra does not provide a complaint resolution service that provides specific outcomes for complainants, but focuses on whether a registered practitioner is practising safely.

A different regulatory framework applies in Queensland and NSW.

22.3.1 Queensland

In Queensland, a co-regulatory system operates, involving the Office of the Health Ombudsman (OHO) and Ahpra. The OHO has jurisdiction and responsibility to receive all complaints and notifications about registered practitioners, unregistered practitioners and health service provider organisations delivering health services in Queensland. Therefore, it is the single front door for all health service complaints in Queensland. Its primary obligation is to protect the health and safety of the public. Functions include assessing, resolving, referring, investigating and prosecuting serious complaints, and undertaking systemic investigations. The OHO has powers to address immediate risk and can take immediate action to suspend or place conditions on the practice of registered and unregistered practitioners.

The OHO jointly considers complaints about registered practitioners with Ahpra [19]. It must refer complaints or notifications indicating an impairment, or possible impairment, of a registered practitioner to Ahpra, and may also refer complaints about the conduct or performance of registered practitioners. Unlike in other jurisdictions, referral of complaints or notifications to Ahpra and the Medical Board is not an escalation. The most serious complaints will usually be dealt with by the OHO.

If it is determined that a matter is indicative of professional misconduct that requires disciplinary action, that action is prosecuted before the Queensland Civil and Administrative Tribunal.

Figure 22.1 Snapshot of Queensland co-regulatory framework

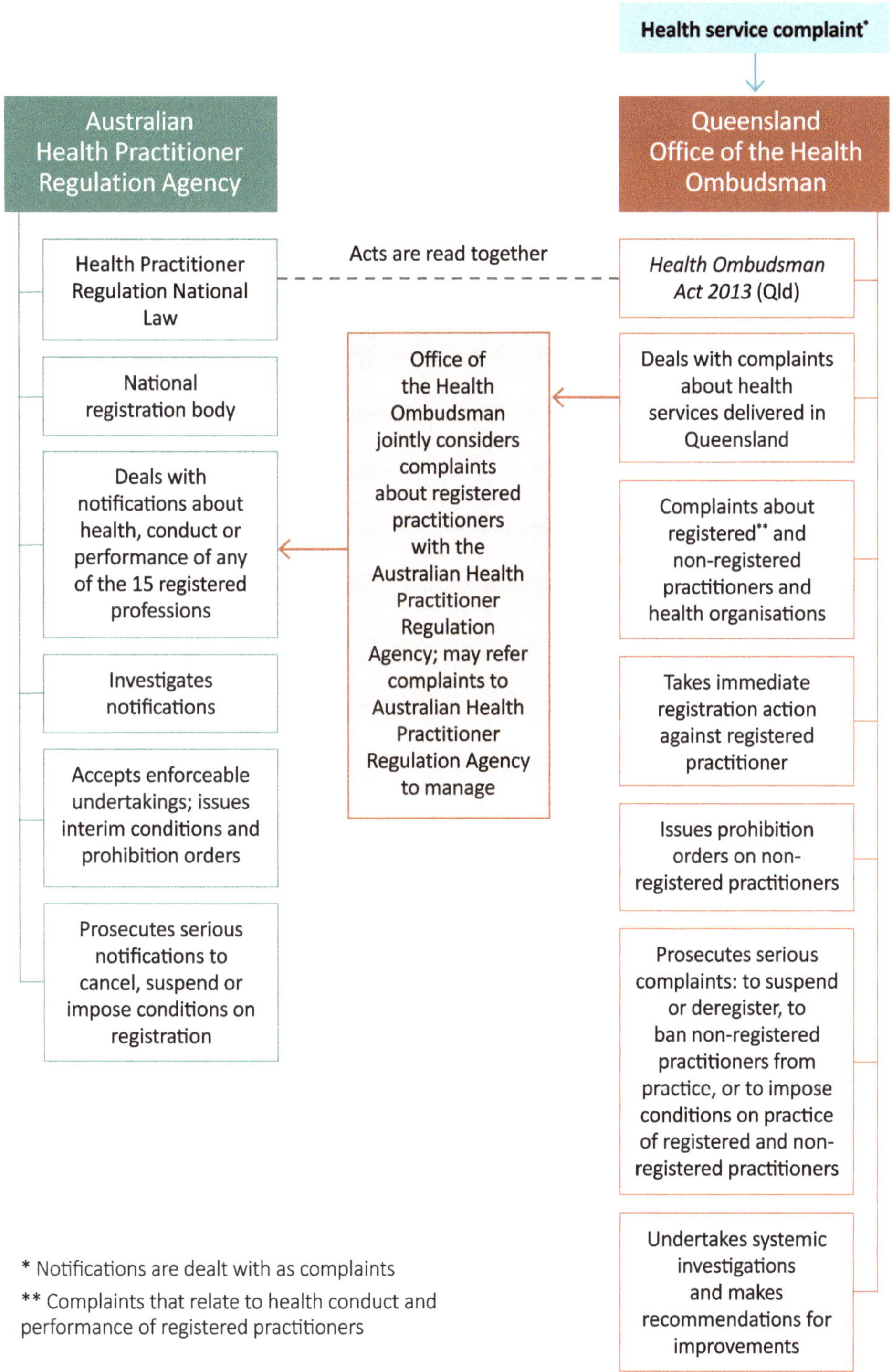

* Notifications are dealt with as complaints

** Complaints that relate to health conduct and performance of registered practitioners

Source: Author.

Figure 22.2 Snapshot of NSW co-regulatory framework

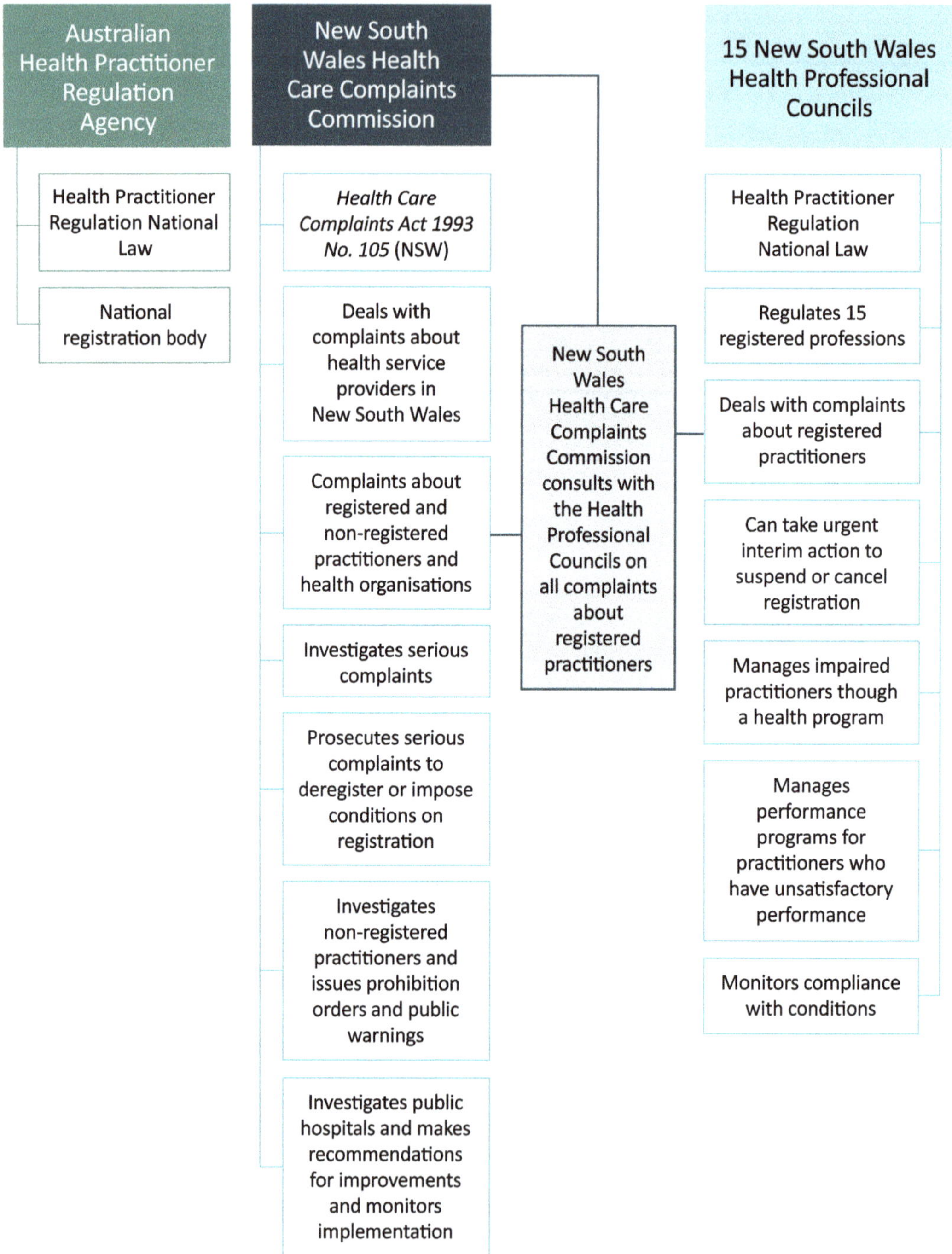

Source: Author.

22.3.2 New South Wales

In NSW, a co-regulatory system also operates, but involves three organisations, each with distinct roles:

- Ahpra and 15 National Boards—the National Registration Body for the 16 registered professions (the Nursing and Midwifery Board of Australia being responsible for two professions). Ahpra and the National Boards manage registration but do not play a role in managing complaints and notifications, with the exception of advertising-related complaints, about registered practitioners in NSW.
- NSW Health Professional Councils (HPCs)—the HPCs' emphasis is on maintaining standards across the 16 registered professions. They have powers to address immediate risk and can take immediate action to protect the public while a matter is being assessed or investigated. The council for the medical profession is the Medical Council of New South Wales.
- The Health Care Complaints Commission (HCCC) co-regulates with the 15 professional councils. It manages complaints about registered practitioners, unregistered practitioners and health service provider organisations. Its primary obligation is to protect the health and safety of the public by resolving, investigating and prosecuting serious complaints.

If it is determined by HCCC that a matter indicates possible professional misconduct that requires disciplinary action, that action is prosecuted before either the NSW Civil and Administrative Tribunal or a Professional Standards Committee.

22.4 The nature of complaints

Medical practitioners should be aware of the range of complaints made against doctors and recognise that most complaints are preventable. The types of serious complaints leading to formal disciplinary hearings are outlined in Chapter 21, Regulation of the medical profession. These include sexual misconduct; gross negligence or gross incompetence; fraudulent documentation; and conviction for serious crimes, offences against drugs of dependence laws, or fraud involving Medicare. Chapter 25, Negligence and professional liability, addresses matters leading to litigation for negligence.

Each health complaints commission or agency publishes an annual report that outlines the number and nature of complaints received during the year in their jurisdiction, or in the case of Ahpra and the Medical Board of Australia, across the country (with the exception of NSW). Website details for each jurisdiction are provided at the end of this chapter.

22.4.1 Common areas of complaint

Common types of complaint are listed below.

Professional performance

- Inadequate competence
- Poor quality, coordination of or delay in treatment
- Missed, delayed, wrong or inadequate diagnosis
- Inadequate care, consultation or treatment
- Unexpected treatment outcome
- Inadequate measures to control sources of infection or to adhere to standard precautions

Access to services

- Access to services—for example, physical access to a facility
- Access to government subsidies—subsidy availability may be affected by a medical practitioner's recommendation
- Refusal to admit or treat where a service is available

Access to records

Patients frequently complain that, when moving to a new area or changing medical practitioners, they have great difficulty in having their records forwarded to their new medical practitioner. Some patients wrongly believe that the entire record is theirs and should be sent in its original form. Sensible medical practitioners will respond professionally (and avoid complaints) by promptly providing relevant photocopied extracts or a summary, by explaining to the patient that the record is owned by the medical practitioner and needs to be retained (for future possible enquiries and purposes), and by offering to respond to any additional enquiries made by their new medical practitioner.

While some medical practitioners charge for this service, the vast majority do not, as they recognise that they also are the beneficiaries of other patients transferring to their practice.

Communication

Communication can play a significant role in whether a patient feels comfortable with and confident in their medical practitioner. It is also vital in determining whether they understand their diagnosis and treatment plan and any costs, and can therefore provide informed consent. The following issues may arise in complaints when a medical practitioner fails to give due regard to the importance of communicating appropriately with their patients:

- manner is rude, discourteous, disrespectful, negative, insensitive, patronising or overbearing
- failure to record/respond appropriately to a complaint
- insensitive or inappropriate comments
- providing wrong, incorrect, inaccurate, misleading or conflicting information
- not providing information, or providing information that is inadequate, incomprehensible, incomplete, or difficult to understand due to jargon or other barriers. This includes inadequate information provided to family, carers or other people.
- failure to communicate openly, honestly and effectively
- failure to gain consent
- failure to warn about adverse effects or costs of treatment
- breaching confidentiality when talking to relatives and friends of the patient without permission.

Professional conduct

Actions that conflict with professional conduct encompass a range of issues, such as:

- verbal or physical assault
- refusal to assist or attend

- boundary violation—medical practitioner commencing an inappropriate personal relationship with a patient that exceeds the bounds of professional practice
- sexual misconduct
- conflicts of interest
- discriminatory conduct
- providing treatments, tests or consultations in excess of what should reasonably be provided in the circumstances
- experimental treatment—the treatment provided was not appropriately authorised or recognised
- inappropriate collection, use or disclosure of information
- National Law breach or offence.

Intimate examinations

Patients will feel particularly vulnerable during consultations involving intimate examinations (see also Chapter 8, Sexual and other professional boundaries: being a doctor in modern society). Doctors should take time to explain the process to their patients—patients may misconstrue professionally appropriate examinations if explanations and procedures are inadequate. To minimise the risk of patients misunderstanding, or feeling uncomfortable or concerned about their examination, medical practitioners should:

- fully explain the reasons for and the nature of any intimate physical examination, and, during history taking, for inquiring about sexual behaviour, performance or dysfunction
- provide privacy while the patient undresses and dresses—direct observation of a patient while the patient is disrobing is likely to be misinterpreted, may increase a patient's anxiety, and may lead to complaint
- provide an appropriate combination of gown and cover sheet, while still conducting a thorough examination
- check if the patient would like somebody else present and consider the use of a chaperone for the examination of particular patients, including those who are young or inexperienced, or from a different cultural background, or otherwise vulnerable
- confirm the patient understands what the doctor has explained to them and check if they have any questions
- confirm the doctor has the patient's consent to proceed with the examination.

Fees and billing

Patients are entitled to open disclosure of anticipated fees, especially for major interventions, admissions to hospital or extensive investigations, and particularly when medical practitioners know that their charges and the charges of the hospital and other professional services will not be adequately covered by the patient's level of health insurance.

22.4.2 Most common complaints for five health professions in Australia

A national cohort study [20] conducted for all complaints received for medicine, nursing/midwifery, dentistry, pharmacy and psychology from 1 July 2012 to 31 December 2013 found that, overall, the risk of complaints is low for registered practitioners, but complaints are most common for medical practitioners and dentists (5% per annum per practitioner) and least common for nurses/midwives (0.5% per annum per practitioner). Gender, age and country of birth were all associated with risk of complaint. Men were more than twice as likely to receive a complaint than women. Another study shows that, with the exception of practitioners from the UK and Ireland, overseas-trained medical practitioners have an increased risk of complaints [21].

In the cohort study, the most common complaints were clinical care, communication, medication and health impairment of the practitioner [20]. Types of complaints varied by profession, gender and age.

22.5 Management of complaints by health complaints agencies

This section describes the management of health complaints by health complaints agencies. Chapter 21, Regulation of the medical profession, deals with the processes applied by Ahpra and the Medical Board of Australia when dealing with notifications of concern about medical practitioners, which differ substantially.

22.5.1 Process

Health complaints agencies will generally gather further information from the person making the complaint to enable them to determine what action, if any, should be taken. Note that a doctor may not always be aware if a complaint has been made about them. For example, if a complaint is not accepted at the initial complaint intake stage or a decision is made to take no further action on initial receipt of the complaint, a medical practitioner may not receive notification of the complaint.

If a doctor is contacted by a health complaints agency and advised a complaint has been made about them, the complaint should be responded to promptly, fully, accurately and thoughtfully. Depending on the potential seriousness of the complaint, advice should be sought from their medical defence organisation. Angry responses, delayed responses or responses that do not address the patient's concerns are of little help to the patient or the responsible agency and show the medical practitioner in an unfavourable light.

22.5.2 Possible complaint outcomes

No further action or the complaint is not accepted by the health complaints agency

Some jurisdictions may decline to deal with certain complaints if the complainant has not attempted to resolve their complaint with the medical practitioner first (e.g. see *Health Ombudsman Act 2013* (Qld) [22]. These decisions not to accept a complaint are informed by such factors as the characteristics of the patient/complainant; for example, vulnerability, age or literacy skills affecting their ability to make a complaint would weigh in favour of the health complaint agency dealing with the complaint, as would the level of seriousness of a complaint. They may decline to deal with a complaint if the medical practitioner has already provided an adequate and reasonable response to the patient or their representative.

Other reasons why no further action may be taken on a complaint include:

- after considering the information it is determined the care and treatment provided was of an appropriate standard and there are no risks to public health and safety that require further action
- the complaint is vexatious, frivolous or not made in good faith
- the complaint is already the subject of legal proceedings, investigation or has been otherwise appropriately dealt with by another person or body.

Complaint resolution

Health complaints agencies provide voluntary informal dispute or complaint resolution processes involving facilitated negotiations between the person making the complaint and the medical practitioner. These processes are generally applied to less complex complaints requiring lower levels of intervention. Potential outcomes include an apology, policy or process improvements, and refunds for out-of-pocket expenses or corrective costs. Often the patient may require ongoing health care, making the local resolution process an important step in rebuilding trust and confidence in the relationship. This may be achieved by sharing information regarding the care received, improving the understanding of clinical treatment, and developing communication protocols for the future [23].

Conciliation

Conciliation is also a voluntary process, but is applied to resolving complex complaints that require detailed explanations or confidential complaint resolution. The process is facilitated by independent conciliators in a confidential and privileged environment. This assists patients, their representatives and medical practitioners to be heard, to identify issues for discussion and to negotiate outcomes. Matters addressed in conciliation tend to be more complex, requiring greater intervention to help parties reach agreement. Information disclosed during a conciliation process—including details relating to any agreements or negotiations—is confidential and privileged, meaning it cannot be discussed outside the process or admitted as evidence in a proceeding before a court, tribunal or disciplinary body. For these reasons, conciliation can be effective in resolving complaints that involve sensitive information or complex clinical issues that require detailed explanations. It provides opportunities for parties to hear each other, ask each other questions and provide responses in a confidential, safe setting [23].

Referral

Complaints may be referred to medical practitioners to deal with locally where there is an ongoing service relationship, the complaint relates to communication issues or local policy matters and there are no risks to the health and safety of the public. Complaints may also be referred to other agencies—for example, police or health departments—that are more appropriate for the complaint subject matter.

Complaints may also be referred to Ahpra and the Medical Board of Australia for management where issues relate to the health, conduct or performance of an individual medical practitioner. In NSW, complaints of this type may be referred to the Medical Council of New South Wales. The Medical Board (supported by Ahpra) and the Medical Council of New South Wales have processes that aim to support safe and ethical practice by improving a practitioner's ability to perform their work, where possible, or to taking regulatory action to reduce the risk to the public going forward.

Investigation

Investigations are generally undertaken where complaints raise issues of public health and safety or systemic issues where recommendations for improvement can be made, and progress implementing them can be monitored. The level and type of investigations undertaken varies in each jurisdiction. In NSW and Queensland, investigations into the conduct or performance of medical practitioners may lead to disciplinary proceedings.

22.5.3 Impacts of complaints on the medical practitioner

There is substantial evidence that complaints in general have significant negative impacts on the health and wellbeing of medical practitioners, although they may also have positive impacts on practice in some cases [13,24]. A study of around 8000 medical practitioners in the UK found that those who experienced professional complaints had a higher risk of anxiety and depression [25].

Medical defence organisations offer varying levels of support including health checks, telephone advice, and advice about claims and complaint processes [26]. This topic is further explored in Chapter 21, Regulation of the medical profession.

Doctors can contact their medical defence organisation or employer for advice and support if a complaint is made about them. In addition, Drs4Drs [27] provides health advisory and referral services that are independent, safe, supportive and confidential, and available in all jurisdictions (see also Chapter 12, Personal health of the doctor: illness and impairment).

Table 22.1 Health complaints commissions or equivalent

Jurisdiction	Title	Website
Australian Capital Territory	ACT Human Rights Commission—Health Services	https://www.hrc.act.gov.au/health
New South Wales	Health Care Complaints Commission	https://www.hccc.nsw.gov.au
Northern Territory	Health and Community Services Complaints Commission	https://hcscc.nt.gov.au
Queensland	Office of the Health Ombudsman	https://www.oho.qld.gov.au
South Australia	Office of the Health and Community Services Complaints Commissioner	https://www.hcscc.sa.gov.au
Tasmania	Health Complaints Commissioner Tasmania	https://www.healthcomplaints.tas.gov.au
Victoria	Health Complaints Commissioner	https://www.hcc.vic.gov.au
	Mental Health and Wellbeing Commission	https://www.mhwc.vic.gov.au
Western Australia	Health and Disability Services Complaints Office	https://www.hadsco.wa.gov.au

Summary

It is never comfortable for a medical practitioner to receive a complaint from a patient, but feedback can be very valuable and handling complaints well is an important skill for all practitioners. Openness to receiving feedback and good management of a complaint at the practice or service level improves relationships with patients; furthermore, complaints are less likely to progress to health complaints agencies or regulatory authorities. Health complaints agencies are present in each jurisdiction, and there are important differences between them, particularly in the states in which there is co-regulation. Common types of complaint include professional performance, access to services or records, communication, professional conduct, issues concerning intimate examinations, and discontent with fees and billing practices. Health complaints agencies provide services such as negotiation and conciliation to assist with complaint resolution, and potential outcomes can include refunds, apologies or practice improvements. Agencies also liaise closely with the professional regulator in all jurisdictions and refer matters that raise concerns about professional performance or conduct of individual medical practitioners to the Medical Board and Ahpra, or the Medical Council of New South Wales. Finally, it is important to recognise the impact on practitioners' health and wellbeing when a complaint is received and take appropriate steps to seek assistance, including from professional indemnity providers.

References

1. Australian Commission on Safety and Quality in Health Care. Partnering with patients in their own care. https://www.safetyandquality.gov.au/standards/nsqhs-standards/partnering-consumers-standard/partnering-patients-their-own-care (accessed Jul 2025).
2. Australian Commission on Safety and Quality in Health Care. National Safety and Quality Health Service Standards – Partnering with consumers standard. https://www.safetyandquality.gov.au/standards/nsqhs-standards/partnering-consumers-standard (accessed Jul 2025).
3. Consumers Health Forum of Australia. Learn about consumer engagement. https://www.chf.org.au/consumer-engagement/learn-more-about-consumer-engagment (accessed Jul 2025).
4. Dalton J, Chambers D, Harden M, et al. Service user engagement and health service reconfiguration: a rapid evidence synthesis. *J Health Serv Res Pol* 2015; 21: 195–205.
5. Johnson A. Consumer and community engagement in health services: a literature review to support the development of an evidence-based consumer and community engagement strategy for the Women's and Children's Health Network, South Australia. Adelaide: Health Consumers Alliance of South Australia and SA Health; 2015.
6. Harding E, Wait S, Scrutton J. The state of play in person-centred care. London: The Health Policy Partnership; 2015. https://www.healthpolicypartnership.com/project/person-centred-care/ (accessed Jul 2025).
7. Australian Commission for Safety and Quality in Health Care. Australian Charter of Healthcare Rights, 2nd edition. https://www.safetyandquality.gov.au/publications-and-resources/resource-library/australian-charter-healthcare-rights-second-edition-all-translations (accessed Jul 2025).
8. International Organization for Standardization. ISO 10002:2018 Quality management—Customer satisfaction—Guidelines for complaint handling in organisations. ISO; 2018. https://www.iso.org/standard/71580.html (accessed Jul 2025).
9. New South Wales Ombudsman. Effective complaint management guidelines 4th ed. Sydney: State of New South Wales; 2024. https://www.ombo.nsw.gov.au/guidance-for-organisations/resources/effective-complaint-management-guide (accessed Jul 2025).
10. Centre for Cultural Diversity in Ageing. Practice guide: culturally inclusive feedback. 2022. https://www.culturaldiversity.com.au/files/Culturally-Inclusive-Feedback.pdf (accessed Jul 2025).
11. Australian Commission on Safety and Quality in Health Care. Complaints management handbook for health care services. 2005. https://www.safetyandquality.gov.au/publications-and-resources/resource-library/complaints-management-handbook-health-care-services (accessed Jul 2025).

12. Nowotny B, Loh E, Lorenz K, Wallace E. Sharing the pain: lessons from missed opportunities for healthcare improvement from patient complaints and litigation in the Australian health system. *Aust Health Rev* 2019; 43: 382–391.
13. Morris J, Canaway R, Bismark M. Reducing, identifying and managing vexatious complaints. Melbourne School of Population and Global Health, Centre for Health Policy; 2017.
14. Bird S. The art of dealing with complaints. *Aust Fam Physician* 2002; 31: 1101–1102.
15. Health Complaints Commissioner (Vic). Complaint handling standards. 2023. https://hcc.vic.gov.au/providers/complaint-handling-standards (accessed Jul 2025).
16. Office of the Health and Community Services Complaints Commissioner (SA). Tips, advice and resources. https://www.hcscc.sa.gov.au/for-service-providers-addressing-complaints/tips-advice-and-resources-2/ (accessed Jul 2025).
17. Australian Health Practitioner Regulation Agency. Health Practitioner Regulation National Law. https://www.ahpra.gov.au/About-Ahpra/What-We-Do/National-Law.aspx (accessed Jul 2025).
18. Medical Board of Australia. Good medical practice: a code of conduct for doctors in Australia. 2020. https://www.medicalboard.gov.au/Codes-Guidelines-Policies/Code-of-conduct.aspx (accessed Jul 2025).
19. *Health Ombudsman Act 2013* (Qld), Pt 3, ss 2A, 2B.
20. Walton M, Kelly PJ, Chiarella EM, et al. Profile of the most common complaints for five health professions in Australia. *Aust Health Rev* 2020; 44: 15–23.
21. Elkin K, Spittal M, Studdert D. Risks of complaints and adverse disciplinary findings against international medical graduates in Victoria and Western Australia. *Med J Aust* 2012; 197: 448–452.
22. *Health Ombudsman Act 2013* (Qld), s 35A.
23. Office of the Health Ombudsman. Annual report 2023–2024. Brisbane: Queensland Government; 2024. https://www.parliament.qld.gov.au/Work-of-the-Assembly/Tabled-Papers/docs/5724t2033/5724t2033-803f.pdf (accessed Jul 2025).
24. Bourne T, Vanderhaegen J, Vranken R, et al. Doctors' experiences and their perception of the most stressful aspects of complaints processes in the UK: an analysis of qualitative survey data. *BMJ Open* 2016; 6: e011711.
25. Bourne T, Wynants L, Peters M, et al. The impact of complaints procedures on the welfare, health and clinical practise of 7926 doctors in the UK: a cross-sectional survey. *BMJ Open* 2015; 5: e006687.
26. Haysom G. The impact of complaints on doctors. *Aust Fam Physician* 2016; 45: 242–244.
27. Doctors' Health Services Pty Ltd. Drs4Drs. https://www.drs4drs.com.au/ (accessed Jul 2025).

23 Patient safety

Anne Tonkin AO, Theanne Walters AM

Introduction

This chapter will focus on the health and safety of members of the public when they access health care—that is, when they become patients or clients of a healthcare practitioner. The Health Practitioner Regulation National Law (the National Law) under which the National Registration and Accreditation Scheme operates refers to 'protection of the public' and 'public confidence in the safety of services by registered health practitioners and students' as paramount elements of the main guiding principle of the scheme [1]. In this chapter, the term 'patient safety' will be used to encompass all elements of a person's experience while accessing health care that have an impact on that person's safety. In addition to physical safety, this includes cultural and psychological safety while under the care of a health practitioner. Psychological and cultural safety while accessing health care are vital elements of ensuring that patients feel comfortable while receiving services, and have a significant impact on whether an individual attends healthcare facilities, undertakes recommended treatments and returns for follow-up. Ensuring the development of a culturally safe and respectful workforce, particularly during interactions with Aboriginal and/or Torres Strait Islander people and their health, is another element of the guiding principles of the National Law [1].

Respectful relationships underlying the teamwork that is so important in contemporary health care also have an impact on the outcomes for patients. It is well established that well-functioning and collaborative clinical teams achieve better results for their patients. The evidence for problems within the current culture of the medical profession will be discussed.

Despite considerable interest in the potential for adverse outcomes of health care for over 25 years, the rates of avoidable physical harm during health care remain uncomfortably high, both in Australia and throughout the developed world [2,3]. Although much has been learned about effective evidence-based approaches to improve safety, the implementation of these remains suboptimal. Similarly, the implementation of approaches to improving psychological and cultural safety for patients remains incomplete and poorly understood by many doctors. These issues will be discussed in this chapter.

23.1 Background

It has long been recognised that health care is associated with complications, sometimes avoidable and due to errors made by healthcare workers. From the 1990s, the safety of care started to be viewed differently, given the high frequency of adverse outcomes, initially recognised in hospital patients [3]. The term 'patient safety' has supplanted previous terms—such as 'medical error'—as systems thinking has been applied to safety in health care, and it has been recognised that when things go wrong it is usually a result of complex interacting factors rather than a single error [2].

23.1.1 Definition of patient safety

The World Health Organization (WHO) definition of patient safety is 'the absence of preventable harm to a patient and reduction of risk of unnecessary harm associated with health care to an acceptable minimum' [3]. WHO expands this within the broader health system context to 'a framework of organized activities that creates cultures, processes, procedures, behaviours, technologies and environments in health care that consistently and sustainably lower risks, reduce the occurrence of avoidable harm, make error less likely and reduce impact of harm when it does occur' [3].

23.1.2 Prevalence of adverse outcomes in health care

The first major study of adverse outcomes in health care in Australia was the Quality in Australian Health Care Study (QAHCS), published in 1995 [4], which showed that the rate of adverse events during hospital admissions in Australia was about 17%, with about half of those events being avoidable. In primary care and outpatient settings, WHO estimates that 40% of patients are harmed, with up to 80% of the harm being judged as preventable [3]. At a global level, it has been estimated that the risk of harm occurring while receiving hospital care in high-income countries is about 1 in 10 patients, and about 30–50% of those events are preventable [2]. The risk of death during health care due to a preventable medical accident was estimated to be about 1 in 300 in high-income countries but may be as high as 4% in low-to-middle income countries [3]. The commonest and most detrimental harms are related to healthcare-associated infections, and the prescription and administration of medicines. Others include diagnostic errors, unsafe surgical procedures, unsafe blood transfusions, and failure to prevent venous thromboembolism [3].

23.2 Factors contributing to patient harm

Multiple interrelated factors contribute to patient harm. Generally, more than one of the following factors is involved in any single incident of patient harm [2]:

- system and organisational factors, including inadequate processes and procedures, disruptions in workflow and care coordination, resource constraints and competency development
- technological factors related to health information systems or medication administration systems
- human factors and behaviour, including communication breakdown between healthcare workers, within healthcare teams and with patients and their families; and fatigue and burnout leading to people taking short cuts
- patient-related factors, including health literacy, cultural safety and engagement with health care
- external factors, including absent or inadequate policies or regulations, and economic and financial pressures.

Three important factors are discussed further in the following subsections.

23.2.1 Inadequate cultural safety for Aboriginal and/or Torres Strait Islander people

It is clear that Aboriginal and/or Torres Strait Islander people have poorer health outcomes, including significantly lower life expectancy and higher burden of chronic disease, when compared with the non-Indigenous population [5]. See also Chapter 17, Culturally safe health care for Aboriginal and/or Torres Strait Islander peoples.

For Aboriginal and/or Torres Strait Islander peoples there are additional factors that contribute to health, including cultural identity, family, community engagement, participation in cultural activities and access to traditional lands and waters [5]. For health care to be safe for Aboriginal and/or Torres Strait Islander people, it must be provided in a culturally sensitive and safe manner. It is well recognised that health outcomes are influenced by a range of social determinants, including institutionalised prejudice, which can reduce access to healthcare programs and discourage individuals from accessing health care even when it is available [5]. Gubhaju et al. report that access to high-quality and culturally secure health care is a key determinant of health for Aboriginal and/or Torres Strait Islander people [6]. The incorporation of cultural safety training into healthcare professional education has increased rapidly over the past 10 years, and its importance has been recognised by inclusion in the Australian Medical Council standards for the accreditation of medical schools and programs [7].

23.2.2 Suboptimal organisational and professional culture

As health care is a complex system, so too is the culture that is expressed within any profession or organisation. Culture defines belief systems and, in turn, how people behave. Two key elements of culture have an impact on safety within health care. One is the attitude of health professionals to risk management and safety guidelines, which influences how assiduously they follow guidelines, such as those for hand hygiene. The other is the interpersonal culture within healthcare teams, which influences the way in which the team functions. A team in which enquiry is punished and uncertainty is belittled is likely to make more errors than one in which intelligent enquiry is encouraged and individuals within the healthcare team feel valued and safe to question. A systematic review of the impact of workplace culture on patient outcomes showed a consistently positive association between culture and outcomes across multiple settings and countries [8]. More recently, a similar association has been demonstrated between clinicians' safety culture and patient-level outcomes within emergency departments across 32 Australian hospitals [9].

Psychological safety, most commonly defined in relation to patient safety as 'a shared belief held by members of a team that the team is safe for interpersonal risk-taking' is a key factor in promoting safe, high-quality health care [10]. Raising concerns when there is a perceived threat to patient safety improves outcomes and is promoted by a psychologically safe workplace with supportive leadership [11].

In Australia, the Medical Training Survey (MTS) has been run annually since 2019, and surveys doctors-in-training about a variety of aspects of their training, including the culture of their workplace and training environment. Results of the MTS have demonstrated consistently that approximately one-third of doctors training in Australian settings report bullying, harassment, discrimination or racism, which in many cases affects the individual's ability to train [12]. This rises to about half of Indigenous doctors-in-training. It seems likely that such experiences contribute to a reduction in psychological safety and thus the ability to focus on the safety of patients. In addition, the MTS indicates that there is variability among trainees in their knowledge and confidence to report potential patient safety concerns. Clearly, there is still much work to be done to improve the culture within the medical profession, and also within healthcare teams more broadly. Such improvement would result in better safety for patients and enhanced wellbeing for healthcare workers and is therefore an important goal for everyone within the healthcare system.

23.2.3 Inequity issues in patient safety

There is a clear association between outcomes of health care and key social determinants of health—such as race, ethnicity, sex, gender identity and disability status—and improving patient safety requires that inequities are acknowledged and addressed [13]. In particular, incident event reporting processes are subject to biases and inequity, leading to under-reporting in some subsets of the patient population and lost opportunities to improve both equity and safety concurrently. Embedding an equity-based approach into safety activities would ensure that harm is reduced equitably for all patients [14]. See also Chapter 16, Achieving full health potential: health equity.

In Australia, the final report of the Royal Commission into Violence, Abuse, Neglect and Exploitation of People with Disability [15] identified that many people with disability are denied access to health care on an equal basis to people without disability. They have worse health outcomes and lower life expectancy than people without disability, and a significant number of deaths each year in people with disability are avoidable [15]. The Royal Commission made several recommendations to improve the training of healthcare workers in providing better health care for people with disability and to embed the right to equitable access to health services in key policy instruments. If enacted, these will help to improve patient safety for this group.

23.3 Improving patient safety by reducing harm during health care

Several key organisations and sectors have been involved in working towards improving patient safety during health care in Australia.

23.3.1 Australian Commission on Safety and Quality in Health Care

In Australia, the publication of the QAHCS was followed by the establishment in 2006 of the Australian Commission on Safety and Quality in Health Care (ACSQHC), which continues its work in the 2020s. The ACSQHC defines patient safety as 'the prevention of error and adverse effects associated with health care' and quality as 'the degree to which health services for individuals and populations increase the likelihood of desired health outcomes and are consistent with current professional knowledge' [16]. The ACSQHC publishes clinical care standards on a wide variety of topics to improve the implementation of evidence-based health care and coordinates work in specific areas to improve outcomes for patients. Further information is available on its website (https://www.safetyandquality.gov.au).

From its early days, the ACSQHC recognised that adverse events are more often the result of system failure rather than the responsibility of an individual healthcare provider, and promoted the idea that healthcare staff should report adverse events and near misses while avoiding the allocation of individual blame wherever possible. Healthcare organisations in Australia have developed best-practice guidelines for patient safety, and national laws supporting patient safety have been enacted. All doctors working in Australia should be aware of the importance of abiding by these laws and guidelines to improve the outcomes for the patients in their care.

23.3.2 World Health Organization

WHO has recognised patient safety as a global health priority, and has taken a global, systems-based approach to improving patient safety. The *Global patient safety action plan 2021–2030* [17] includes an explanation of the contemporary approach to thinking about patient safety and provides some key guiding principles for improving patient safety and reducing avoidable harm in health care.

These are, in summary:

- engage patients and families as partners in safe care
- achieve results through collaborative working
- analyse and share data to generate learning
- translate evidence into actionable and measurable improvement
- base policies and action on the nature of the care setting
- use both scientific expertise and patient experience to improve safety
- instil a safety culture in the design and delivery of health care.

The plan also includes a framework for action, with several strategic objectives to contribute to improving patient safety by eliminating avoidable harm in health care [17].

23.3.3 Medical education and training sector

Safety and quality have also been incorporated into medical education and training. In its standards for the accreditation of medical schools, the Australian Medical Council includes the need for medical students to be taught about systems approaches to healthcare safety and the need to practise health care in a way that maximises patient safety [7]. Similarly, the standards for later phases of education and training also require that the curriculum prepares trainees 'to contribute to the effectiveness and efficiency of the health care system, through knowledge and understanding of the issues associated with the delivery of safe, high-quality and cost-effective health care across a range of health settings within the Australian and/or New Zealand health systems' [18].

The standards also include a requirement that education providers have procedures to inform employers and, where appropriate, regulators where patient safety concerns arise in assessment of trainees. For example, the prevocational framework includes the following: 'providers ... must have clear procedures to immediately address any concerns about patient safety arising from a prevocational doctor's performance' [19]. This demonstrates greater recognition of the importance of the topic and the need for education providers to take action when patient safety is challenged.

23.3.4 Patients and their families

A further development in the person-centred care movement contributing to patient safety is the concept of engaging with the people who receive care, so that responsibility for health and healthcare provision is shared [20]. This has led to the concept of co-production, in which people receiving care are involved in the co-design of systems to promote safety. A systematic overview of 52 reviews of evidence-based strategies to support patient and family engagement in promoting safe care in clinical settings found improved outcomes in a range of safety topics including anticoagulation management, quality of diabetic management, medication safety (adherence to treatment, identification of adverse events and reduced administration errors) and improved compliance with hand hygiene practices by healthcare providers [21].

23.3.5 Individual healthcare workers

Unfortunately, the practical application of evidence-based measures to improve patient safety remains difficult, predominantly because some healthcare workers do not comply with recommendations. For example, hand hygiene has long been recognised as the single most effective way to prevent the spread of healthcare-associated infections [22] but multiple studies have shown that adherence to hand hygiene guidelines is low, particularly among doctors [23].

Doctors have been found to have lower rates of high-level patient safety behavioural intent than other healthcare worker groups, with junior doctors in particular demonstrating a sixfold lower reported intention to engage in safety behaviours compared with senior nurses [24]. Different health professional groups are influenced by different behavioural factors when determining whether to engage in patient safety behaviours, with doctors being most influenced by their colleagues' behaviours. This particularly applies to junior clinicians, who are strongly influenced by the observed behaviour of their seniors [24].

An Australian study of doctors' and medical students' opinions about patient safety behaviours compared doctors, medical students and members of the general public. It found that the three groups had significantly different opinions about the acceptability of potentially unsafe behaviours, such as attendance at a clinic while unwell or failing to report a drug error [25]. The public had a lower tolerance for unsafe behaviours than doctors, while students' opinions varied depending on their stage in the course, as the formation of professional identity during training leads to acceptance of the behavioural norms of their senior colleagues [25].

Awareness of these influences may assist individuals to contribute to patient safety through their own behaviour, which in turn will influence their peers to prioritise patient safety behaviours, such as compliance with guidelines on infection prevention [26]. Behaviours such as reporting adverse events or 'near misses' can contribute significantly to identifying threats to patient safety; all doctors should be aware of the incident reporting system within their workplace and use it when a concern is identified.

23.3.6 Technology

There is great potential in the burgeoning area of digital health and artificial intelligence for improving patient safety, but the challenge lies in how that potential is realised. New technologies can be used to reduce the likelihood of human error, but algorithm-based care can bring with it its own potential for error. The use of technology (such as smartphones) by people receiving care can improve their ability to understand and manage their own care and, if carefully implemented, could contribute significantly to partnerships between providers and receivers of care, and co-production of safety solutions [27]. See also Chapter 29, Professional practice, digital technology and artificial intelligence.

23.3.7 Cultural safety

The Australian Institute of Health and Welfare has developed a monitoring framework that gathers available data to assess progress in achieving cultural safety in the health system for Aboriginal and/or Torres Strait Islander peoples [28]. It demonstrates that, while there have been improvements over the past 20 years, much more action is required. Cultural safety training is becoming more widely available and all doctors would benefit from improving their knowledge and practice, thus contributing to improved health outcomes for Aboriginal and/or Torres Strait Islander people. See also Chapter 17, Culturally safe health care for Aboriginal and/or Torres Strait Islander peoples.

Summary

Many interacting factors contribute to the safety of members of the public when accessing health care, and there has been significant progress in understanding how to reduce preventable harm. However, the rates of avoidable physical harm during health care remain high, partly because of organisational factors, including culture, and partly because of a reluctance of individual healthcare practitioners to embrace evidence-based strategies to reduce harm. Recent attention to human factors within healthcare teams may assist in improving outcomes. Attention to cultural safety, particularly for Aboriginal and/or Torres Strait Islander peoples, is a vital element in improving access to and outcomes of health care in this potentially vulnerable group. It is also becoming apparent that involvement of the people receiving care in co-designing safety strategies can improve outcomes. Such involvement may occur via the use of artificial technology and other digital approaches. The single greatest improvement in patient safety may be derived from better knowledge and attitudes of individual healthcare providers, and a willingness to implement simple strategies, such as for hand hygiene and incident reporting, that are already well known to improve safety.

References

1. *Health Practitioner Regulation National Law (ACT) Act 2010* (ACT), s 3A.
2. Dhingra-Kumar N, Brusaferro S, Arnoldo L. Patient safety in the world. In: Donaldson L, Ricciardi W, Sheridan S, Tartaglia R, editors. Textbook of patient safety and clinical risk management. Springer Cham, 2020. https://doi.org/10.1007/978-3-030-59403-9 (accessed Aug 2025).
3. World Health Organization. Patient safety. Geneva: WHO, 2023. https://www.who.int/news-room/fact-sheets/detail/patient-safety (accessed Aug 2025).
4. Wilson RM, Runciman WB, Gibberd RW, et al. The Quality in Australian Health Care Study. *Med J Aust* 1995; 163: 458–471.
5. Australian Institute of Health and Welfare. Health and wellbeing of First Nations people. Canberra: AIHW, 2024. https://www.aihw.gov.au/reports/australias-health/indigenous-health-and-wellbeing (accessed Aug 2025).
6. Gubhaju L, Williams R, Jones J, et al. 'Cultural security is an on-going journey...' Exploring views from staff members on the quality and cultural security of services for Aboriginal families in Western Australia. *Int J Environ Res Public Health* 2020; 17: 8480.
7. Australian Medical Council. Standards for assessment and accreditation of primary medical programs. Canberra: AMC, 2023. https://www.amc.org.au/wp-content/uploads/2023/08/AMC-Medical_School_Standards-FINAL.pdf (accessed May 2025).
8. Braithwaite J, Herkes J, Ludlow K, et al. Association between organisational and workplace cultures, and patient outcomes: systematic review. *BMJ Open* 2017; 7: e017708.
9. Clay-Williams R, Taylor N, Ting HP, et al. The relationships between quality management systems, safety culture and leadership and patient outcomes in Australian Emergency Departments. *Int J Qual Health Care* 2020; 32(S1): 43–51.
10. Zajac SA, Williams KN, Patel SM, et al. Understanding psychological safety in health care: a qualitative investigation and practical guidance. *Jt Comm J Qual Patient Saf* 2025; Jun 11: S1553-7250(25)00140-0.
11. O'Donovan R, McAuliffe E. A systematic review of factors that enable psychological safety in healthcare teams. Int J Qual Health Care 2020; 32: 240–250.
12. Medical Board of Australia; Australian Health Practitioner Regulation Agency. Medical Training Survey results 2019–2024. https://medicaltrainingsurvey.gov.au/Results/Reports-and-results (accessed Aug 2025).
13. Sivashanker K, Gandhi TK. Advancing safety and equity together. *N Engl J Med* 2020; 382: 301–303.
14. Gandhi TK, Schulson LB, Thomas AD. Bringing the equity lens to patient safety event reporting. *Jt Comm J Qual Patient Saf* 2024; 50: 87–89.
15. Royal Commission into Violence, Abuse, Neglect and Exploitation of People with Disability. Executive Summary, Our vision for an inclusive Australia and recommendations. Commonwealth of Australia, 2023. https://disability.royalcommission.gov.au/publications/final-report (accessed Aug 2025).
16. Australian Commission on Safety and Quality in Health Care. About us – what is safety and quality? https://www.safetyandquality.gov.au/about-us (accessed Aug 2025).
17. World Health Organization. Global patient safety action plan 2021-2030: towards eliminating avoidable harm in health care. Geneva: WHO, 2021. https://www.who.int/teams/integrated-health-services/patient-safety/policy/global-patient-safety-action-plan (accessed Aug 2025).

18. Australian Medical Council. Standards for assessment and accreditation of specialist medical programs by the Australian Medical Council 2023. Canberra: AMC, 2023. https://www.amc.org.au/wp-content/uploads/2023/08/Standards-for-Assessment-and-Accreditation-of-Specialist-Medical-Programs-by-the-Australian-Medical-Council-2023-secured.pdf (accessed Aug 2025).
19. Australian Medical Council. National framework for prevocational (PGY1 And PGY2) medical training. Canberra: AMC, 2024. https://www.amc.org.au/accredited-organisations/prevocational-training/new-national-framework-for-prevocational-pgy1-and-pgy2-medical-training-2024/ (accessed Aug 2025).
20. Sheridan S, Sherman H, Kooijman A, et al. Patients for patient safety. In: Donaldson L, Ricciardi W, Sheridan S, Tartaglia R, editors. Textbook of patient safety and clinical risk management. Springer Cham, 2020. https://doi.org/10.1007/978-3-030-59403-9 (accessed Aug 2025).
21. Sharma AE, Rivadeneira NA, Barr-Walker J, et al. Patient engagement in health care safety: an overview of mixed-quality evidence. *Health Aff (Millwood)* 2018; 37: 1813–1820.
22. World Health Organization. Guidelines on core components of infection prevention and control programmes at the national and acute health care facility level. Geneva: WHO, 2016. https://www.who.int/publications/i/item/9789241549929 (accessed Aug 2025).
23. Costa AL, Privitera GP, Tulli G, Toccafondi G. Infection prevention and control. In: Donaldson L, Ricciardi W, Sheridan S, Tartaglia R, editors. Textbook of patient safety and clinical risk management. Springer Cham, 2020. https://doi.org/10.1007/978-3-030-59403-9 (accessed Aug 2025).
24. Wakefield JG, McLaws M-L, Whitby M, Patton L. Patient safety culture: factors that influence clinician involvement in patient safety behaviours. *Qual Saf Health Care* 2010; 19: 585–591.
25. McGurgan PM, Calvert KL, Nathan EA, et al. Why is patient safety a challenge? Insights from the professionalism opinions of medical students' research. *J Patient Saf* 2022; 18: e1124–e1134.
26. National Health and Medical Research Council; Australian Commission on Safety and Quality in Health Care. Australian guidelines for the prevention and control of infection in healthcare. 2019. https://www.safetyandquality.gov.au/publications-and-resources/resource-library/australian-guidelines-prevention-and-control-infection-healthcare (accessed Aug 2025).
27. Lachman P. Looking to the future. In: Donaldson L, Ricciardi W, Sheridan S, Tartaglia R, editors. Textbook of patient safety and clinical risk management. Springer Cham, 2020. https://doi.org/10.1007/978-3-030-59403-9 (accessed Aug 2025).
28. Australian Institute of Health and Welfare. Cultural safety in health care for Indigenous Australians: monitoring framework. Canberra: AIHW, 2023. https://www.aihw.gov.au/reports/indigenous-australians/cultural-safety-health-care-framework/contents/background-material (accessed Aug 2025).

Further reading

Donaldson L, Ricciardi W, Sheridan S, Tartaglia R, editors. Textbook of patient safety and clinical risk management. Springer Cham, 2020. https://doi.org/10.1007/978-3-030-59403-9

Taylor K, Thompson Guerin P. Health care and Indigenous Australians: Cultural safety in practice (3rd edition). Bloomsbury, 2019.

World Health Organization. Global patient safety action plan 2021-2030: towards eliminating avoidable harm in health care. Geneva: WHO, 2021. https://www.who.int/teams/integrated-health-services/patient-safety/policy/global-patient-safety-action-plan

24 Resource allocation and rationing in health care

Bernadette Tobin AO

Introduction

This chapter canvasses some of the key ethical issues in resource allocation in health care, in particular (a) the responsibility of doctors to steward resources, (b) rival conceptions of justice in allocation, (c) other ethical aspects of resource allocation, (d) ethical issues in evidence-based medicine, (e) levels of decision making in resource allocation, (f) approaches taken overseas and in Australia to the allocation of resources, (g) rationing in a pandemic, and (h) the law and resource allocation.

The success of modern medicine has brought many resourcing challenges. The cost of health care as a proportion of gross domestic product (GDP) in developed countries continues to rise, a development which is exacerbated by ageing populations [1]. In the United States, it is now 17.6% of GDP [2]. In Australia, the rise as a proportion of GDP has been more restrained—from 8.4% in the 2001–02 financial year to 10% in 2022–23 [3]. However, the resources available for the health care of a country's population, even in wealthy countries, are finite and some forms of rationing are inevitable [4,5]. Even affluent countries are not able to provide all the health care that individuals need, let alone want.

Prior to recognition of the need to address the growth in public (tax-funded) expenditure on health care, and in adhering to the ethical precept of putting the interests of their patients as their first concern, doctors were seldom constrained by resource considerations. Indeed, the notion that a decision to treat one patient might limit the treatment available to another patient was rarely foremost in a doctor's mind.

This is changing, and the change is reflected in the relevant sections of the Medical Board of Australia's *Good medical practice: a code of conduct for doctors in Australia* [6]. It confirms that good medical practice involves 'giving priority to investigating and treating patients on the basis of clinical need and the effectiveness of the proposed investigations or treatment' (section 3.4.4), 'supporting the transparent and equitable allocation of healthcare resources' (section 7.2.3), and 'understanding that your use of resources can affect the access other patients have to healthcare resources' (section 7.2.4) [6].

The change is also reflected in the current version (2017) of the Australian Medical Association's *Code of ethics*, which states that while doctors have a primary duty to individual patients, they also have responsibilities to other patients and the wider community (section 1.6 [7]).

The recognition of both the doctor's primary duty to the individual patient and their simultaneous responsibilities to other patients captures perfectly one challenge for today's doctor. In this chapter, the central ethical issues raised by this challenge are explored. Responses designed to assist the community and the medical profession to respond to this age-old but newly appreciated reality are described. The focus is on the ethical principles involved so that practising doctors can be more engaged in debate and decision making, and can more fully understand how strong are the links between resources used in treating individual patients and the resources available to the entire community.

24.1 Ethical considerations

The ethical principle of justice, particularly 'distributive justice', is central to the allocation of healthcare resources at government, institutional or individual practitioner level. As early as 1990, in a discussion paper on ethics and resource allocation, the National Health and Medical Research Council made it clear that arbitrarily differential treatment of people with the same needs is not justifiable:

> In the allocation of any public resources our concern should be primarily with justice. This involves giving to each person his or her due. In allocating health care resources our concern is largely with distributive justice—to distribute amongst members of the community those benefits and burdens due to them. The basis of distributive justice is the notion of fairness. The most appropriate criterion for a fair distribution of resources would appear to be those of equity and need. More specifically, a just allocation should offer equal treatment for those whose needs are similar. In other words, each person is entitled to enjoy an appropriate share of the sum total of the resources available according to their need. However, the need which justifies one person's entitlement must be a need which can be fulfilled in a way compatible with fulfilling the similar needs of others [8].

24.1.1 Competing conceptions of justice in allocating healthcare resources

There are competing views as to how considerations of justice in the allocation of healthcare resources should be applied. Libertarians argue that an allocation of health care is just if it represents what individuals choose to spend their own resources on and what health professionals choose to devote their own resources to. Utilitarians argue that an allocation is just if it results in the greatest good for the greatest number. Egalitarians argue an allocation is just if it ensures that each person, irrespective of wealth or position, has equal access to an adequate level of health care which is—contingent on social resources—sufficient to ensure 'equality of opportunity'. Communitarians argue that an allocation is just if it is based on healthcare need, where the satisfaction of that need is compatible with the fulfilment of similar and equally important needs of others, in particular the needs of the poorest, most marginalised, most vulnerable members of the community [9].

Medical need is thus a common, though not universally accepted, basis for discussions of justice in the distribution of healthcare resources. This raises the question of how and by whom such need is identified and compared. Since bringing considerations of justice into practice is not easy, doctors are tempted to focus on meeting the immediate needs of individual patients in front of them. In so doing, they may be tacitly accepting broader allocation decisions taken by others and thus ignoring the emerging central problem of finite resources [10].

In addition, the ethical theories that address questions of justice in the distribution of healthcare resources are themselves controversial. For example, libertarian theory pays little regard to the provision of health care to the poor and otherwise disadvantaged. Utilitarian theory deprioritises basic care for terminally ill patients, elderly people and people with disabilities. Egalitarian theory deprioritises the autonomy of the healthcare provider, as arguably does strict communitarian theory. Not surprisingly, but at the cost of consistency, corrective considerations are often smuggled into the theories themselves.

Whatever theoretical framework is thought best to explain distributive justice in practice, some key considerations should be noted. First, on any plausible conception of justice in the allocation of healthcare resources, some categories of patients will be unwitting rivals with other categories of patients for scarce healthcare resources. Thus, a moral assessment of the priorities among competing claims to health care must be made by a rationally defensible process that recognises the reality of an individual's need, the finite nature of resources and the importance of excluding morally irrelevant factors such as chance, social worth or race [11]. Second, that assessment should be sensitive to the different criteria by which people can be said to 'need' health care; for instance, urgency, likelihood of greater or longer benefit, likelihood to suffer lesser burdens of treatment, likelihood to suffer greater harms without treatment, less at risk of ill effects of treatment, and likelihood to need treatment for a shorter time or less frequently [12]. Third, different people have different conceptions of the meaning of 'benefit', 'burden', 'harm', etc. Fourth, what constitutes a benefit for (or a burden on) one patient may not be a benefit for (or burden on) another.

24.1.2 Other ethical values in the allocation of healthcare resources

The determination of justice in the distribution of healthcare resources is complicated by the finite nature of the resources. Increasingly, implicit or explicit rationing of health care is necessary, bringing with it a need to identify values that can be used to show that rationing is just and fair. Weale has identified three such values:

- Effectiveness implies the use of health care means that are medically effective. This is unarguable in principle and its acceptance is supported by the widespread embrace of evidence-based medicine. The latter, in turn, raises ethical issues around the application of evidence to resource allocation.
- Efficiency requires the ideas of reducing inefficient management and clinical work practices and avoiding the use of therapeutically ineffective treatment of high expense and of little or no benefit.
- Democratic responsiveness refers to a process whereby society, via representative government, can express a collective opinion about the type of healthcare system the society agrees to support [13].

However, these values have generally not been applied systematically in the varying responses of nations as to how best to allocate healthcare resources. Critics have suggested that too often de facto rationing is hidden by implicit decisions [14]. The approaches taken appear to be influenced by the existing healthcare funding systems. In the United Kingdom, where health care is nationalised, governments have used a variety of instruments including a purchaser–provider split, general practitioner fund-holding and national expert committees to advise on clinical practice guidelines in trying to make health care more efficient [15]. In the US, where only elderly and indigent people are covered by a truly national and truly comprehensive healthcare funding framework, the government had, until 2010, mostly left 'rationing' to the marketplace: for-profit managed care was the dominant model for healthcare provision. There were exceptions to this model—including longstanding not-for-profit health maintenance organisations exemplified by Kaiser Permanente, and the Oregon Health Plan, which was designed to improve access to health care to low-income citizens while also containing costs [16,17]. That said, the passing of the *Patient Protection and Affordable Care Act* (US) in 2010 had by 2016 reduced the uninsured proportion of the population by 50% and had enacted a range of reforms designed to improve healthcare delivery and effectiveness while constraining costs [18].

In Australia, state public healthcare systems apply casemix funding tools to motivate doctors and hospitals to become more efficient, and they combine this with annual efficiency targets. Other 'rationing' tools in use in Australia include measures such as limiting which drugs are subsidised under the Pharmaceutical Benefits Scheme, limiting subsidies for a range of investigations and keeping patient reimbursements for doctors' fees below the annual rise in the consumer price index. Outside the public hospital system, Australian medicine is based predominantly on 'fee for service'. In the past, doctors were generally able to adapt to changes in reimbursements, and thus maintain income, by changing their practices rather than by reducing services. Now, however, the level of reimbursements can adversely affect those who cannot afford to pay an additional 'gap' fee. In the US, it has been observed that the fee-for-service model does not promote good management of resources, partly because the doctor being asked to restrict the use of marginally effective investigations or treatment has no assurance that any savings would go towards more effective health care [19].

24.1.3 Ethical issues in applying evidence to healthcare resource allocation

Though an independent movement, the rise of the evidence-based medicine (EBM) movement has influenced discussion within the profession about the rising cost of health care. Most doctors long believed that their practice was based on available evidence, but EBM formalised the effort to engage in 'best practice'. Now, however, health administrators have sought to bring EBM into their methods of allocating resources [20]. Such an approach brings its own set of ethical difficulties. Some critics argue that many important results of treatment cannot be measured, that EBM is unable to resolve competing claims of different interest groups, and that a crude application of the results of clinical trials may disadvantage some patients [21]. They criticise those charged with making these decisions (about resource allocation) for 'seeking simplistic solutions to inherently complex problems' [22]. Other critics have observed that EBM provides less than desirable guidance for general practice: the ambiguity of early presenting symptoms favours reliance on experience rather than on evidence, and there has been a paucity of research conducted on primary care practices. Similarly, in the management of chronic disease and multi-morbidity, critics note that a 'complex calculus' is needed to incorporate several factors not readily dealt with from the evidence base. They also point out that, in specialist practice, applying the evidence base requires first having made the correct diagnosis [20]. Additional concerns have arisen about the inflexible application of EBM and the management of an excessive volume of guidelines [22]. It is also argued that EBM insufficiently acknowledges the variables of patients' choices, the uncertainties regarding diagnosis, and the undervaluing of evidence for cultural reasons (together with the limited inclusion of some cultural groups in clinical trials).

24.2 Where resource allocation decisions are made

There are broadly three levels of decision making about the allocation of resources, namely the macro-, meso- and micro-levels.

24.2.1 Macro-level allocation

Macro-allocation of resources is outside the experience of most doctors. The Australian Government is first involved in deciding what proportion of the budget will be spent on health (rather than on, say, education, welfare or defence). After this allocation, health departments, federal and state/territory, receive their allocations. Government has traditionally directed how the health budget will be divided, for example, between hospital and community care or between treatment and prevention. More recently, some governments have tended to shift this decision making to regional authorities: they claim that the local community is better placed to identify its own healthcare needs (though some sceptics wonder if this trend is designed to protect governments from being directly associated with unpopular decisions).

24.2.2 Meso-level allocation

The allocation of medical resources at a regional, institutional or local level moves into the intermediate level of decision making, or meso-allocation. At this level, decisions may be influenced by politicians, administrators, boards and committees interacting with institutions and hospitals. Meso-level allocation also includes the role of hospital managers, who are responsible for allocating resources to competing services and specialties [23].

24.2.3 Micro-level allocation

Doctors in their daily clinical work participate in the micro-level allocation of resources when, for example, they allocate the use of their own time and of other resources to patients via the use of appointments, waiting lists, triage, and their decisions about diagnosis, treatment and referral to other health professionals. The impact that such micro-allocation decisions have cumulatively on expenditure on health care is now widely recognised and, together with cost pressures, is a key factor behind such innovations as the introduction of clinician managers, clinical practice guidelines and managed care.

24.3 The doctor and resource allocation

Doctors have traditionally seen themselves as helping individual patients access appropriate health care. This view was understandable in an earlier era when the major resources to be allocated were the doctor's time and expertise. Any persistence of this view may reflect denial of the difficult issues involved in making priority judgements between treatment of patients with similar needs if resources are limited. Even so, the traditional medical principle of 'first (or above all) do no harm' has inherent resource implications: excessive time with, or attention to, one patient has an effect on time with, or attention to, other patients. A more defensible view—that doctors have responsibilities to patients in the wider community as well as to their individual patients—is now found in the Australian Medical Association's *Code of ethics* (as has already been noted). However, this is still not adequately recognised in the latest version of the World Medical Association Declaration of Geneva [24].

In a publicly funded, fee-for-service healthcare system as represented by Medicare Australia, resources are wasted by doctors who provide unnecessary services to patients. Attention to such overservicing should focus not only on the pecuniary motives (and thus the character) of the doctor but also on the harm done to the community by poor use of resources. Doctors can also waste resources when they fail to use their professional knowledge to evaluate claims about new treatments, when they allow themselves to be swayed by marketing [25], or when they (wittingly or unwittingly) participate in disease mongering [26]. In public hospitals, resources can also be wasted by doctors in numerous ways, including: ordering unnecessary tests (or, indeed, ordering any tests before an initial—even if tentative—diagnosis has been made); delaying or cancelling procedures through lack of punctuality; failing to notify planned leave; failing to arrange pre-admission assessment; and failing to communicate previous investigative results. The source of such inefficiencies can now be measured and their impact costed; this allows for the creation of an effective motivational tool when used appropriately. Hospital managers, in response to three decades of budget restriction, recognise that it is desirable to include those responsible for clinical decisions in the meso-allocation of resources in the hospital; hence, the advent of clinician managers [27]. This involvement in the meso-allocation of resources may, however, produce conflict with doctor colleagues, as the clinician manager strives to meet the hospital's financial targets and still provide sufficient resources for fellow clinicians to meet their patient's needs.

Some have argued that it is nearly impossible for the individual doctor to be both champion for the individual patient and keeper of the community healthcare budget because of the conflict of the two roles [28]. Others have excused the doctor from the latter responsibility on the basis that, in a fee-for-service model of health funding, doctors cannot influence where savings will be directed. This lack of influence is likely to be more marked in a for-profit managed care system, where doctors might imagine savings going to corporate profit and not to other needy patients [19].

Doctors in European countries with universal healthcare coverage appear to be more ready to accept the need for cost containment and already participate in bedside rationing, despite the difficult moral dilemmas so posed [29]. In Australia, doctors are increasingly required to consider carefully whether a treatment offered to a patient is likely to be therapeutically effective. As already noted, the introduction in 2010 of a single national Medical Board of Australia brought with it a national code of conduct called *Good medical practice*, which specifically addresses the issue of resource allocation [6].

Decisions about the use of resources will at times produce ethical concern for doctors, and at times family and patient dissatisfaction, especially when the doctor is basing a decision on an assessment of patient need (or the lack of genuine need) for a treatment to which the patient feels they have an entitlement. Jennett has suggested the following criteria for deeming a specific treatment to be inappropriate:

- unnecessary—because the patient is not seriously enough affected to need it or the desired objective can be achieved by simpler means
- unsuccessful—because the patient has a condition too advanced to respond to or benefit from treatment
- unsafe—because the risks outweigh the probable benefits
- unkind—because the 'quality of life' following the treatment is not likely to be good enough or long enough to justify such treatment
- unwise—because it diverts resources from activities which would benefit others to a greater extent [30].

To these criteria may be added terms such as 'not clinically indicated' and 'therapeutically ineffective' or 'futile'. Doctors who advise against treatment, particularly in elderly people, on the grounds that treatment is not clinically indicated may be confusing two ethical questions, namely (1) whether the treatment will be of sufficient therapeutic benefit to the patient and (2) whether resources should be allocated to this patient ahead of others [31]. A treatment can be reasonably judged to be 'futile' if, relative to some agreed goal such as improvement in the patient's prognosis, comfort, wellbeing or general state of health, it is unlikely to work. That said, when speaking to patients and family, doctors need to ensure that their assessment of futility ('therapeutic ineffectiveness') pertains to a specific treatment's likelihood of realising a therapeutic goal and not to a patient's life. Indeed, decisions by doctors that treatments would be ineffective ('futile') are open to misunderstanding without adequate and sensitive explanation to the patient and family.

Hurst and Danis have proposed six minimal requisites for rationing by clinical judgement: a closed system that offers reciprocity; attention to general concerns of justice; respect for individual variations; application of a consistent process; explicitness; and review of decisions [32].

24.4 Approaches taken to resource allocation and rationing

Nearly all of the changes taking place in the organisation and delivery of health care in the developed world involve issues of resource allocation.

At the level of macro-allocation of resources, the most striking innovation has been the development of the Oregon Health Plan in the US. Oregon, like all other US states, provides medical care to the uninsured population with funds derived predominantly from the US Government Medicaid program and, to a lesser extent, from the state itself. The Oregon legislature consulted the entire community (both insured and uninsured) about what medical interventions should be prioritised and, if funds were available, funded. Initially, some 709 medical interventions were ranked according to 'social values' and costed: it was said that only the first 587 services could be afforded. Initially, interventions excluded from funding were: cancer where treatment would not provide a 10% 5-year survival, the stripping of varicose veins, liver transplantation for alcoholic liver disease and ventilatory support for extremely low birthweight babies. However, the latter two were restored when it emerged that their exclusion would breach federal laws, and a revised ranking system of 696 items was produced, of which the first 565 were to be funded. This revised plan commenced operation in 1994. While its development and progress is of interest, the importance and ethical defensibility of the Oregon Health Plan can be overstated. For one thing, the plan related to rationing of treatment only to the uninsured and thus did not limit the health care available to insured citizens. For another, since the passage of the *Patient Protection and Affordable Care Act* (US) in 2010, the proportion of the population in Oregon lacking healthcare insurance decreased from 14.7% in 2013 to 6.2% in 2016 [33].

Other changes in healthcare delivery driven primarily by issues of resource allocation include:

- the development of clinical practice guidelines, at a local or national level, by groups of doctors and others who attempt to combine objective evidence about effectiveness of treatment with the most efficient use of available resources
- the development, usually within hospitals, of care paths or care maps, to guide multidisciplinary patient care teams in the most effective and efficient use of resources to achieve desired patient outcomes
- in the US, the introduction of managed care where the healthcare budget holder (the insurer) determines, to a preset formula, what resources will be made available to the doctor for the treatment of a particular medical condition.

24.4.1 Rationing of health care

Discussion of the 'rationing' of health care has often been inhibited by the connotations of the word itself. This is particularly so in the US, despite the long acceptance of a form of rationing in deciding priorities for recipients of renal transplantation. These connotations are apparent even in the explanations given for the word 'rationing': it has been defined as 'explicit or implicit withholding and allocation of beneficial resources from some patients for the sake of others' [34] and as having the 'central idea [of] denying a potentially beneficial treatment to a patient on the grounds of scarcity' [4]. Resource allocation, effectively a synonym for rationing, seems to have less emotional baggage.

To delay the inevitability of rationing in the US, the medical profession developed an enthusiasm for identifying and ridding the healthcare system of wasteful interventions that do not benefit patients. Some authorities claim that 30% of the healthcare budget could be saved by this means [34,35]. Some doctors are inclined to expect other providers of health care to contribute to costs savings, while being reluctant to commit themselves to a similar approach. This is despite indications that 60% of costs are controlled or influenced by doctors [1].

Rationing has been described as 'necessary, unavoidable and ethically complex' [4]. It is easier to undertake rationing in healthcare systems with a central funding body (e.g. the UK National Health Service [NHS]), as any savings are returned to the system. In a market-dominated system, savings are often seen as being returned to shareholders. For explicit rationing to be fair, seen to be fair, and accepted by all stakeholders, it should be overseen by a legitimate committee or agency. Whatever the mechanism, it should use transparent decision-making processes; offer rational justification based on ethical principle and accurate, comprehensive information; and have an appeals mechanism [16,36]. The membership of the committee or agency also needs careful consideration as to balance and fairness [37]. Even the best rationing systems can be undermined by illegitimate uses of the legitimate 'principle of rescue' in which, for example, public emotions and political response lead to the overruling of legitimate rationing decisions [4].

24.4.2 Rationing of health care in a pandemic

In everyday circumstances as well as in pandemic circumstances, the fundamental principle of medical ethics—that is, respect for the equal worth of every human being—is consistent with the recognition that there may be good reasons to withhold or withdraw medical treatment, either because the treatment does not serve its purpose (is 'futile') or because the treatment is excessively burdensome (that is, it promises too little benefit relative to the burdens it will likely impose). Benefits and burdens are relative to the individual's particular circumstances. Benefits may include the preservation of life, the maintenance or improvement of health, or the relief of discomfort. Burdens may include pain, discomfort, loss of lucidity, breathlessness, agitation, or cost to the patient or to others.

In circumstances of a pandemic, however, it may not be possible to provide a treatment to everyone who could benefit from that treatment. That is, in order to avoid the injustice of treatment being provided unfairly to people because they are wealthy or powerful, treatment may have to be rationed. As already noted, fairness requires the distribution of healthcare resources on the basis of healthcare need (see, for example, *An ethics framework for making resource allocation decisions within clinical care: responding to Covid-19* by Sydney Health Ethics [38]).

Prior to assessing the relative needs of individuals, doctors are required do two things. First, they should ask patients (or their substitute decision makers) about their preferences with regard to specific medical treatments such as intensive care, CPR and intubation; informed refusals of these interventions should be respected (consistent with relevant law in a jurisdiction). Second, before rationing of resources is contemplated, doctors should pursue all reasonable alternatives, which may include therapies that are equivalent or nearly equivalent, the sharing of equipment, transfer to another facility, or (with consent) therapeutic innovation with a reasonable prospect of success.

Over recent years, and in particular during COVID-19, an enormous literature has blossomed on the topic of fairness in allocating finite healthcare resources. This literature is marked by large areas of agreement about what would constitute fairness—as well as unfairness—in allocation. There is widespread agreement that, in a pandemic, decisions should be based on urgency, prognosis and the prospect of success for therapy, and that such decisions should be made on objective clinical criteria (such as the patient's premorbid condition and their pandemic-specific health status) [23]. There is also widespread agreement that, in a pandemic, unjust discrimination—on the basis of age, ethnicity, disability, religion, sexual orientation, gender identity, criminal history, social standing, etc.—should be avoided. That said, it is also recognised that age or disabling premorbid conditions might count among a number of factors in the assessment of prognosis or prospects of therapy. In addition, there is also widespread agreement on the following:

- Allocation decisions should be made by a small triage team with both clinical and ethical expertise, the members of which should be independent of the patient's prior caregivers.
- Life-sustaining treatments should be withdrawn only in accordance with good medical practice; that is, either (a) based on medical judgement that (to a reasonable degree of certainty) the patient will not survive to hospital discharge even if life-sustaining treatment is continued, or (b) after a discussion and agreement with the patient or substitute decision maker that the burdens of treatment outweigh the benefits.
- Patients who are not expected to survive should continue to receive appropriate care relevant to their condition.

In all these matters, doctors should pay due regard to guidelines issued by their professional body, the institution in which they work, and by their local health department.

That said, there are areas of disagreement in the literature. There is disagreement about the legitimacy of implementing arrangements according to the principle of maximising total life-years or maximising total quality-adjusted life-years. It is argued that the former unfairly disadvantages the older patient and the latter unfairly disadvantages the person with a disability [39–41].

24.5 The law and resource allocation

It is theoretically possible for patients to sue hospitals and doctors for not providing treatment to which they believe they are entitled, or to seek a court order that a treatment be provided. Precedents exist in other countries [42]. Courts faced with such claims are likely to conclude that there is an issue they can resolve (a 'justiciable' issue) only where the allegation is that an established policy has been wrongly administered. Where the allegation is that the policy itself is unsound, courts have traditionally kept out of what are essentially political issues [43].

Since the primary responsibility for the administration of hospital services in Australia lies with the states and territories, it is reasonable to expect that their health authorities would have publicly available triage policies. Yet only one state, New South Wales, has publicly available documentation that mentions the need for triage policies [44]. There seems to be a reluctance, politically understandable but ethically regrettable, on the part of health authorities to develop, or at least to issue, triage policies.

Health departments have wide discretion in making resource allocation decisions, and these are generally accepted by the courts [44]. Nonetheless, the publication of both ethical guidelines and specific triage policies, which rely on appropriate evidence and comply with jurisdictional laws, would provide doctors with confidence in implementing their institution's protocols [45]. Such publications would not only promote quality and consistency in decision making, but they would also act as a reminder to the community that healthcare resources are finite, and that, in some circumstances, there will likely be constraints on what forms of health care even an affluent society can provide [46].

Summary

This chapter explored some of the key ethical aspects of issues in resource allocation in health care, in particular: (a) the responsibility of doctors to steward resources; (b) rival conceptions of justice in allocation; (c) other ethical aspects of resource allocation; (d) ethical issues in EBM; (e) levels of allocation decision making (and the role of the doctor at each level); (f) various approaches taken overseas and in Australia to the allocation of resources; (g) the challenge of rationing in a pandemic; and (h) the law and resource allocation.

References

1. Agrawal S, Taitsman J, Cassel C. Educating physicians about responsible management of finite resources. *JAMA* 2013; 309: 1115–1116.
2. Centers for Medicare and Medicaid Services. https://www.cms.gov/data-research/statistics-trends-and-reports/national-health-expenditure-data/historical (accessed Jul 2025).
3. Australian Institute of Health and Welfare. Health expenditure Australia. 2024 [latest update]. https://www.aihw.gov.au/reports/australias-health/health-expenditure (accessed Jul 2025).
4. Scheunemann LP, White DP. The ethics and reality of rationing in medicine. *Chest* 2011; 140: 1625–1632.
5. Meulen R. Is rationing the inevitable consequence of medical advance? *Med Law* 2008; 27: 71–82.
6. Medical Board of Australia. Good medical practice: a code of conduct for doctors in Australia. 2020. https://www.medicalboard.gov.au/codes-guidelines-policies/code-of-conduct.aspx (accessed Jun 2023).
7. Australian Medical Association. Code of ethics 2004. Editorially revised 2006. Revised 2016. Canberra (ACT): AMA Ltd, 2017. https://www.ama.com.au/articles/code-ethics-2004-editorially-revised-2006-revised-2016 (accessed Mar 2022).
8. National Health and Medical Research Council. Discussion paper on ethics and resource allocation in health care. Canberra: AGPS, 1990.
9. Tobin B. The principle of justice: a bioethical perspective. *Bioethics Outlook* 2001; 12.
10. Gillon R. Philosophical medical ethics. Chichester: Wiley, 1986.
11. Lowe M, Kerridge IH, Mitchell KR. 'These sorts of people don't do very well': race and allocation of health care resources. *J Med Ethics* 1995; 21: 356–360.
12. Fisher A, Gormally L. Healthcare allocation: an ethical framework for public policy. London: Linacre Centre, 2001.
13. Weale A. The ethics of rationing. *Br Med Bull* 1995; 51: 831–841.
14. Lauridson SM, Norup MS, Rossel PJ. The secret art of managing healthcare expenses: investigating implicit rationing and autonomy in public healthcare systems. *J Med Ethics* 2007; 33: 704–707.
15. Bryan S, Williams I, McIver S. Seeing the NICE side of cost-effectiveness analysis: a qualitative investigation of the use of CEA in NICE technology appraisals. *Health Econ* 2007; 6: 179–193.
16. Daniels N. Is the Oregon rationing plan fair? JAMA 1991; 265: 2232–2235.
17. Dixon J, Welch HG. Priority setting: lessons from Oregon. *Lancet* 1991; 337: 891–894.
18. Levine DM, Chalasani R, Linder JA, Landon BE. Association of the Patient Protection and Affordable Care Act with ambulatory quality, patient experience, utilization, and cost, 2014–2016. *JAMA Netw Open* 2022; 5: e2218167.
19. Cassel CK, Brennan TE. Managing medical resources: return to the commons? *JAMA* 2007; 297: 2518–2521.
20. Culpepper L, Gilbert TT. Evidence and ethics. Lancet 1999; 353: 829–831.
21. Kerridge I, Lowe M, Henry D. Ethics and evidence based medicine. *BMJ* 1998; 316: 1151–1153.
22. Greenhalgh T, Howick J, Maskrey N; Evidence Based Medicine Renaissance Group. Evidence based medicine: a movement in crisis? *BMJ* 2014; 348: g3725.
23. Pellegrino Center for Clinical Bioethics. Ethical principles for resource allocation in the event of an overwhelming surge of COVID-19 patients. Washington, DC: Georgetown University, 2020. https://repository.digital.georgetown.edu/handle/10822/1059549 (accessed May 2025).
24. World Medical Association. Declaration of Geneva. Revised 2017. https://www.wma.net/policies-post/wma-declaration-of-geneva/ (accessed Mar 2022).
25. Breen KJ. The medical profession and the pharmaceutical industry: when will we open our eyes? *Med J Aust* 2004; 180: 409–410.
26. Heath I. Combating disease mongering: daunting but nonetheless essential. *PLoS Med* 2006; 3: e146.
27. Chantler C. Be a manager. BMJ 1989; 278: 1505–1508.
28. Hiatt HH. Protecting the medical commons: who is responsible? *N Engl J Med* 1975; 293: 235–241.
29. Hurst SA, Slowther AM, Forde R, et al. Prevalence and determinants of physician bedside rationing: data from Europe. *J Gen Intern Med* 2006; 21: 1138–1143.
30. Jennett B. High technology medicine: benefits and burdens. Oxford: Oxford University Press, 1986.

31. Hope T, Sprigings S, Crisp R. 'Not clinically indicated': patients' interests or resource allocation? *BMJ* 1993; 306: 379–387.
32. Hurst SA, Danis M. A framework for rationing by clinical judgment. *Kennedy Inst Ethics J* 2007; 17: 247–266.
33. Ballotpedia. Effect of the Affordable Care Act in Oregon (2009-2017). 2017. https://ballotpedia.org/Effect_of_the_Affordable_Care_Act_in_Oregon_(2009-2017) (accessed Aug 2025).
34. Tilburt JC, Cassel CK. Why the ethics of parsimonious medicine is not the ethics of rationing. *JAMA* 2013; 309: 773–774.
35. Brody H. From an ethics of rationing to an ethics of waste avoidance. *N Engl J Med* 2012, 366: 1949–1951.
36. O'Donnell JL, Smyth D, Frampton C. Prioritizing health-care funding. *Intern Med J* 2005; 35: 409–412.
37. Singer PA, Martin DK, Giacomini M, Purdy L. Priority setting for new technologies in medicine: qualitative case study. *BMJ* 2000; 321: 1316–1319.
38. Sydney Health Ethics. An ethics framework for making resource allocation decisions within clinical care: responding to Covid-19. Sydney (NSW): University of Sydney, 2020. https://www.sydney.edu.au/medicine-health/our-research/research-networks/sydney-health-ethics.html (accessed Apr 2022).
39. University of Pittsburgh, Department of Critical Care Medicine. Allocation of scarce critical care resources during a public health emergency. Pittsburgh, PA (US): University of Pittsburgh, 2021. https://www.ccm.pitt.edu/sites/default/files/2023-05/Allocation_of_Critical_Care_in_Public_Health_Emergency_June2021-FINAL.pdf (accessed Mar 2022).
40. Emanuel E, Persad G, Upshur R, et al. Fair allocation of scarce medical resources in the time of Covid-19. *N Engl J Med* 2020; 382: 2049–2055.
41. Haas LEM, de Lange DW, van Dijk D, van Delden JJM. Should we deny ICU admission to the elderly? Ethical considerations in times of COVID-19. *Crit Care* 2020; 24: 321.
42. Brahams D. Judicial review of refusal to fund treatment. *Lancet* 1995; 345: 717.
43. *Shortland v Northland Health Ltd* (1998) 1 NZLR 433.
44. Close E, Willmott L, Cockburn T, et al. Transparent triage policies during the COVID-19 pandemic: a critical part of medico-legal risk management for clinicians. *Med J Aust* 2021; 215: 71–74.e1.
45. Liddell K, Skopek JM, Palmer S, et al. Who gets the ventilator? Important legal rights in a pandemic. *J Med Ethics* 2020; 46: 421–426.
46. Close E, Young S, Cockburn T, et al. Legal challenges to ICU triage decisions in the Covid-19 pandemic: how effectively does the law regulate bedside rationing decisions in Australia? *UNSW Law J* 2021; 44: 9–59.

Further reading

Beckstead N, Ord T. Bubbles under the wallpaper: healthcare rationing and discrimination. In Udo Schüklenk, Peter Singer, editors. Bioethics: an anthology, 4th edition. London: Wiley-Blackwell, 2021: 413–419.

Emanuel E, Steinmetz A, Schmidt H, editors. Rationing and resource allocation in healthcare: essential readings. New York: Oxford University Press, 2018.

Harris J. The value of life. In Udo Schüklenk, Peter Singer, editors. Bioethics: an anthology, 4th edition. London: Wiley-Blackwell, 2021: 403–412.

Kilner JF. Who lives? Who dies? Ethical criteria in patient selection. New Haven, CT: Yale University Press, 1990.

Leget C, Hoedemakers R. Teaching medical students about fair distribution of healthcare resources. *J Med Ethics* 2007; 33: 737–741.

Little JM. Ethics of resource allocation. In: Fearnside MR, Dooley BJ, Gorton MW, editors. Surgery, ethics and the law. Melbourne: Blackwell Science Asia, 2000.

Maxwell R, editor. Rationing health care. London: Churchill Livingstone, 1995.

Pellegrino ED. Rationing health care: the ethics of medical gatekeeping. *J Contemp Health Law Policy* 1986; 2: 23–45.

Smith GP. Distributive justice and the new medicine. Cheltenham, UK: Edward Elgar Publishing, 2008.

25 Medical negligence and professional liability

Roy Donnelly

Introduction

Being sued or subject to a medical negligence claim is commonly considered by doctors to be 'a moral blight or stigma' [1] upon their competence as a doctor. However, despite the notion of 'fault' or 'error' inherent in an allegation of negligence, the practical purpose of a claim is to seek a financial compensation for an injury resulting from a doctor's care and treatment. Compensation will be payable where that injury has been caused by a medical practitioner providing care below a standard that is considered by a court to be reasonable.

For care and treatment cases (as opposed to consent cases, discussed in section 25.4) the care must also be outside of competent medical practice as defined by peer professional opinion. In most cases, the court's decision about what is a 'reasonable standard' of care, or 'competent medical practice' will be decided by referring to the opinions of medical experts in the relevant specialty (discussed in section 25.6).

In the vast majority of cases, claims for medical negligence are resolved by settlement or discontinuation though mediation or other alternative dispute resolution procedures outside of a court hearing.

25.1 Actions for negligence against medical practitioners

As stated in the case of *Rogers v Whitaker*:

> The law imposes on a medical practitioner a duty to exercise reasonable care and skill in the provision of advice and treatment. That duty is a 'single comprehensive duty covering all the ways in which a doctor is called upon to exercise his [sic] skill and judgement'; it extends to the examination, diagnosis, and treatment of the patient and the provision of information in an appropriate case [2].

25.1.1 Elements of a medical negligence claim

In order to be successful in a claim for medical negligence, a patient (plaintiff or claimant) must prove *liability* of the doctor or health service (defendant), as well as prove the amount or *quantum* of damages to which they are entitled as a result of the defendant's negligence. The elements that need to be proved to find liability are:

1. duty of care—that the patient was owed a duty of care
2. breach—that the required standard of care was not provided
3. causation—the care provided, or not provided, caused the harm suffered by the patient.

In terms of quantum or amount of damages, the patient must also prove that they are entitled to compensation by payment of damages and the amount of those damages.

In medical negligence claims, arguments about quantum of damages and causation are often interlinked. Often the cause of injuries or complications can be multifactorial. In general, the patient must prove that the quantum claimed reflects the severity and impact of the injury as caused by the doctor's negligence, excluding other causes or factors that might have caused or worsened the injury.

25.1.2 Case law and civil liability legislation

In making decisions as to liability and quantum, courts have primarily relied upon the principles of case law—that is, the decisions of past courts as evolved since the decision of *Donoghue v Stevenson* (see section 25.2.1).

A major review of Australian negligence law, known as the Ipp Report, was published in 2002 [3]. The report was commissioned largely in response to a so-called medical indemnity crisis caused by escalating insurance premiums, and possible concerns about the financial viability of certain medical indemnity providers. In response to the Ipp Report, all states and territories across Australia implemented legislative changes that impacted upon certain aspects of medical negligence claims. These were mostly aimed at limiting claims and the potential damages payable, especially for small and medium claims.

The various state-based civil liability Acts are now the starting point used by the courts to assess a claim. This chapter will focus on the principles as defined by the relevant case law, with references to the civil liability legislative provisions where relevant.

25.1.3 Standard of proof

The elements of liability, and the quantum of damages, needs to be proved 'on the balance of probabilities'. This means that the court only needs to be persuaded by the evidence, including any medical expert evidence, that the probability of each element is more than 50%.

25.1.4 Statute of limitations

Statutes of limitations within each state or territory define the period within which a claim for negligence must be commenced before the patient loses their entitlement to bring proceedings. This part of the law is complex and varies between jurisdictions. In general, the period is three years in New South Wales, Victoria, Queensland, South Australia, Western Australia, Tasmania and the Northern Territory. However, there are varying rules and definitions between the jurisdictions as to when the three-year period commences, and how it may be extended in certain circumstances.

Legal advice should be sought relevant to each jurisdiction.

25.2 Duty of care

25.2.1 When does the duty arise?

The original description of the duty of care comes from the landmark English case of *Donoghue v Stevenson* [4] where Ms Donoghue discovered the remains of a dead snail within a bottle of ginger beer she was consuming. That case in 1932 established the modern law of negligence that persons could hold a duty of care to others (and therefore may be required to compensate them for injury).

In *Donoghue*, the duty of care required the person (in the case of Stevenson—a manufacturer of ginger beer) to 'take reasonable care to avoid acts or omissions which you can reasonably foresee would be likely to injure your neighbour' (being Ms Donoghue—the consumer of his ginger beer). The duty of care was owed to 'persons who are so closely and directly affected by my act that I ought reasonably to have them in contemplation ...' (Donoghue [4] at page 580).

The duty of care that exists between a doctor and patient is one of the most well recognised in negligence law. In the overwhelming number of cases, the fact that a duty of care exists for the relevant patient is not called into question. However, there are a few circumstances where the existence of a duty becomes an important question. These are described on the following pages.

25.2.2 Duty of care in an emergency/good Samaritan laws

Traditionally there has been no obligation to provide care to any person where an existing patient care relationship does not exist. However, professional obligations do require doctors to provide assistance in an emergency within the scope of their clinical skills, and some jurisdictions contain laws that require such assistance. All jurisdictions have laws that provide varying protections from a negligence claim in such circumstances—so-called good Samaritan protections.

In general, the case law has not imposed a duty to assist a person in peril, even where it is foreseeable that the consequence of a failure to assist will be the injury or death of the person imperilled. However, in the case of *Woods v Lowns* [5] the court found that a doctor did hold a duty of care to respond to requests for urgent medical assistance to a stranger.

Woods v Lowns involved a claim of negligence against a general practitioner who was allegedly asked to attend a child who was having a seizure about 300 metres away from his practice. On appeal in *Lowns & Anor v Woods & Ors* [6], the NSW Court of Appeal accepted there was no obligation to assist. Nevertheless, the court (agreeing with the decision at first instance) found the doctor negligent in the particular circumstances for failure to assist. The court relied upon the legal principle of 'proximity' and determined that the doctor held a duty of care for the child because he was physically close to the child, there was a direct request to the doctor for help, and there was nothing to prevent the doctor responding. Existing legislation on medical regulation also influenced the outcome of the case.

Outside of the risks of a claim in negligence, there is also an ethical responsibility to provide care in an emergency to the level to which one is trained and experienced. This is included in the Medical Board of Australia's code of conduct [7], which states at section 3.5:

> Treating patients in emergencies requires doctors to consider a range of issues, in addition to the patient's best care. Good medical practice involves offering assistance in an emergency that takes account of your own safety, your skills, the availability of other options and the impact on any other patients under your care; and continuing to provide that assistance until your services are no longer required.

Legislative provisions exist in some jurisdictions that provide an obligation to assist. For example, in NSW, section 139C of the *Health Practitioner Regulation National Law* (NSW) provides that failure to assist a person in urgent need of medical care (unless reasonable steps are taken to ensure another practitioner attends) is considered unsatisfactory professional conduct, stating that:

> [r]efusing or failing, without reasonable cause, to attend (within a reasonable time after being requested to do so) on a person for the purpose of rendering professional services in the capacity of a medical practitioner if the practitioner has reasonable cause to believe the person is in need of urgent attention by a medical practitioner, unless the practitioner has

> taken all reasonable steps to ensure that another medical practitioner attends instead within a reasonable time [8].

In the NT, section 155 of the *Criminal Code Act 1983* makes it a criminal offence to 'callously' fail to provide assistance to a person urgently in need of help including medical assistance or resuscitation:

> Any person who, being able to provide rescue, resuscitation, medical treatment, first aid or succour of any kind to a person urgently in need of it and whose life may be endangered if it is not provided, callously fails to do so is guilty of an offence and is liable to imprisonment for 7 years [9].

Some doctors may have been reluctant to render emergency assistance in the case of accidents for fear of being sued if their attempts were unsuccessful or the patient otherwise suffered an adverse outcome. However, all jurisdictions have enacted some form of legislative protections or good Samaritan laws. These laws prevent doctors being sued for negligence when providing voluntary care to a person in need of emergency assistance. The exact legislative provisions differ between the jurisdictions.

25.2.3 Duty of care to referred or future patients

It is usually clear when a doctor–patient relationship has been established. However, it is important to recognise that a duty of care can arise before a consultation.

In the 1979 case of *Albrighton v Royal Prince Alfred Hospital* [10], a specialist was held to have a duty of care at the time he reviewed the referral, *before* he had reviewed the patient, whom he did not see until later in the week. In this case, the decision was in part based on the neurosurgeon's knowledge of risks to the patient and his failure to intervene sooner to prevent a major complication.

These principles may apply to other circumstances where a doctor is aware of a referral but found to have negligently delayed assessing or providing care while being aware that the patient may suffer harm because of the delay in assessment. However, the outcome in any case will depend on the particular factual circumstances.

25.2.4 Duty of care to third parties

The duty of care of a doctor may extend beyond their patient to third parties (non-patients) who suffer injury because of the doctor's acts or omissions. There are a number of different classes of case where claims have been made by third parties. The principles that apply differ between the classes, the particular facts of each case and, in some cases, the application of specific laws. Some important examples are provided below.

Nervous shock (pure mental harm)

The most common category of claims by third parties are the so-called 'nervous shock' claims by close relatives of a patient who has suffered a serious injury or died as a result of alleged negligence.

A close relative of an injured or deceased patient may claim 'pure mental harm' for the psychological impact on them caused by the death or injury to their close relative. These claims rely upon a duty of care that the doctor holds towards close relatives of their patient, and the foreseeable risk of psychological trauma being experienced by the relatives upon the death or serious injury to the patient.

Civil liability legislation in most jurisdictions (i.e. all except Queensland and the NT) includes provisions applying to claims for pure mental harm. These provisions include a more restrictive definition of the duty of care and foreseeability, limitations on claims to close relatives, and damages only being payable where the claimant suffers a recognised psychiatric injury—generally understood to be a condition listed in the *Diagnostic and statistical manual of mental disorders* (though this is not absolute—see the case of *Whayman v The Motor Accidents Insurance Board* [11]).

Because of the nature of medicine, nervous shock claims are very common. Doctors may be able to reduce the risk of such claims by applying principles of good medical practice. This includes good communication and engagement with family members, working to develop trust, and managing expectations about the risks and possible outcomes of treatment. This is particularly relevant for patients who are very sick and at risk of a poor outcome.

Sexually transmitted diseases

A duty of care has been upheld towards partners of a doctor's patient where there is a risk of acquiring a sexually transmitted disease. In the case of *BT v Oei* [12] the claimant BT contracted HIV from her partner. The partner's general practitioner knew that he was infected with hepatitis B and had previously engaged in high-risk sexual activity. Notwithstanding that BT was not the patient of the doctor, the court found that the doctor owed her a duty of care. A general practitioner exercising a reasonable standard of care in 1992 should have considered a diagnosis of HIV and counselled the husband on the need for an HIV test.

In *Harvey & 1 Ors v PD* [13], another case of HIV transmission, a general practitioner was found liable for failing to provide proper pre-test counselling to a couple who had attended for pre-marriage HIV testing. In that case, one of the partners returned a positive HIV test, the news of which was not disclosed to the other person. On appeal the court found that if proper pre-test counselling had occurred, including the requirement to consent to disclose each other's HIV results, the plaintiff would have avoided contracting HIV by either obtaining her partner's consent to release his results, or terminating the relationship upon his refusal to provide consent.

In sexually transmitted disease cases, there is often a perceived conflict between the duty of confidentiality or privacy owed to the patient versus the duty of care owed to the sexual partner who may be at risk if the information is not disclosed. This is more imperative for life-threatening diseases such as HIV, but in theory can apply to other sexually transmitted diseases. For doctors who find themselves confronted with similar conflicting obligations as to their duties, it is important to seek legal advice so that all available legal options for resolution are considered, such as referral to a relevant public health authority, or where existing privacy law or other legislation allows for disclosure, such to prevent imminent harm to others.

Mental health cases

Claims have been made against doctors and hospitals for alleged failures in the treatment of mental health patients leading to some harm to a third party. However, it has also been found that a duty will not exist if it conflicts with obligations under mental health laws (such as restrictions on the ability to detain someone against their will).

The case of *McKenna v Hunter & New England Local Health District* [14] involved a mental health patient who killed a friend after being discharged from Manning Base Hospital. The friend had agreed to drive the patient to Victoria after his discharge. Relatives of the deceased sued the hospital for nervous shock, alleging that discharging the patient was negligent and caused the death of their relative.

On appeal, the NSW Court of Appeal found that a duty of care was owed to the deceased who was the friend of the patient [15]. Importantly, the court of appeal considered that a duty of care applied to the deceased because of the particular factual circumstances. The duty of care of the hospital did not extend to prevent harm to the general public at large.

McKenna was appealed by the hospital to the High Court, which found that the duty of care alleged was inconsistent with the obligations of the hospital and its doctors under the *Mental Health Act 1990* (NSW) [16]. This Act places legislative restrictions on the ability of doctors to hold a person with a suspected mental illness against their will.

The outcome of *McKenna* should be reassuring to doctors, who will not normally be liable in negligence for decisions to detain or release patients made in accordance with their obligations under the various mental health laws across Australia.

Other cases have confirmed that a duty of care may exist to protect third parties from the foreseeable risks of harm from mental health patients. These are generally in circumstances where the injured person is also under the care or responsibility of the doctor or health service; for example, other hospital patients or hospital staff who are injured by the actions of mental health patients.

Other categories

In the past, the courts have been reluctant to extend the duty of care owed under negligence to third parties who seek damages for effects of injuries on other people. Where a claimed duty of care to third parties gives rise to inconsistent obligations (such as in *McKenna* where the statutory obligations conflicted with the claimed duty of care), it may mean that the duty does not exist. Another example limiting the scope of a duty may include where the duty cannot be limited to a reasonably well defined group of people; for example, if the duty of care might extend to an unlimited number of persons [17,18].

25.2.5 Duty of care of hospitals and private facilities—implications for medical indemnity cover

Hospitals and other organisations providing medical services may be found liable for the negligent actions of their employed medical staff, contracted medical staff or other persons providing clinical services. The legal principles are either based upon the principle of vicarious liability, or the separate principle of non-delegable duty of care.

Vicarious liability is a principle that applies to certain relationships whereby a person or organisation is held liable for the actions of another. The relevant relationship in the circumstances of health care is that of employer and employee, such as between hospitals (public and private) and their employed medical staff. The relationship does not normally include contracted medical staff. Note that employers may not be held responsible where the employee is acting outside of their role as an employee, or outside the authority of their employer; however, these circumstances are generally rare.

Non-delegable duty of care is the principle that applies to persons or organisations who are deemed to hold a responsibility to protect from harm persons who are in some way dependent upon that person or organisation. Within health care, hospitals are deemed to hold a non-delegable duty of care towards their patients. They therefore have a positive duty to ensure reasonable care is provided to their patients, whether that care is provided by employees, contractors or other agents. However, it is generally accepted that a medical consultant providing services to their own private patients in a private hospital will be liable for the care they provide, and not the private hospital.

Implications for medical indemnity insurance

Medical registration in Australia carries a requirement to have in place medical indemnity cover with an approved insurer for every aspect of the doctor's clinical practice.

The above principle means that, normally, doctors who work in private hospitals, private health services, general practice or in other forms of private practice will require their own private indemnity insurance. Doctors who work solely as employees within public hospitals and do not undertake any billing of private patients will be fully indemnified for their work by their employing hospital or health service. However, it is generally recommended that all medical staff, including those working solely in public hospitals with no private patient billings, carry some form of private indemnity cover. The reasons for this recommendation include the following:

- There may be a risk of withdrawal of indemnity from the public hospital or government insurer. This is very rare; however, it is theoretically possible where the employee is found to be acting outside of their employed role or outside of the authority of the employer. It can also occur in other rare circumstances such as conduct found to be reckless or a wilful breach of duty, or criminal conduct (though a private indemnifier may have similar exclusions).
- The public hospital cover may not extend to representation or advice in coronial matters, especially where there may be conflict between the interests of the hospital and the doctor. Public hospital cover is very unlikely to extend to advice in professional disciplinary matters.
- Private indemnity cover usually carries the benefit of provision of independent legal advice that extends beyond civil liability to coronial matters, patient complaints, professional disciplinary matters and general health law advice. Hospital indemnity covers civil claims for damages, but any legal advice provided will be on the basis of protecting the interests of the insured party being the hospital.
- Private indemnity cover will extend to potential liabilities that may be incurred outside of the doctor's employed role. While all states have good Samaritan provisions protecting against liability in the treatment of emergencies (see section 25.2.2), doctors may still find themselves in circumstances of giving medical advice or care outside of their employment and not covered by such provisions.

25.3 Negligence in care and treatment

The main concern of doctors with respect to clinical negligence is usually the element of breach—that is, what defines the reasonable standard of care and how they should practise within that standard.

As described above, once a duty of care is established, a finding of negligence requires proof of a breach of the standard of care, and that the breach was causative of the injury incurred.

There are two distinct categories of breach of standard of care. The first is breach in the provision of care and treatment; the second is breach in the provision of information (consent). This section discusses the breach of duty in care and treatment, and the relevant principles of causation that apply to care and treatment cases.

25.3.1 Breach of the standard of care and treatment

Care and treatment cover the full gamut of services that a medical practitioner may provide to their patients. Claims for medical negligence have been made in almost every aspect of care and treatment, including failure to diagnose, failure to provide proper medical or surgical care, lack of knowledge, failure to attend, failure to refer and/or arrange an appointment, failure of follow-up and failure to provide proper supervision.

What is a reasonable standard of care?

When a claim for negligence is pursued, the court is required to determine whether the practitioner's care and treatment fell below a reasonable standard. Classical descriptions refer to the standard as defined by other competent practitioners. Lord Nathan in 1957 expressed this standard as follows:

> He [sic] will not be judged by the standards of the least qualified member of his class, nor those of the most highly qualified, but by the standard of the ordinary careful and competent practitioner of that class [19].

Assessment of what constitutes a reasonable standard of care therefore relies upon the court receiving expert advice from properly qualified and experienced medical experts as to the care provided by the doctor in the relevant circumstance.

In *Rogers v Whitaker* [2]—probably Australia's most well-known medical negligence case—the High Court ruled that it was ultimately up to the courts to decide whether a doctor had provided a reasonable standard of care. This High Court ruling departed from the longstanding Bolam principle: that the standard of a doctor's care be judged by a responsible body of their medical peers [20]. This caused significant concern among doctors at the time, but since then courts have reverted to their reliance upon the opinions of expert medical witnesses assessing the standard of care and treatment provided by a doctor.

Reinforcing the importance of peer medical opinion was the case of *Lowns & Anor v Woods & Ors* (discussed earlier in section 25.2.2), in which the NSW Court of Appeal stated:

> the courts should be slow to intervene where what is involved is the weighing up of advantages and disadvantages, medical necessities and the like by the profession ... [There must be] strong reasons why a clinical judgement properly arrived at is to be put aside as wrong [6].

Peer professional opinion

A comprehensive review of medical negligence laws was undertaken in the early 2000s and published as the Ipp Report [3]. Following this report, new laws were introduced that prevented a finding of negligence where the doctor acted in accordance with a standard of care that was considered competent by a body of properly qualified and experienced practitioners. For example, section 50 of the NSW *Civil Liability Act 2002* states:

1. A person practising a profession ('a professional') does not incur a liability in negligence arising from the provision of a professional service if it is established that the professional acted in a manner that (at the time the service was provided) was widely accepted in Australia by peer professional opinion as competent professional practice.
2. However, peer professional opinion cannot be relied on for the purposes of this section if the court considers that the opinion is irrational.
3. The fact that there are differing peer professional opinions widely accepted in Australia concerning a matter does not prevent any one or more (or all) of those opinions being relied on for the purposes of this section.
4. Peer professional opinion does not have to be universally accepted to be considered widely accepted [20].

Similar legislation applies in other jurisdictions. For example, in Victoria, the term 'unreasonable' replaces 'irrational' in regard to the peer opinion [21]. In Western Australia, the notion is expanded by the words 'so unreasonable that no reasonable health professional in the health professional's position could have acted or omitted to do something in accordance with that practice' [22].

There have been various decisions considering the meaning of the term 'competent professional practice'. These have been described as advocating for either a narrow or broad interpretation of the term [23]. The law in most jurisdictions has moved towards a broader definition whereby professional practice refers to the manner in which professionals practise their profession, and does not require identification of a particular accepted practice. With respect to the NSW Civil Liability Act, in *Dean v Pope* [24] Brereton JA stated:

> The question posed by s 50 is whether 'the professional acted in a manner that (at the time the service was provided) was widely accepted in Australia by peer professional opinion as competent professional practice'. This requires identifying the manner in which the professional acted, and asking whether it was at the time widely accepted as competent professional practice.

Summary of principles in care and treatment cases

The principles applied by courts in determining whether a reasonable standard of care and treatment has been provided by a doctor may be summarised in general terms as follows:

- Courts are required to decide whether the care and treatment provided was below a reasonable standard. This needs to be proven on the balance of probabilities—that is, more than 50% likely.
- While the courts maintain discretion to determine whether a doctor has provided a reasonable standard of care, decisions will almost always be based upon the court's assessment of competing medical expert reports.
- Courts are legislatively required not to find negligence where the defendant doctor is able to prove that the manner in which they acted was widely accepted as competent professional practice in Australia at the time the care was provided.

25.3.2 Causation in care and treatment cases

In addition to establishing a breach of the duty of care, a patient or claimant in medical negligence is also required to establish that the breach of care caused, or materially contributed to, the injury sustained. This can often be one of the most complex and difficult elements of a claim to establish.

The various civil liability Acts define causation in terms of *factual causation* and *scope of liability*.

Factual causation

Factual causation follows from the common-law 'but for' test. That is, the court finds on the balance of probabilities, *but for* the negligence of the doctor, the patient's injury would not have occurred. It follows that a doctor's care may be clearly below the standard expected; however, a failure to prove causation will mean that the claim will fail. This is often difficult for claimants to accept when they feel there should be some recompense for clear failures in care. An English case often cited is *Barnett v Chelsea & Kensington Hospital Management Committee* [26] whereupon a doctor failed to attend a patient who presented to hospital feeling unwell. The doctor was found not negligent despite the subsequent death of the patient. The patient died from arsenic poisoning for which there was no cure, such that no matter what care was provided at the time, the patient's death was likely unavoidable.

The 'but for' test is intuitively simple. However, there are many cases where such a simple test is not a fair manner in which to determine liability. A common example cited is where there are multiple causative factors leading to a person's injury, and it is therefore difficult to determine the exact contribution of each element.

An English case commonly quoted is *Fairchild v Glenhaven Funeral Services Ltd* (though being a claim against an employer rather than a doctor) [27]. In Fairchild, the claimant suffered mesothelioma secondary to asbestos exposure. The claimant had been exposed to asbestos at multiple different workplaces. A strict application of the 'but for' test in relation to the current employer would fail as the claimant had been exposed within many different jobs. The court found that the current employer's negligence in allowing exposure to asbestos *materially increased* the risk of developing mesothelioma. The employer was therefore liable.

The civil liability laws across Australia allow for such cases where strict factual causation has not been established—often described as 'exceptional' cases. For example, the NSW Civil Liability Act states:

> [i]n determining in an exceptional case, in accordance with established principles, whether negligence that cannot be established as a necessary condition of the occurrence of harm should be accepted as establishing factual causation, the court is to consider (amongst other relevant things) whether or not and why responsibility for the harm should be imposed on the negligent party [28].

As for findings of breach of duty, the court only needs to find that causation is proven on the balance of probabilities (that is, more than 50% likely).

Scope of liability

The scope of liability test must be applied in addition to the test of factual causation. In practice, this means that where factual causation is established, a further so-called 'normative' assessment is made by the court to consider whether or not liability should be imposed upon the doctor. This may result in a finding of no liability, even where factual causation has been established.

A commonly quoted example demonstrating the scope of liability is the case of *Paul v Cooke* [29]. In that case, a neurosurgeon failed to diagnose a patient's cerebral aneurysm, which was then left untreated for a number of years. When it was ultimately diagnosed, the patient underwent attempted coiling which was complicated by rupture of the aneurysm. The neurosurgeon admitted failure to diagnose at the earlier time. It was then argued that an earlier diagnosis, on the balance of probabilities, would have resulted in a successful clipping of the aneurysm. However, the court found that even if factual causation was proven, the risk of rupture during the delayed coiling had not changed.

The failure to diagnose had led to a foreseeable risk of rupture in the period before the diagnosis was ultimately made. However, the aneurysm did not rupture during this period, and the delay did not increase the risk of rupture during the eventual coiling procedure. It was therefore found not appropriate for the scope of liability of the neurosurgeon to extend to the rupture that occurred during the coiling procedure.

Another example where the scope of liability resulted in a finding of no negligence, despite factual causation being established, is the consent case of *Wallace v Kam* [30] discussed in section 25.4.2.

Practical application—mediation of claims

Debates around how the legal principles of causation apply to particular cases of medical negligence results in the production of many volumes of pages of case law, as well as academic analysis. Notwithstanding, for the vast majority of credible medical negligence claims which are settled at mediation, attention focuses primarily on the first test of factual causation.

Where there are doubts as to the strength of causation arguments, such as where there are other contributing factors to the patient's injury, or other intervening circumstances in relation to the claimed injuries, this results in a greater compromise at mediation with respect to the settlement amount agreed.

The rare matters that progress to hearing (and don't settle during the hearing) are assessed on their particular factual circumstances and application of the principles above.

25.4 Negligence in consent

A second and distinct category of negligence applies to 'failure to warn' or consent cases. There are separate considerations in establishing breach of duty and causation in consent cases, which are discussed in this section.

25.4.1 Breach of duty in consent cases

The seminal case regarding consent in Australia is *Rogers v Whitaker* [2], decided by the High Court in 1992. A patient sued an ophthalmic surgeon for failing to warn her of the risk of sympathetic ophthalmia in her good eye when proposing surgery to improve the appearance and sight in her other eye, which had been injured many years earlier. The High Court decision expressly rejected the longstanding Bolam test, which relied upon the opinion of other specialists in deciding whether the doctor was negligent [25]. The court did not accept as decisive evidence from other ophthalmic surgeons that they would not have warned the patient of the risk of sympathetic ophthalmia. In *Rogers*, the High Court stated:

> There is a fundamental difference between, on the one hand, diagnosis and treatment and, on the other hand, the provision of advice or information to a patient. ... except in cases of emergency or necessity, all medical treatment is preceded by the patient's choice to undergo it ... But the choice is, in reality, meaningless unless it is made on the basis of relevant information and advice. ... it would be illogical to hold that the amount of information to be provided by the medical practitioner can be determined from the perspective of the practitioner alone or, for that matter, of the medical profession. ... whether the patient has been given all the relevant information to choose between undergoing and not undergoing the treatment ... is not a question the answer to which depends upon medical standards or practices [2].

The court found that a doctor has a duty to disclose risks that might influence a reasonable person in the position of the patient whether to proceed with the proposed treatment. These are defined as the 'material risks' of the treatment.

The later case of *Rosenberg v Percival* (2001) [31] clarified what comprised a material risk. A risk was considered material in two circumstances, as follows:

- a reasonable person in the patient's position would be likely to attach significance to it ('the objective limb')
- the medical practitioner was, or should have been, aware that the particular patient would be likely to attach significance to it ('the subjective limb').

In *Rogers v Whitaker* [2], Mrs Whitaker alleged that she repeatedly sought information from Dr Rogers regarding any risks associated with the surgery, and in particular the risks to her good eye. In other words, she successfully argued that the 'subjective' limb of the test for material risk disclosure was not met.

In some jurisdictions, the definitions of material risks are specifically included within their respective civil liability laws.

The proper provision of information to patients is an important and complex topic, in particular for procedural specialists, but it is also relevant to all practising doctors. Please refer to Chapter 7, Consent and informed decision making, for more detailed information and guidance.

25.4.2 Causation in failure to warn/consent cases

Factual causation in failure to warn/consent cases

Causation is an important element in consent cases. Even where a doctor is found to have failed to advise about the material risks, they will not be found negligent unless the patient can prove that, had they been told about the risks, they would not have proceeded with the treatment.

In *Rosenberg v Percival* [31], the patient, an experienced health professional, sought damages for chronic pain caused by a temporomandibular joint disorder that followed surgery to realign a fractured jaw. Her claim failed ultimately because the trial judge did not accept her evidence that she would not have had the surgery if she had been warned of this possible outcome. On appeal to the High Court, Chief Justice Gleeson stated:

> The more remote a contingency which a doctor is required to bring to the notice of a patient, the more difficult it may be for the patient to convince a court that the existence of the contingency would have caused the patient to decide against surgery [31].

The outcome of the case was decided primarily on the credibility of the patient's claim that she would not have proceeded with treatment if she had been warned of a particular risk.

In failure to warn cases, the element of causation depends upon the patient proving they would not have proceeded with the procedure if the relevant material risks had been disclosed. The test is subjective to the particular patient rather than an objective assessment of what a 'reasonable person' would do.

Courts are aware of the risks of hindsight bias in that a patient, having experienced a complication of their treatment, may state a belief that they would have refused the treatment if warned of the risk. Courts will generally give low weight to such statements or require other evidence to support such a contention. In some jurisdictions, legislative reforms have rendered any such retrospective statements made by the plaintiff not admissible in negligence proceedings.

Scope of liability in consent cases

As discussed previously, a finding of causation depends on two tests being satisfied: the first being factual causation and the second being the scope of liability (see section 25.3.2).

The issue of scope of liability was central to the High Court case of *Wallace v Kam* [30]. That case involved a patient who suffered the complication of neuropraxia to his femoral nerve, which caused an extended period of postoperative pain. It was found that the surgeon had failed to warn the patient both of the possibility of the complication of neuropraxia as well as the complication of permanent paralysis from damage to his spinal cord.

In *Wallace v Kam*, a key issue was that the trial judge found that the patient would not have proceeded with the operation if warned of the risk of permanent paralysis (which did not eventuate). In its analysis, the High Court determined that the test of factual causation may have been met—but for the failures to warn, the patient would not have undergone the procedure. However, in terms of scope of liability, causation was not established because the patient should not be compensated for a complication that he was willing to accept if warned of the risk. The full court stated that '[h]e is not to be compensated for the occurrence of physical injury the risk of which he was prepared to accept.'

25.4.3 Therapeutic privilege

The judgement in *Rogers v Whitaker* also recognised that the duty to disclose was subject to the longstanding concept of 'therapeutic privilege'. This privilege entitles a doctor to withhold information if the doctor believes disclosure might be harmful to the patient. Reliance on the privilege is rare and, if not carefully applied, may easily be construed as paternalistic and interfering with the ability of the patient to act autonomously. An example of a case where the therapeutic privilege was upheld is *Battersby v Tottman* [32] where a doctor was held to have been entitled to withhold telling a patient that there was a risk of blindness from prolonged treatment for her severe mental illness.

25.4.4 Trespass to the person/civil assault

The requirements of a valid consent are discussed in detail in Chapter 7, Consent and informed decision making. If a doctor undertakes a medical procedure without the consent of the patient (excluding in emergencies or other specific circumstances) the doctor may be guilty of a civil assault or a battery for which an action in trespass to the person may be brought. No action for trespass arises once the patient is informed of the broad nature of what treatment is proposed and consents to that treatment—advising of material risks is not required. Being a civil action, the remedy is damages rather than a criminal penalty.

Trespass to the person is uncommon because of the recognition of the need for consent. A failure to warn of material risks of a treatment procedure is the more common claim for damages. However, there are some cases where the patient may pursue a claim for a trespass to the person because of a fundamental failure to obtain a consent as opposed to a failure to warn of material risks. Examples of cases where a trespass was found include *Murray v McMurchy* [33] where a surgeon performing a caesarean section also performed a sterilisation procedure, which had not been discussed with the patient. Other examples of trespass include cases where the doctor undertook procedures for a non-therapeutic purpose such as in *Dean v Phung* [34]. In that case, a dentist performed $76,000 worth of elective dental work on a patient who initially presented for a minor work-related injury to his front teeth.

The impact of civil liability legislation can create an incentive to pursue a trespass to the person rather than a negligence claim where available. This is because the damages in a trespass case may not be limited by some of the legislative provisions that apply to limit damages in negligence claims. There is also no need to prove causation as an element to the action of trespass.

25.5 Quantum: assessment of damages

Actions for negligence can succeed only if the plaintiff has suffered damage. The courts accept that damage may be physical or psychological and include other impacts of the injury, such as inconvenience or stress of requiring additional treatment, and financial loss caused by the injury.

The award of damages is related to the degree of harm or loss and not to the degree of negligence. The compensation is intended to restore the plaintiff to the position in which they would have been if negligence had not occurred. Damages are assessed and awarded in respect of specific 'heads of damages' based upon past case law. The various jurisdictional civil liability Acts have modified the criteria and amount payable for many categories of damage.

The types of damages payable may be considered under the categories of non-economic loss (general damages), and financial or pecuniary loss.

25.5.1 Non-economic loss (general damages)

This includes compensation for pain, suffering and loss of enjoyment (or amenities) of life. This is referred to as non-economic loss or general damages. In some overseas jurisdictions, the definitions may be different, with 'general damages' referring to any unliquidated losses (including pain and suffering and estimated future pecuniary losses).

Maximum damages payable under this head of damage are limited under civil liability legislation. Generally, damages are payable based upon the court's assessment of the impact of the claimant's injury relative to a most extreme or severe case.

25.5.2 Financial or pecuniary loss

The term 'economic loss' is commonly used to refer to loss of income. In the context of this chapter, 'pecuniary loss' includes compensation for actual financial loss caused by the injury. The main classes of pecuniary loss are:

- out-of-pocket expenses for additional care and treatment related to the injury, such as medical and hospital expenses, allied health care, medications, equipment and transport costs
- the cost of providing supportive care and assistance to the injured person; this can include payment for commercial care where required, and also compensation for so-called gratuitous care provided by relatives of the injured person
- the cost of providing domestic support or care to dependants of the injured person's relatives where the person can no longer provide that care because of the injury
- loss of income or income-earning capacity.

Most pecuniary losses will be divided into past costs actually incurred (prior to the date of mediation or hearing) and estimates of future losses based on the injury and life expectancy, where relevant.

The types of damages payable will depend on the particular circumstances and impact of the injury. Considerations of causation will often overlap with the assessment of damages in medical negligence cases.

Relevantly, where a claimant is awarded damages for care and treatment or income loss, there may be a requirement to repay government-funded benefits that were received because of the injury. These include Medicare benefits paid to treating doctors, social security or Centrelink income support payments, and payments made under the National Disability Insurance Scheme.

25.6 Expert reports

As highlighted in section 25.3.1, *Rogers v Whitaker* [2] affirmed the role of the court to determine the relevant standard of care. Notwithstanding, in practice courts remain highly dependent upon the opinions of experts in determining whether the standard of care has been breached, as well as deciding issues of causation and making assessments of damages.

In contested hearings, the courts are called upon to assess the merits of competing expert opinions presented by both the claimant patient and the defendant doctor or health service. This can lead to the appearance of experts being on the side of one party or the other. However, for doctors providing expert reports, it is important to understand that their primary duty is to the court. They are not advocates for the party who instructs them.

Various codes of conduct and guidelines exist that reinforce the duties of experts to provide opinions that are properly based upon the facts and require an unbiased application of the expert's specialised knowledge to those facts. Courts can be critical of experts where they perceive that the expert has not complied with their duties or has become an advocate for their client's case. In extreme cases, doctors may be subject to disciplinary action for failing to provide opinions that are not properly evidence based or are outside their area of expertise. For example, see the English case of *GMC v Professor Sir Roy Meadow* [35], in which Professor Meadow was initially struck off the GMC register for applying statistical analysis outside his area of expertise to comment on the probability of two occurrences of sudden infant death syndrome in the same family; this was repealed when his evidence assisted in the criminal conviction of the children's mother. However, it has been uncommon for such disciplinary action to be pursued in Australia.

Courts have attempted to deal with the risks of expert bias and to improve the efficiency of trials by introducing various procedures, such as ordering all relevant experts to meet before a trial and produce a report identifying areas of agreement and disagreement (known as an expert conclave), or requiring experts to give evidence in court concurrently (so-called 'hot tubbing') where they are questioned and cross-examined at the same time. For more on expert evidence, see Chapter 26, Medicolegal examinations and reports, court procedures and expert evidence.

25.7 Criminal negligence and manslaughter

While most actions for negligence are processed as civil claims, doctors should be aware that in instances of gross negligence leading to death or serious injury to a patient, criminal actions can in theory be pursued by the police for charges such as gross negligence manslaughter or negligently causing serious injury. This has happened relatively infrequently in Australia. However, numerous cases have been reported from the United Kingdom, where the legal system is similar, though arguably characterised by a greater propensity to pursue doctors for disciplinary matters and sometimes criminal charges. For a high-profile Australian case, see *Patel v The Queen* [36,37]. For high-profile and controversial UK cases, see *Bawa-Garba v R* [38], *Sellu v The Crown* [39] and *R v Misra* [40].

The legal test in Australia for manslaughter includes a requirement to find moral culpability (see *Wilson v The Queen* [41]). This may explain the rarity of such cases being brought against doctors. By contrast, in the UK, the test applied in medical manslaughter cases has been articulated as conduct that is 'truly exceptionally bad' [38–40], which arguably does not import the same concept of moral culpability.

An Australian example that demonstrates the need for moral culpability before the finding of a criminal conviction is *R v Peters* [42]. That case concerned an anaesthetist with drug dependence who infected 55 patients with hepatitis C by injecting himself with fentanyl prior to administering the drug to the patient using the same needle. The court described the doctor's conduct as 'truly reprehensible', which justified a long prison sentence (14 years, with a 10-year non-parole period).

25.8 Risk management and preventing claims for negligence

Reasons commonly considered responsible for medical negligence claims include:

- poor-quality communication with patients
- increased expectations of patients
- increased awareness of patients' rights

- increased range and use of medical services
- advertising by lawyers regarding personal injury and negligence claims
- media coverage of poor medical practice and negligence actions
- increasing importance of the early diagnosis of cancer.

Medical indemnity insurers focus attention on risk-reduction strategies and educating doctors in behaviour and practices that may reduce the incidence of claims. Much of the advice given in this regard revolves around improved communication and maintaining high standards of care. It also includes risk assessment of the physical environment (e.g. disposal of sharps and reduction in infection risks), good record keeping and follow-up of laboratory results.

Advice is directed at avoiding problems that may arise if a doctor does not pay attention to good communication, is not reasonably available or not seen to be caring and sympathetic. Care should be taken in managing unrealistic patient expectations in regard to the expected outcomes of treatment, especially in such areas as cosmetic surgery. Obtaining proper consent is crucial and if complications develop, proper management and open communication should be given priority.

Specific advice given by medical indemnity insurers, based on their experience of recurring problems, includes:

- keep clear, detailed and contemporaneous clinical records
- carefully elicit and record any history of allergies or other important drug reactions
- have a failsafe system of reading, noting and filing investigation reports and following up patients
- avoid making gratuitous and often ill-informed remarks to patients about treatment provided by other doctors
- for surgeons, avoid errors such as those relating to operative site, instrument and pack count and care with the use of diathermy
- give careful instructions about the use of plaster casts
- be aware of the regulations and be alert to the problems of patients with drug dependence and those exhibiting drug-seeking behaviour
- ensure that the release of confidential patient information is done in compliance with relevant privacy laws and guidelines.

It is generally considered that only a relatively small percentage of patients who suffer complications or unexpected outcomes sue their doctors. Surveys have shown that the reasons patients sue include a failure of the doctor to communicate, especially to warn regarding potential complications; a feeling that the doctor has ignored them or will not adequately discuss matters when something goes wrong; feelings of anger and humiliation combined with a need for the doctor to indicate recognition of the patient's problem; a wish that doctors should be accountable; and last and generally of least importance, significant financial loss.

When something unexpected and undesired happens following treatment, the best approach is usually open and frank discussion with the patient, including with any relatives or friends the patient wishes to be involved. Consideration should be given to open disclosure guidelines, which are discussed in Chapter 5, Communication in clinical practice. Encouraging discussion of the facts and making apologies without attributing blame should not represent an admission of liability. If a doctor is uncertain about the correct approach in certain circumstances, advice should be sought from their medical indemnity insurer.

Summary

The fact that a patient suffers a complication of treatment or a poor outcome does not mean that a case in medical negligence will be commenced or will succeed. The law accepts that complications occur and clinical outcomes are not always ideal. Such cases do not necessarily indicate that the care provided was negligent.

For a medical negligence claim to be successful, there must be a breach of the established duty of care. Such a breach occurs where the care and treatment provided is proven on the balance of probabilities to have been below a reasonable standard (and where relevant, not consistent with a recognised practice as defined by peer professional opinion). Alternatively, in consent cases, breach occurs where there has been a failure to warn of material risks—both objective and subjective.

In addition to proving breach of duty, the patient must also prove that the failure to provide a reasonable standard of care caused, or materially contributed to, the injury sustained. In consent cases, the patient must prove that they would have avoided the injury if they had been properly warned—generally because they would not have consented to the treatment.

Finally, the patient must show the injury caused has resulted in damages that are compensable as defined by case law and the civil liability laws in the relevant jurisdictions.

Despite the many references to complex past medical negligence cases fought in the higher courts of Australia, the vast majority of medical negligence claims settle out of court, either by a mediated settlement, or sometimes discontinuation by the patient.

In Australia, all doctors must hold current medical indemnity insurance cover with an approved provider for every aspect of their medical practice. Doctors covered under the insurance policies of their employing hospital should carefully consider the option of taking out separate private indemnity insurance to cover possible claims arising outside the cover of their employment; they should also have access to independent legal advice if required.

References

1. Kirby M. Patients' rights—why the Australian courts have rejected 'Bolam'. *J Med Ethics* 1995; 21: 5–8.
2. *Rogers v Whitaker* (1992) 175 CLR 479.
3. Ipp DA; Law of Negligence Review Panel. Review of the law of negligence. Final report. Canberra: Commonwealth of Australia, 2002. https://treasury.gov.au/review/review-of-the-law-of-negligence (accessed Oct 2015).
4. *Donoghue v Stevenson* [1932] UKHL 100.
5. *Woods v Lowns* (1995) 36 NSWLR 344.
6. *Lowns & Anor v Woods & Ors* (1996) Aust Torts Reports 81-376.
7. Medical Board of Australia. Good medical practice: a code of conduct for doctors in Australia. 2020. https://www.medicalboard.gov.au/Codes-Guidelines-Policies/Code-of-conduct.aspx (accessed May 2025).
8. *Health Practitioner Regulation National Law (NSW) No 86a of 2009*, s 193C.
9. *Criminal Code Act 1983* (NT), s 155.
10. *Albrighton v Royal Prince Alfred Hospital* (1979) 2 NSWLR 165-175.
11. *Whayman v The Motor Accidents Insurance Board* [2003] TASSC 149 at [27].
12. *BT v Oei* (1999) NSWSC 1082.
13. *Harvey & 1 Ors v PD* [2004] NSWCA 97.
14. *McKenna v Hunter & New England Local Health District* [2012] NSWDC 19.
15. *McKenna v Hunter & New England Local Health District* [2013] NSWCA 476.

16. *Hunter and New England Local Health District v McKenna*; *Hunter and New England Local Health District v Simon* [2014] HCA 44.
17. *Sullivan v Moody* [2001] HCA 59.
18. Madden B, McIlwraith J, Madden B. Australian medical liability, 4th ed. Chatswood (NSW): LexisNexis, 2021.
19. Nathan HLN. Medical negligence: being the law of negligence in relation to the medical profession and hospitals. London: Butterworth, 1957.
20. *Civil Liability Act 2002* (NSW), s 5O.
21. *Wrongs Act 1958* (Vic), s 59(2).
22. *Civil Liability Act 2002* (WA), s 5PB.
23. Cameron S, Kim P. The standard of care test revisited: competing approaches to defining competent profession practice in Australia. *J Law Med* 2023; 30: 278–285.
24. *Dean v Pope* [2022] NSWCA 260 at [314].
25. *Bolam v Friern Hospital Management Committee* (1957) 2 All ER 118, at 121 per McNair J.
26. *Barnett v Chelsea & Kensington Hospital Management Committee* [1969] 1 QB 428.
27. *Fairchild v Glenhaven Funeral Services Ltd* (2003) 1 AC 32.
28. *Civil Liability Act 2002* (NSW), s 5D(2).
29. *Paul v Cooke* [2012] NSWSC 840.
30. *Wallace v Kam* [2013] HCA 19.
31. *Rosenberg v Percival* (2001) 205 CLR 434.
32. *Battersby v Tottman* (1985) 37 SASR 524.
33. *Murray v McMurchy* [1949] 2 DLR 442.
34. *Dean v Phung* [2012] NSWCA 223.
35. *GMC v Professor Sir Roy Meadow with HM Attorney General* [2006] EWCA Civ 1390.
36. *Patel v The Queen* [2012] HCA 29.
37. Callaghan D. Conviction for medical manslaughter in Queensland: the decision in R v Patel. *Health Law Bulletin* 2010; 18: 124–126.
38. *Bawa-Garba v R* [2016] EWCA Crim 1841.
39. *Sellu v The Crown* [2016] EWCA Crim 1716.
40. *R v Misra* [2004] EWCA Crim 2375.
41. *Wilson v The Queen* [1992] HCA 31.
42. *R v Peters* [2013] VSC 93.

Further reading

Mathur R. Avant podcast series: Medical manslaughter—could it happen here? Avant Media, 2018; 28 Aug. https://soundcloud.com/user-853393772/sets/medical-manslaughter-series

26 Medicolegal examinations and reports, court procedures and expert evidence

John Quinn AM

Introduction

This chapter is designed to help doctors conduct medicolegal examinations and prepare medicolegal reports, and to advise doctors about appearing in court as ordinary or as expert witnesses. Problems that may arise at medicolegal examinations are identified, and advice is provided about the content and scope of medicolegal reports. After briefly describing the adversarial system used in Australian courts, the chapter then provides broad advice about doctors appearing in courts as ordinary (lay) witnesses or as expert witnesses, and briefly discusses issues facing doctors called to jury duty.

26.1 Medicolegal reports

26.1.1 Request for medical records and documents

For doctors who are primarily in general practice, the most common involvement with the judicial system will be requests to provide copies of documents or clinical notes, and attendance dates of a patient. These usually relate to a matter being assessed for a compensation or insurance claim, or being prepared for legal proceedings involving a court or tribunal appearance. To provide any of these documents, the doctor usually requires the written consent of the patient or their authorised representative. Lawyers should provide this consent letter; without it, doctors should refuse to provide any documents. However, if documents are requested via a subpoena or an order of a court, tribunal, or other 'authority to produce', then the documents must be provided. The doctor does not need to provide an opinion; instead, the requested documents are used by others to piece together a history of pre-existing conditions or progress after an injury or illness. It is reasonable to charge a fee for such work, which should be based on the time taken to provide the documents.

For employed doctors working in hospitals, such as resident medical officers or registrars, requests for clinical records or documents are usually managed by the relevant medical records or medicolegal departments. Any requests made directly to those doctors should be referred to the relevant hospital department for action.

26.1.2 Request for medicolegal reports

Occasionally, a doctor is asked for a medicolegal report about a current or past patient, most often in the context of an insurance or workers compensation claim. The request must be accompanied by a signed authority from the patient to release the medical information and by a letter from the solicitor describing what is requested. These reports are requesting factual information based upon the clinical notes of the treating doctor rather than an opinion on the merits of a claim or potential compensation payable (see section 26.2 for a discussion about medical expert reports). Doctors should follow the request or instructions articulated by the solicitor's letter of request. Again, it is reasonable to charge a fee, based on the time taken, the complexity of the request, and the level of skills and qualifications of the doctor or specialist.

A treating doctor's medicolegal report should contain the patient's history; relevant physical findings; investigations undertaken, with their results; any diagnoses made; and the treatment provided. The doctor should make it clear whether they personally performed the physical examination or if they are relying upon a reported examination performed by a different doctor or clinician. If the patient was referred to another doctor, this should be noted, but it is not the task of the treating doctor to provide any report of the findings of another doctor. If the medicolegal report identifies to whom the patient was referred and when, the requesting solicitor will be able to make a decision about approaching that doctor for a report.

In preparing medicolegal reports about the diagnosis, care and treatment of a patient, doctors should take care to answer the questions asked of them and to make the report concise, factual, objective and complete. Material in the patient's records that is irrelevant to the request should not be included in the report. If the doctor has any doubt in this regard, advice should be sought from the doctor's medical defence organisation. A well-constructed medicolegal report may be sufficient for the solicitor and the court or tribunal, and may avoid the need for the doctor to be called to give oral evidence.

A treating doctor's report is not required to contain an opinion regarding the merits of the patient's claim, although some solicitors may request comments that may be relevant to the patient's claim, such as on aetiology or prognosis. A treating doctor should decline to answer such questions if they feel unqualified to give such an opinion. Doctors should also be aware that any opinions they provide on merits may be open to challenge by expert reports from the insurer or defendant.

Above all, no matter how much compassion the doctor might have for the patient, the report must not be written in a partisan manner. The weight and authority of a doctor's report lies in the professionalism with which it is composed, combining factual accuracy, medical expertise and dispassionate judgement. Some of the advice provided below in relation to expert witness reports is also relevant to treating doctors' reports.

A medicolegal report may be legally privileged and therefore must not be released to any other party without the permission of the solicitor who requested it. Care should be taken to address the report as requested by the solicitor. The lawyers then will determine matters related to privilege. Despite the pressures of medical practice, requests for reports should be handled promptly, so that a patient's claim is not jeopardised and that the administration of justice is not delayed. Undue and excessive delays in providing important medicolegal reports may, in serious cases, result in disciplinary action from the Medical Board of Australia.

Doctors may charge an administrative fee if providing factual information. The cost of medicolegal reports are not covered by Medicare.

26.2 Expert witness reports

An expert witness is someone who possesses particular knowledge or skills that are not expected to be available to the 'average citizen'. Therefore, the expert witness is asked to provide this knowledge in a format that informs the court, tribunal or commission of inquiry, and is understood to inform the decision-making process.

Doctors may be asked to provide expert witness reports for the purpose of potential or actual legal proceedings such as medical negligence claims, medical disciplinary matters or coronial inquests. These reports will ask for an independent opinion from the doctor regarding the standard of care and treatment provided to a patient and/or whether the care provided caused or contributed to the patient's injury or death. In medical negligence claims, these reports are referred to as liability reports and are often prepared based on a review of clinical notes, investigation results and other documents forwarded by the instructing solicitor. Expert witness reports may also be sought from doctors to assist in quantifying the amount of potential damages in a medical negligence claim, which may include a request to undertake a medicolegal examination of the patient and quantify the degree of disability experienced.

Doctors drafting an expert witness report must comply with an expert witness code of conduct or guideline, depending on the jurisdiction, to ensure that their statements are admissible and can be used in court. The instructing solicitors should provide details of the applicable guideline. The paramount duty of an expert witness is to assist the court impartially on matters relevant to the witness's area of expertise. Additional obligations that apply to expert witnesses generally include the following:

- to act honestly and not as an advocate for a particular party
- to cooperate in the conduct of the civil proceeding
- to use reasonable endeavours to assist in the resolution of the dispute, including conferring with other experts to narrow issues in dispute
- to provide a supplementary report if another expert changes their opinion on any material matter.

26.2.1 Content of medical expert witness reports

As discussed above, expert reports drafted for personal injury and negligence cases and general litigation must conform to court codes or guidelines for expert witnesses, which differ between states and territories. These guidelines also include guidance as to the content of the reports. Usually, an expert witness report must clearly state the opinion or opinions of the expert and must also include the items in Box 26.1.

Box 26.1 Components of an expert witness report

1. The name and address of the expert
2. An acknowledgement that the expert has read the code and agrees to be bound by it
3. The qualifications of the expert to prepare the report
4. The assumptions and material facts on which each opinion expressed in the report is based (a letter of instruction may be annexed)
5. The reasons for and any literature or other materials used in support of each such opinion
6. That a particular question, issue or matter falls outside the expert's field of expertise (if applicable)
7. Any examinations, tests or other investigations on which the expert has relied, identifying the person who carried them out and that person's qualifications
8. The extent to which any opinion that the expert has expressed involves the acceptance of another person's opinion, the identification of that other person and the opinion expressed by that other person

Continued over page

9. A declaration that the expert has made all the inquiries that the expert believes are desirable and appropriate (save for any matters identified explicitly in the report), and that no matters of significance that the expert regards as relevant have, to the knowledge of the expert, been withheld from the court
10. Any qualification of an opinion expressed in the report without which the report is, or may be, incomplete or inaccurate
11. Whether any opinion expressed in the report is not a concluded opinion because of insufficient research or insufficient data, or for any other reason
12. Where the report is lengthy or complex, a brief summary of the report is included at the beginning of the report

A solicitor will often disclose and discuss with the client the contents of any medical report received in the course of advising that client. In their reports, doctors should be careful not to make gratuitous remarks about the patient or their professional medical colleagues, but should confine themselves to medical fact and medical opinion.

26.2.2 Medicolegal examinations

Specialist doctors are frequently requested by solicitors or insurers to examine patients for the purpose of providing a report that will be used to assist the solicitor or insurer in determining or pursuing a claim for compensation. This is most commonly to provide information relevant to the determination of quantum or the amount of compensation claimed or payable. The cost of such examinations is not covered by Medicare.

It is usual that appointments for medical examinations are first made by telephone and then confirmed by a solicitor's letter (a 'letter of instruction'). The letter should contain a brief description of the circumstance in which the patient was allegedly harmed or injured; the nature of the harms or injury alleged; copies of relevant medical certificates and other medical reports, imaging and pathology reports; together with details of the alleged disability the patient claims arose out of the harm or injury. There will usually be a series of questions included in the letter of instruction requesting advice on some or all of the items listed in Box 26.2.

Box 26.2 Items commonly addressed in a medicolegal examination

- The patient's description of the event under discussion
- Details of immediate treatment and subsequent management of the injury or harm
- The results of the physical examination
- The patient's current physical condition with particular reference to the alleged injury or disability
- Whether the accident or condition is consistent with the particular injury or disability
- Whether the patient's condition has stabilised, or whether there is any prospect of further improvement or deterioration
- Whether there is any residual disability and if so, the extent of such disability
- Whether there was any existing disability prior to the event in question

Continued over page

- Whether there were any pre-existing conditions contributing to or exacerbated by the event in question
- Whether any further medical treatment is indicated and, if so, an opinion concerning the probable outcome of such treatment
- Whether the patient is fit for any work and, if so, what type of work
- If the patient is unfit for work, the cause of the loss of capacity for work and the degree of incapacitation
- Whether the doctor recommends that the patient be examined by any other specialists
- Whether any further investigations are necessary to inform the specialist's opinion, or assess the degree of impairment
- Whether there are any other matters which the doctor considers relevant

It is important that experts undertaking a consultation for the purposes of providing a report are not providing treatment to the patient. This should be made clear to the patient. Similarly, the expert should refrain from making comments on treatment provided by others.

It is essential that doctors provide reports promptly to solicitors after the medical examination. Court rules put additional pressures of time on solicitors to prepare cases for trial. The courts are very aware of the time pressures on doctors, particularly treating doctors, and generally go out of their way to minimise the interruption involved when doctors attend the court. However, where doctors have agreed to be expert witnesses and have accepted fees to provide an expert report, attendance at court may be required and pressure of clinical work should not be used to delay or avoid such responsibility. Doctors who are unwilling to appear in court should not accept requests to undertake medicolegal examinations.

26.2.3 Problems arising in undertaking medicolegal examinations for expert witness reports

In the usual medical consultation, the doctor acts only in the interests of the patient. In contrast, during a medicolegal consultation, the doctor is a neutral expert employed by a third party and expected to give an impartial opinion to the court or tribunal. To ensure accuracy and validity, the doctor's range of inquiry during history taking must frequently be different from that employed in usual clinical practice. This difference in the purpose of the examination should ideally have been explained to the patient by the solicitor or insurer arranging the appointment, and should be reinforced by the doctor at the beginning of the consultation.

In medical practice, when a patient attends at a doctor's surgery for treatment, mutual honesty is assumed, and this assumption is usually well founded. This mutual trust is not guaranteed in a medicolegal consultation, where the doctor may feel an obligation to minimise the chances of being deceived. However, this should not be translated into an adversarial or aggressive method of questioning, or brusqueness in conducting the physical examination, and respect for the person must be maintained [1]. The patient might also be uncomfortable or reluctant, recognising that the doctor may be employed by another party whose interests are opposed to those of the patient. Of course this is not always the case, as plaintiff's solicitors may also seek opinions and examinations. Doctors should not be surprised if patients undergoing medicolegal examinations consider them to be biased in their medical assessments. For this reason, among others, many doctors do not wish to be involved in medicolegal work.

Doctors can create problems for themselves when composing or attending to requests for medicolegal reports. These include:

- unacceptable delays in responding to requests for reports
- providing poor-quality reports, aggravated by excessive charges
- failing to remain objective
- using judgemental or emotive language
- basing conclusions on inaccurate or incomplete material, or inappropriately implying that the allegations of the patient are false.

At times, medicolegal assessments may lead to the assessor identifying a need for urgent treatment or to recommendations for possibly more effective treatment. Australian Medical Association guidance on this subject advises the independent medical assessor who has serious concerns regarding the management of a patient to contact the treating doctor, with the patient's consent [2].

26.3 Court procedures

Doctors are called to give evidence as expert witnesses in civil and, occasionally, criminal matters, or sometimes Commissions of Inquiry or similar. Doctors may also be asked to give evidence of the facts of their treatment of patients or to give evidence as defendants in civil court actions such as negligence claims. Although the last of these instances is undoubtedly the most stressful, any appearance in court can produce anxiety even in the most experienced doctors. Levels of stress and anxiety may be reduced by having a better understanding of court procedures, being well prepared, and appreciating what is required of the doctor as a witness.

Advice is usually available from the doctor's medical indemnity insurer, which can explain the procedures, guide them through the process and, if required, provide professional, legal or personal support.

26.3.1 The adversarial system

Proceedings in Australian courts are adversarial. The adversarial system prevails in most countries where the legal system was derived from that of the UK. In the adversarial system, trials, whether criminal or civil, are effectively contests between opposing parties with a judge acting as the umpire, deciding on points of law and procedure, and giving legal directions to the jury, which alone decides the issues of fact. Juries are more common in criminal trials, and are very rarely used in civil matters. In civil trials without a jury, the judge decides both issues of law and fact. In the adversarial system, the burden of winning the contest usually rests on the party who initiates the proceedings. In a criminal case, the Crown—in the guise of either a Director of Public Prosecutions or the police—brings the case against an accused person, whereas in a civil case the plaintiff brings an action against a defendant. This structure closely resembles that in medical disciplinary tribunals, although the barrister 'prosecuting' the case against a doctor plays a slightly different role as 'counsel assisting' the tribunal and has a duty to draw the attention of the presiding officer to all relevant matters.

The trial procedure relies heavily on written or oral statements as evidence-in-chief, followed by oral cross-examination by the opposing party. The evidence is established by answers given by witnesses to the questions asked, in turn, by the opposing parties according to the rules of procedure (see section 26.4). The role of presiding judge is that of an umpire, intervening to ensure and enforce these rules only when asked by one of the parties. Judges have only very limited powers to call witnesses in both civil and criminal trials. While judges may ask witnesses questions in the interests of clarifying answers to questions put by counsel, they may not examine witnesses in such a way as to join in the contest or even to appear to do so.

26.4 Giving evidence

The evidence of a witness in both civil and criminal trials falls into three main parts: evidence-in-chief, cross-examination and re-examination.

26.4.1 Evidence-in-chief

Evidence-in-chief is presented through the answers to questions asked by the party who has called the witness. In criminal trials, witnesses called by the Crown are questioned first by the prosecutor; in civil cases, witnesses called by the plaintiff are questioned first by the plaintiff's barrister. Witnesses are asked their names and addresses and, if relevant, their qualifications and experience. Before trials, witnesses are usually asked to prepare statements on the matters on which evidence is sought. These statements are written in conjunction with the lawyers involved, and may be discussed with the barrister prior to appearance of the witness in court. The trend in civil trials is that the witness's statement should represent the majority of the evidence of the witness. This means that, after the identification of the witness as above, the court will then ask the witness to swear as to the truth of their statement. After this, very few questions may be asked of the witness as evidence-in-chief and the process may then move quickly to cross-examination by opposing barristers.

It is standard practice for counsel for one party to request the judge to order all prospective witnesses from the court room to prevent them hearing the evidence or cross-examination of earlier witnesses. The judge usually complies with such a request unless an application is made by counsel to allow a particular witness, such as an expert, to remain in court. Prospective witnesses must remain within the precincts of the court, so that they can respond promptly when called to appear. Witnesses should take the advice of the solicitors involved as to their permitted whereabouts and the expected waiting time periods.

26.4.2 Cross-examination

After evidence-in-chief has been given, the witness is usually examined by counsel for the accused or the defendant. In cross-examination, the witness may be asked questions intended to clarify the evidence-in-chief, or to elicit information that is favourable to the accused or defendant. Questions may also be asked to cast doubt on the accuracy of the evidence previously given by the witness, or to attempt to discredit the witness in the eyes of the judge or jury, and so decrease the weight of the evidence given during the examination-in-chief.

Cross-examination often takes the form of leading questions to which there can be no objection in this stage of the proceedings. The evidence of medical witnesses may be tested by rigorous cross-examination, particularly if the evidence-in-chief has been unfavourable to the cross-examiner's client.

The process of cross-examination can be stressful, especially for doctors with little experience as witnesses. Counsel for the party instructing the doctor should provide general advice about what to expect and how to manage the process of cross-examination (see also sections 26.7 and 26.7.1).

26.4.3 Re-examination

After cross-examination, counsel for the party that called the witness can ask further questions, usually to clarify any ambiguities which may have arisen from the cross-examination. Under the rules of evidence, no new material may be introduced at this stage and re-examination is usually relatively brief.

26.5 Evidence of fact

The law distinguishes between evidence of *fact* and evidence of *opinion*.

26.5.1 Ordinary or lay evidence

Ordinary or 'lay' witnesses are normally only permitted to give evidence of fact—that is, what they saw, heard or otherwise perceived. They are not allowed in most circumstances to provide an opinion, and any such opinions are inadmissible to prove an issue of fact. A doctor, like any other citizen, is an ordinary witness to facts if they witnessed a road accident or a crime or as witness to what they have done in their work as a medical practitioner. The doctor in these circumstances is in exactly the same position as any other witness and is required to state what they saw, heard or did, and not give an opinion about events, except for commonplace observations such as age or general appearance of those involved.

26.5.2 Expert evidence

Expert witnesses are set apart from ordinary or lay witnesses in that they are permitted to express opinions that can be admitted as expert evidence. The privilege of the expert witness to give such evidence of opinion is dependent on the court deciding that an issue before it requires expert evidence. The court must also accept that the witness has the appropriate expertise to give that opinion.

In order to be an expert witness, the witness must have 'specialised knowledge based on the person's training, study or experience' [3]. Doctors are one of the most commonly used experts in hearings.

Expert evidence is usually called in matters concerned with an organised branch of learning, such as medicine or science, where a judge or jury would generally lack the training necessary to understand the significance of certain findings. It may also be admitted where a special occupational knowledge or skill is helpful. For example, a jeweller could express an opinion about the value or authenticity of a certain piece of jewellery, this being an opinion that probably all members of a jury would be unqualified to express. Before admission of such evidence of opinion, the expert witness proffered to the court must be qualified as such. Whether the area in which the expert is called to give evidence is an area of expertise and whether the qualifications and/or expertise of the expert witness are sufficient are matters for the judge to decide [4].

Consistent with the practices of the adversarial system, experts are called by one or the other party to the proceedings. However, as the guidelines noted above require, the primary function of an expert witness is to assist the court by putting it in possession of information essential to its decision. While such evidence may be expected to favour the arguments of the party calling the expert, it is not the expert's task to undertake any partisan presentation of the medical issues. The doctor should be an expert, but not an advocate. Regardless of who called them, experts must maintain their impartiality and be aware that their overriding duty is to assist the court.

Doctors need to remain mindful of the scope of their specialised knowledge and advise the court if they are being asked for opinions that fall outside their area of expertise. Journeys outside the doctor's particular field of expertise may be encouraged by experienced counsel with the aim of discrediting or lessening the weight that may be given to the evidence. Such temptation is to be resisted. When called to court, doctors should seek advice from their professional bodies, senior colleagues, medical indemnity insurers or the lawyers involved.

26.6 Subpoena or other court order

A subpoena is a summons issued by a court that is served on a witness to attend a court at a specified time and place, for a specific purpose. Failure to respond to a valid subpoena without good cause is contempt of court, and a judge may order that the absent witness be arrested, or brought before the court. When witnesses cannot attend, they should advise the party calling them of the circumstances. Strictly, witnesses are required to remain in the precincts of the court for the duration of the trial, although professional witnesses such as doctors can usually make arrangements with the prosecutor or lawyers calling them so that they are not required to wait too long at court before appearing.

Documents, including medical records, may also be the subject of a subpoena or other order of a court and may also be requested by some tribunals. Such a subpoena must also be answered. The subpoena should indicate whether the original record or a photocopy is requested. If the original file is requested, a copy should be kept by the doctor [5]. It is in the interests of patients that material in their files not relevant to the issues in the case to which the subpoena relates be withheld from disclosure. Subpoenas are orders of the court and documents are produced to the court, not to either party's lawyers. The judge has power to decide what material is relevant and should be disclosed. In responding to a subpoena for a patient's complete file, doctors should be willing to inform the lawyers acting for patients of material that appears irrelevant to the issues in the case, disclosure of which would be detrimental to the patient's interests.

In public hospitals, subpoenas are sometimes issued to junior medical staff, who may be asked to attend court with the hospital records, even though they may have had limited or no contact with the particular patient. In such situations, it is important that the doctor involved should notify and discuss the subpoena with the hospital administration or medicolegal department for advice.

26.7 The doctor as a witness

As discussed earlier, in their professional capacity doctors will usually appear in courts as a witness, either as a treating doctor or as an expert witness, and, less commonly, as a defendant in a medical negligence claim or other action. As treating doctors, they may give medical evidence about the condition of a plaintiff, injuries received in a motor vehicle accident, injuries suffered by a victim of an assault, or sometimes in Family Court matters.

Once notified of the possibility of being called as a witness, good preparation should include, as a minimum:

- making contact with the solicitor calling you as a witness to clarify what is required, to check the date and venue, to ensure that you will be readily contactable in case of delays or adjournments, and to clarify who is responsible for notifying whom if changes occur
- re-reading all the relevant material
- collecting the relevant medical records and copies of any statements you have prepared (and in the case of expert witnesses, any reference material to be relied on) to take with you to the court.

In addition, at any hearing, the doctor should dress professionally, as appearances may affect the assessment of the evidence provided.

The expectations of the court reflect the nature of the evidence to be provided. For treating doctors who are not specialists or experts in the field in question, the evidence should be restricted to the care provided to the patient and the history and examination findings of relevance. At times, barristers may try to elicit expert evidence from such witnesses, and doctors must be careful not to be tempted to answer questions beyond the scope of their expertise. Apart from this qualification, much of the advice in section 26.7.1 for expert witnesses is applicable to the role of the treating doctor as a witness. The Australian Medical Association has issued a detailed guide to the professional and ethical obligations of doctors who are asked to give evidence [5].

26.7.1 The experience of being a medical witness

Medical witnesses, whether lay or expert, may be upset by the adversarial nature of courts. A doctor-witness should not react in a hostile manner to this environment, and the cross-examination should not be regarded as a reflection on, or challenge to, the competence or integrity of the doctor. More usefully, the process should be viewed as one in which the doctor is made accountable in public for the views that they express. This fact should be in the doctor's mind at the time a report is prepared. A medical expert witness should not attempt to verbally competitively engage with counsel, who are usually much more versed in and used to such encounters. Sarcasm is out of place and any humour, if attempted at all, should be respectful, relevant and limited. A calm demeanour will add to the credibility of the evidence. Lawyers preparing for an important case are likely to have gone to considerable lengths to inform themselves on the subject matter of the case, and medical witnesses should not assume that they alone have all the medical knowledge.

Courts and tribunals increasingly are taking expert evidence by video link or telephone. While this saves time for doctors, it brings with it less sense of the formality of the court/hearing room. Doctors who give evidence by this means need to be just as well prepared (e.g. by having all the relevant records and reports at hand) and conduct themselves just as professionally as if they were attending in person.

Doctors need to recognise that the scope of what is relevant to the strategy of lawyers in court may be quite different to that which the doctor would consider relevant to the patient's condition. The lawyers' strategic needs govern the questions they ask and the answers they seek. Doctors may find it frustrating that they are not given the opportunity to contribute all that they know of the facts or all of their opinions as experts.

Every time doctors step into the witness box to give evidence, whether as a young doctor working in an emergency department, an experienced general practitioner or a senior specialist, they should make a determined effort to perform well and appear to the court as being professional, well informed, objective and impartial. This involves not taking sides, not arguing or becoming personally hostile with counsel and being tolerant of apparently ill-informed questions. Witnesses should only answer the question asked, should not volunteer information beyond that and should not normally speak directly to the judge unless the judge addresses them directly. If counsel objects to a question put to the witness, a witness should not attempt to answer the question until the judge has ruled on the objection. If the witness feels that important evidence or views are not being sought or are being misconstrued, the witness may address these concerns to the judge.

To be of greatest assistance to the court, medical witnesses should familiarise themselves with the relevant facts of the case and with the relevant professional literature in relation to the area in which they will be giving evidence. Preparation should include conferring with the barrister calling them prior to their appearance in court. When attending court, they should bring all relevant medical documents such as clinical notes, results of investigations, imaging and pathology reports. They are generally able to refer to medical or scientific literature to substantiate their opinions. This literature should be available to be produced in court if required. Medical and scientific evidence should be stated clearly and accurately in terms likely to be understandable to the court, so medical and scientific jargon must be avoided whenever possible. Answers to questions should generally be brief and to the point. Medical witnesses should also avoid trying to second-guess barristers or engage in debate or gamesmanship. The expert witness must be honest and attempt to make known to the court the limits of reliability of the evidence and the inferences that may be properly drawn from it. It is always acceptable to say 'I don't know' (if that is so), or to state that a specific matter is outside one's area of expertise.

Re-examination normally concludes the matter for expert medical witnesses, who are usually formally excused from further attendance. If not excused, they may be required to remain in the court precincts and may be called back to the witness box. The lawyers will advise in this regard.

Finally, doctors appearing as expert witnesses need to appreciate that they are participating in a process that society has developed over centuries, and one which is very different from the scientific and experimental approach used to finding the 'truth' in science or medicine. Court procedures change gradually. For example, both the Federal Court and the Federal Administrative Appeals Tribunal now provide the opportunity in selected cases for expert witnesses to confer for the purpose of narrowing the contested evidence and then to give their evidence and be cross-examined in front of each other, and to be questioned by the presiding officer. This process is known as concurrent evidence, or informally by lawyers as a 'hot tub' [6].

26.7.2 Fees for court appearances

In civil cases, doctors who have given evidence to the court should send an account for their services to the solicitor on whose behalf the doctor was called. Under legislation, courts and tribunals set scales of fees for court attendance, which are updated from time to time, but these are not binding on doctors. When giving evidence upon request from a statutory agency, witness fees are normally prescribed, although they are reviewed from time to time with input from medical professional associations. Information regarding the recommended fee scales may be obtained from a doctor's medical defence organisation.

26.8 Doctors and jury duty

In general, doctors are not automatically excused from jury duty simply because of their profession, but when called for duty may be excused if they provide 'good reason'. This covers more obvious matters such as ill health or incapacity and, for rural doctors, undue time lost travelling, but also includes severe financial or personal hardship. On this last ground, prolonged absence from a medical practice might be argued as likely to cause hardship to current patients or financial hardship to a self-employed doctor [7].

However, doctors should always consider accepting invitations to participate in jury duty. The effectiveness of the legal system, and in particular the criminal trial, relies heavily on participation and involvement of jurors who are representative of the broad spectrum of societal members. Doctors can play an important role in ensuring that goal is met, and that their particular skills and experiences contribute to the effective functioning of juries.

Summary

It is a professional responsibility of doctors to assist the justice system, allowing our society to function with appropriate safeguards for everyone. Such participation should not be feared or seen as a burden, or a challenge to a doctor's professionalism or expert knowledge. Rather, it is best regarded as appropriate participation in society and maintaining justice and protection of our societal standards and expectations.

If doctors as lay witnesses or expert witnesses are well prepared and understand the processes and expectations, participation in the justice system should provide a modicum of pride for the contribution the individual has made.

References

1. Australian Medical Association. Ethical guidelines for conducting independent medical assessments 2010. Revised 2015. https://www.ama.com.au/position-statement/ethical-guidelines-independent-medical-assessments-2010-revised-2015 (accessed Aug 2025).
2. Australian Medical Association. Guidelines for report preparation and court attendance in relation to independent medical assessments 2010. https://ama.com.au/sites/default/files/documents/Guidelines_for_Report_Preparation_and_Court_Attendance_in_Relation_to_Independent_Medical_Assessments_2010.pdf (accessed Aug 2025).
3. *Evidence Act 1995* (NSW), s 79(1).
4. Freckleton I, Selby H, editors. Expert evidence: law, practice, procedure and advocacy. 4th ed. Sydney: Law Book Company, 2009.
5. Australian Medical Association. Ethical guidelines for doctors acting as medical witnesses—2011. https://ama.com.au/sites/default/files/documents/Doctors_Acting_as_Medical_Witnesses_0.pdf (accessed Aug 2025).
6. Administrative Review Tribunal. Administrative Review Tribunal (Expert Evidence) Practice Direction. 2024. https://www.art.gov.au/about/news-and-updates/new-practice-direction-giving-expert-evidence (accessed Aug 2025).
7. Jury duty. *Medical Observer* 2006; Dec 8: 45–46.

Further reading

Beran RG. The role of the expert witness in the adversarial legal system. *J Law Med* 2009; 17: 133–137.

Freckleton I, Selby H, editors. Expert evidence: law, practice, procedure and advocacy. 5th ed. Sydney: Law Book Company, 2013.

27 Medical records, reports and certificates

Ruanne Brell

Introduction

It is essential to make and retain clear and contemporaneous medical records. They ensure safe and efficient ongoing patient care and are also crucial when investigating a claim or complaint in relation to any medical care provided. This chapter discusses the importance of medical records, the essential components, and the position regarding matters such as ownership of and access to medical records. Issues related to information technology and its application to medical records are also discussed.

27.1 The importance of medical records

Medical records are an important component of good medical care and must be complete, accurate and up to date. Primarily, their purpose is to record clinical information for use in patient management and as a means of communication with other doctors and health professionals. Therefore, the medical record should contain sufficient information to enable another doctor to take over the care and management of the patient. This applies in all contexts where a medical record is being maintained for a patient, whether doctors are in solo practice, a group specialist or general practice, or private or public hospital settings.

Medical records can also be important for clinical and epidemiological research, teaching and health administration, and in litigation. Lawyers and medical defence organisations often stress the importance of documentation. Requests for information about patients come not only from other doctors, but also from insurers, employers, police, lawyers and government agencies, for legal, financial or other reasons. Accurate medical records are essential for all of these. (See also Chapter 15, Family violence, child maltreatment and elder abuse, and Chapter 26, Medicolegal examinations and reports, court procedures and expert evidence.)

Incomplete, inadequate or illegible records carry risks for both practitioners and patients. Medical records will be scrutinised by regulators and judicial bodies in the context of a claim or complaint, and failure to meet the required standard will be criticised.

When entering information in medical records, doctors should also ensure they remember the importance of good patient communication and strike the right balance between this and the need to make accurate and complete contemporaneous notes. Communication is addressed in Chapter 5, Communication in clinical practice.

Another professional responsibility closely related to good medical record keeping is the need to keep those records confidential. Doctors should appreciate the ethical principles and laws related to the release of any information from the medical record; these are discussed in section 27.9. Confidentiality and privacy are discussed in Chapter 6, Confidentiality, privacy and disclosure.

27.2 What is a medical record?

The term 'medical record' is used to refer to many different types of data about a person's health. It is used interchangeably with terms such as clinical record, clinical notes, medical notes and others. The term is encompassed but not adopted in the terminology of the privacy laws, which refer instead to 'personal information' and 'health information'.

Essentially, the medical record includes information about the medical history, findings on physical examination, possible diagnoses, investigations ordered, treatment provided and follow-up advice. The record also includes correspondence to and from other doctors, hospitals and health professionals, as well as imaging, test results, videos, photographs, reports, and certificates and other forms completed for or about the patient.

Normally, copies of medicolegal reports, such as those requested by and provided to lawyers and insurers, are held within the patient's medical record, but these should not be released without the permission of the requesting party. (See also Chapter 6, Confidentiality, privacy and disclosure, and Chapter 26, Medicolegal examinations and reports, court procedures and expert evidence.)

Documentation about a patient complaint or claim and correspondence with a medical indemnity organisation about a patient do not form part of the patient's medical record.

27.3 Guidelines for medical records

Section 10.5 of the Medical Board of Australia's *Good medical practice: a code of conduct for doctors in Australia* [1] advises that good practice includes:

> 10.5.1 Keeping accurate, up to date and legible records that report relevant details of clinical history, clinical findings, investigations, diagnosis, information given to patients, medication, referral and other management in a form that can be understood by other health practitioners.
>
> 10.5.2 Ensuring that your medical records are held securely and are protected against unauthorised access.
>
> 10.5.3 Ensuring that your medical records show respect for your patients and do not include demeaning or derogatory remarks.
>
> 10.5.4 Ensuring that the records are sufficient to facilitate continuity of patient care.
>
> 10.5.5 Making records at the time of the events, or as soon as possible afterwards.
>
> 10.5.6 Dating any changes and additions to medical records, including when the record is electronic.
>
> 10.5.7 Recognising patients' right to access information contained in their medical records and facilitating that access.
>
> 10.5.8 Promptly facilitating the transfer of health information when requested by the patient or third party with requisite authority.
>
> 10.5.9 Retaining records for the period required by law and ensuring they are destroyed securely when they are no longer required.

Medicare Australia has also issued advice about the need to maintain adequate and contemporaneous records in relation to the payment of Medicare benefits to patients and has defined its meaning of *adequate* and *contemporaneous* [2].

The professional college or society for certain specialties may also have specific guidance regarding medical records.

27.4 The content of medical records

27.4.1 What should be documented?

Some state and territory laws and regulations govern what must be included in the medical record, for example, in New South Wales [3], Victoria [4] and the Australian Capital Territory [5]. However, these are not replicated across all jurisdictions.

Generally, the medical record should include any information relevant to the diagnosis or treatment of the patient. Any entry in the record needs to be clear, accurate and legible, and contain clinical findings, decisions made, information given to patients, treatment prescribed, investigation(s) requested, and sufficient information to enable another doctor to continue the care of the patient.

The record should be made contemporaneously with the consultation, or as soon as practicable after it (e.g. in emergencies). If the record is not being made at the same time as the consultation or treatment, the entry should include the date and time it is being made.

The Royal Australian College of General Practitioners (RACGP) 'Standards for general practices' (the RACGP Standards) emphasise that patient demographic information should include the full name of the patient, date of birth and contact details to ensure the patient can be correctly identified [6]. The RACGP Standards encourage doctors to record the contact information of the person the patient nominates to be notified in an emergency.

Records should be legible and contemporaneous and contain:

- the history obtained from the patient, including positive and relevant negative features
- examination findings, including both positive and negative findings that impact the differential diagnosis
- the provisional diagnosis reached
- any differential diagnosis considered
- the management plan, including the options discussed with the patient, treatment recommended, prescriptions and tests
- the information provided to the patient and the patient's consent to any treatments.

Records should also include the following details of any medical treatment:

- the date of the treatment
- the nature of the treatment
- where a drug is prescribed, the name and dose including duration and route
- information or advice given to the patient (including diagrams and information sheets), for example, about material risks
- documentation of patient consent to treatment

- the name of any person involved in the treatment
- details of any anaesthetic given to the patient
- details of any tissue sent to pathology
- the results or findings made in relation to the treatment.

A good rule of thumb is to think about what another doctor would want to know from the medical records if they were taking over the patient's care without having the opportunity to speak to the previous doctor [7].

Correspondence to, from or about a patient's clinical care should be kept in the patient's medical record. All telephone calls and telephone messages should be documented in the patient's medical record, including the time and date of the call and what was included in the message.

27.4.2 What should not be documented?

Medical records should always be made keeping in mind that others can and will read them. It should be remembered that patients are entitled to request access to their medical records (see sections 27.8 and 27.9 for more information about ownership and access to medical records).

Avoid any thoughtless, unnecessary or disparaging remarks about the patient or their treatment, or about colleagues. Avoid non-standard abbreviations or obscure shorthand as this can lack clarity and hinder continuity of care.

On occasion, patients may request that sensitive information about them is not documented in their medical record. These requests should be carefully managed. If the information is clinically relevant, then it must be included in the record. Patients can be reassured about the confidentiality of the medical record.

Situations might also arise where a patient requests that information in the medical records be corrected or deleted.

27.4.3 Correcting or deleting information in the medical record

The question of correcting or deleting information in the medical record may arise when:

1. *a patient states that information in their medical record is incorrect and requests that it be corrected; or*
2. *a doctor becomes aware the information is incorrect.*

Generally, patients have the right to request correction of their health information and should do so in writing. The doctor or practice receiving such a request should consider it and respond within a reasonable timeframe (usually 30 days) by either correcting the information or informing the patient that the request has been declined.

If a patient requests that information be corrected or deleted, it is important to first establish that there is in fact an error, and not just a difference of opinion. This involves considering whether the information is inaccurate, out of date, incomplete, irrelevant or misleading. This is rarely the case given the requirements for contemporaneous medical records to be made as discussed above. Also, the retention requirements that apply to medical records (discussed in section 27.7) generally prevent information from being deleted from the medical record.

Errors in demographic information can simply be updated. Otherwise, previous records should generally not be changed; the new or additional information from patients can be documented in a separate entry.

If the request is declined, the patient must be notified in writing, setting out the reasons for refusal (unless unreasonable to do so) and the complaints mechanism available to the individual making the request. That letter can be saved in the medical record.

If a correction is made, other entities should be notified of the correction; this will usually mean other doctors or health practitioners involved in the patient's care.

More information about managing requests from patients for correction or deletion of information in their medical record is available from the Office of the Australian Information Commissioner (OAIC) [8,9]. Examples of situations in which a patient may request a correction or deletion are shown in Box 27.1.

Box 27.1 Examples of situations in which a patient may request a correction or deletion

Example 1: A patient becomes aware that the medical practice has incorrectly recorded their middle name (Pauline instead of Paula) in the notes after seeing it on a referral for pathology investigations. The patient raises it with the practice and shows a copy of their photo identification confirming the correct name. The practice can correct the patient's middle name in the medical record as this is simple demographic information, and it is important that this is correct so there is no confusion about patient identity.

Example 2: At a patient's first consultation with a cardiologist, they reported a family history including persistent low blood pressure on their mother's side. This was documented in the consultation notes on that day. At a subsequent consultation many months later, the patient reports that they were incorrect and in fact their mother had high blood pressure. They also report additional information that their maternal grandfather had high blood pressure and died from a stroke. The doctor should include this new information in the consultation note of the date the information is given, with reference to the consultation date of the previous incorrect information. They should also correct the information in the patient's health summary to note the mother's high blood pressure, not low blood pressure. No additions or deletions should be made to the original consultation note where low blood pressure was mentioned. The information about the maternal grandfather can be added to the health summary as well.

Example 3: The patient asks their general practitioner to delete a copy of a psychiatrist's report diagnosing the patient with personality disorder from their medical record and delete the diagnosis from the list of conditions on the patient's health summary, as the patient does not accept this diagnosis. The doctor considers the request and determines it is a difference of opinion and that the information is accurate, up to date and not misleading. A letter is sent to the patient informing them of the refusal to delete the report and informing them of the complaints process if they wish to pursue it. An entry is also made in the patient's medical record along the lines of: 'The patient has requested that the report of Dr X dated X be deleted because the patient believes the information contained is untrue. This request has been declined—see letter to the patient dated X.'

The key steps in responding to a request from a patient for correction of personal information are summarised in Figure 27.1.

Figure 27.1 Dealing with a patient's correction request

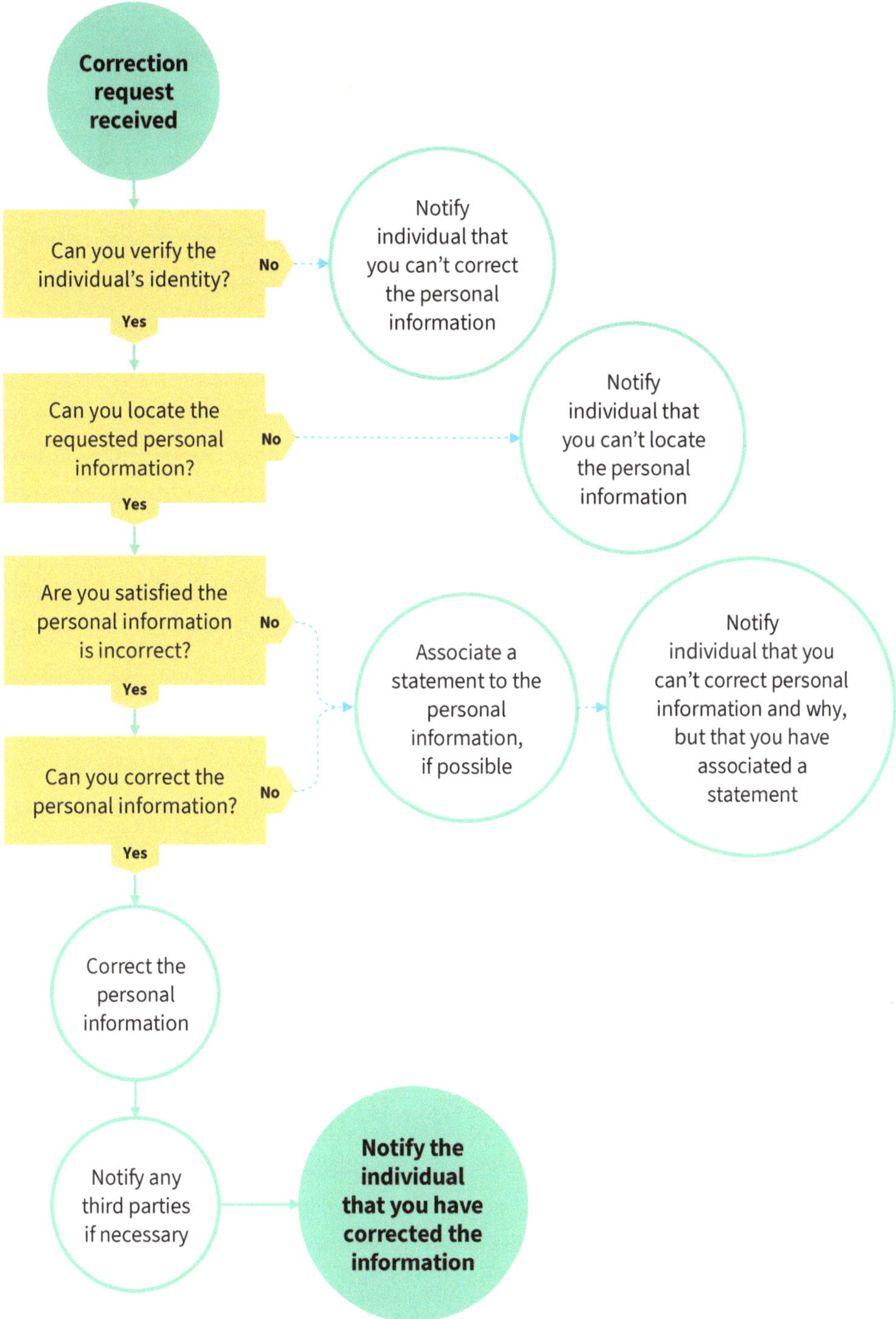

Source: Office of the Australian Information Commissioner, reproduced with permission (https://www.oaic.gov.au/privacy/privacy-guidance-for-organisations-and-government-agencies/health-service-providers/guide-to-health-privacy/chapter-5-correcting-health-information).

27.5 Medical certificates

Medical certificates are legal documents. Doctors must always prepare certificates accurately and truthfully and within the scope of their skills and expertise. It is also important to have considered any supporting documentation and the findings from a thorough and appropriate physical examination where necessary.

A copy of the certificate should always be kept in the patient's medical record in case there is ever a dispute, and as a proper record of the document issued to the patient. The consultation on which the certificate is based should also be documented in the patient's medical record.

Most commonly, medical certificates are requested by patients to certify illness as required by the patient's employer. Certificates might also be requested to confirm a patient's fitness for a certain activity, or recovery from an illness or injury. This is separate from documents requested in relation to statutory schemes such as workers' compensation or other legislative schemes, which must be prepared in accordance with the requirements of the relevant scheme.

27.5.1 Legal requirements of medical certificates

A medical certificate should be clear and legible and include:

- the doctor's name and practice address
- the name of the patient
- the date the patient was examined
- the date the certificate was issued
- the matter being certified and the relevant time period.

Generally, the certificate should not include details of the patient's diagnosis as it is not required for the certificate to be valid and this protects the patient's privacy. In some circumstances, including a diagnosis is required. This should only be done with the patient's consent. If the patient does not authorise release of any details regarding their diagnosis, this should be documented on the certificate and in the medical record. Doctors should also advise the patient that more information may be required. This may ultimately be something the patient needs to address with the organisation requiring the certificate.

Certificates should always be dated the day that the patient was examined and the certificate is issued. They should never be backdated. If the time period being certified starts before the date of the certificate, it should be clearly stated that this is based on the history from the patient together with any findings on examination.

27.5.2 Medical certificates certifying illness

A certificate certifying illness may be issued where a patient has a medical condition that requires time away from work. Most commonly this is because that person is too ill to work, but on occasion (e.g. an infectious disease) it may be because the person should not be at work because of risks to others.

The requirements for a medical certificate regarding illness for work are listed in section 27.5.1.

Even if an employer expects the certificate to include a diagnosis, this is not required, although it can be provided with consent of the patient. For some patients and some illnesses, the patient may not readily appreciate the significance of revealing that information to their employer, and it may fall to the doctor to confirm that it is not mandatory to state the diagnosis on the certificate.

There may be situations where the patient attends late in the course of an illness or the doctor otherwise feels unable to certify an illness following an examination. This should be carefully explained to the patient and documented in the patient's medical record. The RACGP encourages doctors to have a system for documenting these types of ethical dilemmas [10].

One option in this situation is to provide a letter instead of a medical certificate. That letter can state the history given by the patient and any findings on examination, and the patient can then choose to present that to their employer. It should be noted that there are no strict rules about the types of evidence that can be given to substantiate a claim for sick or carer's leave. Statutory declarations from the employee or another person may also be acceptable [11,12]. Given the professional responsibility involved, doctors should decline to provide a certificate if not convinced that it is warranted based on the patient's presentation.

From time to time, employers may contact the doctor who issued a medical certificate for more information about the patient's illness. In this situation, the doctor or practice should verify the identity of the person making the request and ask to see a copy of the certificate being queried. It can then be confirmed whether or not the certificate was provided by the doctor. No other information should be given without express consent from the patient.

The Australian Medical Association states that patients also have responsibilities when requesting certificates of unfitness to work, including attending in a timely manner, being honest in the description of their incapacity and not altering the certificate in any way [13]. If a patient does alter a medical certificate, it may be warranted for the doctor to consider the ongoing therapeutic relationship with that patient. This will depend on the circumstances [14].

27.5.3 Certificates for carer's leave

Under federal workplace legislation, employees can also take leave to care for an immediate family or household member who is sick or injured, or help during a family emergency [15]. The requirements outlined in section 27.5.2 also apply when issuing a carer's certificate.

Doctors may issue a certificate for a patient's family member for this purpose, ensuring the patient (who is not the employee and may not be a patient of the doctor providing the certificate) consents to the certificate being issued if possible. Additional care should be taken to ensure no confidential or sensitive health information is released.

27.5.4 Other certificates

A patient may ask their doctor to complete a certificate to support an application for early release of superannuation benefits to fund their treatment. This is only available in very limited circumstances determined by the Australian Taxation Office [16].

With requests for these certificates and any other certificate or form doctors are asked to complete, it is important to be accurate and truthful at all times. Sometimes it can be difficult to separate the patient's desires and plans from the clinical realities, or the requirements of the document. If in doubt in a particular situation, referral to a relevant specialist or discussion with a medical indemnity provider may be appropriate.

Certification of births is done under state and territory requirements and is usually carried out by a parent of the child. Certification of deaths is covered in Chapter 28, Diagnosing and certifying death and the role of the coroner. Chapter 32, Legal frameworks: rights, responsibilities and protections, covers the notification of infectious diseases and certification of fitness to drive. Doctors are in certain cases bound by law to give certificates, notifications, reports and similar documents for use either in courts of justice or for administrative purposes.

27.6 Electronic medical records

Electronic medical records are now widely used instead of paper-based records, usually as the sole form of the medical record. Regardless of the form of the record, the same requirements regarding content, privacy and confidentiality apply. Some regulations for the content of medical records also require that medical records stored electronically are capable of being printed [17].

There are some specific forms of electronic records, as well as digital content within the record.

27.6.1 My Health Record

My Health Record (previously known as the personally controlled electronic health record) was developed by the federal government and is operated by the Australian Digital Health Agency (ADHA). It is best described as an online summary of a patient's health information. It is not the patient's complete medical record for any healthcare provider or organisation. It does not replace the need to create an appropriate patient medical record and keep it updated and communicate with patients or other practitioners about clinically significant results.

The My Health Record system was designed to improve communication between healthcare providers, and the quality and availability of information between healthcare providers. It remains an opt-in system for healthcare providers but an opt-out system for patients.

Doctors considering opting in to using My Health Record should weigh up the benefits to their patients against the risks. The ADHA has developed resources to assist with this assessment and when using the system [18], and a mobile phone app is also available.

27.6.2 Email and other electronic communication

Email is an increasingly prevalent and convenient method of communication. There has been persistent uncertainty about whether email can be used in clinical practice and, if so, how to do it safely. See Chapter 6, Confidentiality, privacy and disclosure, and Chapter 29, Professional practice, digital technology and artificial intelligence, for a detailed discussion of these issues. As with any communication with or about a patient's clinical care, emails need to be documented in or saved to the patient's medical record. The same applies to text messages, as these form part of the medical record and need to be included in the patient's record. Some electronic health record systems do this automatically.

27.6.3 Digital images

Images may be taken for various purposes in clinical and medicolegal practice, and their use is increasing. Chapter 29, Professional practice, digital technology and artificial intelligence, discusses these developments in more detail. Issues regarding consent for taking and using images are discussed in Chapter 7, Consent and informed decision making.

When taking or using digital images for clinical care, the image should be stored in the patient's medical record. This applies even if the image is of a document that is already part of the patient's medical record, as it is important that there is a record of what was included in the image itself. Consent for the image being taken, and shared, should also be documented in the patient's medical record.

In addition to privacy legislation and professional guidelines, health organisations may also have their own policies about how clinical images should be used and stored in the context of the medical record. This includes private practices and hospitals, and is particularly the case for public hospitals, where there may also be additional requirements arising from state records legislation. See Chapter 6, Confidentiality, privacy and disclosure, for more detail.

27.6.4 Messaging apps

Online communication and messaging platforms are increasingly being used in clinical practice, mainly using popular general applications, and some applications are being developed specifically for use in a health context.

When messages are sent about patient care using messaging apps, these are written records in the same way as other communication about patients and should be treated as such. This means that privacy and confidentiality obligations will apply, as will any legislative requirements regarding the messages being stored in the patient's medical record and how long they must be kept for. Organisations may also have policies about when and how these messages are kept [19].

The doctor who sends the clinical information using a messaging app is the person responsible for ensuring it is saved into the patient's medical record. If it is not clear from the message itself, the participants in the communication and when it took place should also be documented in the medical record.

27.6.5 Artificial intelligence scribe tools

Medical scribe tools using artificial intelligence (AI) are being developed and implemented to assist doctors with the creation of clinical notes. These scribing tools generate a draft clinical note from the consultation. It is important that these drafts are checked for accuracy, and corrected and added to before being saved to the patient's medical record, as it is the doctor's responsibility to ensure that their records are accurate. This is a developing and rapidly changing area. More information is included in Chapter 29, Professional practice, digital technology and artificial intelligence.

27.7 Storage and security of records

It is important that medical records are stored in a way that facilitates reasonable access to the records for continuity of the patient's treatment. In addition, privacy law demands that reasonable steps are taken to protect personal information from misuse, loss, unauthorised access, modification or disclosure.

27.7.1 Security requirements

In practice, this means that measures must be in place for how medical records are stored and who has access to them. Hardcopy medical records should be stored securely, such as in a locked cabinet or room, or secure storage facility. For electronic records, security requirements include password protection, regular backup and offsite storage of backed-up records. Antivirus software and encryption should also be used where possible.

It is prudent to have policies and procedures outlining these security measures, and also confirming that staff should only access medical records for legitimate clinical purposes. This will often also be stated in employment contracts and applicable codes of conduct in public health facilities, and in private employment contracts.

27.7.2 Retention requirements

Requirements for retaining medical records differ across organisations and jurisdictions within Australia. The retention requirements outlined by specific legislation in the ACT, NSW and Victoria [20–23] are consistent. These requirements are:

- For adult patients, records should be kept for seven years from the date of the last entry in the records.
- For children, records should be kept until the child would have turned or will turn 25 years old.

In the states and territories where there is no legislation, it is recommended that medical records are kept for the same time periods.

There are no specific requirements for obstetric records, but it is recommended that the records of the mother and the child are retained for 25 years from the birth of the child.

If a practitioner dies before the time periods above have passed, the obligation to retain the records transfers to the practitioner's estate.

In the public sector, there are specific authorities, policies and guidelines to manage medical records. Record management requirements can depend on a range of factors, particularly the state or territory where the patient sought care, their illness and their age. If the hospital or facility holds the medical record, it will be managed by that facility and covered by its policies. It is important for doctors to be familiar with any specific requirements relating to medical records in the hospitals or organisations in which they work.

27.8 Ownership of medical records

Ownership of the medical record is a separate matter from access to the information contained in the record. Under the common law, medical records are owned by the individual or entity responsible for making the record, usually an individual practitioner, a private practice, or a public or private hospital [24]. Subsequent legislation introduced regimes for access to medical records, discussed in section 27.9.

In public hospitals or facilities, the medical records will be owned by the hospital or facility. It is not always straightforward in private settings. While the common law settled the issue of ownership between patients and doctors, it did not address the issue of ownership between groups of private professionals, or an individual doctor and a private practice. The privacy legislation may also impact these issues of ownership, as could specific contractual terms or, absent that, the intention of the parties in any dispute. An example of a legal dispute concerning ownership of records is outlined in Box 27.2.

Box 27.2 *Health Services for Men Pty Ltd & Ors v D'Souza & Ors* [2000] NSWCA 56

The appellants owned and operated 21 clinics in different states and had 10 different doctors who worked across those clinics. The doctors had agreements with the appellants about how payments were to be made, but the agreements did not include terms about ownership of the medical records. When three doctors parted ways with the appellant, they removed patient files from the premises, consisting primarily of examination sheets and pathology reports. The appellants sought orders from the NSW Court of Appeal to ensure the return of those patient medical records.

In the absence of any specific contractual terms, the Court of Appeal looked at the specific circumstances, including the way patients came to see the doctors at the clinics, the administrative support provided by the clinic and the role of the doctors. It determined that the appellant owned the records and the respondent doctors had no property in the medical records. In doing so, the Court of Appeal commented that the pathology reports may be in a different category—that is, at the time it is prepared, the report is the property of the pathology provider. When it is sent to the doctor who requested it, the report becomes the property of that doctor. However, in the particular circumstances of this case, the pathology reports were determined to be the property of the clinic.

Increasingly, both doctors and practices include terms about the ownership of medical records in written agreements. This would be the starting position if a dispute arose, together with anything else in writing between the parties on the issue. It is important to note that a written agreement between two private parties cannot override legislation. This usually means that even if a practice and practitioner, or individual practitioners, agreed that an individual practitioner could take a copy of all or certain records with them when they left the practice, that practitioner would still need patient consent before disclosing that information to a new practice, for example, so that a new practice could contact those patients.

While cases like the one described in Box 27.2 help establish some general principles, each case turns on its facts, and the individual circumstances will determine the outcome of any dispute.

27.9 Access to medical records

As mentioned above, privacy legislation now covers the right of patients to access their own records. It also sets out principles about who else may be able to access medical records, and how. The legislation and the associated privacy principles are discussed in greater detail in Chapter 6, Confidentiality, privacy and disclosure. The discussion in the following subsections addresses the principles related to patients accessing their own records and others getting access to those records.

27.9.1 Access by patients

Subject to some limited exceptions, privacy legislation gives patients a right to access their own medical records, which includes:

- getting a copy of their medical records
- reviewing their medical records
- requesting that someone else is provided with a copy of their records.

Ideally, a patient should request their medical records in writing. If the request is verbal, it should be documented by the doctor or staff member in the patient's records. The scope of the request should also be clear, as well as how the patient would like to receive the copy of their records.

A patient does not have to give a reason for their request. Enquiries can be made regarding the reason, but if the patient refuses to give one, this is not a sufficient reason to decline the request. Reasonable fees can be charged for facilitating access, but refusal to pay should not be a reason to withhold the records.

The limited exceptions to providing access are set out under the Commonwealth privacy legislation and the applicable state and territory laws, where they exist. Exceptions include where there may be a serious threat to the life, health or safety of the individual or another person, or it might prejudice an investigation.

In all states and territories, freedom of information legislation may also give right of access to health information held by public sector authorities such as public hospitals. Typically, this legislation provides similar exceptions to those in health privacy acts. Given the legislative frameworks in place, doctors are advised to first seek advice from their medical indemnity organisation or from the relevant health privacy office (see Table 6.1 in Chapter 6, Confidentiality, privacy and disclosure).

27.9.2 Access by other health professionals and staff

Under the privacy laws, it is permissible for another doctor or health professional to obtain a patient's medical records without specific consent where they are involved in the patient's treatment for the same condition. This is derived from the wording of the privacy legislation regarding the primary and secondary purposes for which the record was made, and is discussed in detail in Chapter 6, Confidentiality, privacy and disclosure.

Other staff who may physically have access to patients' medical records should only ever access them for legitimate clinical purposes. Medical practices, individual practitioners, hospitals and the like must ensure that their privacy policy covers issues regarding access to medical records, and that all staff are adequately instructed in that policy (see Chapter 6, Confidentiality, privacy and disclosure).

27.9.3 Access by third parties

In some situations, release of medical records is compelled by law. This may be in the form of a summons, subpoena, or warrant from the police, or may be required under legislation. In these situations, patient consent is not required and access should be provided. In the case of a subpoena or summons, the patient or their representatives will usually be aware of the request and can address any concerns about the scope of the request, its relevance and who has access to the documents. Where release is compelled under legislation, the correspondence outlining the request should make clear reference to the legislation, and may also make it clear whether or not the patient is aware of the request or can be told.

Outside of those situations, generally all requests for records should be made with patient consent. Doctors will receive requests for access to medical records from a variety of sources including solicitors, insurers, compensation agencies and even family members. Ideally, the patient's consent should be in writing and signed and dated. If in any doubt about the scope or validity of the consent, it is important to contact the patient to clarify these aspects.

While release of records is often routine, doctors should not hesitate to seek advice from their indemnity insurer or professional association when any uncertainty exists.

A flowchart for decision making about the release of medical records to a third party is provided in Figure 27.2.

Figure 27.2 Providing medical records to a third party

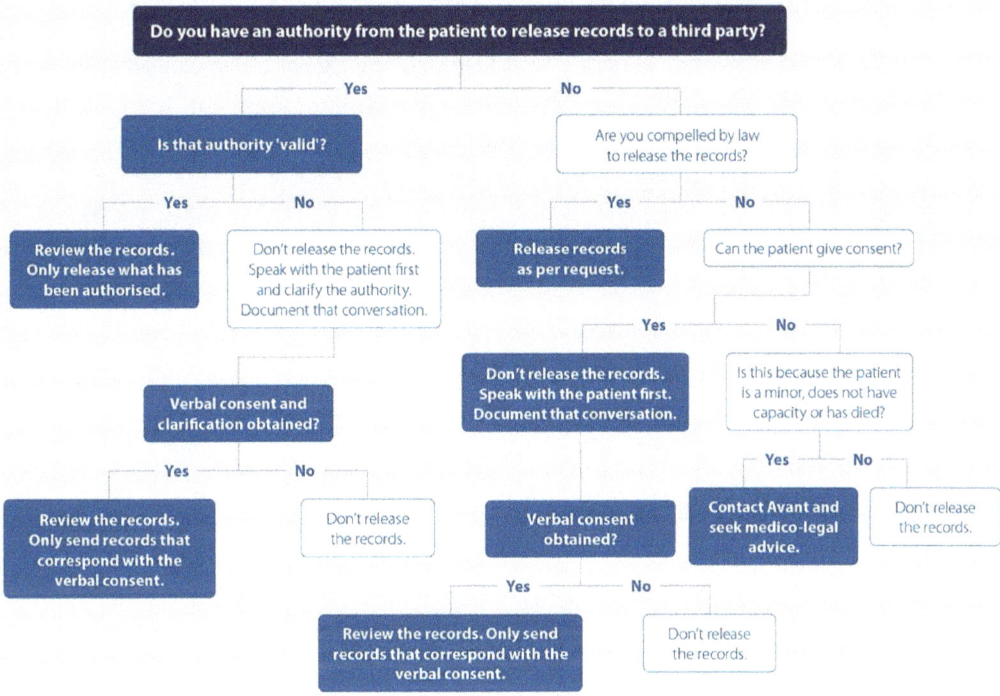

Source: Avant, reproduced with permission (https://avant.org.au/resources/providing-medical-records-to-a-third-party).

27.9.4 Access to medical records of deceased patients

The duty of confidentiality survives a patient's death. Once a patient dies, the executor or administrator of their estate is usually able to access the patient's records, or can authorise a third party to have access to their records. The executor is the person a patient appoints in their will as their representative. An administrator is someone appointed by the court if a patient dies without a will in place. The appropriate authorised person will not always be the patient's 'next of kin' or substitute decision maker. It is therefore important to check the status of the person requesting access to a deceased patient's records before disclosing any information. Once those checks have been made, the deceased's medical records can be released to the authorised person who stands in the place of the patient.

Public hospitals and facilities will have specific policies regarding the management of deceased patients' medical records.

27.9.5 Access to medical records for research

Using medical records for research, whether or not the records contain identifying information about the participants, has legal and ethical ramifications. The use of medical records in research is covered by federal privacy legislation and in some state privacy regimes. It is important that doctors are aware of and understand the limitations that privacy laws impose on the use of medical records for research and the processes that need to be followed. More details are provided in Chapter 31, Medical research.

27.10 Destruction of medical records

There is no specific legislation that requires medical records to be destroyed at a certain time. The effect of the Commonwealth privacy legislation (*Privacy Act 1988* [Cth]) is that medical records should be destroyed or permanently de-identified once they are no longer needed for the purpose for which they were created. This generally means that once records have been retained for the periods discussed in section 27.7.2 they should be securely destroyed. This may change if it is known that the medical records may be relevant to ongoing clinical management, a current claim or complaint, or future action.

When medical records are destroyed, a record of the destruction should be kept. Again, not all states and territories have legislation that addresses this, but it is recommended that all states and territories adopt the same approach. Therefore, at the time of destruction, a record should be made of the name of the patient, their date of birth, the period of time covered by the records and the date of destruction.

Records should be destroyed securely to ensure the confidentiality of the records is maintained. In practice, this is usually arranged through companies providing this specific service or through the facility that owns and controls the records. For electronic records, this can be done by securely deleting the device or file, often in discussion with an IT provider or software company.

Most states have subordinate legislation or guidelines concerning the disposal of medical records in public facilities.

Summary

Medical records are an essential part of clinical practice. It is important for doctors to understand the relevant legislative and professional requirements and become familiar with these to ensure compliance. Good medical records enhance the continuity and quality of patient care. They are also invaluable when responding to claims or complaints as the quality of the doctor's medical record will be a significant factor in the outcome of the matter.

References

1. Medical Board of Australia. Good medical practice: a code of conduct for doctors in Australia. 2020. https://www.medicalboard.gov.au/Codes-Guidelines-Policies/Code-of-conduct.aspx (accessed Jan 2025).
2. Australian Government Department of Health. Medicare Benefits Schedule book – Category 5: operating from 1 March 2021 (GN.15.39, p. 32–33). 2021. http://www.mbsonline.gov.au/internet/mbsonline/publishing.nsf/Content/4EFCF78281A91736CA258654001138AF/$File/202103-cat5.pdf (accessed Jun 2025).
3. Health Practitioner Regulation (New South Wales) Regulation 2016 (NSW), ss 1, 3 of Sch 4. https://legislation.nsw.gov.au/view/html/inforce/current/sl-2016-0543#sch.4 (accessed Jan 2025).
4. *Health Records Act 2001* (Vic), s 3.
5. *Health Records (Privacy and Access) Act 1997* (ACT), Dictionary.
6. Core Standard 7 – Content of patient health records. In: Royal Australian College of General Practitioners. Standards for general practices. 5th ed. 2020. https://www.racgp.org.au/getattachment/ece472a7-9a15-4441-b8e5-be892d4ffd77/Standards-for-general-practices-5th-edition.aspx (accessed Jan 2025).
7. Jammal W. 10 keys to good patient-centred record keeping. 2018. https://www.mcnsw.org.au/10-keys-good-patient-centred-record-keeping (accessed Jan 2025).
8. Office of the Australian Information Commissioner. Chapter 13: APP13 Correction of personal information. 2019. https://www.oaic.gov.au/privacy/australian-privacy-principles/australian-privacy-principles-guidelines/chapter-13-app-13-correction-of-personal-information (accessed Jun 2025).

9. Office of the Australian Information Commissioner. Chapter 5: Correcting health information. 2019. https://www.oaic.gov.au/privacy/privacy-guidance-for-organisations-and-government-agencies/health-service-providers/guide-to-health-privacy/chapter-5-correcting-health-information (accessed Jun 2025).
10. Criterion C2.1 – Respectful and culturally appropriate care. In: Royal Australian College of General Practitioners. Standards for general practices. 5th ed. 2020. https://www.racgp.org.au/getattachment/ece472a7-9a15-4441-b8e5-be892d4ffd77/Standards-for-general-practices-5th-edition.aspx (accessed Jan 2025).
11. *Fair Work Act 2009* (Cth), s 107.
12. Fair Work Ombudsman. Types of evidence needed for sick/carer's leave. https://www.fairwork.gov.au/leave/sick-and-carers-leave/paid-sick-and-carers-leave/notice-and-medical-certificates (accessed Jun 2025).
13. Australian Medical Association. AMA guidelines on medical certificates 2011, revised 2016. 2016. https://ama.com.au/sites/default/files/documents/AMA_Guidelines_on_Medical_Certificates_2011._Revised_2016_0.pdf (accessed Apr 2022).
14. Avant. Medical certificates: your responsibilities. 2025. https://www.avant.org.au/Resources/Public/Medical-certificates-and-your-responsibilities (accessed Jun 2025).
15. *Fair Work Act 2009* (Cth), ss 96, 97, 107.
16. Australian Taxation Office. Early access to super. https://www.ato.gov.au/individuals/super/withdrawing-and-using-your-super/Early-access-to-your-super/ (accessed Jun 2025).
17. Health Practitioner Regulation (New South Wales) Regulation 2016 (NSW), Sch 4, s 4.
18. Australian Government Australian Digital Health Agency. My Health Record: information for healthcare providers and organisations. 2024. https://www.myhealthrecord.gov.au/for-healthcare-professionals (accessed Jun 2025).
19. Avant. Messaging apps: communicating safely in clinical practice. 2021. https://www.avant.org.au/resources/public/messaging-apps-communicating-safely-in-clinical-practice (accessed Jun 2025).
20. *Health Records (Privacy and Access) Act 1997* (ACT), Sch 1, Principle 4.1(2).
21. *Health Records and Information Privacy Act 2002* (NSW), s 25.
22. Health Practitioner Regulation (New South Wales) Regulation 2016 (NSW), Pt 3, s 9.
23. *Health Records Act 2001* (Vic), Sch 1, Principle 4.2.
24. *Breen v Williams* (1995) 186 CLR 71.

Further reading

Avant. Medical records: what you need to know [selected resources prepared by Avant]. https://avant.org.au/medical-records-what-you-need-to-know

Brell R, Gibson E. Here's the right way to correct medical records. Avant, 2019. https://www.avant.org.au/news/here-is-the-right-way-to-correct-medical-records

28 Diagnosing and certifying death and the role of the coroner

Felicity Hawker AM

Introduction

There is a growing medical consensus in a unifying concept of human death [1]. All human death involves the irreversible loss of capacity for consciousness, combined with the irreversible loss of the capacity to breathe. Death then is the irreversible loss of these functions of the brain. Three sets of criteria can be used to diagnose human death, each of which clearly establishes the irreversible loss of these two functions combined. The three criteria sets are circulatory (after cardiorespiratory arrest), somatic (features visible on external inspection of the corpse), and neurological (patients in coma undergoing mechanical ventilation) [1]. The most appropriate set of criteria to use is determined by the circumstances in which the medical practitioner is called upon to diagnose death.

This chapter covers the responsibilities of doctors attending a death and outlines the procedures they should follow in diagnosing the fact of death, certifying the cause of death, filling out the necessary forms, documenting the events and reporting particular deaths to the coroner.

28.1 Responsibilities of the doctor attending a death

28.1.1 How do I confirm that a person has died?

In hospital practice, the criteria set used most commonly to diagnose death is circulatory (cardiorespiratory arrest). To confirm circulatory death, you should observe the individual for a minimum of five minutes to establish that irreversible cardiorespiratory arrest has occurred [1]. The absence of mechanical cardiac function is normally confirmed using both the absence of a carotid pulse on palpation and absence of heart sounds on auscultation. You should also confirm that breath sounds are absent on auscultation of the lungs. After five minutes of continued cardiorespiratory arrest, the absence of the pupillary responses to light, the corneal reflexes, and any motor response to supraorbital pressure should be confirmed. The time and date of death is recorded as the time, using the 24-hour clock, at which these criteria are fulfilled [2].

Diagnosis and confirmation of death using somatic criteria is usually made by ambulance officers and police. These criteria include such signs as rigor mortis, decapitation and decomposition. In this situation, there is no requirement to examine the body for signs of life or evidence of internal organ function [1].

Diagnosis and confirmation of death using neurological criteria is a specialised field, undertaken only in areas where mechanical ventilation is available such as intensive care units. It is described briefly at the end of this chapter.

You must always confirm the identity of the person who has died. In hospital you should check the wristband or other patient identification. In the community you may confirm with family or carers. If you cannot confirm the identity of the person then the death is reportable to the coroner and to the police and you cannot write a death certificate (see section 28.1.4).

28.1.2 Can I write the death certificate?

The Medical Certificate of Cause of Death (MCCD) is an important, internationally recognised legal document (see Chapter 27, Medical records, reports and certificates). In Australia the MCCD is used to notify deaths to the registrar of births, deaths and marriages in each state or territory. It is slightly different in each jurisdiction but usually contains the following:

- demographic information that is used in collating statistics
- Part I. This is about the disease or condition that has directly caused the death. It also includes any antecedent causes giving rise to the disease or condition leading to death.
- Part II. This is for any other significant condition(s) contributing to death, but not related to the disease or condition causing it.

Parts I and II include an approximate interval between the onset of these conditions and death (see Figure 28.1).

If you were responsible for the patient's care immediately before death, or you saw the deceased after death and you are able to form an opinion as to a probable cause of death, you can complete and sign the death certificate. Sometimes you will be asked to sign a death certificate for a patient you don't know or haven't seen recently. This may happen when you are covering other doctors' patients on nights or weekends. There is no legal requirement for you to have had recent contact with the patient, but you do need sufficient information about the history (based on medical records and/or a discussion with the treating doctor) or an examination to be able to provide the cause of death. Sometimes you will also be asked to provide a cremation certificate (see section 28.1.5). When completing these certificates, you should write clearly in block letters. In some states the MCCD and cremation certificate can be completed online. Information on advance care planning and end-of-life care can be found in Chapter 19.

Once the MCCD is completed, it should be forwarded to the registry of births, deaths and marriages in your state or territory (except in Western Australia, where this is done by the funeral director or the person organising disposal of the body).

Before you complete and sign a MCCD, you must check that the death is not reportable to the coroner (see section 28.1.4). If the death is reportable, you *must not* complete or sign the MCCD and you *must* report the death to the coroner.

Perinatal deaths

Perinatal deaths [3] require a separate Medical Certificate of Cause of Perinatal Death (MCCPD). This certificate should be used for a stillborn child of at least 20 weeks' gestation or at least 440 g birth weight. A perinatal death certificate is also required for a live-born child who dies within 28 days of birth. The perinatal death certificate should be completed by or under the supervision of the senior medical officer responsible for the care of the child.

28.1.3 What do I write as the cause of death?

Medical practitioners have a professional responsibility to ensure they complete the MCCD accurately [4]. Complete, accurate and detailed cause of death information is important for:

- legal reasons (e.g. determining the validity of a will or insurance payment)
- statistical and public health purposes [5]
- family members—to know what caused the death and to be aware of conditions that may occur in other family members.

The underlying cause of death is defined as 'the disease or injury which initiated the train of morbid events leading directly to death, or the circumstances of the accident or violence which produced the fatal injury' [6].

The general format of the cause of death component of a MCCD is shown in Figure 28.1.

Figure 28.1 Format of the cause of death component of a death certificate

International Medical Certificate of Cause of Death		
Part I Disease or condition directly leading to death* Antecedent causes Morbid conditions, if any, giving rise to the above cause	**Cause of death** (a)________ Due to (or as a consequence of) (b)________ Due to (or as a consequence of) (c)________ Due to (or as a consequence of) (d)________	**Approximate interval between onset and death**
Part II Other significant conditions contributing to the death but not related to the disease or condition causing it		

*This means the disease, injury or complication which caused the death, NOT ONLY, for example, the mode of dying such as heart failure or asthenia.

The sequence of events you enter in Part I should be your best medical opinion. It is important that you avoid abbreviations and write clearly in block letters.

On line I(a) of the certificate, write the direct cause of death; that is, the disease or complication that led directly to death. There must always be an entry on line I(a). This condition may be the only condition reported in Part I of the certificate, but only if it was not due to, or did not arise as a consequence of, any other disease or injury that occurred before the direct cause of death. That is, the condition entered on line I(a) should have a shorter duration than any diseases mentioned on lines I(b), I(c) and I(d). Always use consecutive lines, never leave blank lines in the sequence. In the instance that death is the result of a tumour/growth, the site should be identified if known (if proven by histopathology) and whether its behaviour is benign, malignant primary, malignant secondary or unknown. For infections, where possible, give the name of the causative agent if the disease name does not imply this. The site of the infection should also be provided (e.g. urinary tract, respiratory tract). Where the causative organism is unknown, document this on the death certificate as 'organism unknown'. In general, terms that signify the mode of death rather than the cause of death (e.g. anoxia, coma, syncope) should be avoided.

If the direct cause of death written on line I(a) was due to or arose as a consequence of another disease, this disease should be entered on line I(b). If the condition entered on line I(b) was itself due to another condition or disease, this other condition should be reported on line I(c). Similarly, a condition antecedent to that reported on line I(c) should be reported on line I(d). Enter any additional antecedent conditions in Part I(d). A condition should be regarded as being antecedent not only in an aetiological or pathological sense, but also where it is believed that this condition prepared the way for the direct cause of death by damage of tissues or impairment of function, even after a long interval.

After completing Part I, you must consider whether there were any other significant conditions which, though not included in the sequence in Part I, contributed to the fatal outcome. If so, these conditions should be entered in Part II. For example, these may be diseases that did not directly cause the death but prevented the person from recovering from or overcoming the disease that did cause death.

The estimated duration between the onset of each condition entered on the certificate and the date of death should be entered in the column provided. The unit of time should be entered in each case. If the time of onset is unknown or cannot be determined, write 'unknown'.

Figure 28.2 Example of a correctly completed cause of death section of the MCCD

International Medical Certificate of Cause of Death		
Part I	**Cause of death**	**Approximate interval between onset and death**
Disease or condition directly leading to death*	(a) Myocardial infarction and arrest	2 hours
	Due to (or as a consequence of)	
Antecedent causes	(b) Hypertensive cardiomyopathy	5 years
Morbid conditions, if any, giving rise to the above cause	Due to (or as a consequence of)	
	(c) Hypertension	40 years
	Due to (or as a consequence of)	
	(d)	
Part II		
Other significant conditions contributing to the death but not related to the disease or condition causing it	Obesity	40 years
	Osteoarthritis right hip	10 years

*This means the disease, injury or complication which caused the death, NOT ONLY, for example, the mode of dying such as heart failure or asthenia.

28.1.4 When must I notify the coroner?

Reportable deaths must be notified to the coroner or police, and a death certificate must not be issued [7,8]. There are significant differences in the definitions of reportable deaths in each state and territory, but generally they include:

- cause of death unknown
- cause of death not certified
- identity of person who has died is unknown
- violent or unnatural death, including death by suicide
- death caused by an accident or injury
- death in police or other lawful custody or where person was held in care (e.g. mental health facility)
- death not a reasonably expected outcome of health-related procedure (definition varies in each jurisdiction).

If in doubt it is always best to phone your jurisdictional coroner's office to discuss the case and ask whether the coroner wishes to be involved. They will provide you with a checklist that you should follow in the event of a reportable death. You could also review the legislative definition of a reportable death in the state or territory in which you work.

Most hospitals will have protocols on referring a death to the coroner. It is usual for all deaths in hospital to be attended by the senior nurse on duty (often called the supervisor or coordinator) and they will be able to advise on the relevant hospital protocols and procedures if they are unfamiliar to you. Ideally, you should make the referral to the coroner shortly after the time of death. Delayed referral may result in loss of relevant information for the coroner, such as removal of medical equipment (see section 28.2).

Deaths from falls may be reportable to the coroner

Elderly and frail patients are often admitted to hospital after a fall at home or in the community. It is important to remember that in some states and territories, the death of such a patient must be reported to the coroner even when many months may have elapsed between the fall and the death.

28.1.5 When do I complete a cremation certificate?

The body of a deceased person cannot lawfully be cremated unless the necessary certificates and permits have been obtained. In all jurisdictions, there are strict limitations on when cremation can take place. Generally, two practitioners need to complete a cremation certificate: the practitioner who attended the deceased patient and usually also examined the body and provided the MCCD ('attending practitioner') and a second independent practitioner, who must first certify the cause of death and secondly believe that it is appropriate for the body to be cremated. The coroner can also give permission for the body to be cremated.

The form of the certification varies depending on the jurisdiction, as do the regulations regarding who qualifies as an attending practitioner or independent practitioner.

You should only sign the attending practitioner's cremation certificate if you are satisfied that the probable cause of death has been identified and there are no circumstances that require the coroner to investigate. In some states and territories, you must view the body before you sign the attending practitioner's cremation certificate.

If you are acting as the second or independent practitioner (also referred to as the authorising practitioner or medical referee), you may provide a certificate if you are appropriately credentialled and if you have carried out the investigations required for your state or territory. Generally, this will include an examination of the body, reviewing the relevant medical records and being satisfied that the cause of death recorded by the attending practitioner is correct and that there is no need for further investigation. You also need to check that the cremation doesn't pose a risk to anyone by certifying that there is no pacemaker or other battery-powered device present in the body.

A cremation certificate must never be signed if:

- there is a possibility that further investigations into the cause of death are required
- you are aware that the deceased did not want to be cremated
- you are aware that someone such as a personal representative or close family member of the deceased has objected to the cremation.

You cannot provide both the attending practitioner's certificate and an independent practitioner's certificate for the same death.

28.1.6 How do I report a death to the coroner?

When you have reported a death to the coroner you may be asked to fill out a medical form or deposition, which in some states and territories is online.

The form will normally ask for:

- identification details of the deceased
- identification details of the certifying doctor
- where the death occurred
- admission diagnosis (if the person was in hospital)
- medical details
- opinion as to cause of death.

The coroner will use this information in their investigation and may request further information if they deem it to be necessary.

28.1.7 What do I write in the medical record?

You should document all aspects of the death certificate and cremation certificate in the medical record, separate to the certificates (see also Chapter 27, Medical records, reports and certificates).

You should also include a reference to any discussions you may have had with the coroner's office about whether the death should or should not be reported and also with the police, who will be responsible for organising the transport of the body to the coronial services mortuary.

In non-coronial cases, you should also document discussions with the family/next of kin and the arrangements for dealing with the body including contacting the funeral director. The funeral director will require a signed printed copy of the MCCD before the body can be released from the hospital (for deaths occurring in hospital).

If the death has been unexpected or the result of a serious adverse event it will be necessary to follow the open disclosure framework and document the discussions that occurred with the family, carers and other persons. When it is not possible for the most senior clinician responsible for the clinical care of the patient to lead the open disclosure, an appropriately senior person who is trained in open disclosure processes should lead the disclosure.

Moreover, if the death was the result of one of the 10 Sentinel Events [9], as identified by the Australian Commission on Safety and Quality in Health Care (ACSQHC) and listed on their website, the death will need to be reported to the appropriate jurisdictional authority or the ACSQHC. Sentinel events are serious incidents that were wholly preventable, and include surgical procedures performed on the wrong patient or the wrong site, unintentional retention of a foreign object in a patient after surgery, ABO blood group incompatible transfusion, and medication error.

28.1.8 What do I do if I am made aware of an error on a death certificate?

An error on a death certificate is not uncommon. It can occur when the legal name of the patient is different from the name they commonly use, when there has been a typographical error as a result of bad handwriting or if an error is discovered with the time and/or cause of death.

The certificate can be corrected and the process depends upon the nature of the error and the stage the death certificate process has reached.

If the cause of death has changed to a cause that is reportable to the coroner, then the incorrect death certificate must be brought to the coroner's attention.

A death certificate should be treated as a medical record, so the incorrect certificate should not be destroyed or altered, even if you have not provided it to anybody. Instead, you should strike through the incorrect entry and mark it 'written in error' followed by your printed name, signature, designation, date and time.

If the MCCD has already been provided to the funeral director and/or family before the error is discovered, they should be notified that the certificate contains an error and asked to return it to the medical practitioner who completed it. The original version should be marked and signed (as above) and kept on file, and a new corrected version is provided to the funeral director and/or family. If the cause of death certificate has already been provided to the registry of births, deaths and marriages before the error is discovered, the registry must be informed. The process of notifying the registry of an error varies for each jurisdiction. Most jurisdictions require the original certifying practitioner, or the coroner, to apply to amend the cause of death. Generally, it is not appropriate for doctors to amend the cause of death on a certificate completed by another practitioner.

28.1.9 What do I do if I am made aware that the deceased person wanted to donate tissue after death?

Some people express a wish to donate their tissues after death, even if organ donation is not possible [10]. There are more opportunities for tissue donations than for organs, because tissues can be retrieved up to 24 hours after cessation of the circulation. Tissues that can be donated include cornea and sclera, skin, heart valves and other cardiovascular tissues, and bone, tendon and cartilage. If you are made aware of a deceased person or their family wanting to donate tissue when you attend them, you should contact the hospital Transplant Coordinator, who will liaise with the family and the relevant tissue banks to arrange the retrieval of tissue. Coronial referral does not exclude tissue donation. Organ donation is discussed briefly at the end of this chapter.

Figure 28.3 outlines the steps you should take when you are asked to attend a patient who has died.

Figure 28.3 Responsibilities of a doctor attending a death

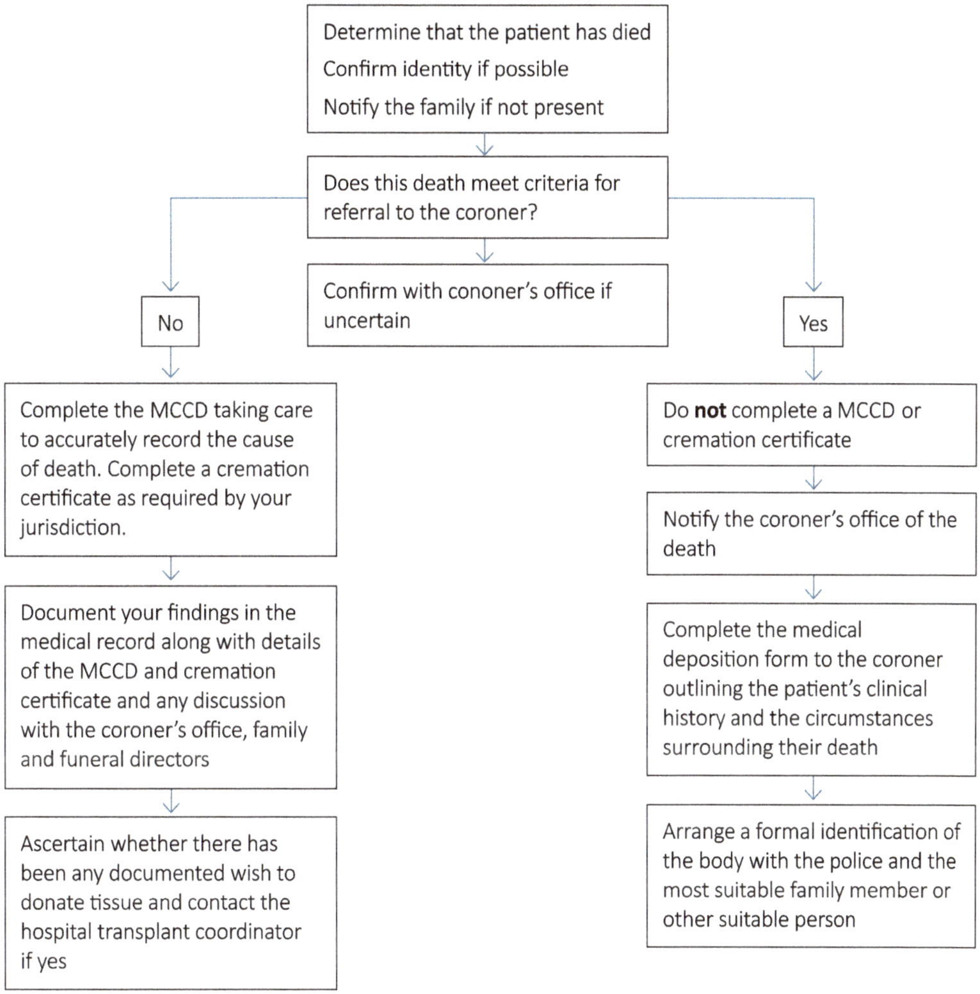

Source: Author.

28.2 What does the coroner do?

The coroner is a judicial officer who is responsible for the independent investigation of reportable deaths (and fires) [11,12]. Coroners are state/territory based. The role of the coroner has been described as 'to speak for the dead to protect the living'. The prime coronial function is to investigate certain deaths to promote public health, to provide preventative advice or to advise on justice. In an investigation into a death, the coroner must find, if possible:

- the identity of the deceased person
- the cause of death.

Deaths that are reportable to the coroner have been discussed under section 28.1.4. You have an obligation to report such a death to the coroner, and failure to do so can result in a fine or other disciplinary action. You may be required to complete a form/deposition for the coroner regarding a reportable death. This is a formal document written on the prescribed form and is based on the patient's clinical records. Police will usually attend a hospital (or a scene of death) on behalf of the coroner to obtain details about the deceased and gather information about the death from healthcare staff, family, friends and other witnesses. The usual obligation to maintain confidentiality regarding patient information under various state/territory privacy and health records acts does not apply to requests for information by someone acting on behalf of the coroner. Hence, if healthcare providers are requested by the coroner (or a police member acting on their behalf) to give any information or assistance for the purposes of a coronial investigation, they must provide it. There are penalties for failing to comply with such a requirement.

Consideration must be given to maintaining the placement of medical apparatus in situ (e.g. cannulas, catheters, central lines, endotracheal and nasogastric tubes), as well as devices attached to these (e.g. IV bags, syringes, drain bottles and bags, urine bags). Ideally, the body should also be left as it was at the time of death and not washed, so as to provide the forensic pathologist with all the relevant information for their medical examination. Exceptions can be made to this general rule if there are special circumstances.

All deaths reported to the coroner require a formal identification to be completed. This can be completed at the hospital or at the scene of the death, if deemed appropriate. Someone who was close to the deceased immediately prior to their death and has known them for a reasonable length of time can complete the formal identification of the deceased person.

The original medical record should be transported to the Coroner's Court as soon as possible after the death.

Approximately 11–14% of all deaths that occur each year in Australia are reported to and investigated by coroners [12]. Only a small proportion (less than 5%) of these deaths result in an inquest. Investigations by coroners, with or without an inquest, result in a changed diagnosis of the cause of death in around 5% of cases. These include changes in findings from natural causes to external causes (e.g. finding unintentional falls or pharmaceutical poisoning) and changes from external to natural causes (e.g. finding cardiovascular or infectious causes of death) [13]. A death that is reported to the coroner will not necessarily lead to an autopsy, let alone an inquest. For example, if a patient dies under anaesthesia during urgent surgery which they are not expected to survive, the death must be reported in most jurisdictions. Commonly, a pathologist will read the medical record and examine the surgeon's operation notes and, provided the clinical situation is clear and the family has not expressed concerns to the coroner, the coroner will usually accept the pathologist's advice that there is nothing to be gained by requiring an autopsy.

If a doctor is able to establish a probable cause of death, but considers that an autopsy may reveal further medically useful information about the patient's illness, including its investigation and treatment, the appropriate course is to issue a MCCD and seek the family's consent for a non-coronial autopsy.

28.3 Neurological determination of death

It is important for all doctors to understand the concepts behind neurological determination of death and how it is determined [14], even though the vast majority will never be involved in certifying death in this way. This is because an individual who is being tested for permanent loss of brain function will always be undergoing mechanical ventilation in an intensive care unit or other high-care area of a hospital. Two doctors are required to determine death by neurological criteria. The qualifications required vary between jurisdictions but one must have a relevant specialist qualification (e.g. intensive care, neurology, neurosurgery). They must not be involved in the removal of organs or tissues for transplantation.

There must be definite clinical or neuroimaging evidence of acute brain pathology consistent with permanent loss of all brain function. All other possible reasons for the person to be totally unresponsive should be excluded (e.g. hypothermia, sedative or neuromuscular-blocking drugs, or severe electrolyte, metabolic or endocrine disturbances) and it must be possible to examine all of the brainstem reflexes.

After a four-hour waiting period, during which the patient must be unresponsive to stimuli, each doctor completes a set of tests (see Table 28.1). These examinations may be consecutive but not simultaneous.

Table 28.1 Process for neurological determination of death (abridged)

Responsiveness		
Apply noxious stimuli in the cranial nerve distribution	There should be no response	
Brainstem reflexes		**Cranial nerve**
Pupillary light reflex—shine a light into both eyes and observe for pupillary constriction	No pupillary constriction response	II and III
Corneal reflex—touch each cornea with cotton wool	No blinking or other response	V and VII
Reflex response to pain in the trigeminal region e.g. pressure over supraorbital nerve	No facial or limb movement	V and VII
Vestibulo-ocular reflex—instil 50 ml ice-cold water into both ear canals using a syringe	No eye movement in relation to the cold water	III, IV, VI and VIII
Gag reflex—touch the posterior pharynx with a tongue depressor or similar	No gag response	IX and X
Cough/tracheal reflex—insert suction catheter through the endotracheal tube so that it touches the tracheal mucosa	No cough response	X
Breathing		
No attempts at breathing when removed from the ventilator despite there being a $PaCO_2$ of > 60 mmHg measured by blood gas analysis while removed from the ventilator during the test		

Source: Adapted from Australian and NZ Intensive Care Society (https://www.anzics.org/wp-content/uploads/2022/04/Appendix-1.pdf)

Please refer to the Statement on Death and Organ Donation [14] for more detail on the process for neurological determination of death.

If there is absence of responsiveness *and* absence of brain stem reflexes *and* absence of spontaneous breathing then the person meets the criteria for neurological determination of death by clinical examination.

28.3.1 Demonstrating the absence of brain perfusion

In some circumstances, clinical examination cannot be relied upon for neurological determination of death. Examples include inability to access both eyes because of swelling and skull fractures involving the external auditory meatus. In these situations, the absence of brain perfusion on imaging is synonymous with neurological determination of death. Although the absence of brain perfusion is determined by a radiologist or nuclear physician, it is the responsibility of the two medical practitioners who have clinically examined the patient to determine that the patient has died. The three acceptable imaging techniques for demonstrating absent brain perfusion are intra-arterial catheter angiography, radionuclide imaging and computed tomography angiography.

Although not a reason for performing these perfusion studies, a picture of an empty skull with blood flow ceasing at the carotid siphon may help family members accept that there is permanent loss of brain function and therefore that death has occurred.

28.3.2 Organ donation

Whether permanent loss of brain function has occurred should always be determined regardless of whether organ donation is being considered. The rigour of neurological determination of death provides certainty to the patient's family that an individual who meets the criteria is dead irrespective of organ donation. However, persons who have been pronounced dead using neurological criteria are ideal organ donors since the circulation persists and vital organs remain perfused. In Australia, potential donors are referred to Donate Life. It is usual for the Intensive Care Specialist who has been involved in determining neurological death to initiate the conversation with the family regarding organ donation, along with the Donation Specialist Nurse. If the family agrees to donation, the Donation Specialist Nurse undertakes the next steps in the donation process.

Summary

The death of a patient is a relatively common event for hospital doctors—less so for those working in the community. Even when expected, it is an emotional time for family and friends. This chapter outlines the responsibilities of doctors and the procedures they should undertake after the death of a patient. The paperwork is necessarily stringent, as death triggers events such as insurance claims and inheritances among so many other things. It is important to get it right in the first instance so as not to trouble grieving families with inadequate or missing paperwork.

Remember also that if you are unsure, you can turn to a senior colleague for help. In many instances, senior medical staff are closely involved in the deaths of their patients and often share the workload of completing the tasks outlined in this chapter.

References

1. Gardiner D, Shemie S, Manara A, Opdam H. International perspective on the diagnosis of death. *BJA* 2012; 108.
2. Oram J, Murphy P. Diagnosis of death. *Continuing Education in Anaesthesia, Critical Care and Pain* 2011; 11: 77–81.
3. Australian Institute of Health and Welfare. Stillbirths and neonatal deaths in Australia: definitions used in reporting. Canberra: AIHW, 2020. https://www.aihw.gov.au/reports/mothers-babies/stillbirths-and-neonatal-deaths-in-australia/contents/technical-notes/definitions-used-in-reporting (accessed Oct 2024).
4. Bird S. How to complete a death certificate: a guide for GPs. *Aust Fam Physician* 2011; 40: 446–449.
5. Australian Bureau of Statistics. Cause of death certification guide. Canberra: ABS. https://www.abs.gov.au/statistics/detailed-methodology-information/cause-death-certification-guide/latest-release (accessed Mar 2025).
6. World Health Organization. Cause of death. Geneva: WHO. https://www.who.int/standards/classifications/classification-of-diseases/cause-of-death (accessed Jul 2025).
7. Neate SL, Bugeja LC, Jelinek, et al. Non-reporting of reportable deaths to the coroner: when in doubt, report. *Med J Aust* 2013; 199: 402–405.
8. Charles A, Ranson D, Bohensky M, Ibrahim J. Under-reporting of deaths to the coroner by doctors: a retrospective review of deaths in two hospitals in Melbourne, Australia. *Int J Qual Health Care* 2007; 19: 232–236.
9. Australian Commission on Safety and Quality in Health Care. Australian Sentinel Events List (version 2). Sydney: ACSQHC, 2020. https://www.safetyandquality.gov.au/sites/default/files/2020-05/australian_sentinel_events_list_version_2_specifications_april_2020.pdf (accessed Oct 2024).
10. Australian Government Organ and Tissue Authority. Donate Life. Canberra: Commonwealth of Australia, 2024. https://www.donatelife.gov.au/ (accessed Oct 2024).
11. Coroners Court of Victoria. Role of a coroner. 2019. https://coronerscourt.vic.gov.au/inquests-findings/2017-bourke-street-inquest/role-coroner (accessed Oct 2024).
12. Coroners Court New South Wales. Role of the coroner. 2023. https://www.coroners.nsw.gov.au/coroners-court/how-the-coroners-court-work/role-of-the-coroner.html (accessed Oct 2024).
13. Studdert DM, Cordner SM. Impact of coronial investigations on manner and cause of death determinations in Australia, 2000–2007. *Med J Aust* 2010; 192: 444–447.
14. Australian and New Zealand Intensive Care Society. The Statement on Death and Organ Donation. 2021. https://www.anzics.com.au/death-and-organ-donation/

29 Professional practice, digital technology and artificial intelligence

Caroline Clarke, Amandeep Hansra, Tim Shaw

Introduction

Health care is in the middle of a digital disruption and transformation. Prior to the global COVID-19 pandemic declared in early 2020, the focus of digital health was largely on improving the functionality and interoperability of electronic health records (EHRs). The response to the COVID-19 pandemic demonstrated that technology can be used to support new ways of delivering health care that can be safe and effective, such as telehealth and remote patient monitoring (RPM). The challenge for the health sector now is to incorporate digital technologies into business-as-usual practices and look forward to how technology can support the development of more personalised and consumer-focused models of care.

Digital technology provides new ways of working for all healthcare providers, including medical practitioners, as well as supporting, enhancing and potentially transforming existing clinical workflows and practices. Digital health goes well beyond EHRs and provides options for improving quality of care and access to services for patients in a patient-centred and culturally safe way. We are in the early days of exploring and understanding how digital health and related new technologies such as artificial intelligence (AI) can improve patient experiences and outcomes. We are yet to realise its full transformative potential.

The targeted use of current, emerging and future technologies will facilitate changes to clinical practice and workflows and can improve clinical outcomes, access to health care and quality of care. These will also be enhanced by the effective use of linked datasets from multiple sources to run analytics or implement AI tools to predict risk and facilitate preventative care in the community. It is essential that all medical practitioners are prepared for the current and future advances in digital health in order to practise in a safe, professional and ethical environment, build their digital health capabilities and provide quality value-based care for patients.

Patients and consumers will also become progressively more digitally literate and confident using technology. They will have increasing access to their own devices and consumer-facing services, collect their own data and manage their own health journey. In fact, 70% of Australians are willing and ready to use virtual health, and over 80% are ready to share their health data in a digitally enabled way. Medical practitioners will need to support their patients in navigating this new environment. Patient support is particularly important for low socioeconomic communities who are less likely to be able to afford and access digitally enabled health care. Removing barriers to access will be integral to the sustainability of digitally enabled health care for all Australians [1].

To help realise this vision of a healthier future for Australians through connected health care, the Australian Government has established the Australian Digital Health Agency (ADHA). The ADHA released a national digital health strategy: *Safe, seamless and secure: evolving health and care to meet the needs of modern Australia* in 2016 [2]. This national strategy proposes seven priority outcomes that focus on secure information exchange, unrestricted access to health care and medicines, ensuring the quality and safety of digitally enabled models of care and a workforce that is capable of delivering these models. In 2021, the Australian Medical Council in collaboration with ADHA developed a *Capability framework on digital health in medicine* [3]. The aim of this framework is to guide how medical education providers throughout the continuum of medical education can play a role in the development of a digitally capable workforce in Australia and Aotearoa New Zealand [4]. (See also Chapter 4, Ethical and legal responsibilities of medical students.)

In addition, all states and territories in Australia have their own digital health strategy and one or more agencies that have carriage of these strategies. This includes the use of centralised EHRs, increased information sharing among the multidisciplinary team and widespread use of telehealth services. All jurisdictions are also exploring patient portals, mobile health applications and RPM. The integration of other digital health technologies, such as AI, is growing but still largely dependent on the initiative of individual practitioners, practices or organisations. (See also Chapter 16, Achieving full health potential: health equity, and section 29.3).

It is challenging to write a comprehensive and up-to-date chapter on digital health, especially post-pandemic, as technology development and implementation are moving so fast. There is also currently a lack of evidence around the implementation of many new technologies into health care and their downstream impact on patient outcomes. In this chapter, we describe the range of current and emerging digital technologies deployed in health care and the implications for medical practice. We emphasise the need to apply sound clinical judgement in the application of any current or future technologies, recognising any impact on clinical safety and quality as well as consideration of the legal and ethical implications of their application in health care. (See also Chapter 3, Ethical principles for the medical profession.)

We start the chapter with a review of EHRs, move through virtual care technologies and then consider the increasing application of AI tools in health care. We conclude with a consideration of a number of key factors impacting across digital health including privacy and cybersecurity.

29.1 Health records and clinical information systems

29.1.1 Electronic health records

EHRs are a digitised version of a patient's clinical record, and are increasingly ubiquitous in health care. Health professionals use EHRs to document patient history and examinations, diagnosis (including laboratory and radiology investigations) and treatments, as well as perform basic functions such as prescribing and ordering. Each jurisdiction has approached the rollout of EHRs differently with some implementing a single EHR, such as Queensland and the Australian Capital Territory, while others have focused on improving the interoperability of existing EHRs across the state/territory. The former approach allows data from individual hospitals to be more easily shared and compared across the state/territory, but there is a reduction in the ability of individual organisations to customise EHRs to their needs and workflow preferences.

In primary care, almost all practices are digitised and use one of a small number of practice management systems, commonly known as clinical information systems. These capture comprehensive patient notes to create a longitudinal record of the patient's health information and improve accessibility and legibility of data in general practice. Most also support basic functionality in primary care such as prescribing, ordering and clinical decision support. These systems do not generally interface with hospital-based EHRs although there is an increasing emphasis on the interoperability of these systems so information can be seamlessly shared. The Royal Australian College of General Practitioners (RACGP) has collaborated with ADHA to document the *Minimum requirements for general practice clinical information systems to improve usability* [5]. (See also Chapter 30, Prescribing and administering medicines.)

The introduction of EHRs provides significant benefits to quality of care, patient safety and clinical outcomes. The cited benefits include:

- accurate and complete patient information being readily available at the point of care
- ability for health information to be securely shared with patients and other clinicians
- built-in clinical decision support which guides evidence-based decision making and decreases clinical variability
- significant reductions in medication errors (discussed further in section 29.1.3)
- legible and complete documentation
- improved workflows and productivity
- improved clinical handover and communication between health professionals
- potential to reduce costs through less paperwork, reduced duplication of testing and improved health outcomes
- increased data quality, accuracy and accessibility.

However, there are also some inherent risks that the use of EHRs may introduce, and which need to be mitigated against, such as:

- increased medical errors due to poorly designed system interfaces or lack of end-user training
- non-adherence to embedded clinical practice guidelines because clinicians are unaware of the guidelines, do not realise a guideline applies to a particular patient, or don't have enough time during a patient visit
- loss of clinician autonomy in making decisions if the EHR blocks ordering of certain tests or medicines
- 'automation bias' where clinicians unquestioningly accept machine advice instead of maintaining vigilance or seeking validation
- alert fatigue where the user may receive so many alerts about drug interactions or contraindications that they ignore them
- planned and unplanned system outages (mitigated via organisational business continuity plans)
- loss of positive personal interactions and eye contact with patients and their carers due to suboptimal room and/or screen set-up
- 'garbage in, garbage out' whereby entry of incomplete or inaccurate patient information will reduce the value of EHRs and other digital technologies that rely on this data
- weak cybersecurity and data breaches.

Box 29.1 Case study: Communication challenges with electronic health records

A well-cited example of failure of communication in the context of an EHR is described by Robert Wachter in his book *The digital doctor* [6].

In 2014, Thomas Duncan was the first patient in the US to be diagnosed with Ebola virus. He presented to the emergency department at a medical centre in Dallas, Texas, with a high fever and symptoms consistent with, but not diagnostic of Ebola. A triage nurse obtained the history that Duncan had recently been in Liberia, the epicentre of an Ebola outbreak, and recorded this information in the EHR. Unfortunately, the doctor who subsequently saw the patient did not see this information and sent him home, exposing dozens of people to the virus.

Duncan was readmitted to hospital and subsequently died of Ebola virus; it was unclear whether the delayed diagnosis made a difference to his outcome or contributed to the spread of the virus.

The hospital initially issued a statement blaming the EHR for the error because of 'separate physician and nursing workflows'. However, this statement was subsequently retracted as the information entered by the nurse was fully accessible by the physician. The problem was that the physician did not look at it, and the nurse did not directly advise the doctor verbally that the patient had a high temperature and had just returned from an overseas trip to Liberia.

The learnings from this scenario are that all users of EHRs need to be aware of how to view the entire patient history, and there is still a role for verbal communication of key pieces of clinical information. (See also Chapter 5, Communication in clinical practice.)

Clinical and administrative data systems

My Health Record (MHR) is a secure online summary of an individual's health information and is available to all Australians. Healthcare providers authorised by their healthcare organisation can access MHR to view and add to their patients' health information. MHR does not replace existing health records, rather it supplements these with a shared source of patient information that can improve care planning and decision making. Information available through MHR can include a patient's health summary, medication prescribing and dispensing history, pathology reports, diagnostic imaging reports and discharge summaries. Patients can control access to information on their MHR, add their own information or opt out of the program altogether if they wish.

Considerable effort is underway to extract data from EHR systems at a local level as well as a jurisdictional level to make data available for decision support, predictive analytics, health planning and research. Being able to extract, clean and compare data across different systems is challenging. It is also clear that a lot of the rich clinical information about patients is found in the free text (uncoded) fields within EHRs which makes it hard to extract, although natural language processing algorithms that can interpret meaning from free text are increasingly having an impact.

Patient administration systems that capture administrative data such as demographic information about patients and patients' interactions with the health system are now used by almost all hospitals. While this data does not include clinical data, it can be a rich source of information about the quality of care delivery such as length of stay, preventable readmissions and so on.

In primary care, the majority of practices use one of a small number of practice management software systems. These collect clinical and administrative data from clinical encounters. A number of external providers work with primary health networks in Australia to extract data from these systems and make it available for benchmarking and quality improvement. A key challenge for the Australian healthcare system regarding data is the divide between primary and acute care data systems that limits the ability to track patients across care contexts. (See also Chapter 27, Medical records, reports and certificates.)

Box 29.2 Case study: Patient Admission and Prediction Tool

The Commonwealth Scientific and Industrial Research Organisation's (CSIRO) Patient Admission and Prediction Tool uses past information about emergency presentations and hospital admissions to predict foot traffic in hospital emergency departments. It collects data about daily and weekly admissions and discharges from the last few years to determine the number of patient presentations throughout the year [7]. Operating at 90% accuracy, the tool is currently used in hospitals across Queensland. The forecasts have particularly helped hospitals in the Gold Coast plan staffing, medical supplies, and beds for schoolies (a high school graduation celebration) [8]. The software is site-specific, highlighting its potential to be adapted for hospitals across Australia. Similar tools are currently being developed and trialled in Victoria and Western Australia. Similar predictive analytics software could potentially also be used for private practices.

Clinical quality registries

There are a number of clinical quality registries (CQRs) available in Australia that collect clinical data from multiple sources. These identify benchmarks and variation in clinical outcomes and feed essential risk-adjusted clinical information back to clinicians, patients, consumers, health service administrators and government to inform clinical practice and quality improvement. The Australian Commission on Safety and Quality in Health Care (ACSQHC) provides standards for the development and application of CQRs. A number of jurisdictions are developing digital CQRs that extract data from multiple sources that can be centrally resourced and managed.

Traditionally, many services, teams and individual clinicians have collected health data relating to their own practice in bespoke platforms that lie outside of centrally managed or resourced systems. While these bespoke systems offer easy access and flexibility, great care must be taken to ensure they meet privacy and governance requirements and are secure from increasing cyber attacks on health data systems.

Patient-reported measures

In recognition that traditional clinical indicators do not accurately capture consumers' views of health care, there has been a recent emphasis on collecting patient-reported experience measures (PREMs) and patient-reported outcome measures (PROMs). PREMs capture patients' perceptions of their experiences of health care and PROMs capture patients' perspectives on how illness and care impact on their health and wellbeing. PROMs and PREMs are now collected by a majority of organisations using surveys and other tools, and this data is increasingly being made available to teams and clinicians. PROMs and PREMs have also been well documented to support clinician decision making and shared care planning. They are a good indicator for overall patient outcomes; especially in those conditions marked by a person's level of health and wellbeing [9]. A number of state governments are developing centralised systems for capturing and integrating PROMs and PREMs into care delivery in a routine and standardised way.

29.1.2 Interoperability

A patient's health data can be stored in many different systems across the healthcare sector but is often not easily shared and therefore might not be accessible to a clinician or the patient when they need it to make decisions. Some of the difficulties with sharing across systems relate to the sensitive nature of the data, which requires a high level of privacy and security. Not having access to a patient's full health data can cause harm when clinicians are faced with making healthcare decisions without full access to all the information they need.

Interoperability is the ability of different EHRs, clinical information and administrative data systems to access, exchange and use data to facilitate seamless and efficient transfer of information. This allows for better coordination of care, with medical practitioners having access to more data from the patient's healthcare journey. This can reduce duplication, improve communication and minimise adverse events from medication interactions. Better coordination of data also allows for high-quality analysis, trend assessment and performance review that ensures improvements in patient care are data driven. Interoperability in health care also reduces the administrative burden for patients and the healthcare workforce as the same information does not need to be communicated repeatedly.

Standards are created to make it easy for healthcare data to be structured, organised and interpreted by different systems to support interoperability. One such standard is *Fast healthcare interoperability resources* (FHIR) which is an open-source standards framework built specifically for healthcare data that has been developed from a previous standard. FHIR was developed in Australia in 2011 and is now used globally, including by Apple for its iPhone health app which allows users to view their FHIR-compliant medical records when medical practitioners choose to make them available. Standards such as FHIR assist Australia in moving towards the goal of interoperability in the healthcare sector so consumers and medical practitioners can access healthcare information from disparate sources across the health system to enable them to make better decisions.

29.1.3 Electronic medication management

Electronic medication management (EMM) has been demonstrated to reduce the number of preventable adverse medication events as well as medication prescribing and administration errors. EMM includes:

- prescribing systems which include electronic ordering and are used in both general practice and hospitals
- decision-support systems such as the use of evidence-based order sets, allergy alerts and flagging of drug interactions
- dispensing systems, including the use of specific software in pharmacies and automated dispensing systems
- ordering and supply solutions such as electronic transfer of prescriptions and inventory solutions.

The ACSQHC provides up-to-date advice on how to safely implement EMM online [10].

Use of EMM supports a number of national medication safety priorities:

- quality use of medicines [11]
- medication reconciliation and best-practice medication histories
- safe use of high-risk medications
- reducing medication-related hospital admissions
- preventing and controlling healthcare-associated infections (antimicrobial stewardship).

29.1.4 Alert fatigue

Alert fatigue associated with clinical decision-support systems is also a well-reported issue particularly in the context of medication allergy alerts. Alert fatigue is defined as clinician desensitisation to a specific notification due to repeated exposure over a period of time [12]. Electronic alert fatigue renders clinical decision-support systems, like EMMs, less effective and presents a serious patient safety issue.

Specific solutions need to be considered to combat alert fatigue, but there is currently no consensus on the optimal approaches. Some suggestions on how to minimise alert fatigue in EHRs and EMM include:

- increasing alert specificity by reducing or eliminating clinically inconsequential alerts
- tailoring alerts to patient characteristics and critical integrated clusters of physiological indicators, e.g. incorporating renal function test results into the alert system so that alerts for nephrotoxic medications are triggered only for patients at high risk
- ranking alerts according to severity with more salient warnings for alerts that are more clinically consequential
- making only high-level (severe) alerts interruptive
- applying human factors principles such as format, content, legibility and colour when designing alerts.

One limitation to addressing alert fatigue is the legal implications of removing alerts. There are concerns about practitioner liability if patients are harmed in the absence of a warning, as exemplified in the case study in Box 29.3.

Box 29.3 Case study: Alert fatigue for paediatric patients

An illustrative case study due to alert fatigue has been described by Carspecken et al. [13]. A 2-year-old patient suffered an adverse drug reaction due to an allergic hypersensitivity to a topical medication. Treating doctors were warned about possible hypersensitivity in an EHR alert. However, these alerts were routinely overridden by the clinical team due to an extended number of non-evidence-based alerts in the EHR. Excessive use of electronic alerts can thus harm patient safety.

29.2 Hybrid health care

During the COVID-19 pandemic there was a rapid shift towards the use of telehealth. While telehealth has been used for decades in supporting rural and remote care in Australia, the COVID-19 pandemic drove the use of telehealth across all care contexts and led to the establishment of multiple virtual care programs across primary and acute care services, regardless of where patients are situated.

While most telehealth during the pandemic was restricted to the use of phone and video consultations, the development and use of multiple other virtual care technologies to support patient–clinician interactions were accelerated. This includes the use of asynchronous text-based consultations, RPM and the use of conversational chatbots and other digital innovations.

As we move beyond the COVID-19 pandemic, it is clear we are entering a new period of hybrid care, where it is likely that many, if not all, of our healthcare interactions will be made up of a mixture of face-to-face and digital-supported communications that may be synchronous or asynchronous. This approach to healthcare delivery supports other principles such as value-based care and new funding models that support outcomes rather than focusing purely on activity. It is likely that much of the research into digital health over the next decade will focus on how these hybrid models of care can be best structured and for which patient and clinician populations.

29.2.1 Telehealth and digital communication

'Telehealth' is the term used to describe the use of telecommunication techniques for the purpose of providing clinical consultations via telemedicine, medical education and health education over a distance. The World Health Organization (WHO) uses the words 'telemedicine' and 'telehealth' synonymously and Scalvini et al. [14] define telemedicine as:

> the delivery of healthcare services, where distance is a critical factor, by all healthcare professionals using information and communication technologies for the exchange of valid information for diagnosis, treatment and prevention of disease and injuries, research and evaluation and for the continuing education of healthcare providers, all in the interests of advancing the health of individuals and their communities.

The WHO describes four elements relevant to telehealth:

1. Its purpose is to provide clinical support.
2. It is intended to overcome geographical barriers, connecting users who are not in the same physical location.
3. It involves the use of various types of ICT.
4. Its goal is to improve health outcomes.

It is worth noting that the COVID-19 pandemic has shifted the emphasis on telehealth from overcoming geographical barriers to providing convenient care, regardless of the location of the practitioner or patient.

Different service elements (including audio communication, RPM, videoconferencing and asynchronous messaging) are used to create telehealth services for particular purposes. Examples include teleconsultations, offline consultations (also known as asynchronous or 'store and forward'), augmented consultations (e.g. using gait analysis or viewing an echocardiogram during a cardiology examination), telepresence consultations, home-based monitoring, remote rehabilitation, remote workforce training and even telesurgery. From a technology perspective, all these elements are available, but the adoption of telehealth into everyday clinical workflows in Australia is still limited.

Most current teleconsultations in Australia are discrete telephone calls between a patient and a practitioner, and these have been driven by COVID-19. ADHA records show that between 13 March 2020 and 31 July 2022, 118.2 million telehealth services were delivered to 18 million patients. Medicare data reveals that 97% of these telehealth consultations were conducted over the telephone [15].

Box 29.4 Case study: Telehealth in the Kimberley

The Visionflex system is a telehealth system (available on desktop computer and tablet) providing accessible and portable health care to remote communities in the Kimberley. Devices included in the system are ultrasounds, digital stethoscopes, endoscopes, blood pressure monitors and more. Doctors can monitor collection of vital signs in real time, and the information is encrypted and saved to the EHR. This is particularly helpful as many clinics in the region do not have doctors on call at night or full-time access to specialist care. Instead, health workers, nurses and family members can help position the equipment to relay accurate health information to doctors for diagnosis and treatment [16].

Telehealth regulations, standards, accountability and funding models

The use of telehealth services can introduce new types of risks and challenges into healthcare delivery and has a potential impact on safety and quality. Australia does not currently have a national telehealth strategy or agreed-upon standards for technology, clinical governance or quality assurance of telehealth services. There is also no formal national accreditation service for telehealth, although organisations like the Australian Council on Healthcare Standards has a quality assessment and improvement program, *EQuIP7 ambulatory care standards*, which includes guidelines and prompt points for telehealth [17].

The widespread use of telehealth during the COVID-19 pandemic highlighted the need for standards and guidelines to be developed to ensure consistency in practice and maintain safety and quality. It is important to maintain the high standards of safety and quality of healthcare services, whether provided in person or by telehealth. Evidence from several studies shows that telehealth consultations are generally safe and adverse outcomes uncommon. However, many of these studies and systematic reviews have been of niche use cases [18]. In some cases, the research has shown that telehealth can be more effective than conventional care in managing some conditions [19]. However, there are also new risks that need to be mitigated or managed including cybersecurity issues, patient data breaches, technology failures and data governance.

Currently, there are no specifications regarding equipment or technology platforms used to conduct telehealth consultations. However, when billing services under the Medicare Benefits Schedule, the Department of Health, Disability and Ageing states that videoconferencing services are preferred over telephone consultations, and some Medicare item numbers are only billable for video consultations. Medical defence organisations (MDOs) generally recommend the use of video over phone when available, as video gives a richer experience.

Both the RACGP and Medical Board have released guidelines for telehealth and videoconferencing [20,21]. These guidelines outline the importance of tailoring technology-based consultations to patients. Some patients may prefer or need a video consultation if they are hard of hearing or deaf or if it is a complex consultation. A video feed can improve the quality and safety of these interactions as medical practitioners can conduct a visual review in lieu of a physical examination; for example, for wound management or determining if patients look unwell. It is also important for doctors to follow the board's *Good medical practice: a code of conduct for doctors in Australia* for telehealth services just as they do in face-to-face consultations [22].

In December 2021, the Australian Government announced further investment into telehealth to ensure funding is made permanent under Medicare [23]. Medical specialist, allied health, nurse, midwifery, nurse practitioner and GP telehealth services will continue to be funded under Medicare to substitute face-to-face care when this is appropriate. For general practice services, patients must have had a face-to-face consultation with their telehealth provider in the previous 12 months to access Medicare-subsidised telehealth services.

Box 29.5 Case study: A virtual hospital

An example of an expanded telehealth service providing virtual care is Royal Prince Alfred's Virtual Hospital. It is a service that was established in February 2020 as an alternative to inpatient care for Sydney Local Health District patients. In March 2020, however, it was used to remotely monitor stable COVID-19 patients in home isolation and hotel quarantine. It included twice-daily video consultations with a registered nurse and RPM of vital signs such as oxygen saturation, heart rate and temperature. Wearable devices allowed data to be shared with the provider team who could assess early if a patient was deteriorating at home and required inpatient admission. This model of caring for COVID-19 patients has been replicated across the state and is a model that can be used for many other conditions in addition to COVID-19. Telehealth models of care into the future will extend beyond simply substituting a face-to-face consultation with a phone or video consultation.

29.2.2 Asynchronous digital communication

Other innovative models of care that come under the broad term of telehealth are direct-to-consumer asynchronous platforms that deliver medical services segregated into disease-specific conditions. These businesses cater to a specific condition, and patients access the services online using messaging platforms and completing forms. The doctor interacts with the patient in an asynchronous manner, responding by providing a prescription or asking further questions. Medications are delivered on a subscription basis to patients' homes, and consumers have a convenient and seamless experience. These models are increasingly popular as consumers seek more convenience and a customer-friendly experience compared with the traditional way of seeing a healthcare provider.

These models have, however, raised safety and clinical governance concerns, as the doctor prescribing the medication may be unfamiliar with the patient, and the model encourages potential fragmentation of care and records. There are also concerns that these models do not provide holistic care and make it difficult for the healthcare provider to complete a thorough consultation without directly interacting with the patient or knowing any of their pre-existing medical history. Currently, these services are not funded by Medicare, and consumers pay privately for these services.

The Medical Board of Australia currently does not support asynchronous care. Doctors should refer to the most recent guidelines when providing these services [21].

These new models of care that use different forms of telehealth provide an opportunity to make health care more convenient, accessible and consumer friendly. They also, however, have the propensity to introduce more clinical risk as described in the above example. It is important for clinicians to ensure they engage with their MDOs prior to commencing work in these new models of care to verify they are covered with their existing medical indemnity policy. The MDOs are still trying to assess some of these new models of care using telehealth and quantify any new risks, if any [24].

These new models allow for care to be provided remotely across not only state/territory borders but international borders as well. This is already taking place with teleradiology and teledermatology where clinicians are located in one country and provide remote services for another country. Consultations via telehealth platforms where clinicians and patients are in different countries are not always covered by existing medical indemnity policies, and MDOs will usually have specific conditions that need to be met to ensure coverage. In addition, any doctor providing services to Australian patients is expected to be registered with the Medical Board of Australia and the Australian Health Practitioner Regulation Agency.

Box 29.6 Case study: My Health Clinic at Home

Feros Care's My Health Clinic at Home (MHCAH) leveraged telehealth services, computers and vital signs monitoring equipment to allow patients with chronic health conditions to take control of their health care. Patients could discuss their results with their nurse on a videoconference or telephone call at any time. MHCAH was a federally funded program, and cost approximately $15 per participant per week [25]. Enrolled patients reported fewer visits to the doctor and emergency department as well as a reduction in non-local hospital admissions over the 2013–14 trial period. This change can be attributed to improvements in patient self-efficacy for health management and lower levels of emotional distress [25]. It should be noted that many providers did struggle to create quiet and protected spaces with dedicated equipment for videoconferencing (e.g. headphones, stable internet connection).

Box 29.7 Key points for practice: Telehealth

Telehealth can be a useful adjunct to face-to-face health care if you:

- create a supportive environment for patients based on their needs, preferences and digital ability
- follow guidelines from organisations such as the RACGP, Medical Board of Australia, MDOs and the Australian Medical Association
- are aware of the risks associated with telehealth, such as cybersecurity issues, data breaches, technology failures and data governance concerns.

29.2.3 Remote patient monitoring

RPM is an extension of telehealth and can augment a telehealth consultation being conducted by a healthcare practitioner. This often involves the use of remote devices to capture key monitoring information about a patient who is usually in an out-of-hospital setting. Patients can be given devices to monitor their heart rate, breathing, blood pressure, oxygen saturation, body weight, temperature, heart rhythm and blood sugar levels or be asked to complete questionnaires. This information is then interpreted and allows healthcare workers to assess changes in a patient's condition remotely and provide appropriate care interventions earlier or help the patient self-manage their condition and prevent a hospital admission or a deterioration.

Many successful pilots of RPM programs have shown success in Australia, including CSIRO's research pilot, which showed the benefits of an RPM trial with 287 participants. The research showed a 53% decrease in hospital admission and a 76% reduction in length of stay if admitted to hospital during the 12-month trial. The researchers calculated a 24% saving to the health system over the year through a reduction in use of healthcare services [26].

Aside from cost savings to the health system, RPM is also useful at times when the health system is overwhelmed and needs to manage resources more efficiently. During the 2021–2022 COVID-19

Omicron outbreak in Australia, RPM was used to keep patients at home for longer and monitor them for any signs of deterioration to free up hospital beds and staff for those who were sickest. RPM enhances the quality of the care delivered in out-of-hospital settings and can also be used to keep the elderly in their homes longer.

Care needs to be exercised when using RPM to ensure that outputs from remote devices are accurate and that appropriate clinical governance standards are applied in managing remote patients, including how to respond to a deteriorating patient. A number of jurisdictions, such as New South Wales, are working to provide access to RPM solutions that include integrated devices and management platforms to overcome these challenges and standardise remote care.

Box 29.8 Key points for practice: Remote patient monitoring

- RPM allows the collection of patient information at home or in the community.
- It's particularly useful for the management of patients with chronic diseases.
- RPM can produce cost savings for patients and the health system by minimising travel costs and reducing hospital presentations and admissions.
- Take care to ensure accuracy of RPM devices.
- Establish and maintain appropriate clinical governance when delivering RPM.

29.2.4 Mobile health applications and consumer wearables

Mobile health (mHealth) applications are health-related apps that are available to the public through app stores. It is estimated that around 350,000 mHealth apps are available to consumers, and deciding what is the most appropriate app to use for consumers can be overwhelming. Consumers and healthcare providers have struggled to assess every mHealth app available for safety, suitability for consumers, effectiveness, and privacy and security. These apps can be used for a multitude of purposes including simple reminders and record keeping of symptoms and medications or management of chronic diseases such as diabetes. They can even help to diagnose medical conditions. Apps can also connect to medical devices via bluetooth to record vital health information or facilitate telehealth consultations through text messaging or video.

There is widespread evidence available that mHealth apps have a promising role in management of many health conditions, through improved patient engagement, adherence and compliance [27]. However, there are also increasing numbers of people engaging with mHealth apps that are not safe or trustworthy and experiencing harm as a result [28]. In Australia currently the mHealth app environment is largely unregulated. While the Therapeutics Goods Administration (TGA) does not regulate mobile apps that are sources of information or tools that manage a healthy lifestyle, they are increasingly regulating mobile apps that could be categorised as a medical device. If the purpose of the mobile app is medical—that is, the intended purpose of the app is to diagnose, monitor, predict, prevent or investigate disease—and it is not on the TGA's excluded list, it may be regulated under the 'software as medical device' regulation and be required to be listed on the Australian Register of Therapeutic Goods [29].

The RACGP has a factsheet [30] that discusses what to consider when discussing health apps with patients. More recently, the ADHA has released its *Assessment framework for mHealth apps* to provide guidance for app developers working on mHealth apps for release in Australia [31].

Consumer devices, wearables and Internet of Things

Aside from devices used in RPM, consumers can also collect information about their own health and wellbeing through consumer-grade wearables and the Internet of Things (IoT). Deloitte Global predicted that 320 million consumer-grade wearable devices would ship worldwide in 2022 alone [32]. Wearable technologies include electronic devices such as Fitbits, smart watches, jewellery, 'smart' patches and clothes. One in five Australians owns a wearable fitness tracker. Apple watches are the most common wearable, making up 43% of all wearables purchased by Australians [33]. Wearables are able to capture all sorts of data from heart rate, steps, blood pressure, body fat levels, sleep patterns, oxygen saturation, and even motion to identify when someone has had a fall. The COVID-19 pandemic saw many consumers start to monitor their health at home using devices. Patients who measured their blood oxygen saturation were alerted to seek medical care when their saturation levels were low.

There are some concerns about the growth in consumer-collected health data. The data collected by different consumer devices have varying levels of accuracy, and it is prudent to calibrate abnormal results from a wearable and investigate further any abnormalities identified. In some cases, wearables can lead to false positive results and cause concern and harm unnecessarily. There are also workflow issues in how a clinician incorporates the vast amounts of patient-collected data into a normal consultation. Some EHRs are now enabling consumers to share data from their wearables and health apps with their treating doctors.

Data privacy and cybersecurity threats remain a concern in this area, as consumers are increasingly willing to share their health data. Hackers have found ways to steal health and fitness records through smart watches and have also been known to hack medical devices such as drug infusion pumps and pacemakers.

29.2.5 Data from devices and remote monitoring

As noted earlier in this chapter, RPM is now relatively common. Data generated from these devices has clear value in terms of understanding a patient's health status and trajectory. Health services are grappling with how to integrate data from devices into electronic health systems in a seamless and secure way.

The emergence of increasingly high-quality and affordable devices and apps that are available direct to consumers, while increasing the ability to monitor patients remotely, is further complicating how to integrate this data effectively into systems of care so it can be accessed and used effectively.

Box 29.9 Key points for practice: Health data

- Consider how data from RPM devices will be used in practice. What data will be collected and how will it be analysed?
- Ensure data collection complies with appropriate governance and privacy standards for use and disclosure, including for personal reflection and practice improvement. Refer to organisational data governance frameworks. Obtain patient consent and ethics approval, if needed, when using patient data for secondary purposes such as research and quality improvement.
- Act in the best interests of patients, and abide by your legal and ethical obligations when disclosing patient data to third parties.
- Make use of predictive tools as they become available for patient populations and consider how these tools can be built into the patient journey.

29.2.6 Secure messaging

Secure messaging supports the delivery of messages containing clinical documents and/or other information between healthcare organisations. This includes e-orders and e-referrals that are sent either directly or through one or more secure messaging providers. This process can replace other forms of exchanging documents and information such as fax, post or email. It ensures the safe, seamless and secure exchange of clinical information between healthcare providers. The kinds of documents most commonly sent and received by secure message delivery include referrals, letters and reports, results, discharge summaries and patient summaries. Secure messaging helps prevent unauthorised interception of messages, reduces reliance on paper, decreases errors associated with transcribing or legibility, notifies senders upon successful receipt of the message and integrates with clinical systems allowing for more seamless workflow.

Secure messaging is a simple process to use, whereby clinicians create documents in their own clinical information system and choose the recipient from an integrated address book. Once the recipient is chosen, the message is encrypted before it leaves the system. The message is decrypted after being received by the intended recipient into their clinical information system as a document that they can view and download.

The use of post, fax and email to share patients' demographic and clinical information puts this information at risk of interception, and therefore healthcare providers are encouraged to invest in secure messaging capabilities. ADHA has extensive materials relating to secure messaging on its website [34].

The ADHA has also been working with the pathology and radiology sectors to encourage the use of e-requesting. This is where pathology or radiology requests are sent from clinical information systems to participating providers via secure electronic communications. It is intended to speed up delivery of reports back to the requesting doctors, streamline the patient experience and decrease the chance of legibility or transcription errors. The diagnostic imaging project is also looking at the digital transfer of diagnostic imaging requests and results. The RACGP and ADHA have a range of resources to support doctors with e-requesting [35].

29.2.7 Use of social media in health care

Social media is defined as any electronic or digital communication tool capable of use as a means of social communication, including but not limited to online and other tools such as:

- social networking sites (e.g. Facebook, Instagram, WeChat, Weibo, Snapchat, TikTok)
- video and photo sharing websites
- professional networking platforms (e.g. LinkedIn)
- discussion forums (e.g. Google groups, WhatsApp, Reddit, Whirlpool, Facebook groups, Signal)
- email and other computer-based messaging (e.g. Slack, MS Teams)
- blogs including corporate, personal and media blogs (and comments sections or 'your say' forums on newspaper sites)
- media sharing (e.g. YouTube, Flickr, Instagram)
- knowledge/information aggregation (e.g. Second Life, Discord)
- appointment booking sites and apps (e.g. HealthEngine, Whitecoat, Podium, HotDoc).

Inappropriate use of social media can result in harm to both patients and the profession. This may be due to confidentiality breaches, unintended sharing of personal information, inappropriate boundary crossing or even defamation. Doctors using social media should be aware that information posted on sites (including those that are password protected) can be shared and circulated easily and rapidly, and it is often difficult to remove or change the content of social media posts.

Doctors should also be cautious about interacting with patients or other members of the public through a social media forum [36]. Medical information or advice posted by a doctor on any social media platform could be seen as establishing a therapeutic relationship with the individual who accesses and relies on the information.

Multiple organisations have released guidelines for social media use in health care including the Medical Board of Australia, the Australian Health Practitioner Regulation Agency and the Australian Medical Association, which has published a comprehensive summary of doctors' rights and obligations when using social medial and common pitfalls when engaging patients on these platforms [37,38]. (See also Chapter 6, Confidentiality, privacy and disclosure, and Chapter 8, Sexual and other professional boundaries: being a doctor in modern society.)

Box 29.10 Key points for practice: Social media

- Be aware of social media policies set by your employer and professional associations. You may be prohibited from posting content even with patient consent.
- Obtain written and specific patient consent before posting patient information or images online. Protect patients by de-identifying the information and/or image in a post.
- Give careful thought to publishing something on social media. Consider whether you would be comfortable with your patients, colleagues and/or employers seeing it.
- Avoid posting images or comments that might endorse activities or behaviour that could damage your professional reputation or be in breach of professional obligations. This includes liking or following groups whose content could reflect poorly on you and/or the medical profession.
- Be aware that the content of a post may be discoverable even if deleted. Never assume that something that has been posted online can be deleted.
- Respond to friend requests from a patient by directing them to a professional social networking page. Do not extend friend requests to patients.

29.3 Data, artificial intelligence and personalised health care

29.3.1 Big data and analytics

Today, approximately 30% of the world's data volume is being generated by the healthcare industry. Traditionally, health data has been used to support direct patient care, health planning, quality improvement and research. The increasing availability of linked and identified health datasets has opened the door to using data to predict patient risk in near real time. It has also put actionable data in the hands of clinicians and medical administrators so they can continuously monitor performance and outcomes.

This increasing reliance on data in health care requires clinicians to be aware of the different datasets that are available to them and how to analyse this data to support their practice. At a minimum, clinicians need to be able to understand the lifecycle of health data and be able to assess the accuracy and robustness of any datasets they use in their practice.

The term 'big data' is now ubiquitous and refers to the aggregation of large amounts of data that surpass traditional storage, management and analytic capabilities. The application of AI and other analytic tools on big datasets is reaping rewards in industries such as finance, travel and engineering. However, while health is rich in clinical and administrative data and emerging datasets such as genomics information, the health industry has been slow to harness this data to transform care and care delivery. The ability to combine clinical data with genomics data and data derived from apps and devices presents the promise of developing precision medicine in terms of targeted therapies and personalised medicine to deliver tailored health and wellness pathways. (See also Chapter 31, Medical research.)

29.3.2 Artificial intelligence and machine learning

The impact that AI and machine learning (ML) are having on healthcare delivery is growing rapidly [39]. AI can be described as the capability of a computer system to mimic human cognitive functions such as problem solving and learning. It involves training computers to undertake tasks which, at present, humans can do better. ML is a subset of AI and refers to the process of using mathematical data models to help computer algorithms learn from datasets without every step being explicitly programmed by a human.

Not surprisingly, given the repetitive nature of image interpretation and the ability of computer algorithms to learn from analysing multiple image sets of the same condition or presentation, an early focus of AI and ML has been in pathology and radiology.

Box 29.11 Case study: Imaging and radiology

Misinterpretation of chest X-rays has contributed to many cases of missed lung cancer diagnosis. These human errors are often unavoidable, but can be significantly reduced by using ML to assist interpretation, especially for junior doctors [40]. For example, Annalise.ai is a decision-support AI tool that assists radiologists to accurately diagnose medical conditions. Annalise.ai is currently being used across 300 sites in Australia, with Sonic Healthcare Australia deciding to implement the tool in its radiology clinics across the country. It is also available for use in other countries, including Aotearoa New Zealand, Malaysia, the UK and the European Union [41]. A recent study found diagnostic accuracy of radiologists assisted by Annalise.ai was significantly improved compared to unassisted radiologists. The tool improved decision making by reducing human error and making more information available to radiologists, especially for complex cases with multiple findings [42].

Annalise.ai was trained using over 750,000 chest X-rays from three continents. Each X-ray was labelled by a radiologist using a standardised label and compared to the diagnosis reached by the AI tool.

AI is increasingly being applied to predict risk in healthcare settings, such as a patient's chance of a preventable hospital readmission. AI is also being deployed into many EHRs and other clinician-facing platforms and tools to enhance clinical decision making. AI has the potential to reduce the burden of repetitive decision making and improve accuracy as well as provide much deeper insights into health trajectories.

Box 29.12 Case study: Risk of Hospitalisation algorithm

NSW Health's Risk of Hospitalisation (RoH) score predicts patients' clinical deterioration. The score is derived from a validated algorithm that makes a prediction based on demographic and socioeconomic factors and the medical history of the patient. NSW Health has built this algorithm into its Patient Flow System allowing clinical teams to access daily risk predictions. The score is also used to determine the care each patient needs, such as daily medical reviews or recommendations for at-home care. This score was used extensively in triaging patients with COVID-19 during the pandemic.

Multiple resources are available that provide information on the growing impact of AI and ML in health care from a range of organisations including the WHO, CSIRO and the Royal Australian and New Zealand College of Radiologists [43–45].

While the potential benefits of AI and ML in health care are substantial, there are significant issues that need to be addressed and monitored, including how AI tools are developed and deployed as well as how health professionals apply AI in their practice.

As AI algorithms become increasingly sophisticated, they will inevitably challenge autonomy of practice, with machines rather than humans making decisions regarding care delivery. Already computer algorithms can perform as well as, if not better than, humans in repetitive tasks such as plain X-ray reading. As increasing amounts of health data become available and decision-support tools become more sophisticated, computers will start to be able to make independent decisions around care. These developments will challenge regulators, decision makers and clinicians to ensure that humans ultimately control the decision-making process and that AI is developed in an understandable and transparent way.

In the development of tools that use AI, there is a significant risk of building bias into the algorithms as they only learn from the data they are given. This can substantially impact on their accuracy. If, for example, a biased sample of training data is not representative of patient characteristics such as age, gender or ethnicity, then this will potentially reduce the impact of the algorithms for patients not represented. This has significant implications for the ethical development of AI and ML tools as well as their accuracy in certain patient populations.

In addition to bias in the data used in the development of AI algorithms, significant challenges remain in Australia and internationally in accessing robust and high-quality data across the care continuum. Australia is particularly challenged with linking acute and primary care datasets. This significantly reduces the effectiveness of algorithms in cases where a patient's complete data across acute and primary care is required to make predictions about outcomes such as likelihood of hospital readmission. In this instance, while the algorithm may be applied in an acute care context, a detailed understanding of data related to a patient's comorbidities and interactions with primary care is vital to make robust predictions.

The 'black-box' issue in AI refers to the inability of those using or reviewing tools that use AI to fully understand how the inputs and processes of algorithm development relate to the algorithm outputs. This may be due to the sheer complexity of algorithm development, particularly in the case of deep neural networks where it becomes virtually impossible to trace how their millions (and sometimes billions) of parameters combine within the algorithm to make decisions. The lack of understanding of the algorithm development process can also result from private organisations withholding information to protect their intellectual property rights. There is growing recognition that the development of AI or

ML solutions needs to be explicable and transparent, while acknowledging that many algorithms are developed by private corporations who have the right to protect their intellectual property.

The development and implementation of tools and devices that use AI in Australia are regulated under the TGA as long as their purpose is diagnosing, monitoring, predicting or preventing disease. These tools are often referred to as 'software as a medical device' and details of relevant inclusion and exclusion criteria can be found on the TGA website. If an AI-based tool is listed in the Australian Register of Therapeutic Goods, this can provide some comfort to Australian clinicians that these tools and devices that they use in their practice and that may influence their decision making will likely have been through the TGA approval process.

The introduction of web-accessible generative AI tools such as ChatGPT has brought new opportunities and challenges for the use of AI in health care. These tools now place sophisticated AI algorithms directly into the hands of consumers and health professionals via their mobile devices. While this will allow for the widescale adoption of these tools, it raises serious issues regarding how clinical governance standards are applied to the use of these tools. It is imperative that health professionals apply sound clinical judgement in the application of these technologies and comply with local clinical governance standards.

Box 29.13 Key points for practice: Artificial intelligence and machine learning

With the rapid development of AI-driven tools and devices, clinicians should exercise caution and consider the following points, especially when using an AI-supported tool or device for the first time:

- Review how the AI/ML tool was developed. Ask whether the algorithms have been published and if the development is transparent or explicable.
- If using AI tools to inform decision making, explore whether the population that was used to train the models is relevant to the population that you are treating.
- Consider whether the tools may have inherent bias because of the data used to train the algorithms and if this will impact the tool's accuracy if used in a specific patient population. Consider factors such as patient gender, ethnicity and socioeconomic status.
- Make sure you are sufficiently trained to use AI tools effectively and safely.
- Apply clinical judgement when using tools powered by AI/ML, especially if they are new or making recommendations about how care should be delivered. If the recommendations do not appear sound, then do not use them until you have explored the underlying development of the tools.
- Provide feedback to the developers of AI tools as feedback is critical for them to improve accuracy and usefulness in clinical settings.

29.3.3 Personalised medicine and health care

There is a growing number of examples where health services are looking at how they can improve the value of care through redesigning care models and using digital technologies to substantially change how care is delivered and by whom. The use of these models allows for a more personalised experience for the patient rather than a one-size-fits-all approach which is traditionally how the system is structured.

These new models typically:

- apply ML or AI to health data to identify patients at risk of poor outcomes
- place the identified patients on a personalised care program using digital tools to change their behaviour and reduce their risk
- include a virtual navigator, who may or may not be a health professional, who remotely communicates with a cohort of patients and coordinates issues such as referrals or changes in medication with specialist services
- have inbuilt monitoring of patients to assess risk and include escalation flags.

In a number of instances, these new models have improved outcomes while reducing reliance on specialist services.

Box 29.14 Case study: AI for predictive risk assessment

Reducing avoidable hospital readmissions improves patient outcomes and safety while decreasing clinician overload. AI algorithms have been successfully used to examine existing datasets (e.g. EHRs) to identify patients at risk of unplanned re-hospitalisations [46]. For example, the Australian Government Health Care Homes trial linked general practitioner, hospital and death registry data to create a predictive risk model algorithm for patients with chronic health conditions. The algorithm assessed patient demographics, pathology test results, medications and lifestyle factors to identify patients likely to be hospitalised over the next year [47]. At-risk patients were then contacted by the Health Care Homes team to receive proactive evidence-based care from their preferred physician.

Enrolled primary care practices have reported improvements in patient monitoring and care management due to proactive communication with patients. One barrier to implementation was staff turnover in enrolled practices. AI-driven risk assessment relies on high-quality data, and practices need to dedicate time and resources to familiarise new staff members with the algorithm, especially inputting complete data [47].

Box 29.15 Key points for practice: Risk identification

There are a number of issues that need to be considered by healthcare professionals engaged in AI risk identification programs, including how they should:

- maintain a therapeutic relationship with patients
- work and communicate in a virtual team with new members who may be delivering aspects of care that were previously someone else's responsibility or fulfilling entirely new roles
- ensure that the risk assessment algorithms used by the program are sound and not biased.

29.4 Important considerations

29.4.1 Cybersecurity

Cybersecurity is defined as the protection of computer systems and networks from information disclosure or theft of or damage to hardware, software or electronic data, as well as from the disruption or misdirection of services they provide. As health care moves further into the digital space, cybersecurity becomes increasingly critical and is the responsibility of all medical practitioners. All healthcare organisations using EHRs need to be aware of the risks of cybersecurity attacks and ensure they have a cybersecurity plan in place to address these risks.

There are six practical steps that can be taken:

1. Build security awareness.
2. Keep software up to date.
3. Use strong passwords or phrases and implement multifactor authentication.
4. Back up data regularly with an offsite option for backup storage.
5. Do not respond to phishing emails, texts and calls. Workforce education is critical here.
6. Do not pay ransom on ransomware attacks.

ADHA has developed a comprehensive set of resources providing more details about cybersecurity fundamentals and awareness and how to manage cybersecurity threats [48].

The use of these emerging technologies to automate, augment and introduce new possibilities into the way health care is delivered will begin to drive real benefits in health care. This will require new workflows to be introduced and have an impact on the requirements of certain roles of healthcare workers, including doctors. Many of the technologies mentioned already exist today and are being deployed in small-scale projects. However, few are used at scale across the health system to maximise their benefits.

29.4.2 Data governance, privacy and appropriate use

With increasing access to patient data comes increasing responsibility to ensure this data is used appropriately and in the best interest of the patient. This is particularly challenging as the access to diverse and new datasets can sometimes run ahead of existing governance and privacy frameworks.

Regarding privacy, legal obligations are set out in the 13 Australian Privacy Principles (APPs), outlined in the Privacy Act 1988 (Cth). The APPs determine how health information should be collected, used, stored and disclosed. The APPs are designed to be technology-neutral and flexible to developed and emerging technologies. Please refer to Chapter 6, Confidentiality, privacy and disclosure, and the independent national regulator, the Office of the Australian Information Commissioner, for a summary of APPs and how they apply to health care.

APPs apply to the acts of third parties, based in Australia or overseas, if the health information is collected from an individual who is physically present in Australia [49]. It is the responsibility of the health service provider to inform the individual of this risk when the technology is recommended or used by the provider's organisation [49]. This will likely involve checking privacy settings of technologies used to provide a health service or collect or hold health information. It is also important that doctors keep themselves updated on their organisation's privacy policy.

Many digital health technologies are developed or hosted by organisations overseas. Health information collected or stored on these technologies may be disclosed or made available to overseas recipients for a range of activities such as error reporting or advertisements. For example, mHealth apps transmit user data outside of the app to third parties who often reserve the right to use the de-identified data for their own commercial purposes [50]. Unfortunately, many mHealth apps only provide the privacy policies of the developer, while almost half of those on Google Play either do not provide any privacy policy text or violate their privacy policies [51].

When using health data, clinicians must consider whether that usage is in the best interest of the patient and also if the consent of the patient is required and/or if permission must be sought in terms of ethical or organisational approval. Increasingly, data legislation internationally is heading towards ownership of health data by the patient and giving patients full control of their data. This includes legislation such as the General Data Protection Regulation in Europe. Increasingly, health data is seen as a valuable asset and clinicians must be careful regarding how data they collect or contribute to may potentially be onsold or commercialised downstream.

Another key aspect of managing health data is understanding where it is stored. Increasingly, data systems live on the cloud, meaning the data is stored in data centres and accessed via the internet rather than being stored on a local server which is managed locally. An individual can also be tracked across multiple applications indefinitely. Unique identifiers are used to track individuals across telecommunications networks, operating systems and web browsers. When information can be collected from multiple sources, an individual could potentially be re-identified using the aggregated data. While cloud-based data centres offer many advantages in terms of efficiency and cost, they can be hosted anywhere in the world, potentially exposing the data to different governance and privacy standards. In recognition of this, state, territory and federal governments and regulators have strict rules regarding whether or not data can be stored offshore. This also applies to data that may be collected from consumer-facing apps and devices.

29.4.3 Equity and access

Access to technology is not equal with almost 2.5 million Australians not online and another 4 million people being limited internet users. This digital divide is influenced by a range of factors including age, location, socioeconomic status, language and digital health literacy of patients and healthcare professionals alike. For example, older patients may not understand how to use digital platforms, while patients from lower socioeconomic backgrounds may not have the equipment to access health information or care. These factors, along with other social determinants of health, should be taken into consideration before recommending digital solutions, as digital inclusion often follows and reinforces existing patterns of health-related vulnerabilities and socioeconomic disadvantage. (See also Chapter 16, Achieving full health potential: health equity.)

Digital inclusion is influenced by three factors: ability, affordability and access [52]. Mobile connectivity is only available for one-third of Australia's total land area, limiting access to the internet for rural and/or remote areas. Affordability of internet and other devices also contributes to the digital divide with half of low-income households struggling to pay for internet access and being more likely to be limited to their mobiles only. Australians who can afford internet access may not have the digital literacy to navigate online information and digital platforms. Less than 40% of Australians feel they have the digital skills to navigate changes in technology, with the majority concerned about privacy invasion and misinformation.

Questions to consider when recommending digital solutions:

- Does the patient need internet access?
- Does the patient have good mobile coverage at their location?
- What level of knowledge does the patient require to successfully use this digital solution?

Indigenous health can benefit enormously from the introduction of digital solutions especially as many Aboriginal and Torres Strait Islander communities are remote or very remote. Initiatives such as MHR have enabled Aboriginal and Torres Strait Islander communities to take greater control over their health care and better direct conversations about their health [53]. In particular, older Aboriginal and/or Torres Strait Islander adults (aged 65 years and over) are seeking telehealth technologies to assist with access, equity and cost-effectiveness of health services [54]. More importantly, equal digital inclusion has been identified as one of the national targets in the National agreement on Closing the Gap to ensure Aboriginal and Torres Strait Islander communities can make informed decisions about their own lives [55].

Despite the benefits of digital health initiatives, there are several barriers that remain for these populations [54]. These initiatives need to acknowledge unequal internet access for Aboriginal and/or Torres Strait Islander people and cultural sensitivities surrounding data ownership. Almost a third of Aboriginal and Torres Strait Islander communities in remote areas have no household internet or phone connection due to a lack of affordability [51]. Lack of access to digital health initiatives is compounded by lower levels of digital literacy among these communities, as well as lower interest in digital solutions compared to the national average [52]. These barriers need to be acknowledged, and trust needs to be built into digital solutions before recommending a transition to remote care. The National Indigenous Australians Agency has compiled an Indigenous digital inclusion plan that provides greater detail about the challenges faced by Aboriginal and/or Torres Strait Islander communities, as well as information on digital inclusion programs [56].

Indigenous data sovereignty refers to the right of Aboriginal and/or Torres Strait Islander communities to determine how their information should be managed in accordance with their practices and customs [56]. This right extends to the ability to govern the collection, ownership and application of Indigenous data. These movements have developed in response to the historic use of data for state monitoring and control of Aboriginal and/or Torres Strait Islander peoples [56]. The Maiam nayri Wingara Indigenous Data Sovereignty collective was formed in 2017 to develop data sovereignty and governance principles [57]. A summit conducted by the collective held that Aboriginal and Torres Strait Islander people have a right to:

- data governance or control over data creation, analysis, dissemination and infrastructure
- data that is accessible and available at an individual and community level
- data that empowers self-determination and self-governance
- a data ecosystem that is accountable to the Aboriginal and/or Torres Strait Islander community
- data that protects and respects Aboriginal and/or Torres Strait Islander interests [54].

The *National best practice guidelines for collecting Indigenous status in health data sets* provide advice on how to implement best practice and improve data quality when collecting Indigenous status in health data [58]. Data quality is important, as any under-identification of Indigenous status can create difficulties in measuring progress made towards closing the gap.

Box 29.16 Case study: Telstra's Communicare software supporting Indigenous health

Telstra Health's Communicare software was developed in 1994 and provides a digital care solution for primary and community health services. It supports over 50% of Aboriginal Medical Services (AMSs).

It enables multidisciplinary teams to access configurable workflow and clinical items to support specific programs and conditions such as renal disease, and assists healthcare teams in implementing preventable healthcare measures. This helps to support patients in the long term as well as the short term.

It can provide a holistic, patient-centric view across a patient's entire journey through the health service, enabling healthcare providers to analyse and evaluate outcomes and equipping them with information and insights to help make more informed decisions to improve health care in Aboriginal and/or Torres Strait Islander communities.

Aboriginal and/or Torres Strait Islander communities are highly unique and often require digital health software that is culturally specific. Communicare is configured with many fields that are specific to supporting health and care for Aboriginal and/or Torres Strait Islander peoples, such as culturally sensitive mourning replacement terms, cardiotocography status and skin groups. It has been built with the capability to make continuity of care as simple as possible. For example, its integrated transport management system enables an AMS to schedule transport for patients who require this, enabling continuity of care.

Summary

This chapter has provided a high-level overview of many examples of digital health technologies and the impact of these technologies on the current and future delivery of healthcare services. The chapter does not cover every possible technology that is currently being developed or innovations not yet imagined. It is expected that digital health will remain a dynamic and changing environment, such that any guidelines on using digital health in clinical practice will have to be sufficiently broad and flexible to accommodate future transformations. It is important to continue to use sound clinical judgement and decision making when using any digital health technology in everyday clinical practice. High levels of quality and safety of care must be maintained regardless of what technology is used, and practitioners should consider any equity, access, privacy and ethical implications that may arise. Digital health is, after all, health care.

References

1. Baxby L, Bennett S, Watson P, et al. Australia's health reimagined: the journey to a connected and confident consumer. 2022. https://www2.deloitte.com/au/en/pages/life-sciences-and-healthcare/articles/australias-health-reimagined.html (accessed Jun 2023).
2. Australian Digital Health Agency. Safe, seamless and secure: evolving health and care to meet the needs of modern Australia. 2016. https://www.digitalhealth.gov.au/sites/default/files/2020-11/Australia%27s%20National%20Digital%20Health%20Strategy%20-%20Safe%2C%20seamless%20and%20secure.pdf (accessed Jun 2023).
3. Australian Digital Health Agency; Australian Medical Council. Synthesis of evidence and recommendations for a capability framework in digital health in medicine. 2021. https://www.amc.org.au/wp-content/uploads/2021/05/Milestone-6-Synthesis-of-Evidence-and-Recommendations-Digital-Health-in-Medicine-Capability-Framework-2021-Final-Version.pdf (accessed Jun 2023).
4. Brunner M, McGregor D, Keep M, et al. An eHealth capabilities framework for graduates and health professionals: mixed-methods study *J Med Int Res*; 2018: 20: e10229.
5. Royal Australian College of General Practitioners. Minimum requirements for general practice clinical information systems to improve usability. 2019. https://www.racgp.org.au/FSDEDEV/media/documents/Running%20a%20practice/Support%20and%20tools/Minimum-requirements-for-general-practice-CIS.pdf (accessed Jun 2023).
6. Wachter RM. The digital doctor: hope, hype and harm at the dawn of medicine's computer age. New York: McGraw Hill, 2017.
7. Commonwealth Scientific and Industrial Research Organisation. Cutting hospital waiting times. 2021. https://www.csiro.au/en/research/technology-space/data/waiting-times (accessed Jun 2023).
8. Smith P. Patient Admission Prediction Tool – the one toolie that's welcome at Schoolies. *Hospital and Healthcare*. 2013. https://www.hospitalhealth.com.au/content/nursing/article/patient-admission-prediction-tool-the-one-toolie-that-s-welcome-at-schoolies-148875692 (accessed Jun 2023).
9. Agency for Clinical Innovation. Patient-reported measures. https://aci.health.nsw.gov.au/statewide-programs/prms (accessed Jun 2023).
10. Australian Commission on Safety and Quality in Health Care. Electronic medication management. https://www.safetyandquality.gov.au/our-work/medication-safety/electronic-medication-management (accessed Jun 2023).
11. Department of Health and Aged Care. Safe use of medicines. 2022. https://www1.health.gov.au/internet/main/publishing.nsf/Content/nmp-quality.htm-copy2 (accessed Jun 2023).
12. Embi PJ, Leonard AC. Evaluating alert fatigue over time to HER-based clinical trial alerts: findings from a randomized controlled study. *J Am Med Inform Assoc* 2012; 19: e145–e148.
13. Carspecken GW, Sharek PJ, Longhurst C, et al. A clinical case of electronic health record drug alert fatigue: consequences for patient outcome. *Pediatrics* 2013; 131: e1970–e1973.
14. Scalvini S, Vitacca M, Paletta L, et al. Telemedicine: a new frontier for effective healthcare services. *Monaldi Arch Chest Dis* 2004; 61(4): 226–233.
15. Australian Digital Health Agency. Telehealth. 2024. https://www.digitalhealth.gov.au/healthcare-providers/initiatives-and-programs/telehealth (accessed Jun 2025).
16. Visionflex. A community-based solution for Indigenous healthcare. 2021. https://www.visionflex.com/community-based-solution-for-indigenous-healthcare/ (accessed Jun 2023).
17. Australian Council on Healthcare Standards. Evaluation and Quality Improvement Program. https://www.achsi.org/services/standards-overview/see-all-standards (accessed Jun 2023).
18. McKenzie R, Kanhutu KN. Telehealth quality check: is it time for national standards? *AJGP* 2021; 50: 778–781.
19. Snoswell CL, Chelberg G, Guzman KRD, et al. The clinical effectiveness of telehealth: a systematic review of meta-analyses from 2010 to 2019. *J Telemed Telecare* 2021; 29: 669–684.
20. Royal Australian College of General Practitioners. Guide to providing telephone and video consultations in general practice. https://www.racgp.org.au/clinical-resources/covid-19-resources/telehealth/guide-to-provide-phone-and-video-consultation (accessed Jun 2023).
21. Medical Board of Australia. Telehealth consultations with patients. 2023. https://www.medicalboard.gov.au/codes-guidelines-policies/telehealth-consultations-with-patients.aspx (accessed Jun 2023).

22. Medical Board of Australia. Good medical practice: a code of conduct for doctors in Australia. 2020. https://www.medicalboard.gov.au/codes-guidelines-policies/code-of-conduct.aspx (accessed Jun 2023).

23. Department of Health and Aged Care. COVID-19 advice for health professionals. 2021. https://www.health.gov.au/news/permanent-telehealth-for-all-australians (accessed Jun 2023).

24. Avant. Telehealth – medico-legal risk for GPs. 2020. https://www.avant.org.au/Resources/Public/Telehealth-medico-legal-risk-for-GPs/ (accessed Jun 2023).

25. Southern Cross University. Feros Care's My Health Clinic at Home Pilot: final report. 2014. https://www.feroscare.com.au/wp-content/uploads/docs/default-source/default-document-library/mhcah-pilot-full-report-jan15.pdf (accessed Jun 2023).

26. Commonwealth Scientific and Industrial Research Organisation. Home monitoring of chronic diseases. 2021. https://www.csiro.au/en/research/health-medical/diagnostics/home-monitoring (accessed Jun 2023).

27. Volpi SS, Biduski D, Bellei EA, et al. Using a mobile health app to improve patients' adherence to hypertension treatment: a non-randomised clinical trial. *PeerJ* 2021; 9: e11491.

28. Akbar S, Coiera E, Magrabi F. Safety concerns with consumer-facing mobile health applications and their consequences: a scoping review. *J Am Med Inform Assoc* 2020; 27: 330–340.

29. Therapeutic Goods Administration. Regulation of software based medical devices. 2023. https://www.tga.gov.au/regulation-software-based-medical-devices (accessed Jun 2023).

30. Royal Australian College of General Practitioners. Factsheet: health apps. https://www.racgp.org.au/FSDEDEV/media/documents/Patient%20information/Recommending-Health-Apps-Factsheet.pdf

31. Australian Digital Health Agency. Assessment framework for mHealth apps. 2022. https://www.digitalhealth.gov.au/sites/default/files/documents/adha-mhealth-assessment-framework-dec.pdf

32. Loucks J, Stewart D, Bucaille A, et al. Wearable technology in health care: getting better all the time. 2021. https://www2.deloitte.com/xe/en/insights/industry/technology/technology-media-and-telecom-predictions/2022/wearable-technology-healthcare.html (accessed Jun 2023).

33. Singh B, Maher C. Why wearable fitness trackers aren't as useless as some make them out to be. 2021. https://www.abc.net.au/news/2021-12-13/wearable-fitness-trackers-do-they-work/100691444 (accessed Jun 2023).

34. Australian Digital Health Agency. Secure messaging. 2024. https://www.digitalhealth.gov.au/healthcare-providers/initiatives-and-programs/secure-messaging (accessed May 2025).

35. Royal Australian College of General Practitioners. Using personal mobile devices for clinical photos in general practice. 2019. https://www.racgp.org.au/FSDEDEV/media/documents/Running%20a%20practice/Practice%20resources/Using-personal-mobile-devices-for-clinical-photos.pdf (accessed Jun 2023).

36. Mansfield SJ, Morrison SG, Stephens HO, et al. Social media and the medical profession *Med J Aust* 2011; 194: 642–644.

37. Medical Board of Australia. Social media: how to meet your obligations under the national law. 2019. https://www.medicalboard.gov.au/Codes-Guidelines-Policies/Social-media-guidance.aspx (accessed Jun 2023).

38. Australian Medical Association. A guide to social media and medical professionalism: the tips and traps every doctor and medical student should know. 2020. https://ama.com.au/sites/default/files/documents/2020%20AMA%20Social%20Media%20Guide%20FINAL_0.pdf (accessed Jun 2023).

39. Commonwealth Scientific and Industrial Research Organisation. Artificial intelligence and machine learning. https://research.csiro.au/cor/machine-learning/ (accessed May 2025).

40. Seah JCY, Tang CHM, Buchlak QD, et al. Effect of a comprehensive deep-learning model on the accuracy of chest x-ray interpretation by radiologists: a retrospective, multireader multicase study *Lancet Digit Health* 2021; 3: e496–4506.

41. Annalise.ai. Annalise.ai. https://annalise.ai/ (accessed Jun 2023).

42. Annalise.ai. Uncertainty and confidence in medical imaging AI. 2021. https://annalise.ai/2021/06/uncertainty-confidence-medical-imaging-ai/ (accessed Jun 2023).

43. World Health Organization. Ethics and governance of artificial intelligence for health. 2021. https://www.who.int/publications/i/item/9789240029200

44. Koopman B, Bradford D, Hansen D. Exemplars of artificial intelligence and machine learning in health care: improving the safety, quality, efficiency and accessibility of Australia's healthcare system. 2021. Commonwealth Scientific and Industrial Research Organisation. https://aehrc.csiro.au/wp-content/uploads/2021/10/Exemplars-AI-in-Health-July-2020.pdf

45. Royal Australian and New Zealand College of Radiologists. RANZCR position statement on the regulation of artificial intelligence in medicine. 2022. https://www.ranzcr.com/documents/5579-ranzcr-position-statement-on-the-regulation-of-artificial-intelligence-in-medicine/file (accessed May 2025).

46. Davis S, Zhang J, Lee I, et al. Effective hospital readmission prediction models using machine-learned features. *BMC Health Serv Res* 2022; 22: 1415.

47. Department of Health and Aged Care. Health Care Homes trial – evaluation reports collection. 2022. https://www.health.gov.au/resources/collections/health-care-homes-trial-evaluation-reports-collection (accessed May 2025).

48. Australian Digital Health Agency. Cyber security. https://www.digitalhealth.gov.au/healthcare-providers/cyber-security (accessed Jun 2023).

49. Office of the Australian Information Commissioner. Australian privacy principles guidelines: Privacy Act 1988. 2014. https://www.oaic.gov.au/__data/assets/pdf_file/0009/1125/app-guidelines-july-2019.pdf (accessed Jun 2023).

50. Grundy Q, Chiu K, Held F, et al. Data sharing practices of medicines related apps and the mobile ecosystem: traffic, content, and network analysis. *BMJ* 2019; 364: l920.

51. Tangari G, Muhammed I, Ijaz K, et al. Mobile health and privacy: cross-sectional study. *BMJ* 2021; 373: n1248.

52. Good Things Foundation Australia. Digital nation Australia 2021. 2021. https://www.goodthingsfoundation.org.au/news/digital-nation-australia-2021/ (accessed Jun 2023).

53. Australian Digital Health Agency. Gurriny Yealamucka connects Yarrabah community with technology for better healthcare. 2021. https://www.digitalhealth.gov.au/newsroom/media-releases/gurriny-yealamucka-connects-yarrabah-community-with-technology-for-better-healthcare

54. Choukou M, Maddah A, Polyvana A, et al. Digital health technology for Indigenous older adults: a scoping review. *Int J Med Informatics* 2021; 148: 104408.

55. Department of Prime Minister and Cabinet. National agreement on closing the gap. 2020. https://www.closingthegap.gov.au/sites/default/files/2021-05/ctg-national-agreement_apr-21.pdf

56. Lovett R, Lee V, Kukutai T, et al. Good data practices for Indigenous data sovereignty and governance. In Daly A, Devitt SK, Mann M, editors. Good data. Amsterdam: Institute of Network Cultures, 2019.

57. Maiam nayri Wingara Indigenous Data Sovereignty Collective. About us. https://www.maiamnayriwingara.org/about-us (accessed Jun 2023).

58. Australian Institute of Health and Welfare. National best practice guidelines for collecting Indigenous status in health data sets. 2010. https://www.aihw.gov.au/getmedia/ad54c4a7-4e03-4604-a0f3-ccb13c6d4260/11052.pdf.aspx?inline=true (accessed Jun 2023).

30 Prescribing and administering medicines

Jeremy Hayllar

Introduction

This chapter focuses on the regulatory framework for the prescription of medicines by doctors in their daily practice and discusses some of the specific situations that prescribing doctors may face. It also examines the ethical and professional issues around the important relationship that should exist between doctors and pharmacists (see also Chapter 11, The doctor and interprofessional relationships). The chapter does not attempt to provide details about the manufacture, approval and distribution processes for medicinal products or how the regulatory framework affects pharmacists, dentists, nurses and others. The clinical knowledge, skills and judgement required to prescribe medicines effectively and efficiently are also beyond the scope of this book.

30.1 Regulatory framework for prescribing

30.1.1 Therapeutic goods

For a doctor to prescribe a medicine within Australia, it must usually be approved for supply in Australia (as determined by the Therapeutic Goods Administration [TGA]), and either registered or listed on the Australian Register of Therapeutic Goods (ARTG). Special arrangements can sometimes be made to import medicines that are not on the ARTG. In most cases, the medicine is subsidised on the Pharmaceutical Benefits Scheme (PBS) so that the patient pays a capped contribution, which is often far less than the actual cost of the medicine. Some PBS-subsidised medicines are restricted to being prescribed by specific specialists or for limited indications for which there is a positive benefit–cost ratio. The Medical Board of Australia's *Good medical practice: a code of conduct for doctors in Australia* also includes the need for doctors to ensure that they have adequate knowledge and skills to provide safe clinical care, and this includes knowledge about the medicines they prescribe.

Through the *Therapeutic Goods Act 1989* (Cth), administered by the TGA of the Department of Health, Disability and Ageing, the Australian Government is responsible for overseeing the national system that controls the safety, quality, efficacy and availability of therapeutic goods (drugs and devices), whether produced here or abroad. Through the *National Health Act 1953* (Cth), it is also responsible for the PBS, which is designed to ensure community access to affordable prescription medicines when they meet cost–benefit criteria. This chapter covers the aspects of the PBS that regulate or control medical practitioners' prescribing of medicines included in the PBS. The TGA provides a useful overview of this regulatory system [1].

While the registration of medicines (therapeutic goods) is a federal responsibility, controlling access to those medicines is constitutionally the responsibility of the states and territories. Each jurisdiction has its own legislation to regulate the availability and use of medicines (and poisons). In particular, jurisdictions vary in their approaches to self-prescribing, although it is well understood that self-treatment may result in suboptimal care (see also Chapter 12, Personal health of the doctor: illness and impairment). The controls exist primarily to protect the public, and to a lesser extent to protect doctors from the dangers of self-administration. The legislation provides for criminal penalties for breaches; any convictions of doctors by the courts usually result in a notification to the Medical Board of Australia to determine whether unprofessional conduct was involved, and whether the doctor's practice or prescribing rights should be restricted (see Chapter 21, Regulation of the medical profession). The relevant state and territory Acts are listed in Table 30.1. Contact details for the medicines and poisons agencies, which regulate access to medicines and particularly drugs of dependence in each jurisdiction, are available on the TGA website [2].

Table 30.1 Legislation controlling prescription and access to medicines

State or territory	Name of legislation
Australian Capital Territory	*Medicines, Poisons and Therapeutic Goods Act 2008* Medicines, Poisons and Therapeutic Goods Regulations 2008
New South Wales	*Poisons and Therapeutic Goods Act 1966* (amended 1996) Poisons and Therapeutic Goods Regulation 2008
Northern Territory	*Medicines, Poisons and Therapeutic Goods Act 2012*
Queensland	*Medicines and Poisons Act 2019* Medicines and Poisons (Medicines) Regulations 2021
South Australia	*Controlled Substances Act 1984* Controlled Substances (Poisons) Regulations 2011
Tasmania	*Poisons Act 1971* *Misuse of Drugs Act 2001* Poisons Regulations 2018
Victoria	*Drugs, Poisons and Controlled Substances Act 1981* Drugs, Poisons and Controlled Substances Regulations 2017
Western Australia	*Medicines and Poisons Act 2014* Medicines and Poisons Regulations 2016

30.1.2 Standard scheduling of medicines and poisons

Medicines approved for use in Australia are subjected to jurisdictional rules restricting their availability (e.g. prescription only or over the counter). To ensure the states and territories are substantially uniform in their approach to regulating the availability of medicines, the Advisory Committee on Medicines Scheduling was established by the Therapeutic Goods Act. Comprising relevant state and territory representatives, a key task of this committee is advising and making recommendations to the Secretary of the Department of Health to maintain the Standard for the Uniform Scheduling of Medicines and

Poisons (SUSMP) [3] which lists all the drugs contained in each schedule (available on the department's website). The schedules are given below, with some examples of the drugs included in each. The schedules of most relevance to medical practice are Schedules 2 and 3 (over-the-counter medicines that may be recommended by medical practitioners but do not require a prescription), Schedule 4 (prescription-only medicines) and Schedule 8 (controlled medicines, including drugs of dependence).

Table 30.2 Schedules of medicines and poisons in Australia

Schedule	Classification	Description
Schedule 1	Not currently in use	–
Schedule 2	Pharmacy Medicine	Substances, the safe use of which may require advice from a pharmacist and which should be available from a pharmacy or, where a pharmacy service is not available, from a licensed person.' No prescription is required and these medicines may be advertised direct to the public. Examples include aspirin and paracetamol; limited quantities of a range of antihistamines, both sedating and non-sedating; various topical antifungal and steroid products; limited quantities of histamine H2 blockers and proton pump inhibitors; benzocaine and lignocaine lozenges and suppositories; some non-steroidal anti-inflammatory medicines.
Schedule 3	Pharmacist Only Medicine	'Substances, the safe use of which requires professional advice, but which should be available to the public from a pharmacist without a prescription.' No prescription is required for the public to obtain Schedule 3 medicines from a pharmacist. Examples include cannabidiol up to 150 mg daily (with 1% or less tetrahydrocannabinol content) although at the time of writing no relevant products are available; emergency post-coital contraception; melatonin tablets up to 2 mg; orlistat; pseudoephedrine (other than preparations for stimulant, appetite suppression or weight-control purposes); some antihistamines; salbutamol metered aerosol inhalers; various triptans for migraine.
Schedule 4	Prescription Only Medicine	'Substances, the use or supply of which should be by or on the order of persons permitted by State or Territory legislation to prescribe and should be available from a pharmacist on prescription.' This schedule covers most of the common medicines prescribed by doctors, and also includes anabolic steroidal agents, local anaesthetics, most benzodiazepines (although benzodiazepines are classified as 'monitored' or 'high risk' medicines, see section 30.3.2), codeine in doses of up to 30 mg in combination with another substance (also 'monitored' medicines), chemotherapeutic agents, gabapentinoids, sex hormones, tramadol (also a 'monitored' medicine), and vaccines for human use.

Continued over page

Schedule	Classification	Description
Schedule 5	Caution	'Substances with a low potential for causing harm, the extent of which can be reduced through the use of appropriate packaging with simple warnings and safety directions on the label.' These include many domestic poisons, such as acetic acid, kerosene, methylated spirits and mineral turpentine.
Schedule 6	Poison	'Substances with a moderate potential for causing harm, the extent of which can be reduced through the use of distinctive packaging with strong warnings and safety directions on the label.' These include industrial and agricultural poisons, eucalyptus oil and formaldehyde.
Schedule 7	Dangerous Poison	'Substances with a high potential for causing harm at low exposure and which require special precautions during manufacture, handling or use.' Special regulations restricting their availability, possession, storage or use may apply. These include strychnine, cyanides and agricultural poisons such as paraquat.
Schedule 8	Controlled Drug	'Substances which should be available for use but require restriction of manufacture, supply, distribution, possession and use to reduce abuse, misuse and physical or psychological dependence.' These include barbiturates, two benzodiazepines (alprazolam and flunitrazepam), buprenorphine, cocaine, codeine when presented as the sole active ingredient, dexamphetamine, fentanyl and derivatives, hydromorphone, ketamine, methadone, methylphenidate, morphine, oxycodone, pentazocine, pethidine, tapentadol, and tetrahydrocannabinol-based products.
Schedule 9	Prohibited Substance	'Substances which may be abused or misused, the manufacture, possession, sale or use of which should be prohibited by law except when required for medical or scientific research, or for analytical, teaching or training purposes with approval of Commonwealth and/or State or Territory Health Authorities.' These include heroin, lysergic acid, phencyclidine and tetrahydrocannabinols (except where included in Schedule 4 or 8).
Schedule 10		Substances of such danger to health as to warrant prohibition of sale, supply and use.

Although Schedule 8 refers to drugs of dependence, it must be noted that some Schedule 4 medicines can also induce dependence. For this reason, and because some Schedule 4 drugs are subject to misuse and trafficking, several such drugs are regulated and monitored as if they were Schedule 8 Controlled Drugs. These include benzodiazepines, anorectic medicines and anabolic steroids. In addition, there are a small number of specified Schedule 4 drugs that may only be prescribed by a doctor who is authorised to do so: these include retinoids, ovulatory stimulants, prostaglandins and thalidomide. Minor variations in scheduling between the states and territories are recorded by the TGA and available on the website [4].

30.1.3 Some relevant terminology

The legislation controlling prescribing by doctors refers to drugs, therapeutic goods, poisons and drug dependence. These terms are explained as follows:

- A *drug* is any chemical substance, synthetic or extracted from plant or animal tissue, that has a physiological effect on the body; drugs are the active constituents of prescription medicines and also of recreational drug products.
- A *medicine* (sometimes termed medication) is a medicinal product containing an active ingredient or drug, presented in a specific formulation (e.g. tablet, capsule, liquid) of known composition, and intended for use as a treatment to prevent, alleviate or cure disease.
- *Therapeutic goods* are defined as goods that are represented to be, or are likely to be, taken or used for therapeutic purposes. They include medicines, therapeutic devices and materials used in pregnancy testing, and testing for susceptibility to diseases.
- A *poison* is any substance that, when absorbed into the blood, adversely affects health or destroys life. The resulting effect from the ingestion, absorption or inhalation of a poison is called poisoning.
- The World Health Organization has discarded the terms *addiction* and *habituation* in favour of the single term *drug dependence*. This is defined as a syndrome comprising a cluster of behavioural, cognitive and physiological phenomena that develop after repeated use of some substances. Typically, this includes a strong desire to take the drug, difficulties in controlling its use, persisting in its use despite harmful consequences, a higher priority given to drug use than other activities and obligations, increased tolerance, and sometimes a physical withdrawal state if use is interrupted [5].

As some state and territory legislation in Australia still refers to, and differentiates between, drugs of addiction and drugs of dependence, some additional relevant terms are defined below:

- A *drug addict* is a person who has acquired an overpowering desire for the continued administration of any drug of dependence and in whom the cessation of the administration of such drug leads to definite symptoms of mental or physical distress or disorder.
- *Drug abuse* (also referred to as *drug misuse*) [6] or *harmful use* have specific definitions and are used to describe behaviours that occur in individuals who are taking drugs of dependence with resultant problems, but who do not meet the criteria for drug dependence. These descriptions may be relevant to the problems that occur in some individuals, including some medical practitioners, who use prescribed drugs for non-medical purposes or use prescription drugs obtained illegally.
- *Drug tolerance* involves the adaptation of body tissues, predominantly the brain, to steadily increasing dosages of a drug to achieve a constant physical or psychological effect. When the drug being used is withdrawn, an illness of variable intensity usually follows. Both tolerance and withdrawal symptoms are physical phenomena that respond to physical treatment.

30.2 Prescribing medicines

30.2.1 Prescribing medicines: general requirements

Doctors can prescribe medicines containing drugs in Schedules 2, 3, 4 and 8 for the medical treatment of their patients, although a pharmacist may also supply Schedule 2 and 3 drugs without a doctor's prescription. Being mindful that some medicines should not be stopped abruptly, if a patient runs out of their medication and their prescriber cannot be contacted, a pharmacy can issue a 3-day emergency supply of some prescription medicines (not including controlled substances like benzodiazepines or opioids).

The use of electronic prescriptions (e-scripts) is rapidly becoming the standard of care, both for face-to-face and telehealth consultations. The prescriber sends an electronic prescription by SMS or email, which is downloaded to a patient's smartphone and read electronically by a pharmacy (more detail in section 30.2.2). Some doctors use prescribing software to generate printed prescriptions. If writing by hand, doctors always need to take care with their prescriptions as errors and/or illegibility have been known to cause serious adverse effects, including deaths. Doctors should not prescribe for themselves (see Chapter 12, Personal health of the doctor: illness and impairment); self-prescribing is illegal in Victoria and the Northern Territory and strongly discouraged elsewhere. Prescribing for family and relatives should be avoided whenever possible. This is discussed in more detail in Chapter 8, Sexual and other professional boundaries: being a doctor in modern society, and Chapter 21, Regulation of the medical profession.

The following advice about prescribing combines the statutory requirements with sensible precautions to protect community interests and the interests of pharmacists and doctors:

- Prescription pads should be stored securely and should only be accessible to authorised persons. If stolen, the police and the state or territory department of health must be notified. Similarly, computer passwords that give access to prescribing software must be kept secure and not shared with anyone else.
- The prescription must clearly show the doctor's name, address, prescriber number and telephone number; the last item being particularly important to enable prompt contact from the dispensing pharmacist.
- The date the prescription was written must be shown.
- The patient's name and address must be shown. In the case of Schedule 8 medicines, the patient's date of birth must also be written on the prescription. The prescription may only be written for the medical treatment of the person named on the prescription.
- The prescription must be legible and include the generic name of the active component (drug) in the preparation. It is illegal for a pharmacist to dispense a prescription if the pharmacist is uncertain of the name of the drug or the directions written on the prescription.
- Pharmacists may become concerned that there is an error on the prescription that could cause serious harm to a patient (e.g. methotrexate intended for weekly dosing for arthritis may inadvertently be written as a daily dose, which has caused death). In this case, the pharmacist is expected to contact the doctor by telephone, and it is essential for the doctor to take their advice seriously (see section 30.2.8).
- Prescribing by doctors is for the medical treatment of patients; hence, prescribing for other purposes, such as anabolic steroids for bodybuilding, other cosmetic reasons, or enhanced sporting performance is not permitted.
- A precise dose of the active drug should be specified and in general the frequency of administration specified. A doctor who uses the term 'as directed' needs to be especially careful that the patient is fully informed of those directions, preferably in writing.
- Non-standard abbreviations should be avoided to reduce error; a list of accepted abbreviations is published by the Australian Commission on Safety and Quality in Health Care [7].
- The quantity of medication and number of repeat authorisations must be shown. For Schedule 8 medicines, the quantity and number of repeats must be given in both figures and words.
- Where an unusually large dose is prescribed, the drug and the dose should be underlined and initialled or signed in ink.

- The full details on the prescription must be in the doctor's own handwriting (unless computer-generated or an e-script—see section 30.2.2).
- No space should be left between the last item on the prescription and the doctor's signature, to reduce the risk of forged additions.
- For medicines that are prescribed and funded under the PBS, the requirements outlined in the *Schedule of pharmaceutical benefits* [8] must be followed.
- For PBS prescriptions, only three items may be prescribed on one prescription page. Only one prescription per day for any specific medicine may be written for a patient, and back-dating and forward-dating of prescriptions is not permitted. Under Regulation 49 of the *Schedule of pharmaceutical benefits*, where patients may experience hardship (e.g. if they are travelling long distances or overseas), pharmacists are permitted to fill repeat prescriptions ahead of the due date, provided the doctor has initialled the prescription with the symbol 'R49' (previously R24) (see also section 30.3.5) [8].
- In the case of public hospitals participating in pharmaceutical reforms, a specific prescription pad (in triplicate) allows up to 10 items on one prescription form. The prescriber's name, prescriber number and contact number (phone number or pager) must be included. Authority medicines may also be included on this single prescription form, with the approval number or the STREAMLINED authority code recorded in the approval column on the prescription form.
- Where a prescriber has concerns about a patient receiving the full quantity of a prescription at one time, they may specify 'staged supply', indicating on the prescription how often the patient may collect the medicine (e.g. daily or weekly). Pharmacies often charge for this service.

Prescribers should recognise that it is common for treatment not to be taken as prescribed, causing significant avoidable morbidity and mortality, particularly in chronic disease management. A range of factors may contribute to this, including drug side effects, lack of a shared goal of the aim of treatment, misunderstanding or lack of information, depression, financial hardship and in some instances lower socioeconomic status. Recognising these may help overcome potential barriers to effective treatment with medicines [9]. Two federal health department programs are designed to improve effective and safe use of medicines. Under the Home Medicines Review program, a pharmacist visits patients at home, helps them understand all their medicines, and makes recommendations to help prescribers and patients develop medicine management plans to increase the quality use of medicines and decrease adverse events. The Dose Administration Aids Program supports pharmacies to provide medicines to their patients in a well-sealed, tamper-proof device, to help patients take their medicines at the right dose and time.

30.2.2 Computer-generated and electronic prescriptions

There are additional legal requirements placed on doctors who generate prescriptions by computer, primarily because of the risk of fraud. Only doctors may have access to the prescription-writing computer program. All the information described above for handwritten prescriptions must be included on the computer-generated prescription. The prescribing doctor's name must appear immediately beneath the last item on the prescription, followed by their handwritten signature. Any space below the signature must either be electronically blocked out or the number of items prescribed must be specified on that prescription. The computer program must ensure that the details of each prescription are kept with the records of the patient and preserved for at least 1 year. No handwritten amendments may be made to a printed computer-generated prescription; if a change or amendment is needed, a new prescription must be generated. Under recent medicine regulations, active-ingredient prescribing requires the generic name of the drug to be used, rather than a trade name, although handwritten prescriptions are currently exempted. For drugs of dependence, only one item per prescription is permitted and the doctor must confirm *in handwriting* all the particulars including the name of the medicine, the strength (amount of active drug in each dosage unit), quantity and repeats.

Electronic prescribing is also available, where the prescriber can create an electronic prescription (an e-script) that is linked to a unique electronic token in the form of a QR code, which is sent to the patient as an SMS or email. The token is a key that can be read by appropriately equipped pharmacies to unlock the electronic prescription. Tokens also allow use of the Active Script List, which can display all active eligible barcoded paper and electronic prescriptions for the information of prescribers and pharmacists, with the consent of the patient.

With advances in technology, there has been an increase in the availability of prescribing via telehealth (video, telephone or online) instead of an in-person consultation. When this is done as part of an ongoing treating relationship and includes an interaction between the patient and practitioner, it can offer the advantages of convenience and ready access. However, when prescribing is carried out without any interaction other than through a brief online questionnaire, the risks of adverse effects is increased, and routine use of this form of prescribing is not supported by relevant colleges or the Medical Board of Australia [10].

30.2.3 Authority prescriptions

Nearly 1000 medicines are subsidised on the PBS at a cost of over $12 billion annually. These medicines are placed in one of three categories: unrestricted, restricted to specific therapeutic indications, or authority required. The third category—requiring the authority of Medicare under the PBS to prescribe the drugs concerned—is designed primarily to contain costs, and in some cases to improve safety of highly toxic preparations. Authority required benefits fall into two categories: Authority required and Authority required (STREAMLINED). Authority required prescriptions must be approved by Services Australia (by post, telephone or via its website) prior to being issued. Authority required (STREAMLINED) prescriptions require a specific code to be recorded in place of an approval. The code corresponds to the medicine and its approved indication—for example, gabapentin 300 mg capsules is an Authority required (STREAMLINED) medicine for partial epileptic seizures which have failed to be controlled satisfactorily by other antiepileptic drugs (code 1834M). When gabapentin is used for refractory neuropathic pain, unable to be controlled by other drugs, the code is different (4592Q). Drugs requiring an authority include newer, expensive medicines, although authority may also be sought to prescribe an increased quantity of a particular medicine or to provide an increased number of repeat prescriptions.

Prescribing practitioners apply on a combined application/authority prescription form available as personalised pre-printed prescription pads from the PBS. Applications may also be made by telephone (1800 888 333) or online [8]. The triplicate copy of the prescription must be retained in the patient record for a minimum of 12 months, and must include the details of the indication for which the drug is being prescribed. Only one item can be prescribed on each authority prescription form. The maximum quantity of a drug of dependence authorised at any one time will generally not exceed 1 month's therapy. Where supply for a longer period is warranted, authorised quantities will normally not exceed 3 months' supply. Some highly specialised medicines require a written authority, after a written request for approval has been made, in some cases accompanied by specific test results.

Similar arrangements exist for authority prescriptions for veterans, but the authority is sought from the Department of Veterans' Affairs.

30.2.4 Storage and record keeping of drugs of dependence

Under the legislation, doctors are obliged to store drugs of dependence in a locked steel cabinet fixed to the wall or the floor, and to transport them securely in a locked doctor's bag or similar locked receptacle. If the locked bag or receptacle is out of the doctor's immediate possession, it should be stored out of sight in a locked cupboard or a locked vehicle. In addition, a written record must be kept for a minimum of 3 years, showing to whom any such drug has been administered or supplied. The unaltered record must also show for each such medicine an accurate balance of the stock at hand. Any supplies given to patients must be labelled with the medicine details, the name of the patient, the date of supply, the directions for use and the doctor's name and address.

Each year, doctors are prosecuted in courts and/or disciplined by the Medical Board of Australia for offences relating to drugs of dependence. Ignorance of the regulations is not a defence. Common offences include prescribing for a person with drug dependence without a permit, prescribing for a continuous period longer than that specified in the permit, prescribing in excess of the quantity specified in the permit, failing to notify the health department of a patient that the doctor has reason to believe is drug dependent, and prescribing methadone liquid without an approval. These offences appear to be based upon several failings, including:

- ignorance of the regulations that govern chronic prescribing of drugs of dependence
- ignorance of the dangers of prolonged prescribing of Schedule 8 drugs
- naivety in dealing with people with obvious drug dependence
- ignorance of the generic and trade names of some Schedule 8 drugs (that is, not recognising a drug to be a narcotic).

30.2.5 Storage of Schedule 4 medicines

Schedule 4 medicines (including 'starter packs') and Schedule 4 vaccines held at a doctor's practice must also be handled in a way that reduces the chance of unauthorised persons gaining access to them. This means that they must be stored in a lockable cabinet or room to which only authorised persons have access. The labelling regulations referred to in section 30.2.4 when supplying drugs of dependence also apply when supplying Schedule 4 drugs (including pharmaceutical 'starter packs')—an obligation often overlooked.

The *National vaccine storage guidelines* ('Strive for 5') provide information and advice for vaccine storage management for Australian immunisation service providers, including medical practices [11]. 'Strive for 5' refers to 5°C, the point midway between 2 and 8°C, which is the temperature range recommended for vaccine storage.

30.2.6 Use of generic versus trade names

The PBS authorises pharmacists to dispense a cheaper generic alternative for some medicines prescribed by their trade name unless the doctor indicates on the prescription that generic substitution is not permitted. All prescriptions, including electronic scripts, must now use the generic name of the active drug in the medicine being prescribed. Using generic names reduces the risk of inadvertent prescribing of more than one product containing the same drug or class of drug, which leads to an increased risk of adverse effects.

30.2.7 Prescribing and dispensing

As discussed in Chapter 11, The doctor and interprofessional relationships, there are good reasons for the separation of prescribing by doctors from dispensing by pharmacists. However, in rural and remote regions of Australia where communities are small and local pharmacies do not exist, general practitioners may apply for government authorisation to stock and dispense medications. Despite observations of overprescribing in other countries, this authorisation has not been misused by rural and remote general practitioners in Australia [12].

30.2.8 Relationship of doctors with pharmacists

Professional relationships between doctors and pharmacists deserve special attention. As both professions are regulated to protect the public, mutual cooperation will only enhance the level of that protection and the quality of medical care. In these relationships, prompt and courteous receipt or return of a telephone call from a pharmacist is good medical practice and a sign of a competent professional. Ensuring the prescription and the doctor's signature are legible and providing a contact telephone number for the pharmacist is also good medical practice. The professional training and the responsibilities of pharmacists, and more detail about doctors' relationships with pharmacists, are provided in Chapter 11, The doctor and interprofessional relationships. It is important to acknowledge that pharmacists have specialised knowledge about the effects, side effects, potential drug interactions and appropriate dosing of drugs and can support the prescriber to avoid potentially damaging errors. Essentially, the dispensing pharmacist provides a 'safety net' for patients when prescribing errors are made. In the context of prescribing drugs of dependence, doctors must be aware that:

- pharmacists' handling of these drugs is also subject to strict regulations
- regular inspections of prescriptions held by pharmacists are undertaken, which help identify doctors who self-prescribe and patients who 'doctor shop' to gain additional supplies of drugs
- real-time prescription monitoring [13] (e.g. QScript in Queensland or SafeScript in New South Wales and Victoria) requires both prescriber and pharmacist to consult their state online system prior to prescribing or dispensing Schedule 8 and some Schedule 4 medicines—'monitored or high-risk medicines' (see section 30.3.2 for more details).

30.3 Prescribing in particular situations

30.3.1 Prescribing for special populations

Special care is needed when prescribing for children, to ensure the medication is appropriate and the correct dose is given. This applies in particular to psychotropic medicines and 'off-label' use. A child's absorption, distribution, metabolism and excretion of medications may all differ from adults. Doses should be obtained from a paediatric dosage reference text; these are generally calculated on the basis of body weight. The prescription should contain the total prescribed dose, and the weight of the child should be noted to allow the pharmacist to check the dose on the prescription. All medicines should be kept out of reach of children and, where possible, provided in child-resistant containers.

Prescribing for older patients may present a range of challenges. Premarketing trials often exclude older patients, thus medication doses may not be appropriate. Age-related changes should be considered, both pharmacokinetic (i.e. the way in which the body handles the drug, including absorption, distribution, metabolism and excretion) and pharmacodynamic (i.e. the effects of the drug on the individual patient). For example, the pharmacokinetics of diazepam and lithium are altered in older adults, so that a given dose of either medication leads to higher plasma concentrations and possible toxicity in an older compared with a younger patient [14]. Where possible, avoiding polypharmacy is essential because the greater the number of medications a person takes, the greater is their risk of an adverse drug reaction or interaction and hospital admission. The Beers criteria provide guidance on potentially inappropriate medication use, in particular medicines or combinations of medicines that are best avoided in older adults, and give advice on deprescribing (ceasing unnecessary prescriptions) according to clinical need [15].

Particularly in rural and remote locations, doctors need to be aware of the circumstances of those for whom they are prescribing, the safety of medicines in the home (especially where children are present), and the possibility of diversion. In remote communities, including Aboriginal and/or Torres Strait Islander communities, there may be overcrowding with no safe lockable cupboards. Some older people carry their medications with them for safety, but exposure to high temperatures may compromise the efficacy or viability of some medications, such as thyroxine and aspirin. Lack of refrigeration may also be an issue. Supplying smaller amounts or using alternative local storage facilities—for example, at a local health service—may increase both safety and medication adherence.

30.3.2 Prescribing drugs of dependence

A doctor prescribing drugs of dependence, including opioids, benzodiazepines and certain stimulants, needs to be aware of the regulations (see below), sensitive to the possibility of inducing dependence and alert to the manipulative and deceptive behaviour of some drug-dependent patients. The vast majority of patients who visit doctors are cooperative and want to be truthful. It takes a heightened awareness on the part of the doctor to be alert to drug-seeking behaviour. An example of a drug-seeking person could be a patient who:

- is new to your practice and seeks a drug of dependence at the first visit
- claims to be travelling interstate and has run out of supplies or has lost a prescription
- claims that their regular doctor is unavailable
- produces a letter from another doctor purporting to authorise the administration of an opioid. It may be appropriate for a doctor to provide such a letter to a patient in genuine need, but the onus to confirm the provenance of the letter is on the new doctor, who, if in doubt, should contact the apparent author of the letter. (Note that there have been instances where the fraudulent letter contained an after-hours number that was answered by an accomplice of the fraudster). The phone number on any letter should be independently verified where possible; for example, through a search engine using the name and clinic of the other doctor.

Other strategies to reduce risk include:

- avoiding rushed consultations in which a proper history and examination are not completed. The examination should include checking for signs of drug use, such as pupillary constriction or dilatation, injection marks, or features of intoxication or withdrawal.
- strictly limiting the amounts prescribed and directing the patient back to their own doctor if the patient is unknown to you but you believe an opioid is justified on clinical grounds.

Doctors also need to be aware that dependence is a characteristic of the drug and not necessarily the patient. The possibility of dependence should be kept in mind for all patients to whom such medicines are prescribed. The essential feature of a substance use disorder is a cluster of cognitive, behavioural and physiological symptoms, meaning that the individual continues using the substance despite significant substance-related problems [6]. The *Diagnostic and statistical manual of mental disorders, fifth edition* (DSM-5) lists 11 criteria which vary across 10 classes of substances under the broad heading of Substance Use Disorder [6]. Included in these criteria are tolerance (needing more of a substance to achieve the same effect) and withdrawal (symptoms resulting from stopping or significantly reducing the substance, relieved by taking more of the substance). In the case of prescribed opioids, taken as directed, the presence of tolerance or withdrawal does not contribute to a diagnosis of substance use disorder. The word addiction (or addict) is omitted from the official DSM-5 substance use disorder diagnostic terminology because of its uncertain definition and its potentially negative connotations [6].

Doctors should be aware of the increased risk of prescribed drugs of dependence being diverted for non-medical use (e.g. injected rather than ingested, or used by another person). One example is the treatment of ADHD with stimulants such as dexamphetamine. One study examined medical and non-medical use of stimulants, showing a positive correlation between rates of prescribing and non-medical use and related harms; it suggested that for each secondary school student prescribed dexamphetamine for ADHD, about 2.5 students had used it for non-medical purposes [16]. Similarly, higher rates of prescribing for adults with ADHD correlated with higher rates of non-medical amphetamine use. More broadly, pharmaceutical opioids, sedatives and stimulants for non-medical use are primarily sourced from friends and family, while prescription shopping and forgery are relatively uncommon [17]. Prescribers need to be alert to the possibility of medication diversion.

Doctors should not hesitate to use the services of the relevant state or territory health department for general advice, as well as for specific advice about whether a particular patient is already known to the health department. The contact details for these services are available on the TGA website [2]. In addition, Medicare runs a Prescription Shopping Information Service (1800 631 181) which allows doctors to determine whether a particular patient is already of concern to Medicare staff who audit prescribing information [18]. This service operates 24 hours a day, 7 days a week. To access information, doctors need to register with the service.

Real-time monitoring of the prescribing and dispensing of drugs of dependence (known as 'monitored' or 'high-risk' medicines) has been introduced across several states; for example, SafeScript in Victoria and NSW, or QScript in Queensland. This is in response to a growing number of overdose deaths involving prescription medicines, typically combinations of drugs of dependence. Where these systems are in place, compliance is mandatory. Any health practitioner prescribing a 'monitored medicine' must refer to their state's online prescription monitoring service (which gives the prescriber read-only access). The pharmacist receiving the script must enter dispensing details. Prescribers should consult with their local state or territory legislation for details of which Schedule 4 medicines are included—for example, not all services include gabapentinoids, while all real-time prescription monitoring systems include Schedule 8 medicines. The service provides an invaluable reference and decision-making tool to the prescriber about 'monitored medicines' that have been prescribed, including the prescriber, date, dose, quantity and any repeats, as well as recording the details of other health practitioners consulting the system about that patient [13]. Patients commit criminal offences by forging or altering prescriptions or by attending several practitioners to obtain drugs for themselves or to sell to others. In Victoria, patients are obliged to inform doctors if they have received drugs of dependence from other doctors in the previous 8 weeks. Real-time prescribing systems now require both the prescriber and the pharmacist to check the patient's Schedule 8 and Schedule 4 'monitored medicine' prescribing history.

Doctors have at times been severely criticised by coroners for contributing to the death of drug-dependent patients by failing to heed the following principles of prescribing.

The regulations vary between states and territories, but share the following principles:

- The drug must be necessary for the treatment of a medical condition.
- The doctor must make a genuine attempt to check the patient's identity and the details of recent treatment by other doctors or hospitals (greatly facilitated by the introduction of real-time prescription monitoring services).
- The doctor must attempt to ascertain if the patient is drug dependent. If so, it may be an offence to prescribe further drugs of dependence.
- All required details must be written on a prescription by the doctor; these provisions exist to reduce the opportunity for drug-dependent patients to alter the prescription.
- The doctor must also comply with the state or territory regulations regarding the need for a permit if a drug of dependence is required for prolonged periods.
- If a doctor has reason to believe that a person has obtained drugs under false pretences, the doctor must notify the state or territory drugs and poisons office (see Table 30.1) or the police.
- There is a total prohibition on self-prescribing or self-administering drugs of dependence.
- Where narcotic drugs are stored in a clinic, surgery or hospital, there must be adequate security and records.
- The requirements of the PBS must also be met. A permit from a state or territory health department drugs of dependence section to continue prescribing does not absolve the doctor from separately obtaining PBS authority for increased quantities if these are needed.

30.3.3 Prescribing for family and relatives

It is not uncommon for doctors to be approached by family members, relatives and close friends for medical advice and prescriptions. In general, taking on the medical care of such people does not represent good medical practice (see also Chapter 8, Sexual and other professional boundaries: being a doctor in modern society) [19]. The Medical Board of Australia's advice on this topic states:

> Whenever possible, avoid providing medical care to anyone with whom you have a close personal relationship. In most cases, providing care to close friends, those you work with and family members is inappropriate because of the lack of objectivity, possible discontinuity of care, and risks to the doctor and patient. In some cases, providing care to those close to you is unavoidable. Whenever this is the case, good medical practice requires recognition and careful management of these issues [20].

Prescribing psychoactive drugs or drugs of dependence (including providing repeat prescriptions of drugs prescribed by another doctor) is especially problematic, as such clinical decisions require careful evaluation, objectivity and appropriate record keeping. Some medical indemnity policies exclude cover for elective care of a doctor's immediate family members.

30.3.4 Prescribing in an emergency

Verbal prescriptions, in person or via telephone, or prescriptions by fax are acceptable in an emergency and may be made to a pharmacist; in a hospital or nursing home, an order to administer a drug can be made to a nurse. (In the NT, Schedule 8 drugs are excluded from these provisions, while in Victoria the patient must present the original prescription with the faxed prescription to a pharmacist before the medicine is dispensed, unless the fax was accompanied by a phone call). In all instances, the verbal instructions must be confirmed in writing within 24 hours or as soon as is practicable. Telephoned prescriptions to pharmacists should also be written and mailed that day.

30.3.5 Prescribing for patients travelling abroad

The PBS website has detailed advice for patients [21] about travelling with medications. From a regulatory perspective, doctors need to be aware that medicines subsidised by the PBS can be taken or sent out of Australia only for the personal use of the traveller or someone they are accompanying, such as a child. In addition, there are legal restrictions on the quantity of PBS medications that a traveller can take or send overseas. Some countries have restrictions on taking specific drugs across their borders, including the need for a written prescription and sometimes a letter from the prescriber [22].

30.3.6 Prescribing in hospitals and nursing homes

Patient medication charts must be written and signed by a doctor to authorise the *administration* of most medicines by a registered nurse; that is, a single dose of the medicine is given to be consumed at that time. A brief list of nurse-initiated medicines (e.g. simple analgesics and laxatives) is usually available in such institutions. In practice, a letter from the doctor referring the patient to hospital which includes instructions regarding drugs, or a telephone call from the doctor, will be accepted, provided the medication chart is subsequently completed within 24 hours. Medication orders or medication charts are not to be confused with prescriptions, which are an authorised prescriber's instructions to a registered pharmacist to *supply* a medication (e.g. a month's treatment). In some facilities the patient medication chart may also be used by the pharmacist to *supply* medications for discharge.

30.3.7 Prescribing or dispensing unregistered medicines

The Therapeutic Goods Act maintains the ARTG and makes it unlawful to supply therapeutic goods that are not *registered* or *listed* therein.

The distinction between 'registered' and 'listed' refers to the different levels of evidence in regard to safety and efficacy required for a drug to be so entered; most complementary medicines are listed on the ARTG.

However, it is becoming more common for a doctor to access unregistered medicines, outside the context of clinical trials (which are regulated through the combination of the Therapeutic Goods Act and associated guidelines issued by the National Health and Medical Research Council—see Chapter 31, Medical research). Unregistered medicines can be obtained through the Special Access Scheme, the Authorised Prescriber Scheme or by personal importation; that is, if a patient attends with a drug that has been personally imported without authorisation. Almost any medication can be accessed through these schemes if it is considered clinically justified. Such use of unregistered medicines should be considered experimental; therefore, written informed consent from the patient is required and any adverse events should be reported to the TGA. Most medicinal cannabis products are currently unapproved and not included on the ARTG, although they are listed and can be prescribed with TGA approval through the Special Access Scheme (see section 30.5). The two exceptions that are approved are Epidiolex (cannabidiol) and Sativex (nabiximols, containing a mixture of tetrahydrocannabinol and cannabidiol).

30.3.8 Prescribing drugs outside their approved indications

Another aspect of the ARTG, which is at times overlooked by doctors, is that drugs are registered for approved indications. These indications are documented in the prescribing information issued by the manufacturer after approval by the TGA. Use of any registered drug for conditions not covered by the indication is permitted in the context of a clinical trial or on compassionate grounds. Use for other conditions not listed in the prescribing information is known as 'off-label' prescribing. Such use in Australia is not in breach of the Therapeutic Goods Act. Depending on the clinical situation and the availability of any safety and efficacy data, doctors who choose to use drugs in this manner must adequately inform patients, who may become concerned that their condition is not listed in the consumer medicine information [23,24]. In addition, when used outside the approved indications, the drug may not be covered by the PBS [23]. Research demonstrates that off-label use of medications is more likely to be associated with adverse effects, therefore special caution is required [25].

30.4 Prescribing particular drugs of interest

30.4.1 Prescribing benzodiazepines

Since the 1980s, most doctors have become aware of the dangers of prescribing benzodiazepines and in particular their long-term use. Any patient risks becoming dependent, and withdrawal symptoms have been reported after only 1 week's use of a normal dose of a benzodiazepine. It is probable that 45% of long-term users in Australia are dependent, and most of these people gain little from their treatment because of tolerance [26]. The long-term use of benzodiazepines, the absence of clear indications for such use, and their association with memory loss, falls and cognitive impairment in older people remains a problem [27,28]. In addition, doctors need to keep in mind the risk of diversion of benzodiazepines to be sold on the street. Most of the benzodiazepines used by drug-dependent people in this way originate as prescription items [29], although the use of cryptomarkets on the dark web for supplies of psychoactive prescription medicines is growing [30].

30.4.2 Prescribing antibiotics

With increasing concern about antimicrobial resistance, the concept of antibiotic stewardship has emerged in recent years 'to improve the safe and appropriate use of antimicrobials, reduce patient harm and prevent and contain antimicrobial resistance' [31], as promoted by the Australian Commission on Safety and Quality in Health Care (ACSQHC). This goal now forms part of the ACSQHC Preventing and Controlling Infections Standard [32]. A range of resources is available to support rational antibiotic prescribing, including the Antibiotic Therapeutic Guidelines [33]. Any doctor prescribing antimicrobials is advised to familiarise themselves with these guidelines and use antibiotics only when there is a demonstrable need.

30.4.3 Prescribing drugs of dependence for chronic non-malignant conditions

Australia, like many developed countries, has seen a marked growth in opioid prescribing over the past 20 years [34,35]. A significant proportion of the prescribing has been for self-limiting or non-chronic conditions [36]. This growth, observed for morphine, oxycodone, fentanyl and compound paracetamol–codeine preparations, has been associated with increases in misuse, diversion, overdose and deaths [35]. Doctors should exercise great caution in prescribing these drugs for chronic non-terminal illnesses, consider alternative treatment options and closely monitor those for whom they are prescribed [37]. When opioids are prescribed, doctors should consider co-prescribing the opioid antagonist naloxone (available both as a nasal spray and for administration by injection). This is particularly important where higher doses of opioid are involved, or other neurological depressants are also prescribed [38]. The goal is to raise awareness of the risks from these medications for the patient and their family, and to help prevent unintentional overdose. State and territory legislation limits the duration of treatment with an opioid and requires application for a permit to prescribe after specific durations. Every doctor should be familiar with the rules in their jurisdiction. Where an opioid is prescribed for more than 12 months, the PBS requires a review by a second medical practitioner. The ACSQHC has issued an Opioid Analgesic Stewardship in Acute Pain Clinical Care Standard, which describes the key components of care that patients can expect when they are prescribed opioid analgesics for acute pain in acute care settings. It contains nine quality statements with related indicators that align with key principles, which are the foundation for achieving safe, high-quality care [39].

30.5 Changes in prescribing medicines: a dynamic and challenging area

Aside from expected updates such as new medications being listed on the PBS, scheduling changes (e.g. codeine products being up-scheduled from Schedule 3 to Schedule 4 on 1 February 2018) and changes to PBS requirements (e.g. tighter restrictions around prescription opioids introduced in 2020), doctors must be equipped for other arising challenges. A recent example is the promotion of ivermectin and/or hydroxychloroquine for the prevention or treatment of COVID-19. Although both treatments have been shown repeatedly to be ineffective in controlled trials, they have been heavily promoted in certain sections of the community, and doctors have been subjected to pressure to prescribe them [40,41].

In the area of mental health, there is growing interest in the therapeutic potential of psychoactive substances, many of which (gamma-hydroxybutyrate [GHB], methylenedioxymethamphetamine [MDMA, also known as ecstasy], lysergic acid [LSD], and cannabis products not listed in Schedules 3, 4 or 8) are Schedule 9 Prohibited Substances. The TGA's introduction in 2016 of a medicinal cannabis Special Access Scheme approval process (both for individual patients and for particular classes of patients), and the growing uptake of these products, shows how medical and community perceptions of 'illegal drugs' may be evolving, supported by some evidence from clinical trials.

Indications for medicinal cannabis products (currently numbering more than 500 being used by more than a million Australians) include a range of conditions (epilepsy, spasticity due to multiple sclerosis, nausea and vomiting related to AIDS or cancer, palliative care and chronic non-cancer pain). A range of guidance documents prepared by the National Drug and Alcohol Research Centre reviews the clinical evidence for the use of medicinal cannabis [42]. Psilocybine (magic mushrooms) has recently been rescheduled from Schedule 9 to Schedule 8, and can be used in specific circumstances to treat psychiatric conditions [43]. The prescribing of medicinal cannabis products and other drugs sometimes used for recreational purposes has increased dramatically over the past few years with the development of online prescribing services that provide consumers with drugs on demand, in many cases without the benefit of a real-time doctor–patient consultation. The Medical Board of Australia has issued revised telehealth guidelines [10] that make it very clear that asynchronous prescribing without any direct doctor–patient interaction is not regarded as good medical practice. This includes prescribing platforms that provide a specific product to all consumers who request it, without any consideration of the patient's medical or psychiatric history. There have been cases of practitioners working for these companies who have had regulatory action taken against them when patients have suffered serious outcomes, including death (Medical Board of Australia, unpublished information).

Summary

Prescribing is a key skill for all medical practitioners, and an understanding of the regulations that govern prescribing is crucial for good medical practice, as well as to avoid serious adverse outcomes for patients and practitioners themselves. Each practitioner should become familiar with the rules (particularly scheduling and PBS requirements) that govern the prescribing of the medicines that they most commonly use, within the state or territory in which they are working. All prescribers should also ensure that they have ready access to the online resources provided by the PBS and by state, territory and Commonwealth governments. The Therapeutic Guidelines website also provides excellent guidelines for the safe and effective use of drugs. It is also important to remember that most pharmacists know more detail about medicines and prescribing than most doctors, and doctors should utilise that source of information and advice when needed. Most public hospitals have a Drug Information Service, run by highly skilled pharmacists with specific training, and available by telephone to all practitioners as well as members of the public.

References

1. Therapeutic Goods Administration. Health professional information and education. 2018. https://www.tga.gov.au/health-professional-information-and-education (accessed Oct 2021).
2. Therapeutic Goods Administration. Contacts for state/territory medicines & poisons regulations units. 2021. https://www.tga.gov.au/contacts-stateterritory-medicines-poisons-regulation-units (accessed Oct 2021).
3. Therapeutic Goods Administration. Standard for the Uniform Scheduling of Medicines and Poisons (the SUSMP). No.35 (Poisons Standard February 2022). https://www.tga.gov.au/publication/poisons-standard-susmp (accessed Sep 2024).
4. Therapeutic Goods Administration. Australian state and territory variations from Part 4 of the Poisons Standard. 2021. https://www.tga.gov.au/how-we-regulate/ingredients-and-scheduling-medicines-and-chemicals/poisons-standard-and-scheduling-medicines-and-chemicals/scheduling/australian-state-territory-variations-part-4-poisons-standard (accessed Oct 2021).
5. World Health Organization. International classification of diseases 11th Revision. https://icd.who.int/en (accessed Sep 2024).
6. American Psychiatric Association. Diagnostic and statistical manual of mental disorders. 5th ed. Washington, DC: APA Press, 2013. https://www.psychiatry.org/dsm5 (accessed Oct 2021).
7. Australian Commission on Safety and Quality in Health Care. Recommendations for safe use of medicines terminology. 2024. https://www.safetyandquality.gov.au/publications-and-resources/resource-library/recommendations-safe-use-medicines-terminology (accessed Jul 2025).
8. Pharmaceutical Benefits Scheme. Schedule of pharmaceutical benefits. http://www.pbs.gov.au/browse/publications (accessed Oct 2021).
9. Gast A, Mathes T. Medication adherence influencing factors – an (updated) overview of systematic reviews. *Syst Rev* 2019; 8: 112.
10. Medical Board of Australia. Telehealth consultations with patients. 2023. https://www.medicalboard.gov.au/Codes-Guidelines-Policies/Telehealth-consultations-with-patients.aspx (accessed Sep 2024).
11. National Immunisation Program. National Vaccine Storage Guidelines – 'Strive for 5'. 3rd edition. Commonwealth of Australia as represented by the Department of Health, 2019. https://www.health.gov.au/resources/publications/national-vaccine-storage-guidelines-strive-for-5 (accessed Sep 2024).
12. Lim D, Emery JD, Lewis J, Sunderland VB. Australian dispensing doctors' prescribing: quantitative and qualitative analysis. *Med J Aust* 2011; 195: 172–175.
13. Australian Department of Health. National real time prescription monitoring. 2024. https://www.health.gov.au/initiatives-and-programs/national-real-time-prescription-monitoring-rtpm (accessed Sep 2024).
14. Rochon PA. Drug prescribing for older adults. In: UpToDate, Connor RF (Ed), Wolters Kluwer. https://www.uptodate.com/contents/drug-prescribing-for-older-adults (accessed Oct 2022).

15. American Geriatrics Society Beers Criteria Update Expert Panel. American Geriatrics Society 2019 updated AGS Beers criteria for potentially inappropriate medication use in older adults. *J Am Geriatr Soc* 2019; 67: 674–694.
16. Whitely M, Allsop S. Look west for Australian evidence of the relationship between amphetamine-type stimulant prescribing and meth/amphetamine use. *Drug Alcohol Rev* 2020; 39: 519–524.
17. Hulme S, Bright D, Nielsen S. The source and diversions of pharmaceutical drugs for non-medical use: a systematic review and meta-analysis. *Drug Alcohol Depend* 2018; 186: 242–256.
18. Australian Government Services Australia. Prescription Shopping Program. 2024. https://www.servicesaustralia.gov.au/prescription-shopping-program (accessed Sep 2024).
19. Bird S. The pitfalls of prescribing for family and friends. *Aust Prescr* 2016; 39: 11–13.
20. Medical Board of Australia. Good medical practice: a code of conduct for doctors in Australia. 2020. https://www.medicalboard.gov.au/Codes-Guidelines-Policies/Code-of-conduct.aspx (accessed Sep 2024).
21. Australian Government Services Australia. How to manage your PBS medicine overseas. 2022. https://www.servicesaustralia.gov.au/how-to-manage-your-pbs-medicine-overseas (accessed Sep 2024).
22. Zwar N. Travelling with medicines in 2018. *Aust Prescr* 2018; 41: 102–104.
23. Day RO. Ongoing challenges of off-label prescribing. *Aust Prescr* 2023; 46: 86–89.
24. Gazarian M, Kelly M, McPhee JR, et al. Off-label use of medicines: consensus recommendations for evaluating appropriateness. *Med J Aust* 2006; 185: 544–548.
25. Eguale T, Buckeridge DL, Verma A, et al. Association of off-label drug use and adverse drug events in an adult population. *JAMA Intern Med* 2016; 176: 55–63.
26. Brett J, Murnion B. Management of benzodiazepine misuse and dependence. *Aust Prescr* 2015; 38: 152–155.
27. Smith AJ, Sketris I, Cooke C, et al. A comparison of benzodiazepine and related drug use in Nova Scotia and Australia. *Can J Psychiatry* 2008; 53: 545–552.
28. Pariente A, Dartigues JF, Benichou J, et al. Benzodiazepines and injurious falls in community dwelling elders. *Drugs Aging* 2008; 25: 61–70.
29. Nielsen S, Bruno R, Degenhardt L, et al. The sources of pharmaceuticals for problematic users of benzodiazepines and prescription opioids. *Med J Aust* 2013; 199: 696–699.
30. Aldridge J, Stevens A, Barratt MJ. Will growth in cryptomarket drug buying increase the harms of illicit drugs? *Addiction* 2018; 113: 789–796.
31. Australian Commission on Safety and Quality in Health Care. Antimicrobial Stewardship in Australian Health Care. Sydney: ACSQHC, 2023. https://www.safetyandquality.gov.au/publications-and-resources/resource-library/antimicrobial-stewardship-australian-health-care (accessed Sep 2024).
32. Australian Commission on Safety and Quality in Health Care. NSQHS Standards 2021 Preventing and Controlling Infections Standard. Sydney: ACSQHC, 2021. https://www.safetyandquality.gov.au/standards/nsqhs-standards/preventing-and-controlling-infections-standard (accessed Sep 2024).
33. Antibiotic. In: Therapeutic Guidelines. Melbourne: Therapeutic Guidelines Limited; accessed Sep 2024. https://www.tg.org.au
34. Dunlop AJ, Lokuge B, Lintzeris N. Opioid prescribing in Australia: too much and not enough. *Med J Aust* 2021; 215: 117–118.
35. Roxburgh A, Bruno R, Larance B, Burns L. Prescription of opioid analgesics and related harms in Australia. *Med J Aust* 2011; 195: 280–284.
36. Harrison CM, Charles J, Henderson J, Britt H. Opioid prescribing in Australian general practice. *Med J Aust* 2012; 196: 380–381.
37. Currow DC, Phillips J, Clark K. Using opioids in general practice for chronic non-cancer pain: an overview of current evidence. *Med J Aust* 2016; 204: 305–309.
38. Coe MA, Walsh SL. Distribution of naloxone for overdose prevention to chronic pain patients. *Prev Med* 2015; 80: 41–43.
39. Australian Commission on Safety and Quality in Health Care. Opioid Analgesic Stewardship in Acute Pain Clinical Care Standard. Sydney: ACSQHC, 2022. https://www.safetyandquality.gov.au/standards/clinical-care-standards/opioid-analgesic-stewardship-acute-pain-clinical-care-standard (accessed Sep 2024).
40. Singh B, Ryan H, Kredo T, et al. Chloroquine or hydroxychloroquine for prevention and treatment of COVID-19 (review). *Cochrane Database Syst Rev* 2021; 2: CD013587.

41. Popp M, Stegemann M, Metzendorf M-I, et al. Ivermectin for preventing and treating COVID-19. *Cochrane Database Syst Rev* 2021; 7: CD015017.
42. Therapeutic Goods Administration. Medicinal cannabis – guidance documents. 2023. https://www.tga.gov.au/medicinal-cannabis-guidance-documents (accessed Sep 2024).
43. Therapeutic Goods Administration. Re-scheduling of psilocybin and MDMA in the Poisons Standard: questions and answers. 2023. https://www.tga.gov.au/resources/publication/scheduling-decisions-final/notice-final-decision-amend-or-not-amend-current-poisons-standard-june-2022-acms-38-psilocybine-and-mdma/re-scheduling-psilocybin-and-mdma-poisons-standard-questions-and-answers (accessed Sep 2024).

31 Medical research

Michael Franco

Introduction

This chapter summarises the ethical principles of human research, the governance of research, the expected standards of good clinical research practice, the responsibilities of researchers, and research misconduct involving doctors. Overlapping with research are clinical audit and quality assurance studies, in which doctors are increasingly expected to participate, and which can raise similar ethical issues. A clear understanding of research-related issues is essential not only for doctors actively conducting research but also for those who may be called upon, even indirectly, to support research efforts.

31.1 The place of clinical research

Medical research is generally welcomed by society, especially where it is conducted with altruistic motives and with the aim to improve the health and wellbeing of the entire populace. Specifically in Australia, health and medical research is of increasing priority for the general public [1] and is supported by government at the state/territory and national level. In the modern medical era, research is no longer the domain of a select few doctors and academics. Many undergraduate medical school degrees and vocational specialist training programs require undertaking a research project for successful completion. Therefore, it is critical that all doctors understand the ethical issues and responsibilities of being involved in medical research.

Research carries inherent risks for human participants, as well as having the potential to cause ethical dilemmas, via the conduct or outcomes of the research. It is common for questions of autonomy, equity, transparency, competency and consent to arise. Experience has shown that even well-motivated researchers may at times pursue their research inappropriately, to the detriment of the research participants. To protect research participants, international and national codes of research ethics have been in place for more than 60 years. In Australia, health and medical research is overseen by nationally accountable ethics and research governance systems in hospitals and medical research institutes [2,3]. The Australian Government provides governance and funding via the National Health and Medical Research Council (NHMRC) and the Medical Research Future Fund [4]. Two key elements of this governance are compliance with the National Clinical Trials Governance Framework (NCTGF) [5] and the prospective ethical review of all research proposals by Human Research Ethics Committees (HRECs).

31.2 Codes of ethics in clinical research

The stimulus for the development of international codes of medical ethics, specifically regarding research, was the gross abrogation of accepted standards of medical research by doctors in Nazi Germany before and during the Second World War. The first international code of research ethics, *Recommendations guiding medical doctors in biomedical research involving human subjects*, was adopted by the World Medical Association in 1964 at its 18th Assembly in Helsinki and is now better known as the *Declaration of Helsinki*. The document has been revised on eight occasions, and the most recent revision was completed in 2024 [6]. While still relevant to Australian health and medical research, the *Declaration of Helsinki* is no longer the key guide in this country, having been supplanted by the *National statement on ethical conduct in human research* (the 'National Statement') [7] and the *Australian code for the responsible conduct of research* ('the Code') [8]. These two documents are issued conjointly by the NHMRC, the Australian Research Council (ARC) and Universities Australia.

The National Statement requires institutions and researchers to have all proposed human research reviewed and approved by an HREC. These processes are designed to ensure that all such research meets the key ethical requirements of research merit and integrity, justice, beneficence and respect for humans, to provide proper protection for the participants. The Code requires institutions and researchers to fulfil responsibilities for issues including researcher training, data storage, intellectual property, authorship, copyright and publication of research findings. The Code also contains definitions of research misconduct and specifies procedures to address allegations of such conduct.

Like the *Declaration of Helsinki*, the National Statement and the Code are revised periodically, in a process that involves broad public consultation. The National Statement is supported by codes for research in specific contexts such as assisted reproductive technology and gene therapy, and codes for research involving specific populations, such as Aboriginal and/or Torres Strait Islander peoples [9]. These documents are available on the NHMRC website (http://www.nhmrc.gov.au). These specific guidelines are consistent with the key ethical principles for medical research drawn from the National Statement and the Code, as described in this chapter.

31.3 Research governance

Research governance is the overarching framework which provides a structure for ensuring organisations (including hospitals, universities and research institutes) conducting research have management strategies in place to minimise risk to participants, researchers, the organisation and broader community. It describes the policies and procedures by which institutions seek to assure the safety, quality and ethical propriety of the research they sponsor or conduct [2,3,10].

Research governance is a much broader subject than research ethics, although the role of HRECs is a core component of governance [2,11]. HREC review is a core component of a sound research governance framework. In the Australian context, a strong emphasis is placed on a robust HREC review, which works in parallel to an organisation's robust governance framework that supports the safe conduct of research.

Research governance in Australia is guided by the National Statement [7] and the Code [8]. For clinical research, these documents derive their authority from the *National Health and Medical Research Council Act 1992* (Cth). Receipt of NHMRC funding of research is dependent on institutions and their staff complying with the guidelines in these two documents. When an institution accepts an NHMRC-funded research grant on behalf of a researcher, a deed of agreement is signed with the NHMRC binding the institution to follow the guidelines. The Commonwealth *Therapeutic Goods Act 1989* makes it illegal for a clinical trial of an unregistered therapeutic agent to begin before the trial protocol has been approved by a properly constituted HREC, as provided for in the National Statement.

Aspects of clinical research may also be governed by a mix of laws, codes of conduct or other guidelines covering aspects such as privacy, consent, biosafety and radiation safety. This mix may include both state/territory and federal requirements. This chapter does not fully canvass these matters.

As provided in the preamble of the National Statement:

> [r]esponsibility for the ethical design, review and conduct of human research is in fact exercised at many levels, by: researchers (and where relevant their supervisors); HRECs and others conducting ethical review of research; institutions that set up the processes of ethical review, and whose employees, resources and facilities are involved in research; funding organizations; agencies that set standards; and governments. While the processes of ethics review are important in this field, individual researchers and the institutions within which they work hold primary responsibility for seeing that their research is ethically acceptable [7].

In 2023, the Australian Commission on Safety and Quality in Health Care implemented the NCTGF. This framework embeds clinical trials into routine health service provision and strengthens the clinical and corporate governance arrangements for governments, hospital administrators, health services, private companies, trial sponsors and trial investigators [5].

All public and private Australian hospitals, day procedure services and public dental services that provide a clinical trials service must comply with and are formally assessed against this framework at least once every three years. Health service organisations are required to demonstrate their compliance through various actions, strategies and evidence.

The framework has five domains that are consistent with the National Safety and Quality Health Service Standards [12]:

- **Governance, leadership and culture:** Establishing clear roles and responsibilities for clinical trial service provision.
- **Patient safety and quality improvement systems:** Ensuring continuous improvement and adherence to safety standards.
- **Clinical performance and effectiveness:** Monitoring and enhancing the effectiveness of clinical trials.
- **Safe environment for the delivery of care:** Creating a secure and supportive environment for trial participants.
- **Partnering with consumers:** Engaging patients and the public in the clinical trial process [5].

31.4 What constitutes clinical research

In the setting of medical practice and healthcare delivery, the term 'research' includes any systematic study or experiment designed to generate new knowledge. Research may involve an individual patient or groups of patients and may include the evaluation of new or unproven medicines, diagnostic tests, therapies, devices, novel technologies or methods of technological deployment, or procedures or studies not necessarily directed primarily towards management or treatment of the patients' conditions. Where a doctor is unsure whether what is proposed to be done represents research, they should seek independent advice, preferably from the institution's research governance body.

Some types of audit and quality assurance studies may be difficult to distinguish from clinical research. Again, in such situations, doctors should consult the institution's research governance office. Most research offices will have a clear algorithm or matrix that distinguishes an activity that requires review by an HREC versus another mechanism of review (such as approval as a quality assurance activity). Ethics approval is likely to be required if the study:

- involves activities outside routine health care
- poses burdens and risks beyond those of routine care
- involves data collection that does not fulfil privacy definitions of related secondary purposes
- is being conducted or funded by a person who has no affiliation as a staff member or a student of the organisation [13].

31.5 Requirements for ethically acceptable research

The ethical principles or values that guide clinical research have much in common with the ethical principles for medical practice (see Chapter 3, Ethical principles for the medical profession). The values include respect for human beings, research merit and integrity, justice and beneficence; these values underpin a relationship of trust and mutual responsibility between the research participant and researcher [7]. Other relevant values include altruism, contributing to societal or community goals, respect for cultural diversity, and the values identified by Aboriginal and/or Torres Strait Islander peoples—reciprocity, respect, equity, responsibility, survival and protection, and spirit and integrity [9].

The value of respect is central to all research involving humans. Respect acknowledges that each human being has intrinsic value and includes the principle of respect for autonomy—for the right to determine one's own life and make one's own decisions. It also involves providing for the protection of those with diminished or no autonomy. Unless proposed research has merit and the researchers who are to carry out the research have integrity, the involvement of human participants cannot be ethically justifiable. In research, justice includes distributive justice and procedural justice. Distributive justice refers to the fair distribution of the benefits and burdens of research participation, and of the outcomes of research, while procedural justice refers to fair treatment in the recruitment of participants and the review of research. Beneficence is demonstrated by establishing that risks of harm are justified by the potential benefits of the research to participants and to others, being alert to the wellbeing of research participants, and reflecting on the social and cultural implications of the research [7].

The requirements for ethically acceptable research involving humans are spelled out in considerable but not exhaustive detail in the National Statement [7]. The statement provides principles and guidelines but is not a prescriptive document, as it is intended to enable the research community to apply the principles in the context of the proposed research study.

The following principles must be considered and adhered to when planning and conducting any type of medical research. This includes clinical research into the aetiology, prevention, screening, diagnosis or therapy of disease; epidemiological research; and laboratory research (using human tissue samples).

- Research should be justified by its potential benefits, including its contribution to knowledge and understanding, to improved social welfare or to the skill and expertise of researchers. Not only must the researcher have this view, but they also must satisfy an HREC that this is the case. Such an HREC must be established and function in accordance with the National Statement and be provided with all the relevant scientific background material and a detailed research protocol, using an appropriate template, such as the National Ethics Application Form.
- Sources of funding and resources should be fully disclosed. Most commonly, research is undertaken with academic, cooperative group, government, non-government organisation, pharmaceutical or other private industry funding.

- All prospective participants must be provided with factual information about proposed treatments or procedures, their risks, costs, inconvenience and discomforts, and the existence of alternative measures, so that they can give informed consent.
- The ethical obligations that doctors owe their patients differ from those that researchers owe to participants [14]. While doctors are required to act in their patients' best interests, researchers are required to act with respect for and to protect participants. To avoid the possibility of coercion, consent should preferably not be obtained by a doctor in a treating relationship with the patient. In any case, the patient must understand that participation is voluntary, that refusal to participate will not affect the doctor–patient relationship or access to care and that, if the patient agrees to participate, they are also free to withdraw at any time in the future (see also Chapter 7, Consent and informed decision making).
- Participants' privacy must be respected at all times, and the confidentiality of information collected in the research that relates to participants must be protected. There is a complex arrangement of federal and state/territory legislation and guidelines covering privacy in health research, which is overseen by HRECs [15–18] (see also Chapter 6, Confidentiality, privacy and disclosure).
- The progress of a research study must be regularly reviewed, and progress reports made to and considered by an independent committee. This is usually the HREC that approved the protocol, but in large-scale therapeutic trials, often conducted at many sites in Australia and internationally, where side effects and endpoints may be difficult for one of many involved researchers to evaluate objectively, a separate central oversight or data and safety monitoring committee may be required.
- The ongoing monitoring of research is a responsibility of multiple parties: the researchers, the HREC that approved the study, the organisation where the research is conducted and, in the instances of commercially sponsored research, the sponsor. Under an organisation's research governance framework, there should be clear policies and procedures detailing the reporting requirements, which include safety reporting, annual reporting, monitoring and auditing. The underlying premise is that monitoring is a joint responsibility to ensure safety.
- Volunteers may be recruited for non-clinical, non-therapeutic biomedical research, but care must be taken to ensure that participation is free of pressure, coercion or inducement. Staff or students of the researcher's institution should not be directly approached or actively recruited to participate, although as individuals, such persons are free to respond to advertisements. The greater the risks of the research, the greater the need to avoid any suggestion of coercion or inducement of staff or students to participate. Volunteers may be reimbursed for reasonable expenses, including loss of wages, travel and meals, but the level of remuneration should not be disproportionate to the contribution, so as to induce participants to expose themselves to risks.
- For research involving Aboriginal and/or Torres Strait Islander people, the dedicated guidelines [9] must be consulted and followed [19]. This may also include using a particular or additional Aboriginal and/or Torres Strait Islander research ethics committee in addition to institutional HRECs.
- For particular fields of research (e.g. clinical trials, use of data or tissue banks, or genetic research) and for particular subsets of participants (e.g. children, pregnant women, persons of diminished competence, or people in other countries), the relevant chapters of the National Statement must be consulted and followed.
- Research should only be performed if there is a realistic possibility of the translation of results into real benefit for health and wellbeing (i.e. avoidance of 'research for the sake of research' which is simply indulging the curiosity of the researchers).

31.6 Special areas in medical research

This section details several problematic areas in the conduct of medical research that deserve specific attention.

31.6.1 Research where capacity to give informed consent is questionable

There are many clinical situations where the purpose or aims of a research project appear to be extremely valuable, but where the potential participant may not be able to provide informed consent. This is most obvious where a candidate has a mental illness, intellectual disability, critical illness or life-limiting chronic illness. Specific chapters in the National Statement identify the ethical matters that need to be addressed so that HRECs can approve appropriate research protocols [7].

Less obvious impediments to obtaining proper consent are also the subject of specific chapters in the National Statement, such as where the person being considered for participation in clinical research is in a dependent relationship with the doctor or is in another comparable situation. These can include elderly people with reduced independence, and hospital and laboratory staff.

31.6.2 Research involving children and young people

Research involving children and young people raises issues about their capacity to understand what the research entails and whether their consent to participate is sufficient for their participation. Because the consent of parents is usually required, issues of possible coercion and of conflicting values and interests of parents versus the child may arise. Researchers must respect the developing capacity of children and young people to be involved in decisions about participation in research. The child or young person's particular level of maturity has implications for whether their consent is necessary and/or sufficient to authorise participation. Different levels of maturity and of the corresponding capacity to be involved exist and will vary from child to child. Even young children with very limited cognitive capacity should be engaged at their level in discussion about the research and its likely outcomes.

The National Statement sets out minimum procedures for consent to participation by children. It avoids specifying numerical ages of maturity to provide informed consent; rather, it advises that a young person's capacity to provide informed consent will be determined by several factors of each individual child. The onus is on the research team to establish processes that determine the level of competency within the proposed research participant group and then develop informed consent processes tailored to various levels of competency.

The central ethical dilemma in research involving children is the tension between the need for knowledge about the effects of treatments or medication with children (rather than extrapolating from research with adults) and the need to minimise risks to children. However, in some projects, researchers may need to justify higher levels of risk by the necessity of seeking results that relate to children. In recognition of this dilemma, the National Statement states:

> When children and young people are not of sufficient maturity to consent to participation in research, it is justifiable to involve them only when:
>
> (a) it is likely to advance knowledge about the health or welfare of, or other matters relevant to, children and young people; or
>
> (b) children's or young people's participation is indispensable to the conduct of the research [7].

31.6.3 Research using human embryos

Research using stored human embryos that have been declared excess to the needs of the parents, and certain other types of embryos, may be undertaken in Australia under licence and under strictly regulated conditions provided for in the *Research Involving Human Embryos Act 2002* (Cth). The Act established the Embryo Research Licensing Committee as a new principal committee of the NHMRC. The committee may not issue a licence for any proposed research unless it is satisfied that the research proposal has been considered and approved by an HREC in accordance with the relevant guidelines, which were developed by the Australian Health Ethics Committee and issued by the NHMRC (https://www.nhmrc.gov.au/research-policy/embryo-research-licensing; see also Chapter 13, Infertility and assisted reproductive treatment).

31.6.4 Research with Aboriginal and/or Torres Strait Islander peoples

Improving the health and wellbeing of Aboriginal and/or Torres Strait Islander peoples is a national priority [9]. With research being key to the advancement of health care, research focusing on Aboriginal and/or Torres Strait Islander populations as well as ensuring access to research more generally for Aboriginal and/or Torres Strait Islander peoples are critical.

The Australian Institute of Aboriginal and Torres Strait Islander Studies (AIATSIS) has published a code of ethics for Aboriginal and Torres Strait Islander research, which outlines four principles that underpin ethical Australian Indigenous research [20]:

- Indigenous self-determination
- Indigenous leadership
- impact and value
- sustainability and accountability.

Each principle frames a set of responsibilities for researchers, institutions and review bodies when conducting research with Aboriginal and/or Torres Strait Islander people. Again, this may also include using a particular or additional Aboriginal and/or Torres Strait Islander research ethics committee in addition to institutional HRECs [20].

31.6.5 Medical records and research

Medical records held by doctors and healthcare institutions, as well as other health records held by government agencies and other similar organisations, are an important resource for clinical, public health and epidemiological research. The basic ethical and legal principle is that such records may not be used for other purposes, such as research, without the consent of the person to whom the record applies. However, public interest in protecting the privacy of the individual can compete with the public interest in seeing important research conducted. To resolve this tension, federal and state/territory legislation and associated guidelines give to HRECs the task of weighing these competing interests.

In planning research involving access to medical records, the feasibility of seeking the consent of each patient should first be assessed, as this is always the preferred method for any research. If this is not feasible, then the second option that should be explored is to only collect data that is fully de-identified and cannot be reassociated with an individual.

As neither approach may be satisfactory or feasible, sections 95 and 95A of the *Privacy Act 1988* (Cth) provide another approach. Under these sections of the Act, the NHMRC is charged with issuing guidelines that, when approved by the Australian Information Commissioner, permit some medical and health research to proceed in ways that would otherwise infringe the Australian Privacy Principles (see Chapter 6, Confidentiality, privacy and disclosure). The current guidelines demand that such research may only be conducted after an HREC has examined the proposal and, following the NHMRC guidelines, carefully weighed the competing interests involved [15,16]. Any doctor considering research involving access to medical records or other stored information, including tissue and genetic samples, will need to be familiar with this legislation and seek appropriate advice from an HREC prior to commencement of any study.

The ongoing move from paper-based to electronic formats of medical records brings both opportunity and novel risks. Data stored in electronic medical records and other large databases (e.g. pathology laboratory information systems), provide an opportunity for research to be greatly improved in quality, accessibility, scale, scope and efficiency. It also enables the use of big data in combination with advanced data analytic techniques such as natural language processing, machine learning and artificial intelligence. The performance of such research has the potential to be revolutionary and accelerate medical and health care at an unprecedented rate—especially in the fields of population health, genetics and personalised medicine. However, this potential for significantly increased access to healthcare data comes with risks of inappropriate access, poor data security and storage, researchers being given access to data beyond the scope of HREC-approved research, and impacts on the ethical principles of personal autonomy and privacy [21]. To mitigate these risks, medical researchers and HRECs should link with their organisational bodies responsible for data governance, informatics and cybersecurity in addition to the areas traditionally considered when assessing a submission for medical research. Chapter 29, Professional practice, digital technology and artificial intelligence, provides further detail on the broader impact of technological developments on the ethical practice of medicine.

31.6.6 Research by medical students and doctors in training

Modern medical education at the level of both undergraduate and vocational training requires learners to undertake significant research projects. The research undertaken by trainees carries unique ethical issues that should be considered, including:

- having an appropriately experienced supervisor
- ensuring any research commenced is either able to be completed in the limited timeframe provided by the training period or there is a clear plan for who will continue the research at the completion of the training period
- ensuring that students or junior doctors are not coerced into ethically inappropriate research, research methodology or publication by more senior staff (see also section 31.7)
- ensuring that the research is of intrinsic value and not performed solely for the purpose of completing a project.

31.6.7 Registration of clinical trials

In Australia, as in many developed countries, it is now mandatory that every clinical trial be registered on a World Health Organization–recognised register such as the Australian New Zealand Clinical Trials Registry or ClinicalTrials.gov. These registers were developed, in part, to be a key protection against publication bias—a bias that occurs due to scientific publications being more likely to publish studies with positive rather than negative results (i.e. studies that do not meet their intended outcome or show benefit). As negative results were frequently not published, or were rejected for publication, this skewed the body of data on which evidence-based medicine was dependent [22].

Importantly, trial registries provide a publicly available database, allowing potential subjects or clinicians to seek out studies that may be of relevance to them, promoting greater equity of access to medical research, particularly for people in rural and regional areas and other poorly served populations. Registration of trials is also a means of transparency and a show of respect for patients who consent to becoming subjects.

31.7 Standards for responsible research conduct

As noted earlier, the standards of professional conduct for researchers, research supervisors and trainee researchers are laid down in the NHMRC Code [8]. The Code sets out the broad principles of responsible and accountable research practice and identifies the responsibilities of institutions and researchers in areas such as data and record management, publication and dissemination of findings, authorship, conflict of interest, supervision of students and research trainees, and the handling of allegations of research misconduct. The document also describes the institutional responsibilities in each of these domains.

The Code defines the principles underpinning good research practice, noting that the Australian and international community expects research to be conducted responsibly, ethically and with integrity, and that the primary responsibility for ensuring the integrity of research lies with individual researchers and institutions, supported by the Code and its associated guides. These provide advice regarding compliance with key principles, including honesty, rigour, transparency, respect for research participants and accountability for the development, undertaking and reporting of research [8].

The Code places an onus on institutions to ensure that researchers are trained in research ethics and research practices according to the Code, the National Statement, and related documents, and places an onus on researchers to familiarise themselves with these documents. One study of the staff of a large research institute suggested that clinician researchers were the group least informed about these documents [23]. A medical student or doctor planning to become involved in research should not rely on this chapter; they should study the Code, the National Statement and any other guidelines specific to the proposed field of research. Chapters of the National Statement of note for doctors include those on publication of results, authorship and conflicts of interest, as summarised below. In addition, for doctors new to research, there are guides to internationally accepted codes of good clinical practice available from the Australian Government [24] and the World Health Organization [25].

A particularly useful document is the International Council for the Harmonisation of Technical Requirements for Pharmaceuticals for Human Use (ICH) *Guideline for good clinical practice* [26]. Originally developed for commercially sponsored drug trials, this guidance has become known as the 'GCP guidelines' (even though the guidelines apply to clinical research rather than clinical practice). The GCP guidelines detail requirements such as trial documentation, protocol amendments, indemnity, reporting lines for adverse events and provision of medical care for trial participants. The Australian Therapeutic Goods Administration has adopted the ICH GCP guidelines in Australia in the Therapeutic Goods Regulations, and compliance with the GCP guidelines is a condition of approval for the conduct of a clinical trial [24,27]. Ongoing updates of ICH guidance are expected, and doctors involved with clinical research should be aware of the most recent version.

31.7.1 Publication and dissemination of research findings

The publication of clinical research serves several purposes, including the opportunity for peer review and independent evaluation by the medical profession and other readers, and the dissemination of advances in scientific and medical knowledge. Publication is also critical in obtaining funding for future research. The National Statement emphasises that researchers have a responsibility to the research and wider community to disseminate, as broadly as possible, an accurate and complete account of their research [7]. Researchers also have an obligation to provide research participants with an appropriate summary of the research results [28].

Researchers must ensure that they cite relevant work of others accurately. Use of the work of other authors without acknowledgement is plagiarism and constitutes research misconduct.

31.7.2 Authorship

The NHMRC Guide to Authorship (which supports the Code) requires that to be named as an author, a researcher must have made a substantial scholarly contribution to the work and be able to take responsibility for at least that contribution. Substantial contributions can be made by way of conception and design of the project, analysis and interpretation of research data, drafting significant parts of the work, or critically revising it so as to contribute to the interpretation. The Guide notes that

> authorship should not be attributed solely on the basis of:
>
> - the provision of funding, data, materials, infrastructure or access to equipment
> - the provision of routine technical support, technical advice or technical assistance
> - the position or profession of an individual, such as their role as the author's supervisor or head of department ('gift authorship')
> - whether the contribution was paid for or voluntary
> - the status of an individual who has not made a significant intellectual or scholarly contribution being such that it would elevate the esteem of the research ('guest authorship') [29].

Unfortunately, the widespread use of citation metrics (whereby authors are rewarded for the number of publications on which they are named and the frequency of citation of those publications) creates incentives to add additional authors whose contributions do not meet these criteria. Junior researchers may have difficulty resisting requests from more senior colleagues to be named as an author when this is not appropriate or conversely to have their work acknowledged appropriately, for example by being named as first author [30].

Where a work has several authors, one should be appointed executive author to take overall responsibility and to manage communication about the work with the publisher. Editors of medical journals normally require that manuscripts be accompanied by several statements, including:

- that the research that involves human participants has been the subject of independent ethical review (including evidence of HREC approval)
- a statement of conflict of interest from all authors (see section 31.7.3)
- a statement of credit, documenting the precise contribution of each author
- that all authors accept responsibility for the contents of the manuscript and veracity of additionally provided information [31]
- disclosure of any funding sources.

Institutions usually issue guidelines to their employees setting down their policies regarding publications. Any publication wherein an individual patient may be identified, such as a case report or a study containing a clinical photograph, requires the written consent of that patient. In collaborative research, it is advisable to document an agreement covering these issues, as well as intellectual property issues, prior to commencing the research.

31.7.3 Conflicts of interest

Conflicts of interest in research occur quite frequently, and are most often related to the sources of research funding. This is more likely to occur when the researcher stands to gain financially from the success or continuation of a research project, or when the funding of the research is provided by an organisation such as a pharmaceutical company that has a financial interest in the outcome (see also Chapter 9, Doctors, industry and conflicts of interest). As defined in the Guide on disclosure of interests, which supports the Code,

> a conflict of interest exists in a situation where an independent observer might reasonably conclude that the professional actions of a person are or may be unduly influenced by other interests [32].

The Guide also emphasises that 'the perception that a conflict of interest exists is a serious matter and can raise concerns about the integrity of individuals or the management practices of the institution' [32]. Therefore, it is important that researchers understand that the mere perception of potential conflicts of interest should be acknowledged, declared and considered both at the point of HREC submission and in any publication of results.

The Guide explains that researchers should manage conflicts of interest by being fully informed of the conflict of interest policy of their institution, maintaining good records of activities that may lead to conflicts (such as consultancies; membership of committees, boards of directors and advisory groups; and receipt of payments, services or equipment from outside bodies), reviewing current activities for actual or apparent conflicts, and bringing possible conflicts of interest to the attention of the research management office.

31.8 Patenting of medical procedures

It is generally accepted that new pharmaceuticals and technological devices may be subject to patent protection. Until recently, doctors had tacitly agreed that clinical procedures (such as new operations, new physical treatments and new ways of performing clinical procedures) would not be subject to such protection. Indeed, under the Hippocratic Oath and subsequent codes of ethics, there is a clear ethical imperative to pass on such advances freely to other doctors. In some jurisdictions, including the United Kingdom, Aotearoa New Zealand and Canada, patent legislation excludes such procedures from patentability. This is not the case in Australia, and although the medical profession at large does not favour the patenting of such procedures, individual doctors have applied for patents for new treatments and it appears that courts will deal with such applications according to the statutory requirements and not be influenced by medical ethics [33].

31.9 Research undertaken in private medical practice

The concept that independent medical practitioners should maintain an intellectual curiosity in their daily clinical practice is worthy of support. This is also supported by the requirement for medical practitioners to engage in documented continuing professional development (CPD) activities via specialty colleges or other CPD providers. Research in private practice is legitimate and ethical, provided the doctor follows the NHMRC guidelines, including the requirement that the research be approved by an HREC. Occasionally, research is undertaken independently of an institution because the ideas of the researcher are unacceptable to mainstream medical thinking or because the personality of the doctor is such that the doctor is unable to work cooperatively within an institutional framework. If such research is done without HREC approval, the doctor is at risk of being disciplined by the Medical Board of Australia for unprofessional conduct.

Doctors, in their private practices, may be involved with new drug or device development in collaboration with sponsor companies, often involving multisite clinical trials; again, such clinical research requires appropriate ethical approval and monitoring.

31.10 Misconduct in medical research

There is no single agreed definition of research misconduct. In 2012, a consensus statement defined research misconduct as follows:

> Research misconduct is defined as behaviour by a researcher, intentional or not, that falls short of good ethical and scientific standards (Edinburgh 1999). Research misconduct includes fabrication, falsification, suppression, or inappropriate manipulation of data; inappropriate image manipulation; plagiarism; misleading reporting; redundant publication; authorship malpractice such as guest or ghost authorship; failure to disclose funding sources or competing interests; misreporting of funder involvement; and unethical research (for example, failure to obtain adequate patient consent) [34].

Almost all clinical research involving human participants or human tissue is conducted in hospitals, research institutions and universities and is subject to scrutiny by HRECs, internal and external funding bodies, peer review, and medical journal editors and their reviewers. Although this extensive system of oversight offers considerable reassurance that clinical research is conducted ethically and responsibly, instances of misrepresentation and fraud and of harm to research participants continue to occur, may be increasing in frequency [35,36], and are probably under-reported and under-recognised [37]. Some types of research misconduct can result in serious injury or the death of research participants [38]. Just as trust of the community in the medical profession can be undermined by the unethical behaviour of one doctor in clinical practice, so too can trust in medical research be undermined by a single instance of research misconduct. There is, therefore, an ethical obligation for doctors who suspect or believe that a colleague is engaged in unethical research practices or research misconduct to notify their suspicions to an appropriate authority.

As noted throughout this chapter, misconduct may be overt or covert, real or perceived, and driven by noble or nefarious motives. Regardless of the intent or lack thereof, all breaches of the NHMRC Code or National Statement should be reported and dealt with promptly, transparently and by an independent body.

The investigation and adjudication of allegations of research misconduct have been problematic in many countries [39–42], and in Australia there have been instances where the outcome has been unsatisfactory for the researcher and the institution [43]. The Code provides a definition of research misconduct and clear guidance on how allegations of misconduct are to be handled by institutions [8].

Institutions in receipt of NHMRC research funding are obliged to notify the NHMRC when allegations of research misconduct arise. The institution retains the responsibility for investigating and assessing such allegations according to the framework laid down in the Code. A person who is dissatisfied with the way an institution has dealt with allegations under the Code may refer the matter to the Australian Research Integrity Committee (ARIC). The ARIC is a joint committee of the NHMRC and the ARC. The ARIC has the power to review the processes followed by an institution and make recommendations to the CEO of NHMRC or the ARC, as appropriate, but it does not conduct a re-hearing of the matters [44]. The Code flags the possibility of a centralised system of handling allegations of misconduct in the future. It should also be noted that any doctor who is alleged to have been involved in research misconduct is at risk of having their conduct examined by the Medical Board of Australia [38].

The rewards of scientific publication are sufficient to tempt some researchers to exaggerate, falsify or invent research data, which may be published and the fraud not detected for lengthy periods of time. When a doctor suspects that research data may be false or fraudulent, they have a clear duty to raise those suspicions with the appropriate authority, as described in the Code [8]. Alternatively, the matter may be referred to the Medical Board as a possible instance of 'professional misconduct'. Any doctor who reports suspicions in good faith deserves adequate support from peers and employers, as such whistleblowers may encounter intimidation and coordinated campaigns of vilification [45] (see also Chapter 25, Negligence and professional liability).

31.11 Biomedical research using animals

As many doctors also undertake research involving experiments with animals, prospective researchers should familiarise themselves with the guidance issued on the use and care of animals used in biomedical research. This comprises the *Australian code of practice for the care and use of animals for scientific purposes* [46] and the state and territory legislative regimes that license institutions to conduct such research, establish periodic inspections to ensure compliance and require prior ethical review of research by animal ethics committees, in conformity with the code of practice [46].

Summary

Clinical research plays a crucial role in the advancement of knowledge and the enhancement of patient care. Nevertheless, it is not without its risks. Whether doctors are actively engaged in research, assisting others in their investigations, or discussing research with patients, it is important for all to be well informed about the protective measures and regulations in effect. These measures are designed to maintain the balance between the greater good of society and the potential harm to individuals.

References

1. Research Australia. 2022 Public Opinion Poll on Health & Medical Research & Innovation, https://researchaustralia.org/reports/public-opinion-polling-2/ (accessed Sep 2024).
2. Walsh MK, McNeil JJ, Breen KJ. Improving the governance of health research. *Med J Aust* 2005; 182: 468–471.
3. Anderson WP, Cordner CD, Breen KJ. Strengthening Australia's framework for research oversight. *Med J Aust* 2006; 184: 261–262.
4. Australian Government Department of Health, Disability and Ageing. Health data and medical research. 2024. https://www.health.gov.au/topics/health-data-and-medical-research (accessed Sep 2024).
5. Australian Commission on Quality and Safety in Health Care. National Clinical Trials Governance Framework. 2023. https://www.safetyandquality.gov.au/standards/national-clinical-trials-governance-framework (accessed Sep 2024).
6. World Medical Association. Declaration of Helsinki – ethical principles for medical research involving human subjects. 1964. Amended 2024. https://www.wma.net/policies-post/wma-declaration-of-helsinki-ethical-principles-for-medical-research-involving-human-subjects/ (accessed Apr 2025).
7. National Health and Medical Research Council. National statement on ethical conduct in human research. 2023. https://www.nhmrc.gov.au/about-us/publications/national-statement-ethical-conduct-human-research-2023 (accessed Sep 2024).
8. National Health and Medical Research Council. Australian code for the responsible conduct of research. 2018. https://www.nhmrc.gov.au/about-us/publications/australian-code-responsible-conduct-research-2018 (accessed Apr 2022).
9. National Health and Medical Research Council. Values and ethics: guidelines for ethical conduct in Aboriginal and Torres Strait Islander research. 2003. Updated 2018. https://www.nhmrc.gov.au/research-policy/ethics/ethical-guidelines-research-aboriginal-and-torres-strait-islander-peoples (accessed Sep 2024).

10. Shaw S, Boynton PM, Greenhalgh T. Research governance: where did it come from, what does it mean? *J R Soc Med* 2005; 98: 496–502.
11. Krastev Y, Grimm M, Metcalfe A. Research governance and change in research ethics practices at a major Australian university. *Monash Bioeth Rev* 2011; 29: 16.1–7.
12. Australian Commission on Safety and Quality in Health Care. The National Safety and Quality Health Service Standards (2nd ed – version 2). Sydney: AHSQHC, 2021. https://www.safetyandquality.gov.au/publications-and-resources/resource-library/national-safety-and-quality-health-service-standards-second-edition (accessed Apr 2025).
13. National Health and Medical Research Council. Ethical considerations in quality assurance and evaluation activities. 2014. https://www.nhmrc.gov.au/about-us/resources/ethical-considerations-quality-assurance-and-evaluation-activities (accessed Sep 2024).
14. Litton P, Miller FG. What physician-investigators owe patients who participate in research. *JAMA* 2010; 304: 1491–1492.
15. National Health and Medical Research Council. Guidelines approved under Section 95A of the *Privacy Act 1988*. Updated 2024. https://www.nhmrc.gov.au/about-us/publications/guidelines-approved-under-section-95a-privacy-act-1988 (accessed Sep 2024).
16. National Health and Medical Research Council. Guidelines under Section 95 of the *Privacy Act 1988*. Updated 2024. https://www.nhmrc.gov.au/about-us/publications/guidelines-under-section-95-privacy-act-1988 (accessed Sep 2024).
17. Office of the Health Services Commissioner (Victoria). Statutory guidelines on research issued for the purposes of Health Privacy Principles 1.1(e)(iii) & 2.2(g)(iii) *Health Records Act 2001* (Vic). Melbourne, 2002. https://hcc.vic.gov.au/sites/default/files/2021-04/guidelines_research_vic_gazette.pdf (accessed Sep 2024).
18. O'Keefe CM, Connolly CJ. Privacy and the use of health data for research. *Med J Aust* 2010; 193: 537–541.
19. Studdert DM, Vu TM, Fox SS, et al. Ethics review of multisite studies: the difficult case of community-based Indigenous health research. *Med J Aust* 2010; 192: 275–280.
20. Australian Institute of Aboriginal and Torres Strait Islander Studies. AIATSIS code of ethics for Aboriginal and Torres Strait Islander research. Canberra: AIATSIS, 2020. https://aiatsis.gov.au/research/ethical-research/code-ethics (accessed Sep 2024).
21. Pastorino R, De Vito C, Migliara G, et al. Benefits and challenges of Big Data in healthcare: an overview of the European initiatives. *Eur J Public Health* 2019; 29: 23–27.
22. Chalmers I, Glasziou P, Godlee F. All trials must be registered and the results published. *BMJ* 2013; 346: f105.
23. Babl FE, Sharwood LN. Research governance: current knowledge among clinical researchers. *Med J Aust* 2008; 188: 649–652.
24. Australian Clinical Trials. Good clinical practice (GCP) for clinical trials in Australia. Canberra: Commonwealth of Australia, 2023. https://www.australianclinicaltrials.gov.au/researchers/good-clinical-practice (accessed Sep 2024).
25. World Health Organization. Handbook for good clinical research practice (GCP): guidance for implementation. Geneva: WHO, 2005. https://iris.who.int/handle/10665/43392 (accessed Sep 2024).
26. International Council for Harmonisation of Technical Requirements for Pharmaceuticals for Human Use. ICH harmonised guideline: Integrated addendum to ICH E6(R1): guideline for good clinical practice E6(R2). 2016. https://database.ich.org/sites/default/files/E6_R2_Addendum.pdf (accessed Sep 2024).
27. Australian Government Department of Health, Disability and Ageing. ICH guideline for good clinical practice. 2018. https://www.tga.gov.au/publication/note-guidance-good-clinical-practice (accessed Sep 2024).
28. National Health and Medical Research Council. Statement on consumer and community participation in health and medical research. 2002. Updated 2016. https://www.nhmrc.gov.au/about-us/publications/statement-consumer-and-community-involvement-health-and-medical-research (accessed Sep 2024).
29. National Health and Medical Research Council. Authorship: a guide supporting the Australian code for the responsible conduct of research. Canberra: NHMRC, 2019. https://www.nhmrc.gov.au/sites/default/files/documents/attachments/Authorship-Guide.pdf (accessed Jul 2025).

30. Kovacs J. Honorary authorship epidemic in scholarly publications? How the current use of citation-based evaluative metrics make (pseudo)honorary authors from honest contributors of every multi-author article. *J Med Ethics* 2013; 39: 509–512.
31. International Committee of Medical Journal Editors. Recommendations for the conduct, reporting, editing and publication of scholarly work in medical journals. Updated 2025. http://www.icmje.org/recommendations (accessed Jun 2025).
32. National Health and Medical Research Council. Disclosure of interests and management of conflicts of interest: A guide supporting the Australian code for the responsible conduct of research. Canberra: NHMRC, 2019. https://www.nhmrc.gov.au/about-us/publications/australian-code-responsible-conduct-research-2018 (accessed Jun 2025).
33. Jones JW, McCullough LB, Richman BW. Ethics of patenting surgical procedures. *J Vasc Surg* 2003; 37: 235–236.
34. A consensus statement on research misconduct in the UK. *BMJ* 2012; 344: e1111.
35. Steen RG. Retractions in the scientific literature: is the incidence of research fraud increasing? *J Med Ethics* 2011; 37: 249–253.
36. Khajuria A, Agha R. Fraud in scientific research – birth of the Concordat to uphold research integrity in the United Kingdom. *J R Soc Med* 2014; 107: 61–65.
37. Fanelli D. How many scientists fabricate or falsify research? A systematic review and meta-analysis of survey data. *PLoS One* 2009; 4: e5738.
38. Breen KJ. Misconduct in medical research: whose responsibility? *Intern Med* J 2003; 33: 186–119.
39. Lock S, Wells F, Farthing M, editors. Fraud and misconduct in biomedical research. 3rd ed. London: BMJ Publishing Group, 2001.
40. Dyer C. Research integrity. The fraud squad. *BMJ* 2011; 342: d4017.
41. Chalmers I, Haines A. Commentary: skilled forensic capacity needed to investigate allegations of research misconduct. *BMJ* 2011; 342: d3977.
42. Wager E. Coping with scientific misconduct. *BMJ* 2011; 343: d6586.
43. Van Der Weyden MB. Managing allegations of scientific misconduct and fraud: lessons from the 'Hall affair'. *Med J Aust* 2004; 180: 149–151.
44. National Health and Medical Research Council. Australian Research Integrity Committee. https://www.nhmrc.gov.au/research-policy/research-integrity/australian-research-integrity-committee-aric (accessed Sep 2024).
45. Faunce TA, Jeffreys S. Whistleblowing and scientific misconduct: renewing legal and virtue ethics foundations. *Med Law* 2007; 26: 567–584.
46. National Health and Medical Research Council. Australian code of practice for the care and use of animals for scientific purposes. 8th ed. 2013. http://www.nhmrc.gov.au/guidelines-publications/ea28 (accessed Sep 2024).

Further reading

Biggs H. Healthcare research ethics and law: regulation, review and responsibility. London: Routledge-Cavendish, 2010.

Emanuel EJ, Grady CG, Crouch RA, et al, editors. The Oxford textbook of clinical research ethics. Oxford: Oxford University Press, 2011.

Goldacre B. Bad science. London: Fourth Estate, 2008.

Judson HJ. The great betrayal. Fraud in science. New York: Harcourt, 2004.

Lock S, Wells F, Farthing M, editors. Fraud and misconduct in biomedical research. 3rd ed. London: BMJ Publishing Group, 2001.

Moynihan R, Cassels A. Selling sickness. How drug companies are turning us all into patients. Sydney: Allen and Unwin, 2005.

32 Legal frameworks: rights, responsibilities and protections

Erwin Loh

Introduction

The bulk of state and Commonwealth legislation that is most often and directly relevant to medical practice has been addressed in previous chapters. The differences in laws between jurisdictions are more often in detail than in principle. This chapter summarises some further laws that may involve practising doctors, and highlights the principles involved in these laws. Doctors wishing to seek more detailed advice concerning their legal responsibilities should consult the department or statutory body established to administer the relevant Act, or the legal advisers associated with their medical defence organisation.

These additional responsibilities emphasise that the community places great trust in the professionalism of doctors. Doctors' legal responsibilities can be divided into four categories:

- statutory duties, such as certifying testamentary capacity, statutory declarations or making mandatory notifications of infectious diseases
- medicolegal reports, such as assessment reports for social security or workers' compensation claims
- forensic medicine, for example, relating to child abuse assessments or the taking of blood samples from people accused of serious crime
- general areas of law, such as anticompetitive legislation, work health and safety laws, and human rights legislation.

Failure by a doctor to fulfil these responsibilities will diminish the community's trust in the medical profession and may lead to censure and/or sanctions by the Medical Board of Australia, a disciplinary tribunal or the Health Care Complaints Commissioner. In some instances, doctors may face fines or even terms of imprisonment for failing to meet these responsibilities without adequate cause.

32.1 Statutory duties

32.1.1 Testamentary capacity and witnessing wills

A will or testament is a legal document that expresses a person's wishes for how their property is to be distributed after their death and who is to manage the property until its final distribution. Doctors may receive a request to assess the testamentary capacity of a patient or to witness a patient's will. A person must have testamentary capacity to make a valid will, and it is important to note that a starting point is the assumption that an adult person does have capacity, as stated in law in each jurisdiction in Australia. The test of whether a person has sufficient capacity to make a will was set out in *Banks v Goodfellow* [1]:

> It is essential to the exercise of such a power that a testator shall understand the nature of the act and its effects; shall understand the extent of the property of which he is disposing; shall be able to comprehend and appreciate the claims to which he ought to give effect; and, with a view to the latter object, that no disorder of the mind shall poison his affections, pervert his sense of right, or prevent the exercise of his natural faculties—that no insane delusion shall influence his will in disposing of his property and bring about a disposal of it which, if the mind had been sound, would not have been made.

Doctors should ensure they have the appropriate skills and experience before assessing a patient for testamentary capacity. If the doctor, or the organisation with which the doctor is associated, has a conflict of interest, or stands to be a beneficiary of the will, then this task must not be accepted.

There are four essential elements in assessing testamentary capacity. The doctor needs to ensure that the person:

- understands that they are giving instructions in regard to the disposal of assets after their death
- is of clear mind and able to state the extent and nature of their assets
- is able to recall and understand the claims of potential heirs
- does not demonstrate any sign of serious mental illness, such as delusions or hallucinations, or the effects of medications, which could impair decision making [2].

There are parallels between assessing capacity and following the principles of informed consent (see Chapter 7, Consent and informed decision making). The standard of testamentary capacity that needs to be established will depend on the complexity of the will (the more complex the will, the higher the standard). A finding of incapacity in one area does not automatically mean capacity is an issue in other areas, including capacity to consent to medical treatment. Patients who are not capable of managing certain parts of their affairs may still be capable of making a will. There is no standardised clinical test for testamentary capacity; for example, the Mini-Mental Standardised Examination is not a good indicator of testamentary capacity.

Statutory rules on the execution of wills are defined in legislation in all Australian jurisdictions: *Wills Act 1968* (ACT); *Succession Act 2006* (NSW); *Wills Act 2000* (NT); *Succession Act 1981* (Qld); *Succession Act 2023* (SA); *Wills Act 2008* (Tas); *Wills Act 1997* (Vic); and *Wills Act 1970* (WA).

The doctor should ensure that the instructions provided by the person are given voluntarily—in other words, there is no undue influence or coercion. It is also important that, when certifying testamentary capacity, the doctor ensures that they have no personal conflict of interest. There have been cases of patients leaving large bequests to their treating doctor, which have led to disciplinary proceedings before the Medical Board and tribunals. Given the capacity of an executor to charge the estate, a doctor should not be involved in will making if it is possible they will be an executor or beneficiary. There will also be a conflict of interest if a member of the doctor's family or their partner is a beneficiary of the will.

32.1.2 Statutory declarations

Registered medical practitioners, along with many other professionals, are authorised to witness statutory declarations. This authorisation is found in legislation about giving evidence or in dedicated legislation; for example, the Commonwealth *Statutory Declarations Act 1959* and the Victorian

Evidence (Miscellaneous Provisions) Act 1958. In responding to such a request, the doctor is not attesting to the content of the declaration, but to the identity of the person and to the fact that they witnessed the person sign the declaration. The wording required for the declaration varies between jurisdictions. For example, in Victoria, the person making the declaration is required to state:

> I, [your full name] of [your address], declare that the contents of this statutory declaration are true and correct [3].

As a witness to the declaration, the doctor must print their full name, sign and date the document, and write their professional qualifications and address, which can be the practice address. In documents of more than one page, every page should be so signed. The possibility of conflict of interest (actual or perceived) should always be considered, and the doctor should not witness a statutory declaration if they may also benefit from the issue being declared.

32.1.3 Statutory immunity and qualified privilege

When medical errors and serious adverse events occur in health care, doctors and other clinicians participate in quality improvement and peer review audit activities. It is important that they are able to do this without worrying about potential litigation if their involvement and the information they share are incorrectly interpreted by the general public or the media. See also Chapter 10, Continuing professional development.

To mitigate these concerns, laws to protect the confidentiality of quality assurance activities and grant immunity from personal liability for clinicians on certain committees have been enacted in all Australian jurisdictions: *Health Act 1993* (ACT); *Health Administration Act 1982* (NSW); *Mental Health and Related Services Act 1998* (NT); *Health Services Act 1991* (Qld); *Health Care Act 2008* (SA); *Health Act 1997* (Tas); *Health Services Act 1988* (Vic); *Health Services (Quality Improvement) Act 1994* (WA); and *Health Insurance Act 1973* (Cth) [4].

These laws create rights and benefits known as 'qualified privilege' or 'statutory immunity'. They seek to achieve a balance between the competing public interests of encouraging clinicians to take part in quality assurance and improvement activities, and the open and transparent access to information about those activities, particularly those related to adverse events. These laws differ between the states and territories, but are all designed to encourage clinician participation in quality assurance and improvement activities. The laws ensure that documents and proceedings of clinical quality committees or activities are confidential; that documents and proceedings are protected from being used in legal actions; and that present and former members of clinical quality committees, acting in good faith in carrying out their duties, are protected from legal liability.

While these laws protect the confidentiality of some quality assurance and improvement information, the protection, once granted, does not cover 'primary' materials such as clinical notes or other records made as part of the ongoing care of a patient. Complaint letters, minutes from other committees referred to the protected committee, and clinical incident forms are also not protected by these laws. It should also be noted that some laws only protect the confidentiality of quality assurance and improvement information that identifies patients or clinicians. Information that does not identify individuals will not be protected by these laws.

Moving forward, the medical profession and regulators will need to ensure that the right balance is achieved between the potentially competing professional and public interests so that qualified privilege and statutory immunity frameworks continue to function in the best interests of the medical profession and the general public [5].

32.1.4 Whistleblower protections

A whistleblower is an insider within an organisation who reports misconduct or dishonest or illegal activity that has occurred within that organisation [6]. Effective protection of whistleblowers from reprisals reduces the risk of fraud and other inappropriate conduct in organisations.

The *Public Interest Disclosure Act 2013* (Cth) enables public officials to raise suspected wrongdoing within the Commonwealth public sector. According to this legislation, Australian government agencies, Commonwealth companies and public authorities have a responsibility to investigate and act on suspected wrongdoing. The Act also offers disclosers protection from reprisal action and certain immunities from liability.

The *Corporations Act 2001* (Cth) outlines obligations for company officers as well as protections for whistleblowers, relating to disclosures made by officers, employees or contractors supplying goods or services to a company. Also, the *Aged Care Act 1997* (Cth) has whistleblower protections in relation to reportable assaults.

In addition, all Australian states and territories have public interest disclosure laws: *Public Interest Disclosure Act 2012* (ACT); *Public Interest Disclosures Act 1994* (NSW); *Independent Commissioner Against Corruption Act 2017* (NT); *Public Interest Disclosure Act 2010* (Qld); *Whistleblowers Protection Act 1993* (SA); *Public Interest Disclosures Act 2002* (Tas); *Protected Disclosure Act 2012* (Vic); and *Public Interest Disclosure Act 2003* (WA). These laws establish:

- reliable means for wrongdoing to be reported
- protections for those who make such reports
- frameworks to address reported matters.

Doctors need to be aware of the whistleblower policies of the organisations they are part of, to ensure that they comply with the process to avoid breaching requirements.

32.1.5 Vulnerable adult or elder abuse mandatory reporting

Note that mandatory reporting of suspected child abuse is addressed in Chapter 15, Family violence, child maltreatment and elder abuse.

Mandatory reporting of suspected cases of abuse or neglect of adults applies if the person involved is living in a residential facility, such as those run by psychiatric, aged care or disability service providers, or other government-run facilities (e.g. suspected elder abuse of residents in nursing homes). These reporting requirements (some in legislation and some in policy) apply to facilities run or funded by government (both federal and state or territory). In the Northern Territory, the requirement extends to any suspicion of adults exposed to domestic or family violence. At the time of writing, there are no other mandatory reporting requirements for doctors in relation to vulnerable adults, elder abuse or domestic violence [7].

Where an adult patient has informed a doctor of past sexual abuse, the doctor's mandatory reporting obligations vary depending on the state or territory. In New South Wales, doctors must make a mandatory report if there is an identifiable group of children at risk of significant harm, such as when an adult patient reports that they know an alleged offender continues to have contact with children, for example, through their occupation [8]. Other states and territories do not have equivalent provisions, but a report of historical sexual abuse by an adult patient may still warrant reporting to the relevant child protection unit if the offender continues to have contact with children, particularly if through their occupation, and there is a risk of harm to the children.

32.1.6 Infectious diseases mandatory reporting

Legislation exists in all states and territories for the purpose of controlling the spread of infectious diseases. It covers such matters as the responsibility of doctors and pathology laboratories to notify authorities about individuals diagnosed with specific infectious diseases; the powers of the state or territory to test, treat or quarantine such individuals; and the responsibility of patients to seek treatment and to avoid behaviour that might result in spread of infection. Broadly, the legislation covers HIV/AIDS, other sexually transmissible infections (STIs) and other infectious diseases.

HIV/AIDS

Public health legislation has been enacted in all Australian jurisdictions in an effort to reduce the spread of HIV. The laws are complex and vary between states and territories; the differences at times reflect the conflict between proponents of traditional coercive public health measures and those who argue that, because of HIV's limited mode of transmission and the risk of discrimination (thus driving the disease 'underground'), the legislation should be framed to encourage behavioural change and voluntary testing. The legislation is far-reaching, covering not only the requirements of notification, but also such matters as counselling prior to testing, powers of detention and isolation, and powers to compel testing and tracing of sexual contracts. In some states, the law creates offences of knowingly transmitting infections or exposing others to the risk of infection. The laws also address the issue of privacy and confidentiality (see Chapter 6, Confidentiality, privacy and disclosure). In all states and territories, doctors who diagnose HIV infection or AIDS have a legal obligation to notify their respective health departments. This responsibility rests also with pathologists and pathology departments in NSW, Victoria, Queensland, Tasmania and the Australian Capital Territory.

Different state and territory Acts prescribe varying other legal obligations, special powers and offences. The relevant Acts are: *Public Health Act 2010* (NSW); *Public Health and Wellbeing Act 2008* (Vic); *Public Health Act 2005* (Qld); *Public Health Act 2011* (SA); *Health Act 1911* (WA); *Public Health Act 1997* (Tas) and Public Health (Miscellaneous Amendments) Bill 2015 (Tas); *Notifiable Diseases Act 1981* (NT); and *Public Health Act 1997* (ACT).

Other sexually transmissible infections

Doctors and pathologists are obliged under law to notify the state or territory health department when certain STIs are diagnosed. In Victoria, Tasmania and the ACT, the patient's full name is not required. STIs other than HIV that are notifiable include chlamydia in Western Australia and the ACT; syphilis and gonorrhoea in NSW and South Australia; and syphilis, gonorrhoea, chancroid, donovanosis, lymphogranuloma venereum and chlamydia in Victoria and Tasmania. Genital herpes is notifiable in the NT. In NSW, it is an offence if a doctor fails to advise a patient with an STI of the patient's responsibilities, under the Public Health Act.

Infectious diseases that are not sexually transmitted

Every state and territory either publishes schedules or regulations in their government gazette or promulgates lists to doctors that specify a large number of infectious diseases that must be notified to the respective health departments. A list of these infections and appropriate notification forms are available from the relevant health departments. The relevant legislation is given earlier in this section. Infectious diseases are also covered by the *Quarantine Act 1908* (Cth), which provides that people, animals, goods and the transport that brought them to Australia may be detained if there is believed to be a risk of quarantinable disease, including smallpox, plague, cholera, yellow fever, typhus and leprosy.

32.1.7 Fitness for firearm licence reporting

A doctor may have to notify the state or territory commissioner of police if a patient has made threats to harm themselves or others, and the doctor believes the person to be a risk to themselves or the public if they possess a firearm. This duty to notify is mandatory in SA (*Firearms Regulations 2017*) [9], NT (*Firearms Act 1997*) [10] and Tasmania (*Firearms Act 1996*) [11], but voluntary in NSW (*Firearms Act 1996*) [12], WA (*Firearms Act 1973*) [13], Queensland (*Weapons Act 1990*) [14], Victoria (*Firearms Act 1996*) [15] and the ACT (*Firearms Act 1996*) [16].

In addition, in SA and Tasmania, it is also mandatory for doctors to notify the police if they treat a patient with a gunshot wound, including the duty to retain any ammunition recovered from the wound.

New legislation enacted in March 2025 in WA requires that anyone buying a firearm in that state will have to undergo mandatory and ongoing mental health checks.

The legislation provides immunity from criminal or civil action for doctors who breach a patient's privacy by disclosing information in good faith to the police [17].

32.2 Medicolegal reports

See also Chapter 26, Medicolegal examinations and reports, court procedures and expert evidence, and Chapter 27, Medical records, reports and certificates.

32.2.1 Social security assessments

Under Commonwealth social security legislation, persons with illness or injury leading to temporary or permanent disability with incapacity to work are entitled to social security income in the form of the Disability Support Pension (DSP) or other payments [18].

DSP entitlement is heavily dependent on the treating doctor completing a medical report form provided by Centrelink (the Commonwealth agency responsible for administering the legislation). This report may be used to decide which payment a patient is entitled to or to determine whether the patient could benefit from vocational rehabilitation. It should be completed promptly, fully, legibly and accurately.

Some applicants for the DSP may be assessed by doctors on behalf of Centrelink, and by Centrelink job capacity assessors, so those doctors and assessors need to be fully informed by the treating doctor of the applicant's illnesses and/or injuries. Centrelink staff may seek additional medical reports from specialists, especially if the treating doctor's report is unclear or insufficient for the assessor to complete their report. Patients may be unfairly discriminated against if the medical information relied on at these independent assessments is based predominantly on the patient's own understanding of their illness or injury and not on a well-prepared report from a treating doctor.

32.2.2 National Disability Insurance Scheme reports

A doctor can support a patient's National Disability Insurance Scheme (NDIS) access request to the National Disability Insurance Agency (NDIA) by completing the supporting evidence section of the NDIS Access Request Form or by documenting that the patient has or is likely to have a permanent disability. The doctor can also provide a report relevant to the diagnosis or condition that details the extent of the functional impact of the disability.

The doctor should summarise the effect of the disability on the patient's day-to-day function in all relevant domains, including mobility, communication, social interaction, learning, self-care or their ability to self-manage. To avoid requests for additional evidence about a patient's disability, the doctor should include information about treatments that have been completed or planned, permanency of the impairment, and the impact the impairment has on the patient's functional capacity [19].

32.2.3 Workers' compensation assessments

Although knowledge of the requirements for workers' compensation insurance is relevant to doctors who are employers (see Chapter 33, Entering and leaving practice and practice management), this section focuses on the role of a doctor in treating injured workers. Workers' compensation schemes are now generally 'no fault' in that entitlement is not conditional on proof of negligence. Compensation is normally paid where a work-related injury or disease is documented and there is evidence that the person was employed. The term 'work related' implies being caused by, contributed to or aggravated by the person's work. In most states and territories, this includes travel to and from work. Stress as a contributing or causative factor to compensable disease or disability under these schemes appears to be handled inconsistently.

The role of a treating doctor in workers' compensation schemes is to objectively assess any person presenting for treatment and to provide accurate certification of the disease or injury and consequent disability. The assessment of disability will include such matters as degree and expected duration of disability, and subsequently, fitness to return to part-time or full-time work. Some understanding of the type of work performed by the injured person should be obtained so that the certificates are meaningful. Objectivity on the part of the doctor must be observed. Some doctors err by acting too strongly as an advocate for the patient and overlooking that there is also a responsibility to the community to ensure that the compensation schemes are not misused. Others may err by too harshly denying certificates to injured workers, or by understating the degree of injury or disability. Doctors who are not the treating doctor may also be asked to examine and report on a person seeking workers' compensation. Aspects of this role, which does not have the dynamics of the usual doctor–patient relationship and frequently leads to complaints against doctors, are covered in Chapter 26, Medicolegal examinations and reports, court procedures and expert evidence.

In most states and territories, when a worker makes a claim for compensation, the treating doctor is required to describe the illness or injury on a certificate provided by the workers' compensation authority. When completing and signing such a certificate, the doctor is simply reporting the relevant medical findings, and is not attesting to any belief formed as to whether the illness or injury is work related. That decision is not one for the doctor to make, although the treating doctor's opinion, as well as the opinions of medical experts, may be considered should an employer contest the claim and the matter come to formal determination.

Some doctors refuse to take on the care of persons presenting with work-related injuries as they find the paperwork tedious and the possibility of a court appearance unappealing. As in any other field of medical practice, there is no ethical obligation to accept such patients, provided it is not an emergency and that alternative sources of medical care are reasonably available. However, treating doctors who refuse to complete workers' compensation reports for existing patients will still have a duty of care to treat these patients for their conditions.

The treating doctor may also be involved in rehabilitation of the injured worker, requiring discussions with the employer or a rehabilitation counsellor or case manager and at times workplace visits. The doctor must obtain the patient's consent for the release of any medical information during these processes. Doctors should be cooperative in answering telephone calls or inquiries from employers and rehabilitation providers, as courteous discussion will serve to identify the issues before seeking the patient's consent to release information (see also Chapter 6, Confidentiality, privacy and disclosure).

In cases where the patient's illness is prolonged, and where recovery from injury appears to be unduly slow, doctors must ensure that the patient is fully reassessed at appropriate intervals and should consider seeking second opinions. A second opinion protects the interests of the patient primarily, but also can protect the doctor from criticism and the community from expensive misuse of the compensation system.

More information about state and federal workers' compensation schemes, including the relevant legislation, is available from Safe Work Australia [20].

32.2.4 Pre-employment medical examinations

Many employers now ask that potential employees submit themselves for pre-employment medical checks. Although many such examinations will be straightforward, doctors need to be alert to the risk of breaching anti-discrimination laws (e.g. the Victorian *Equal Opportunity Act 2010*). The Equal Opportunity and Human Rights Commission in Victoria has issued guidelines in this regard, which emphasise the need for the doctor to be informed by the employer about the genuine and reasonable job requirements for the particular position and the capacities required to perform these [21]. Doctors should be familiar with the process of pre-employment assessments. They need to explain to the job applicant the nature of any assessment and its relationship to the job requirements, and assure the applicant that only health information relevant to their job capacity will be conveyed to the employer.

Questions asked of the applicant must only relate to health issues relevant to the job. Thus, questions about past compensation claims or sick days away from a previous job may not be asked. A preferred approach is to outline the job requirements and ask the applicant, or test the applicant, to see if there are any conditions that will affect their ability to do the job. The report to the employer must not contain information about a disability or impairment unrelated to the job requirements.

32.2.5 Fitness to drive assessments

Persons applying for a licence to drive a motor vehicle are required to inform the licensing authority of any illness or disability (including treatment thereof) that might impair their ability to drive. Doctors may then be approached by the licensing authority to provide a medical report, usually according to a proforma, as to the individual's fitness to drive. Persons holding current licences, or persons whose licences have been suspended or cancelled, also may be asked by the licensing authority to provide a medical report.

Clear, helpful guidelines are available to assist doctors in fulfilling their responsibilities [22]. Doctors in clinical practice should familiarise themselves with these guidelines and refer to them when necessary. These guidelines describe in detail the requirements for obtaining private and commercial driving licences. They contain general advice and guidance in regard to the medical assessment of drivers and cover specific standards for all medical conditions that have the potential to affect driving capacity, as well as the details of the ethical and relevant legal responsibilities of doctors in each state and territory. The guide is sensitive to the difficulty that doctors can meet when counselling patients to give up their driving licence. Sections of the guidelines detail the legal responsibilities of drivers and doctors; showing these to patients being counselled about giving up driving may help to resolve problematic discussions.

In making an assessment of fitness to drive, doctors are performing a duty on behalf of both the community and the patient, and must be objective and honest in their assessment. As the request for assessment is frequently based on observations of police or others who have concern for the safety of the public, the task must be undertaken with care and caution. A treating doctor who forms a view that a patient may be unfit to drive should inform the patient of the legal requirements on both the patient and the doctor and advise the patient to notify the licensing authority of this unfitness.

In the NT and SA, doctors have a mandatory obligation to report a person's unfitness to drive, while in the other jurisdictions, doctors who notify the licensing authority in good faith are immune from civil action [23]. The national guidelines recommend that:

> health professionals should consider reporting directly to the driver licensing authority in situations where a patient is either:
>
> - unable to appreciate the impact of their condition
> - unable to take notice of the health professional's recommendations due to cognitive impairment
> - provides unreliable information on their condition, or
> - continues driving despite appropriate advice and is likely to endanger the public [22].

In this situation, privacy legislation provides protection to the doctor, as does the relevant licensing legislation in all states and territories other than WA. Advice is available from state and territory licensing authorities and their medical advisers who have access to formal testing facilities where ability to drive can be properly assessed in marginal cases.

32.3 Forensic medicine

32.3.1 Blood samples from persons involved in motor vehicle accidents

In all jurisdictions, persons involved in motor vehicle accidents who attend hospital for treatment must provide a blood sample. Testing is permitted without the consent of the person, and the doctor who takes the blood sample is granted protection from legal action. A doctor who fails to take, or fails to arrange the taking of, a blood alcohol sample may be charged with an offence, except where the doctor believes that the taking of the blood would compromise patient care.

Doctors who care for persons involved in motor vehicle accidents need to be familiar with the law in their state or territory pertaining to taking, dividing, labelling and storing of blood samples taken from such individuals.

In most states and territories, the road safety legislation provides police the powers to arrest persons in charge of motor vehicles who may be under the influence of drugs other than alcohol. When this occurs, the driver may be required to allow a doctor to take a blood sample.

Doctors also may be asked to express an opinion as to whether a driver is medically capable of participating in a breath alcohol test. After preliminary breath tests, if the driver requests it or if the breath sample has been insufficient, drivers may be brought by police for blood alcohol testing; this does not require the person's consent other than in Tasmania and the ACT.

The relevant legislation is: *Road Transport Act 2013* (NSW); *Road Safety Act 1986* (Vic); *Transport Operations (Road Use Management) Act 1995* (Qld); *Road Traffic Act 1961* (SA); *Road Traffic Act 1974* (WA); *Road Safety (Alcohol and Drugs) Act 1970* (Tas); *Traffic Act 1987* (NT); and *Road Transport (Alcohol and Drugs) Act 1977* (ACT).

32.3.2 Blood samples from persons accused of serious crime

All Australian states and territories have legislation enabling the collection of biological samples from people suspected of committing a range of criminal offences. Specifics of the legislation vary between jurisdictions but cover the type of sample (e.g. hair, blood or buccal swab), consent, the use of force, and the role of the courts in issuing orders. Doctors requested to draw such samples should establish either that the patient has consented or that there is an appropriate order authorising the collection without patient consent. Junior doctors should seek advice from one of their supervising senior doctors in these circumstances.

32.4 General areas of law

32.4.1 Anti-competitive legislation

Doctors who are in private practice are carrying on a business and subject to the provisions of the *Competition and Consumer Act 2010* (Cth) (which replaced the Commonwealth *Trade Practices Act 1974*). This Act also provides powers for consumer protection from misleading advertising. The Act is administered by the Australian Competition and Consumer Commission (ACCC) [24].

Doctors can cooperate with each other to develop arrangements that better serve their patients, but anti-competitive conduct, such as market sharing or price fixing, is not permitted. The Act also protects doctors' rights if other doctors or hospital systems act in an anti-competitive way towards them. For example, in the case of *ACCC v Ramsay Health Care* [25], the ACCC alleged that Ramsay Health Care Australia told surgeons who were planning to establish a competing private day surgery facility in the same regional locality that their access to operating theatre time at a local Ramsay Health Care private hospital would be substantially reduced or withdrawn.

To ensure fair practice, doctors must be careful not to:

- use unclear criteria for credentialing or admitting rights at hospitals to restrict the trade of other health professionals
- allow competing specialists to threaten boycotts at hospitals to prevent other specialists from being credentialed there
- make agreements with associates or partners operating as separate legal entities on patient fees or joint negotiations with suppliers, financial service providers or landlords, unless they have gained an authorisation from the ACCC
- act unconscionably by using a superior commercial position to subject another party to, or force them to accept, harsh or oppressive behaviour
- employ unfair tactics or attempts to unreasonably extract benefits from another business or professional by using their size or bargaining power.

In addition, to protect consumers, doctors must not:

- mislead patients about fees, procedures or outcomes
- use misleading advertising relating to qualifications, area of expertise, fees, procedures or outcomes
- act unconscionably by acting in bad faith and deliberately taking advantage of patients who are disadvantaged by:
  - ignorance of important facts that the doctor knows but the patient does not understand

- financial problems
- infirmity or age
- lack of understanding of the nature of the transaction
- lack of assistance or explanation when these are necessary
- a special disadvantage that impairs their capacity to judge what is in their best interests, such as English being their second language or situational factors causing a lack of practical alternatives.

32.4.2 Workplace relations

The *Fair Work Act 2009* (Cth) sets up Australia's national workplace relations system, which includes the following key elements [26]:

- a safety net of minimum terms and conditions of employment
- a system of enterprise-level collective bargaining underpinned by bargaining obligations and rules governing industrial action
- provision for individual flexibility arrangements as a way to allow an individual worker and an employer to make flexible work arrangements that meet their genuine needs, provided that the employee is better off overall
- protections against unfair or unlawful termination of employment
- protection of the freedom of both employers and employees to choose whether or not to be represented by a third party in workplace matters and the provision of rules governing the rights and responsibilities of employer and employee representatives.

Doctors should be aware that employers and employees not covered by the federal Fair Work Act remain covered by the applicable state or territory industrial relations system. However, federal entitlements to unpaid parental leave, notice of termination or payment in lieu of notice, and protection from unlawful termination of employment will still apply to employees who are covered by a state industrial relations system.

32.4.3 Workplace health and safety

Hospitals and other healthcare settings may have significant workplace safety risks, including risks of nosocomial infection, environmental and poisoning hazards, and occupational physical and psychological violence. Doctors have an important role to ensure a safe working environment for other medical colleagues, especially junior medical staff, as well as other healthcare workers. This workplace health and safety (WHS) responsibility also extends to safety for visitors to health facilities.

Safe Work Australia is the national body that oversees the development of national WHS and workers' compensation policies, and is responsible for the development and evaluation of the model WHS laws [27]. The model laws have been developed for implementation by the Commonwealth, states and territories, but do not apply in a jurisdiction unless the jurisdiction has separately taken action to implement the laws as their own WHS laws.

Each state and territory is responsible for enforcing their own WHS laws, which establish a framework for prevention, compensation and rehabilitation in relation to workplace-related injury and illness. The primary focus of WHS laws is on fostering safe work environments and systems of work, by eliminating or controlling risks. The Commonwealth, ACT, NSW, NT and Queensland implemented the model WHS laws in their jurisdictions on 1 January 2012. SA and Tasmania implemented the model WHS laws on

1 January 2013. WA implemented their model laws on 1 March 2022. Victoria is the only jurisdiction that has not implemented the model WHS laws [27].

WHS laws impose a duty on employers to take all reasonably practicable steps to protect the health and safety of employees at the workplace. In addition, the laws impose a general duty of care to persons other than employees who are present in the workplace, and to persons outside the workplace who are affected by the operations of the workplace. Employees also have a duty to take care of their own health and safety, as well as the health and safety of others, while in the workplace. Regulations, standards and codes of practice will provide more detailed guidance.

Doctors should be aware that WHS laws also cover workplace issues such as stress, fatigue and burnout in employees, an issue that has become more prominent since the COVID-19 pandemic. This also includes psychological distress arising out of an unsafe workplace environment due to a culture of incivility, bullying, harassment and discrimination. In 2022, the Medical Training Survey found that 34% of junior doctors had experienced and/or witnessed bullying, harassment, discrimination and racism [28]. Sexual harassment of female doctors is also a potential WHS issue for employers [29]. In addition, doctors need to be aware that safety in the workplace includes ensuring safe working hours and rostering practices, especially for junior doctors working shiftwork in hospitals [30].

32.4.4 Human rights legislation

Doctors should be aware that human rights laws may be relevant to healthcare delivery. The right to health is at the core of the 1948 Universal Declaration of Human Rights and other international instruments, and is the focus of the United Nations' work around human rights [31]. Specifically, Article 12(1) of the International Covenant on Economic, Social and Cultural Rights recognises 'the right of everyone to the enjoyment of the highest attainable standard of physical and mental health' [32].

In Australia, human rights protection can be found in the Constitution, our common-law system, and bodies such as the Australian Human Rights Commission. Federal legislation is also in place to protect people from discrimination and breaches of human rights, such as the *Age Discrimination Act 2004*, *Sex Discrimination Act 1984*, *Racial Discrimination Act 1975* and *Disability Discrimination Act 1992*.

Doctors should be aware of their obligations under the Medical Board of Australia's *Good medical practice: a code of conduct for doctors in Australia*, which outlines doctors' right to not provide or directly participate in treatments to which they conscientiously object, while not using their objection to impede access to treatments that are legal, or allowing their own moral or religious views to deny patients access to medical care [33].

Three Australian jurisdictions—Queensland, Victoria and the ACT—have enacted human rights legislation. The Victorian *Charter of Human Rights and Responsibilities Act 2006* and the ACT's *Human Rights Act 2004* both create a limited right to health arising from a right to life. However, these laws do not oblige healthcare providers to provide particular health services. The Victorian legislation does impose obligations on public authorities to consider relevant human rights in decision making, and requires public authorities to act in a manner compatible with human rights.

The Queensland human rights legislation includes an explicit, but limited, right to health services [34], defined in the *Human Rights Act 2019* (Qld) as:

> Every person has the right to access health services without discrimination
>
> A person must not be refused emergency medical treatment that is immediately necessary to save the person's life or to prevent serious impairment to the person [35].

In summary, unlike some other countries, Australia does not have a protected right to health in legislation or in the Constitution. The limited rights arising out of state human rights laws in Australia are designed to hold public authorities to human rights standards, and are not meant to create causes of legal action for individuals to uphold these rights. State-based human rights commissions do not have the power to compel public authorities to provide particular health services or treatments, or invalidate existing legislation, and can only declare that an existing legislation, or a decision made by a public authority, is inconsistent with human rights.

During the COVID-19 pandemic, some individuals claimed a right to freedom and challenged public health measures implemented to restrict movement. The High Court rejected the claim that lockdown public health measures imposed in Victoria infringed on freedom of movement implied in the Australian Constitution, confirming the Constitution provides no basis for an implication of freedom of movement that limits legislative or executive power [36].

Summary

Contemporary medical practice occurs within a complex legal framework that affects the day-to-day practice of many practitioners. Many legal aspects of practice, including the laws relating to prescribing, confidentiality, medical record keeping, certifying birth and death, termination of pregnancy and end-of-life care, have been dealt with in other chapters. This chapter has described additional legal responsibilities that apply in four major areas: statutory duties, medicolegal reports, forensic medicine, and general areas of law including human rights legislation. It is crucial that doctors practising in any area of medicine that is subject to these laws ensure that they are aware of the requirements, both at a federal and state or territory level, and how they may impact on their practice.

References

1. *Banks v Goodfellow* (1870) LR 5 QB 549.
2. Purser K, Rosenfeld T. Evaluation of legal capacity by doctors and lawyers: the need for collaborative assessment. *Med J Aust* 2014; 201: 483–485.
3. Victoria State Government, Justice and Community Safety. Statutory declarations. 2024. https://www.justice.vic.gov.au/statdecs (accessed Jan 2025).
4. Studdert D, Richardson M. Legal aspects of open disclosure: a review of Australian law. *Med J Aust* 2010; 193: 273–276.
5. Ahern S, Hopper I, Loh E. Qualified privilege legislation to support clinician quality assurance: balancing professional and public interests. *Med J Aust* 2019; 210: 343–346.
6. Australian Securities and Investments Commission. Whistleblower rights and protections (Information sheet 238). 2024. https://asic.gov.au/about-asic/asic-investigations-and-enforcement/whistleblowing/whistleblower-rights-and-protections/ (accessed Jan 2025).
7. National Domestic Family and Sexual Violence Counselling Service. Mandatory reporting requirements. https://www.1800respect.org.au/resources-and-tools/reporting-and-protection/mandatory-reporting (accessed Mar 2023).
8. NSW Government Department of Communities and Justice. Mandatory reporters: What to report and when. 2025. https://dcj.nsw.gov.au/children-and-families/protecting-our-kids/mandatory-reporters/mandatory-reporters--what-to-report-and-when.html (accessed Jul 2025).
9. *Firearms Regulations 2017* (SA), s 96.
10. *Firearms Act 2017* (NT), s 101.
11. *Firearms Act 1996* (Tas), ss 148, 158A.
12. *Firearms Act 1996* (NSW), s 79.
13. *Firearms Act 1973* (WA), s 23B.
14. *Weapons Act 1990* (Qld), s 151.

15. *Firearms Act 1996* (Vic), s 183.
16. *Firearms Act 1996* (ACT), s 261.
17. MIGA. Firearms and reporting obligations. 2021. https://www.miga.com.au/Articles/Firearms-and-reporting-obligations-(1) (accessed Mar 2023).
18. Services Australia. Medical evidence. 2024. https://www.servicesaustralia.gov.au/medical-evidence-for-disability-support-pension?context=22276 (accessed Jan 2025).
19. NDIS. A GP and health professional's guide to the NDIS. 2020. https://www.ndis.gov.au/media/332/download (accessed Jan 2025).
20. Safe Work Australia. Workers' compensation. https://www.safeworkaustralia.gov.au/workers-compensation (accessed Jan 2025).
21. Victorian Equal Opportunity and Human Rights Commission. Guideline for the recruitment industry and employers: complying with the *Equal Opportunity Act 2010* in recruitment. 2014. https://www.humanrights.vic.gov.au/resources/recruitment-guideline/ (accessed Oct 2021).
22. Austroads. Assessing fitness to drive. 2022. https://austroads.com.au/drivers-and-vehicles/assessing-fitness-to-drive (accessed Mar 2023).
23. Austroads. Assessing fitness to drive: Appendix 3 Legislation relating to reporting. https://austroads.com.au/publications/assessing-fitness-to-drive/ap-g56/legislation-relating-to-reporting (accessed Mar 2023).
24. Australian Competition and Consumer Commission. Medical professionals. https://www.accc.gov.au/business/associations-and-professional-services/medical-professionals (accessed Mar 2023).
25. *ACCC v Ramsay Health Care* [2020] FCA 308.
26. Fair Work Commission. Fair work legislation. https://www.fwc.gov.au/about-us/legislation-and-regulations (accessed Jun 2025).
27. Safe Work Australia. The model WHS laws: WHS laws in your jurisdiction. https://www.safeworkaustralia.gov.au/law-and-regulation/legislation (accessed Oct 2021).
28. Medical Training Survey. Culture of medical training in the spotlight. 2023. https://www.medicaltrainingsurvey.gov.au/News/Article/Culture-of-medical-training-in-the-spotlight-in-2022 (accessed Mar 2023).
29. Mathews B, Bismark MM. Sexual harassment in the medical profession: legal and ethical responsibilities. *Med J Aust* 2015; 203: 189–192.
30. Australian Medical Association. National code of practice—hours of work, shiftwork and rostering for hospital doctors. 2016. https://ama.com.au/sites/default/files/documents/FINAL_NCP_Hours_of_work_2016.pdf (accessed Jan 2025).
31. United Nations. Universal Declaration of Human Rights. 1948. https://www.un.org/en/universal-declaration-human-rights (accessed Oct 2021).
32. Department of Foreign Affairs, Canberra. International Covenant on Economic, Social and Cultural Rights (New York, 16 December 1966) [Australian Treaty Series 1976 No 5]. http://www.austlii.edu.au/au/other/dfat/treaties/1976/5.html (accessed Oct 2021).
33. Medical Board of Australia. Good medical practice: a code of conduct for doctors in Australia. 2020. https://www.medicalboard.gov.au/Codes-Guidelines-Policies/Code-of-conduct.aspx (accessed Jan 2025).
34. Brolan CE. Queensland's new Human Rights Act and the right to access health services. *Med J Aust* 2020; 213: 158–160.e1.
35. *Human Rights Act 2019* (Qld), s 37.
36. *Gerner v Victoria* [2020] HCA 48.

Further reading

Legal Services Commission South Australia. Medical treatment and related issues. In: Law Handbook. https://www.lawhandbook.sa.gov.au/ch29.php

Samuel S. Medicine and law: health and justice in partnership [editorial]. *Aust J Gen Pract* 2019; 48: 5.

33 Entering and leaving practice and practice management

Antonio Di Dio, Michael Isaacs

Introduction

Most Australian doctors undertake their own full-time or part-time private clinical practice, and are thus effectively running a small business. To successfully manage such an enterprise requires knowledge, some skill, and investment of time and energy. For larger medical groups, a practice manager may be employed to undertake some of this work, or the task may be allocated to a medical member of the group who has the necessary skills and interest. This chapter gives a broad overview of the tasks involved in career planning and establishing, managing and leaving a practice, and directs the reader to more detailed sources of information and professional help. It does not address the management issues specific to services such as radiology, pathology and day procedure centres.

33.1 Choosing your career

Key points

- Deciding on your career trajectory is a dynamic process that occurs during preclinical, clinical and postgraduate years.
- It is important to understand the hurdles (academic, industrial, structural) that may be entailed with these decisions.
- The number of pre-specialty training years are increasing, which has both benefits (broader experience) and detriments (longer time to specialty).

Some medical students are able to determine their career direction at an early stage, but many wait at least until they have experienced their first postgraduate ('intern') year before seriously considering this. The period from the intern year onwards has assumed increased importance as a time for decision making before doctors focus their clinical experience into general practice, medicine, surgery or other fields, in preparation for joining formal training programs. These years are also assuming greater importance within careers: the National Medical Workforce Strategy 2021–2031 [1] notes that junior doctors may now experience more barriers to admission to formal training programs. A growing number of unaccredited training positions coupled with undersupply of certain specialists within accredited facilities is making access to certain training programs increasingly difficult. It is becoming more common for doctors not to be accepted for their chosen specialist training until four or five years after medical school, or after undertaking further higher education.

Despite this, it is very helpful for many doctors that positions providing further broad experience are available. Many successful careers have followed even when doctors-in-training have changed direction part-way through or on completion of a training program in general practice or a specialty. In choosing a career in medicine, an early-career doctor should at least:

- gain some experience in the field(s) being considered, and while doing so, look as objectively as possible at what work in that field of practice will entail
- talk to many people, informally and formally, about career choices, opportunities and the work each person does; attend career expos where available; and seek advice from senior medical staff who are available to counsel early-career doctors on career choice. This latter information is vital, as junior doctors often err in judging only the practical aspect of the work (such as delivering babies) without looking at the totality of the practice (such as the running of an obstetric unit or private practice) and the lifestyle around that practice (such as difficult hours and the potential effect on family).
- observe that most patient care takes place outside major public hospitals, and that hospital training will have given most early-career doctors a narrow view of health care; many specialty areas such as general practice, occupational medicine, public health, Indigenous health, sexual health, travel medicine, forensic medicine and sports medicine will not be encountered during hospital training
- note that in addition to clinical practice, medical graduates' skills are also used in non-clinical settings including administration, academia, teaching, research, industry and even the media
- note that many doctors are now more flexible in their approach to their careers and that some fields of practice provide greater flexibility than others
- note that the positive and negative experiences in hospital training are usually bound in the human interactions and culture of a workplace, and not necessarily in the specific quality of the work. An early-career doctor who enjoyed their work placement in cardiology may have done so because of the wonderful environment they worked in, but could still choose to pursue an alternative career due to interests and passions outside of the practice of cardiology.

While some structural biases persist for traditionally marginalised groups within the medical field, the situation is improving. Women constitute 50% or more of new medical graduates and over 87% of obstetric registrars, and are gradually increasing their presence in all fields of medical practice. Aboriginal and/or Torres Strait Islander communities are also being better served by increasing representation. Addressing issues around part-time training, job-sharing and onsite child care, as well as campaigns such as a single employer model allowing hospital-based doctors a greater financial incentive to enter out-of-hospital practice, are helping to accommodate more varied career trajectories. No career path should be regarded as impossible for graduates, and career advice and encouragement is increasingly available from doctors of similar experiences and backgrounds.

When contemplating career choices, all early-career doctors should examine their strengths and weaknesses as part of the process of making major decisions. This self-knowledge can also assist in personal and professional development. Other sources exist that discuss this in more depth [2].

33.2 Importance of good practice management

Key points

- Good practice management involves the sum of all clinical and non-clinical functions of the practice.
- Resources are available from key bodies to guide managing a practice.

Good practice management is not just an exercise in self-interest. While there are personal benefits, good practice management is a prerequisite to good patient care and is in the best interests of patients. In a well-run practice, appointment systems work, patient records are not misplaced, investigation results are not overlooked, recall systems are efficient and safe, bulk-billing errors to Medicare do not occur and patients are guided efficiently to the help and resources they need. Errors in billing can be extremely costly and lead to stressful processes, and educating oneself in appropriate use of the Medicare Benefits Schedule is the responsibility of all doctors working in private practice. As mentioned in Chapter 5, Communication in clinical practice, better patient outcomes are achieved where there is good communication and a good doctor–patient relationship is established. This relationship begins from the moment a patient first phones the practice for an appointment or first enters the waiting room. Patients may not be able to assess a doctor's medical knowledge or clinical skill, but they can assess waiting times, the friendliness and competence of staff, the appearance of the waiting room and the consultation room and the general ambience of the practice [3]. Even before this, the practice's website and ease of making appointments and identifying practice information can sometimes be the first contact a patient has with the doctor or practice. Effort spent initially in planning, furnishing, equipping, organising and staffing a practice and then in maintaining it with good management will be rewarded.

Extensive guidance is available, especially for general practitioners (GPs), through a series of excellent publications by the Royal Australian College of General Practitioners (RACGP) on its website [4]. The RACGP also offers a practice advisory service and regular educational activities in practice management. The Royal Australasian College of Surgeons produces a guide for recent fellows, *Preparation for practice*, which covers practice establishment and practice management issues in considerable depth [5]. In addition, each state and territory branch of the Australian Medical Association (AMA) provides professional advice and services in aspects of practice management. The *Medical Journal of Australia*'s careers section and the medical newspapers carry regular columns devoted to aspects of practice management. This chapter draws heavily on the RACGP publications and several other sources, including the AMA. The federal Department of Health, Disability and Ageing and Services Australia provide material relevant to a range of Commonwealth services (e.g. Medicare, the Pharmaceutical Benefits Scheme [PBS], Department of Veterans' Affairs [DVA], My Aged Care, and Centrelink). These federal sources provide detailed guidance on the legal obligations of the individual practitioner and their practice.

33.3 Preparing to enter private practice

Key points

- When undertaking clinical training, remain mindful of the processes outside your clinical work, as these skills will be useful should you enter independent practice.
- Broad experiences in multiple different places of practice can solidify this knowledge.

It is important for doctors who decide to enter independent private practice to learn the essentials of good practice management. Having this knowledge is useful when undertaking locum work or entering a group practice on a trial basis, to help evaluate the management of the practice that the doctor may intend to join. It is very challenging and not recommended to take on solo practice without at least some exposure to locum or employee practice work first—there is simply too much to learn and the administrative burden and lack of clinical oversight can be challenging even for experienced practitioners.

For GPs whose postgraduate training is predominantly based in general practice, taking notice of how each practice is managed is one starting point. After completion of training, working as an employee in one or more general practices will also provide insights. For specialists entering private practice, finding opportunities to experience a well-run practice is usually a very informal process; the simple approach of trainees informing mentors and other specialists with whom they have worked that they wish to commence in private practice or are available to provide holiday cover may bring surprising and beneficial results.

33.4 Setting up a medical practice

Key points

- When starting out, consider the benefits and detriments of joining/acquiring an existing practice or establishing somewhere new.
- Engage appropriate professionals: legal counsel, accountants, security, office managers, etc. Consider whether you wish to maintain solo practice or work with other doctors.
- The location of your practice may be influenced by personal circumstance, financial/government incentive, or the particular medical needs of the area.
- The premises itself will need to be appraised to meet financial, legal and practical considerations.

For both GPs and specialists, establishing a medical practice requires considerable preparation and planning. Ideally, this should involve setting of professional, personal and financial priorities, seeking information on practice management and obtaining knowledge about contracts and obligations for locum and assistant work. As much of the planning will involve financial decisions, professional advice should be sought. The relevant college and the AMA are good starting points; non-medical professionals, such as an accountant with experience in medical practice, may also provide contacts with other professionals such as bookkeepers, solicitors and financial experts. Other key aspects to consider are addressed in the following sections.

33.4.1 Starting out

Should a new practitioner start by joining an existing practice run by a mentor or older colleague, buying an existing practice or establishing a new practice? The potential benefits of joining an established practice include the opportunity to receive mentoring and business advice, and to participate in case discussions with more experienced colleagues. In buying and taking over an established practice, there is no guarantee that existing patients will choose to continue to see the new doctor taking over—the style of practice may be quite different from the previous doctor. Ideally, vendor doctors will stay on for an agreed period, from several months to a year, to ensure the best possible 'handover' of clinical and financial concerns, and minimise patient departures.

33.4.2 Financial, business and legal advice

As the owner-manager of a small business, the doctor will require initial and ongoing professional assistance from an accountant, a solicitor and a bank manager. A solicitor will be needed to advise on purchasing or leasing premises, staff contracts, partnership agreements and arranging incorporation or trust funds, while an accountant will advise on matters including taxation, superannuation, workers' compensation, practice insurance and the accounting and billing systems to use. Legal practitioners with knowledge of the issues surrounding medical practice can be difficult to find, so it can be helpful to seek the recommendation of other doctors who can vouch for their ability. Ensure that your relationships with these professionals are positive, as their skills may stay with you in partnership for decades. You should meet with them, annually or quarterly depending on profession, to track your goals and discuss your frustrations and successes. It is additionally important to ensure that you have good filing systems in relation to this—knowing all your contacts and where your leases and key documents are will save you time, over and over again. It is worth seeking out professionals, especially your accountant and bookkeeper, who have other medical clients, as they will have experienced many of the potential pitfalls and assist you in building structures (sole trader, partnership, trust, corporate and so on) that are the best ones for you today and in the future. They will also see potential hurdles on the horizon, such as the current issue of payroll tax and past difficulties with renting to pathology companies, years before they arise, and allow preparation for those uncertainties. In Australia during the COVID-19 pandemic, many doctors running businesses needed complex taxation advice about state and federal business continuity and income loss payments, and the accountant and corporate associates were invaluable resources to practitioners who were very busy in their clinical roles. Many of the most difficult situations for doctors arise in running out of physical space when their practice wants to grow but cannot, or in the departure from a financial agreement with colleagues. Both of these can be avoided or at least minimised by simple planning at the start of running a practice.

Apart from the more obvious considerations, which include financing entry into practice and obtaining legal assistance over contracts and purchases, decisions will need to be made about incorporation or using a service trust to run the medical practice. Self-managed superannuation fund legislation may provide the opportunity to purchase a medical practice through superannuation. Individualised taxation advice and legal advice are essential to guide the choice of the most appropriate financial and organisational structure. This must be stressed—getting those structures optimised at the start of practice can save a great deal of time and effort later on.

33.4.3 Location

When choosing a location, GPs will need to consider factors including population trends, number and location of competing practices, visibility and exposure of potential sites, personal and family choice, their own medical interests and capabilities, and local medical resources. Specialists will need to be aware of matters such as public and private hospital appointments, transport access or parking, and the perceived medical needs of the area being considered. Local planning and zoning regulations must also be considered by both groups. Advice and information may be available from other doctors in the area, but as your arrival may not be welcomed, this may not be totally reliable. For GPs, a more detailed discussion of this critical decision making is provided by the RACGP [4] and it is highly recommended that it be reviewed before major decisions are made. Anti-competitive legislation is covered in Chapter 32, Legal frameworks: rights, responsibilities and protections.

In addition, the federal government offers financial incentives for GPs in underserved areas. These programs are subject to change: information about current incentives and assistance is available from the Department of Health, Disability and Ageing website [6].

33.4.4 Solo or group practice

What type of practice do you wish to work in? Larger group practices may allow greater flexibility of working hours, but each practitioner has proportionally less input about how the practice is managed. Group practices may also differ in their structure, such as partnership versus associateship. A partnership of doctors implies a contract (preferably written) whereby all expenses and income are shared between the partners according to an agreed formula. It also involves a formal structure, which should involve a regular meeting to discuss and deal with the business and practice issues which arise. An associateship of doctors implies an agreement (also preferably written) to share the costs of providing the practice infrastructure but without sharing the practice income. Associates bill in their own names and retain the income, apart from that required to pay the agreed share of overheads.

There are professional pros and cons to these structures as well. Sometimes solo practice is best for logistical reasons, is more strategically nimble, and has easier governance and oversight. At other times group practice is more collegial, easier to arrange and cover each other at times of leave, and colleagues confer support and education and supervision of each other, formally or informally. In some areas of medicine, solo practice is financially unsustainable.

33.4.5 Premises

Whether the premises is purchased, leased/rented, or newly built is a primarily financial decision. Whatever the decision, careful consideration should be given to the location and design of the building. Consider the patient's viewpoint (provisions for car parking, disabled access, comfort, privacy and quietness); the staff's viewpoint (space, lighting, comfort, toilets, staffroom, parking, security and storage); and the doctor's viewpoint (consultation and procedure rooms, access to staff and colleagues, capacity to deal with urgent cases and access to hospitals). Be aware of legislative requirements for the premises, including infection control and accessibility. Relevant legislation varies on a state-by-state basis. Consideration must also be given to heating, cooling and safety, and especially the safety of children. A well-designed practice assists in marketing and adds greatly to staff efficiency and morale. Obviously this is sometimes entirely determined by the practice where you work as an associate, and eventually decide to join long term, but it illustrates how every role you have, even in junior and hospital years, is part of your learning experience about service delivery and, possibly, your own practice.

33.4.6 Security issues

Verbal and physical aggression, primarily from patients and their relatives, is a common experience in both hospital and family practice [7–11]. The risk of physical aggression should be factored into the design of the consulting and waiting areas. In the case of a threat of violence from a patient, having a safety exit for reception staff, a second door to the consulting room (or having the doctor seated closest to the single door), and an alarm system—for example, via the practice computer network—for discreetly alerting another staff member of the need for assistance are all steps to be considered. The practice should have protocols for handling threats of violence appropriate to the nature of the practice and staff should be instructed in these protocols. Depending on the assessed risks, a doctor should not work alone in a practice and a staff member should not be on duty alone when patients are likely to attend.

Another form of aggression is sexual harassment, most often of female doctors by male patients [12,13]. Respondents to a 2013 survey of female Australian GPs reported that over half had experience of such harassment, often on multiple occasions [13]. At present, no training is offered for this aspect of practice and support systems for doctors affected by such harassment have not been developed. This is an area requiring attention, as the experience is often very negative for female doctors and has led to unwanted limitation of their practice [14].

33.4.7 Equipping a practice

A large up-front investment is required to equip a new practice or to purchase a practice that is already equipped. There are also additional costs for a doctor who proposes to provide new services, which may have sophisticated technological requirements. The list of probable requirements includes fittings, furniture, computer and storage systems, and basic medical, office and communication equipment (telephone, photocopier and often also fax machine). For computer systems, practice management, clinical medical records software and security and backup arrangements need to be considered. Computer problems occur often in practice, and like your accountant, strong relationships with computer professionals (hardware and software) are vital. Discuss a service agreement up front: having a professional who you can call at very short notice will pay for itself many times over. See also Chapter 6, Confidentiality, privacy and disclosure; Chapter 27, Medical records, reports and certificates; and Chapter 29, Professional practice, digital technology and artificial intelligence.

Preparation for formal accreditation of general practice requires considerable planning and documentation, and the RACGP *Standards for general practices* should be consulted [15]. Many practices find it motivating for the individual and very time efficient for the doctors for a staff member to be in charge of the accreditation cycle. While some essential stationery such as Medicare stationery, PBS prescription pads and DVA stationery is provided freely by Services Australia and the federal Department of Health, Disability and Ageing, this and other practice stationery should be ordered several months before going into independent practice.

33.4.8 Options to avoid managing your own practice

Companies can establish or purchase medical practices, and this trend has gradually developed in Australia. There are advantages and disadvantages to working in a corporate practice. Practices are becoming increasingly large and complex, often with co-located allied health or pathology services [16]. The arrangement advantages the doctor by allowing more comprehensive management, and frees them from the work and worry of all of the issues that can arise in managing a practice. On the other hand, the doctor is no longer in control of the practice and may find themselves in conflict with the company over the commercial aims of the company and quality and ethical standards. Doctors may feel pressured or incentivised to conduct their care in ways that maximise billable items, rather than for the benefit of their patient. There is variable evidence to suggest that corporate practices deliver less patient satisfaction and poorer patient outcomes as a result. If tied by an inflexible contract, it can be difficult to escape from this mode of practice without a significant financial penalty [16]. The AMA has developed a very helpful aid to assist doctors who are thinking of entering into a contract with a corporation [17].

33.5 Administrative requirements

Key points

- Medicare is an important source of practice funding (through bulk-billing) and supply (through PBS orders).
- Make sure to engage with relevant state or territory bodies to ensure you are kept up to date and are meeting legislative requirements, including continuing professional development (CPD).

33.5.1 Recognition by Medicare

The principles of Medicare and the PBS are described in Chapter 20, The Australian healthcare system. For patients to claim rebates from Medicare and for doctors to bulk-bill Medicare, each doctor must be a registered medical practitioner and be granted a provider number by Medicare. A separate provider number is required for each practice location. Self-education on appropriate billing is available through the RACGP or your medical defence organisation, in addition to ad hoc information from your practice colleagues. It is very important to bill appropriately and to inform yourself of how to do this. Specialist registration grants access to different levels of rebate for services particular to that specialty. This is particularly relevant for practitioners with specialist registration in general practice. A provision also remains for practitioners who were vocationally registered with the Medical Board of Australia prior to June 2021 to claim rebates as a general practitioner without specialist registration. Barring this exception, without specialist registration Medicare rebates will be paid at a lower general rate.

Doctors must also apply to Medicare for a PBS prescriber number and may also order personalised PBS Authority prescription pads from Medicare. Until these are printed, interim PBS prescription pads may be issued. Medicare can also issue a copy of the *Schedule of pharmaceutical benefits*, the doctor's bag order form booklet and the *Medicare benefits schedule book*, and supplies of all the relevant Medicare stationery and direct-billing imprinter. The doctor must approach the DVA separately to be appointed as a local medical officer and to receive their stationery and guidelines.

The relevant state or territory health department should also be contacted by doctors to ensure that they are on mailing lists and receive copies of notices and publications relevant to their fields of practice.

33.5.2 Continuing professional development

Regardless of the type of registration held with the Medical Board of Australia, all practitioners have yearly educational obligations. These are collectively referred to as 'continuing professional development' (CPD), and may be more or less stringent depending on type of registration and specialty. CPD requirements can be met in multiple different ways, including self-directed study, structured courses, specialist training or research. From January 2024, the Medical Board of Australia required all practitioners to have a CPD home—an organisation accredited to provide a CPD program. This may be fulfilled by a relevant specialist college, or by a non-college program for practitioners not affiliated with a college. Chapter 10, Continuing professional development, discusses CPD in more detail.

33.5.3 Medical indemnity

Medical indemnity cover is compulsory for doctors in independent practice. Existing levels of cover will need to be reviewed, especially when entering private practice directly from a training program or when deciding to undertake procedural work. The guidance and services provided by medical indemnity organisations are addressed in other chapters. In Australia, about 5% of Australian practitioners receive a notification to the Australian Health Practitioner Regulation Agency each year. Although most of these do not require any regulatory action, it is vital to ensure that you have appropriate cover and professional support.

33.6 Selecting, employing and training staff

Key points

- Staff selection includes clinical (nurses, allied health, other doctors/registrars) and non-clinical (receptionists, administrative).
- Be aware of the state and federal labour/OHS laws, and ensure you are meeting obligations around safe working conditions, contracts, remuneration, etc.
- Maintain regular communication with your staff to ensure smooth running of the workplace.

33.6.1 Staff selection

Selection of staff requires careful attention, as they represent both the practice's greatest asset and its greatest expense [18,19]. Most early-career doctors have had little involvement in writing job descriptions, interviewing and selecting staff, evaluating references or speaking with former employers, so advice should be sought and professional assistance considered. Before interviewing potential staff, a job description should be written and information obtained on current award conditions and market rates. Be cautious if deciding to employ friends and family. While this may have economic advantages, it does not necessarily provide all the skills required and can create complex and unfavourable social or professional dynamics. Employing patients is also fraught with potential problems, and any individual employed should cease to be a patient of the practice and be referred for their medical care elsewhere. Consideration may also be given to the opportunity to facilitate the training of registrars within a private practice. However, the added responsibility and obligations of the practice to the trainees needs to be carefully addressed.

New staff need to be fully informed of their role and responsibilities, which should be documented, at least in a simple outline. They also need to be informed of the terms and conditions of employment. Their remuneration must cover the required superannuation, workers' compensation and taxation provisions, as penalties for not meeting these provisions are severe. The advice of an experienced accountant should be sought on these matters. It is especially important to ensure that new staff members are aware of the requirement of confidentiality in all matters, how complaints are handled in the practice, and of the fact that the doctor is ultimately responsible for the actions of staff.

33.6.2 Staff training

As employers, doctors should become aware of the range of training courses available for medical practice staff and of the associations they may wish to join. Staff also need support and supervision, and even the smallest practice should develop a practice manual to cover all the information a staff member would need to know about the practice. This manual may then be further developed to include details of available community resources, local hospitals, specialist services and businesses that are commonly approached. This manual would be particularly useful for temporary staff who may cover absences or sick leave.

Just as good communication with patients is vital, so it is with staff. Regular meetings should be held to discuss current issues and problems and to maintain morale and cohesion. When a staff member is performing poorly, fair procedures for performance review and constructive coaching should be implemented. As caring managers, doctors should make time for staff feedback, where they and their staff can discuss how the practice is performing, what difficulties staff may be experiencing and how improvements may be made. Be familiar with relevant industrial legislation regarding disciplinary procedures and dismissal should the need arise.

33.6.3 Caring for staff and staff safety

There are legal requirements to provide workers' compensation insurance and to meet occupational health and safety regulations. This extends to assessing the risks posed by aggressive or violent behaviour of patients and taking sensible precautions to reduce those risks, as well as training staff how to handle such situations [20]. An infection-control strategy should be in place and should be regularly reviewed. Like all the above materials in relation to running a practice, these documents should be clearly identifiable, appropriately filed and located within the space of the practice manager or equivalent person. Annual vaccination against influenza should be encouraged. Depending on the staff member's duties, hepatitis B, COVID-19 and other vaccinations may be sensible.

As the hazards of cross-infection and of transmission of viral infection (COVID-19, hepatitis B, hepatitis C and HIV) are increasingly recognised, and as more procedures are undertaken in private doctors' offices, doctors need to be aware of and take steps to prevent risks to patients. Sharps, disposal containers and hazardous chemicals must not be within reach of children. Compliance with infection-control guidelines [15,21] must be observed, and reference should be made to the National Safety and Quality Health Service Standards around infection prevention and control systems [22].

In general, it is preferable that staff do not become patients of the practice. As with employing friends and family, this can create complex and unfavourable social or professional dynamics (see also Chapter 8, Sexual and other professional boundaries: being a doctor in modern society). There are also significant risks around confidentiality and privacy (as discussed in Chapter 6, Confidentiality, privacy and disclosure), as staff members by necessity have access to practice records.

33.6.4 After-hours arrangements

Options for after-hours service provision include providing your own cover, purchasing cover from an after-hours deputising service or making cooperative arrangements with other practices. Staff and patients need to be made aware of the after-hours cover arrangements. GPs need to meet the requirements of vocational registration in regard to after-hours cover.

33.7 Marketing and advertising a medical practice

Key points

- Be aware of the legal and regulatory restrictions on advertising a practice.
- Consider a variety of media, including word of mouth, social media, meetings with local groups or other health professionals, and print/poster advertisement.

The Medical Board of Australia has issued guidelines about what the Health Practitioner Regulation National Law states about advertising (see Chapter 21, Regulation of the medical profession). The board has also developed specific guidelines (available on the Medical Board of Australia website) for doctors advertising cosmetic procedures, particularly on social media or online. In most areas of practice, word-of-mouth advertising remains the most effective form of generating new patients [23,24]. There are other acceptable means of informing prospective patients and professional colleagues of the establishment of the practice. GPs new to a community should visit local pharmacists, hospitals, hostels, nursing homes, in-home nursing services, hospice services and other doctors, thereby learning about the community while making the practice known. It may be useful to create an information sheet or brochure about the services offered. Specialists in smaller communities can introduce themselves personally to GPs, and in larger communities can offer to participate as speakers at educational events to help make themselves known. Conflicts of interest (see Chapter 9, Doctors, industry and conflicts of interest) should be identified and managed.

Another option to consider is setting up a clear, informative and well-maintained website, which can provide helpful information for patients and offer online appointment booking. Websites of specialists can also offer useful information for referring doctors and their staff. Social media plays a major role for many medical practices by providing a web presence, as well as enhanced opportunities for communication and networking with related medical organisations. The use or misuse of social media by doctors or practice staff can lead to breaches of personal or patient privacy and expose doctors to complaints of unprofessional conduct [24]. This is discussed in more detail in Chapter 8, Sexual and other professional boundaries: being a doctor in modern society, Chapter 27, Medical records, reports and certificates, and Chapter 29, Professional practice, digital technology and artificial intelligence, where several sources of guidance are provided.

33.8 Planning for a healthy approach to work

Key points

- Maintain activities outside work, be they social, family, leisure or otherwise.
- There are options for doctors beyond clinical practice, including academia, research and policy development.

It is important when starting in independent practice to plan for a healthy lifestyle. Approximately 80% of Australians visited a GP in any given year, but that number is less for doctors, especially male doctors. Self-care is a vital part of caring for others. This will include allocating time for social and family activities, leisure or sporting activities, and for continuing professional development. Doctors who do this are less likely to suffer the stress-related problems discussed in Chapter 12, Personal health of the doctor: illness and impairment. In the development and running of a medical practice, where appropriate, doctors should take positive steps to engage with the local community.

Part-time clinical practice is not uncommon. Medical expertise can be used in multiple different domains beyond clinical work, and a practitioner may decide to split their time between their patients and other pursuits. Involvement with a medical school can be valuable to both the students and the teacher, keeping practice current and influencing future practitioners. Many medical schools in Australia have particular interest in engaging clinicians, and may offer recognition via academic title or remuneration. Clinical research can also be considered, as trials often require a registered practitioner to supervise subjects and ensure their safety through the trial.

Medical expertise can also be leveraged in more indirect ways. Involvement in policy or advocacy can also be considered: participation with the AMA or specialist college committees can have influence on a wide scale, while involvement in local health service boards can have a similar effect locally. Involvement with medical regulation through membership of the Medical Board of Australia or one of its decision-making committees contributes to patient safety and the standing of the profession within society. The problem-solving skills of a doctor are often highly sought after in the corporate sector, although anecdotally, these are often high-stress environments even in comparison to clinical practice.

33.9 Closing a medical practice and planning for retirement

Key points

- There are legislative obligations that must be met regarding the closing of a practice, including notifications, data retention and staff redundancies.
- Consider also ethical obligations and minimise where possible the impact on the community served.
- Doctors tend to deny illness and have ill-defined plans for retirement. Planning is key to minimising the stress that may result from this transition, especially if external circumstances necessitate retiring unexpectedly.

There are a large number of matters to be attended to when a medical practice is to be closed or the doctor is retiring from practice. The effect of practice closure on the community should be carefully managed, and minimised where possible. Factors that may be considered include the rurality and socioeconomics of the area the practice serves, or if the practice is serving a particular demographic (such as Aboriginal and/or Torres Strait Islander or LGBTIQ+ communities). In addition to these professional considerations, legislative requirements must be met in relation to keeping or disposing of medical records or notifying patients regarding future access to medical records (see Chapter 27, Medical records, reports and certificates), notifying the medical indemnity organisation of planned retirement, and informing a range of other bodies including the Australian Tax Office, Medicare, the state or territory workers' compensation authority, the public liability insurer and the Australian Health Practitioner Regulation Agency. Advice may also be needed in regard to staff entitlements. Drugs and prescription pads must be disposed of in a manner consistent with the relevant state or territory legislation. The AMA state and territory branches or medical indemnifiers can provide more detailed advice in these matters.

For a range of reasons [25], perhaps related to the tendency of doctors to deny illness (see Chapter 12, Personal health of the doctor: illness and impairment), doctors tend not to plan ahead for retirement, whether financially or generally what they will do after retirement. As a result, many retire to an unhappy or unsatisfying life. Harvard-based psychiatrist George Vaillant, who initially studied the causes of distress in younger doctors, later turned his attention to ageing and retirement [26]. He believes that retirement is only stressful in four situations: if involuntary and unplanned, if finances are limited, if work has been an escape from an unhappy home, or if retirement has been precipitated by ill health.

There could be multiple triggers for a doctor to start considering retirement. This may be as simple as recognising personal change: perhaps the passion for the field has finally subsided, or competing life priorities may take precedence. Ill health can strike without warning [27], and sensible doctors plan for this possibility via such steps as assigning powers of attorney (medical and financial), having an up-to-date will and ensuring that superannuation assets have a current binding nomination. The more gradual biological effects of ageing are discussed in Chapter 12, Personal health of the doctor: illness and impairment. Particular recognition should be paid to the effect of chronic or degenerative illness on the ability of a doctor to continue practice.

Several years before retirement, doctors should find the time to begin planning the process. This can involve reading [26], attending seminars such as those conducted by medical organisations and superannuation funds, and talking to older colleagues about their experiences. It is increasingly common for practitioners to gradually reduce their clinical hours, rather than stop work entirely. An experienced practitioner can consider putting their expertise to use in other, non-clinical domains of medicine, as outlined in section 33.8.

Summary

Many legislative and administrative requirements are involved for a practitioner in commencing or ceasing practice, particularly in the private sector. Advocacy groups such as the AMA and medical indemnity providers are good sources of advice. For recent graduates embarking on establishing a new practice, the advice of an experienced mentor in the same scope of practice may be invaluable. Whatever the source of advice, it is vital that practitioners make themselves aware of the requirements that they need to fulfil, and put effort into planning well before making the change into or out of practice.

References

1. Department of Health. National Medical Workforce Strategy 2021–2031. Commonwealth of Australia, 2021. https://www.health.gov.au/our-work/national-medical-workforce-strategy-2021-2031 (accessed Aug 2025).
2. Breen KJ. So you want to be a doctor? A guide for prospective medical students in Australia. Melbourne: ACER Press, 2012.
3. Bray K. Your guide to choosing a good GP. CHOICE, 2014. http://www.choice.com.au/reviews-and-tests/food-and-health/general-health/health-practitioners/choosing-a-gp.aspx (accessed Jul 2023).
4. Royal Australian College of General Practitioners. General Practice Business Toolkit. https://www.racgp.org.au/running-a-practice/practice-resources/practice-tools/general-practice-business-toolkit (accessed Jul 2023).
5. Royal Australasian College of Surgeons. Preparation for practice. A guide for younger fellows. 5th ed. 2015. https://www.surgeons.org/-/media/Project/RACS/surgeons-org/files/reports-guidelines-publications/manuals-guidelines/p4p-guide-2015_web-version.pdf (accessed July 2023).
6. Department of Health, Disability and Ageing. Rural health workforce initiatives and programs. Commonwealth of Australia, 2023 [latest update]. https://www.health.gov.au/health-topics/rural-health-workforce/programs (accessed Aug 2025).
7. Hills DJ, Joyce CM, Humphries JS. A national study of workplace aggression in Australian clinical medical practice. *Med J Aust* 2012; 197: 336–340.
8. Hills DJ, Joyce CM, Humphreys JS. Workplace aggression prevention and minimisation in Australian clinical medical practice settings – a national study. *Aust Health Rev* 2013; 37: 606–613.
9. Forrest LE, Herath PM, McRae IS, Parker RM. A national survey of general practitioners' experiences of patient-initiated aggression in Australia. *Med J Aust* 2011; 194: 605–608.
10. Rowe L, Kidd MR. Increasing violence in Australian general practice is a public health issue. *Med J Aust* 2007; 337: 118–119.
11. Magin PJ, Joy E, Ireland MC, et al. Experiences of occupational violence in Australian urban general practice: a cross-sectional study of GPs. *Med J Aust* 2005; 183: 352–356.
12. Phillips SP, Schneidner MS. Sexual harassment of female doctors by patients. *N Engl J Med* 1993; 329: 1936–1939.
13. Bratuskins PA, McGarry HA, Wilkinson SJ. Sexual harassment of Australian female general practitioners by patients. *Med J Aust* 2013; 199: 454.
14. Baker L. Sexual harassment by patients forces doctors to alter their practice. *BMJ* 2014; 348: g118.
15. Royal Australian College of General Practitioners. Standards for general practices. 5th edn. 2020. https://www.racgp.org.au/running-a-practice/practice-standards/standards-5th-edition/standards-for-general-practices-5th-ed (accessed Jul 2023).
16. de Moel-Mandel C, Sundararajan V. The impact of practice size and ownership on general practice care in Australia. *Med J Aust* 2021; 214: 408–410.e1.
17. Australian Medical Association. Corporatisation of general practice – decision support kit for doctors. 2015. https://ama.com.au/sites/default/files/documents/Corporatisation_Kit.pdf (accessed Aug 2025).
18. How to hire staff. *MJA Careers* 2010; 193(Number 11/12): C3.
19. McGilvray A. Only the best. *MJA Careers* 2013; 199: C1–C2.
20. Royal Australian College of General Practitioners. General practice Business Toolkit Module 2: Ensuring your practice is safe and secure. https://www.racgp.org.au/running-a-practice/practice-resources/practice-tools/general-practice-business-toolkit/general-practice-tool-kit/module-2/safety-and-security (accessed Aug 2025).
21. National Health and Medical Research Council. Australian guidelines for the prevention and control of infection in healthcare. 2019. https://www.nhmrc.gov.au/about-us/publications/australian-guidelines-prevention-and-control-infection-healthcare-2019 (accessed Aug 2025).
22. Australian Commission on Safety and Quality in Health Care. National Safety and Quality Health Service Standards 2nd edn. 2021. https://www.safetyandquality.gov.au/publications-and-resources/resource-library/national-safety-and-quality-health-service-standards-second-edition (accessed Jul 2023).
23. McGilvray A. Reputation management. *MJA Careers* 2013; 199: C1–C2.

24. Ryan K. Should you advertise your medical practice? *MJA Careers* 2012; 196: C6–C7.
25. Draper BM. Older doctors and retirement. *Med J Aust* 2017; 206: 202–203.
26. Vaillant G. Ageing well. Melbourne: Scribe Publications, 2002: 221.
27. de Campo J. An illness aide-memoire. *MJA Careers* 2012; 196: C9.

Further reading

Australian Government Department of Health, Disability and Ageing. DoctorConnect. https://www.health.gov.au/our-work/doctorconnect

Table of cases

Page numbers are given in **bold**. Where the title of the case is not named on the discussion page but it is in an endnote, the endnote number is given to indicate the position of the discussion on the page. For example, **394n25** means the discussion is on page 394 at the point where endnote 25 is cited.

Table of statutes

Statutes are arranged by jurisdiction. Page numbers are given in **bold** and indicate the location of the discussion; page numbers in the format **203n1** indicate endnotes.

Commonwealth of Australia

Australian Capital Territory

New South Wales

Northern Territory

Queensland

South Australia

Tasmania

Victoria

Western Australia

United States of America

Index

A

B

E

M

N

S

www.ingramcontent.com/pod-product-compliance
Lightning Source LLC
LaVergne TN
LVHW070905210926
848482LV00017B/997
9781923118430